OXFORD MEDICAL PUBLICATIONS

Psychiatric Ethics

# Psychiatric Ethics

## SECOND EDITION

Edited by

### SIDNEY BLOCH
*Associate Professor in Psychiatry, University of Melbourne,*
*Victoria, Australia*

and

### PAUL CHODOFF
*Clinical Professor of Psychiatry,*
*George Washington University,*
*Washington DC*

OXFORD   NEW YORK   MELBOURNE
OXFORD UNIVERSITY PRESS
1991

Oxford University Press, Walton Street, Oxford OX2 6DP

Oxford   New York   Toronto
Delhi   Bombay   Calcutta   Madras   Karachi
Petaling Jaya   Singapore   Hong Kong   Tokyo
Nairobi   Dar es Salaam   Cape Town
Melbourne   Auckland
and associated companies in
Berlin   Ibadan

Oxford is a trade mark of Oxford University Press

Published in the United States
by Oxford University Press, New York

British Library Cataloguing in Publication Data
Psychiatric ethics.—2nd. ed.
1. Medicine. Psychiatry. Ethical aspects
I. Bloch, Sidney 1941–   II. Chodoff, Paul
174.2

ISBN 0–19–261865–2
ISBN 0–19–261864–4 pbk

Library of Congress Cataloging in Publication Data
(Data available)

Set by Footnote Graphics, Warminster, Wiltshire
Printed in Great Britain by
Courier International Ltd
Tiptree, Colchester, Essex

To Felicity and Selma

# Preface

We have been delighted with the response to the first edition of *Psychiatric ethics* by our psychiatric colleagues, and other mental health professionals. The book's publication in 1981 was obviously timely and paralleled the then developing interest among psychiatrists, and related professional groups, in the ethical dimensions of their work. The 1980s have seen a burgeoning of that interest, making the publication of an updated volume essential. This we have sought to do by returning to our original group of contributors. In a small proportion of cases the nature of the topic has not required any major revision; by contrast, other chapters have undergone substantial updating.

We have also identified new topics which warrant readers' attention; they are psychiatry as a profession, the concept of disease and illness, ethical aspects of deinstitutionalization and psychogeriatrics, and two examples of the improper use of psychiatry—in Nazi Germany and contemporary Japan. Some colleagues would obviously have wanted an account of the ethics involved in other areas of psychiatry not covered in the 24 chapters. As editors however we have had to recognize the need to keep the volume within reasonable bounds.

Finally, we would like to acknowledge our gratitude to the contributors, both old and new, without whose cordial and helpful collaboration the second edition could not have been produced. We also thank Kathy Madden for her unstinting secretarial and administrative support, which has proved invaluable. Last, but not least, our thanks go to the staff at Oxford University Press who have given us every encouragement.

*Melbourne and Washington*                                   S.B.
July 1990                                                    P.C.

# Contents

# Contributors

**John Bancroft,** M.D., F.R.C.P., F.R.C.PSYCH., CLINICAL CONSULTANT
MRC Reproductive Biology Unit, Edinburgh.

**Sidney Bloch,** PH.D., F.R.C.PSYCH., F.R.A.N.Z.C.P., ASSOCIATE PROFESSOR
(CLINICAL) AND READER
Department of Psychiatry, University of Melbourne.

**Paul Brown,** M.B., B.S., M.R.C.PSYCH., F.R.A.N.Z.C.P., CONSULTANT
PSYCHIATRIST
St. Vincent's Hospital, Melbourne.

**Paul Chodoff,** M.D., CLINICAL PROFESSOR OF PSYCHIATRY
George Washington University, Washington DC.

**Allen Dyer,** M.D., PH.D., PROFESSOR AND ASSOCIATE CHAIRMAN
Department of Psychiatry, Albany Medical College, Albany, NY
CHIEF MEDICAL OFFICER, Capital District Psychiatric Center, Albany, NY.

**William Fulford,** PH.D., D.PHIL., M.R.C.PSYCH., RESEARCH PSYCHIATRIST
Department of Psychiatry, University of Oxford.

**Philip Graham,** F.R.C.P., F.R.C.PSYCH., PROFESSOR OF CHILD
PSYCHIATRY
Institute of Child Health, University of London, Hospital for Sick
Children, London.

**Timothy Harding,** M.D., F.R.C.PSYCH., CHARGÉ DE COURS
Institut Universitaire de médecine légale, Genève.

**R. M. Hare,** F.B.A., WHITE'S PROFESSOR OF MORAL PHILOSOPHY AND
FELLOW OF CORPUS CHRISTI COLLEGE EMERITUS, University of Oxford;
PROFESSOR OF PHILOSOPHY, University of Florida, Gainsville.

**David Heyd,** PH.D., SENIOR LECTURER IN PHILOSOPHY
The Hebrew University, Jerusalem.

**David I. Joseph,** M.D., CLINICAL PROFESSOR
Department of Psychiatry and Behavioural Sciences, George
Washington University, Washington DC; ASSOCIATE DIRECTOR OF
RESIDENCY TRAINING, St. Elizabeths/District of Columbia Commission on
Mental Health Services, Washington DC.

**T. Byram Karasu,** M.D., PROFESSOR OF PSYCHIATRY
Albert Einstein College of Medicine, New York.

**Kevin Kelly,** M.D., CLINICAL ASSISTANT PROFESSOR
Department of Psychiatry, Cornell University Medical College, New
York.

**David Mechanic,** PH.D., DIRECTOR
Institute for Health, Health Care Policy, and Aging Research,
UNIVERSITY PROFESSOR and RENÉ DUBOS PROFESSOR OF BEHAVIOURAL
SCIENCES, Rutgers University, New Brunswick, New Jersey.

**Harold Merskey,** D.M., F.R.C.PSYCH., PROFESSOR OF PSYCHIATRY
University of Western Ontario, Canada.

**Robert Michels,** M.D., PSYCHIATRIST-IN-CHIEF
The New York Hospital and BARKLIE MCKEE HENRY PROFESSOR AND
CHAIRMAN, Department of Psychiatry, Cornell University Medical
College, New York.

**Robert Miller,** M.D., PH.D., TRAINING DIRECTOR
Forensic Center Mendota Mental Health Institute, Madison, WI;
CLINICAL PROFESSOR OF PSYCHIATRY AND LECTURER IN LAW, University of
Wisconsin–Madison; ASSOCIATE CLINICAL PROFESSOR OF PSYCHIATRY,
Medical College of Wisconsin, Milwaukee.

**Benno Müller-Hill,** DR. RER. NAT., PROFESSOR OF GENETICS
Institute of Genetics, University of Cologne, West Germany.

**David Musto,** M.A., M.D., PROFESSOR OF PSYCHIATRY (CHILD STUDY CENTER)
AND HISTORY OF MEDICINE
Yale University, Newhaven.

**Joseph N. Onek,** ATTORNEY
Onek, Klein & Farr, Washington, DC.

**Catherine Oppenheimer,** M.R.C.P., F.R.C.PSYCH., CONSULTANT IN
PSYCHOGERIATRICS
Warneford Hospital, Oxford.

**Roger Peele,** M.D., CHAIR
Psychiatry Department, Commission on Mental Health Services, Saint
Elizabeth's Campus, Washington, DC; CLINICAL PROFESSOR OF
PSYCHIATRY, George Washington University.

**Jonas Rappeport,** M.D., CHIEF MEDICAL OFFICER
Circuit Court for Baltimore City; CLINICAL PROFESSOR OF PSYCHIATRY,
University of Maryland School of Medicine; ADJUNCT PROFESSOR OF LAW,
University of Maryland School of Law and ASSOCIATE PROFESSOR OF
PSYCHIATRY, Johns Hopkins University, Baltimore.

**Walter Reich,** M.D., PROFESSOR OF PSYCHIATRY
Uniformed Services University of the Health Sciences, Washington, DC;
SENIOR SCHOLAR, Woodrow Wilson International Center for Scholars;
SENIOR RESEARCH PSYCHIATRIST, National Institute of Mental Health;
LECTURER IN PSYCHIATRY, Yale University, New Haven.

**John Wing,** M.D., PH.D., F.R.C.PSYCH., EMERITUS PROFESSOR OF SOCIAL
PSYCHIATRY
Institute of Psychiatry, University of London; DIRECTOR, Research Unit,
Royal College of Psychiatrists, London.

# 1

# Introduction

*Sidney Bloch and Paul Chodoff*

## Why a book on psychiatric ethics?

Some psychiatrists might well pose the question: why is there a need for a book on psychiatric ethics? Indeed, why have the editors bothered with a second edition? The profession after all has existed for centuries and during this time its practitioners have managed to care for the mentally ill without becoming unduly preoccupied with moral questions. They might go further and aver that the psychiatrist's prime and sole interest is in his patients: it is inherent in the nature of his work that their optimal welfare is his *raison d'être*. These psychiatrists could buttress their argument by demonstrating the strong links between psychiatry and its parent profession of medicine, which has an even longer tradition of tending the ill along well-established and self-evident principles of ethical conduct. Thus, the first principle of the American Medical Association's Principles of Medical Ethics,† which originated in 1847, states: 'The principal objective of the medical profession is to render service to humanity with full respect for the dignity of man.'[1] What could be more explicit?

Evidently psychiatrists, along with their medical colleagues, have, throughout the history of their profession, assumed implicitly that they could perform their task without ethical difficulties by serving the best interests of their patients. In the process they have tended by and large to ignore the ethical foundations of their work. One reflection of this state of affairs is the neglect of ethics in the education of psychiatrists. Most programmes have devoted little time to the subject, although the situation appears to be improving in the 1980s, when ethical issues have been introduced into training. To the extent that psychiatric ethics is still relatively understudied, can we discern elements of denial?

This would be partially to be expected: the psychiatrist who had to consider the ethical component of each decision he made would soon be immobilized. Psychiatric practice is characterized by uncertainties and ambiguities which must be kept within bounds.

Thomas Szasz was one of the first psychiatrists to highlight his colleagues'

† The appendix contains codes of medical ethics relevant to psychiatry.

denial: 'Unfortunately these (ethical considerations) are often denied, minimised or merely kept out of focus; for the ideal of the medical profession as well as of the people whom it serves seems to be having a system of medicine (allegedly) free of ethical value.'[2] More specifically in the case of American psychiatrists, Seymour Halleck has argued that they: 'are still convinced that their professional mandate is simply that of healing a form of illness and that their therapeutic activities do not and should not have political consequences'.[3] Halleck believes that a psychiatrist has a political role whether he is prepared to recognize it or not, and that this role has significant social and ethical implications. We would thoroughly agree with these contentions of both Szasz and Halleck. The contemporary psychiatrist, by virtue of his complex professional role, is required to grapple with a broad range of ethical problems. These problems may be relatively simple and direct and susceptible to easy remedies; most, unfortunately, will be far too complex for ready solution. In some instances the ethical dimension of the problem will be obvious; but it will be hidden in others, and require careful disentanglement. It is necessary, however, to remember that not every difficulty a psychiatrist faces is an ethical one. Room must be left for mistakes and errors in judgement made in good faith.

Psychiatrists may be relatively blind to ethical aspects of their profession for several reasons. As was mentioned above, the ethical quality of a situation which a psychiatrist faces may not be easily apparent. Personal qualities within himself may hamper the psychiatrist's perception (denial has already been mentioned), or he may not have acquired a coherent and integrated set of principles with which to guide his conduct. Possibly the most significant barrier is that the psychiatrist, like other people, is necessarily involved in an internal conflict between forces motivating him towards or away from right behaviour.

Unfortunately a psychiatrist cannot rely on 'dedication to his patients' to lessen the immensity of the ethical problems facing him, any more than he can cling to the proposition that psychiatry is basically an objective, scientifically based discipline, and therefore unaffected by values. As we hope will become obvious in the chapters that follow, the need for the psychiatrist to make vital moral decisions is pervasive, infiltrating almost every facet of his work. And his task is made more complicated by the fact that most of the ethical problems he faces have not hitherto been adequately dealt with, let alone resolved. Some problems have not even begun to receive systematic study.

## The contemporary interest in psychiatric ethics

There is evidence in the past two or three decades that interest among psychiatrists (and the medical profession generally) in the ethical foundations of their work has escalated, perhaps more so than in any other period of psychiatry's history. Psychiatric ethics has within a relatively short period become a most respectable subject. For example, its literature has mushroomed, particularly in the 1970s and 1980s. Many psychiatric journals contain papers on ethical topics, and the bibliography is growing rapidly. The 1984 bibliography of the Hastings Center (the Institute of Society, Ethics, and the Life Sciences), for example, lists over 300 references in the section on behaviour-control.[4] The Center's journal and its British counterpart, the *Journal of Medical Ethics*, regularly publish articles pertinent to mental health. The comprehensive *Encyclopaedia of bioethics*[5] published by the Kennedy Institute of Ethics, contains many entries relevant to psychiatry. Conferences and workshops on aspects of psychiatric ethics are becoming commonplace. Ethical topics played an important role in the 1977 Congress of the World Psychiatric Association in Hawaii. The Congress was also noteworthy for its adoption of a set of ethical guidelines for practising psychiatrists. The *Declaration of Hawaii* (see Appendix) was the culmination of several years' concern by the Association about questions concerning the ethical conduct of psychiatry among its member societies. The Congress went further by setting up a framework to implement the investigation of ethical conduct among these member societies. Several national psychiatric organizations have also paid increased attention to ethics and have set up special ethics committees. The British Royal College of Psychiatrists, for instance, established an ethics committee in 1974. A comparable committee in the American Psychiatric Association developed a code of ethics to serve as a guide for American psychiatrists in 1973 (see Appendix). Most district branches of the American Psychiatric Association have actively functioning ethics committees. The Royal Australian and New Zealand College of Psychiatrists has had an Ethics Committee since 1978.

The absence of specific psychiatric codes until the 1970s was perhaps related to the notion that general medical codes such as the Hippocratic Oath, the *Declaration of Geneva*, and the American Medical Association's *Principles of medical ethics* were sufficient to cover the needs of the psychiatric profession. But with the growing focus more specifically on psychiatric ethics has come the recognition that a number of problems are unique to the psychiatrist, and therefore deserve specialized attention.

## The reasons for the psychiatrist's new interest in ethics

Several factors have contributed to the burgeoning of interest in ethical issues among psychiatrists since the 1960s. Among these are:

1. The 'medical consumer movement': recipients of health care have in recent years come to constitute a potent and more or less coherent social

force (see Chapter 21). Perhaps as an example of the sceptical attitude towards authority which is developing as an apparent general cultural trend in the West, the physician no longer compels blind reverence, nor is there unquestioning compliance with his methods. We are now seeing growing demands that the views of the patient and his family be acknowledged and respected. Moore[6] has likened the movement to a 'social egalitarian revolution' in which demands are made that 'the patient be given greater responsibility in determining his or her care, and involving less willingness to accept the opinions of professional experts'. There are calls for greater consumer participation in medical policy-making, and for the medical establishment's recognition of decent health care as a basic civil right. Consider among other developments the formation of a patients' association, community health councils, and the phenomenal proliferation of self-help groups.[7] Although many of the last have arisen because they provide a forum for mutual support, other motives include the disaffection from conventional health care and the determination of patients with particular disabilities to form pressure lobbies to influence government authorities. The psychiatric patient, too, has thus been instrumental in forcing the psychiatrist to scrutinize more closely his professional activities. In the US, the activities of the National Association for Mental Illness (NAMI) have been particularly noteworthy.

2. It is no coincidence that the increased interest in ethics among psychiatrists has been associated with vehement, repeated attacks on their profession by what might be termed broadly the civil liberties approach to mental illness. This movement has been generated largely by psychiatrists themselves, a minority among their colleagues, but under the vigorous and articulate leadership of Thomas Szasz and Ronald Laing; and by lawyers who, especially in the United States, have come to constitute a relatively large and influential group known as the mental health bar.

Although many psychiatrists would dismiss figures like Szasz and Laing as polemicists, there is no doubt that they have been spurred by their critiques to adopt a more self-searching and questioning attitude to their profession. Szasz was the first to spark off widespread controversy with his publication in 1960 of *The myth of mental illness*[2,8] and since that time he has mounted a barrage of books and articles insisting that the psychiatrist is nothing more than a modern-day inquisitor labelling and classifying behaviour in order to limit people's liberties.[9] Ronald Liefer, another psychiatric activist and a leader of the American 'Radical Psychiatry Movement', has argued vociferously that 'the State has assumed most of the traditional social functions of regulating and controlling human conduct. Because all moral codes are not codified in law, and because the power of the State is limited by a rule of law, the State is unable satisfactorily to control and influence individuals. This requires a new social institution that, under the auspices of an acceptable modern authority, can control and guide conduct without conspicuously violating publicly avowed ideals of freedom and respect for the individual. Psychiatry, in medical disguise, has assumed this historical function.'[10]

R. D. Laing,[11] too, added fuel to the fires with his claims that what has been called mental illness is but an anguished protest against intolerable social pressure, and that psychiatrists, rather than treating this condition with drugs and confinement, should examine their role in perpetuating it. J. Robitscher[12] has made similar cogent criticisms in his book *The powers of psychiatry*.

Faced with these criticisms from both colleagues and the legal profession psychiatrists have been provoked into considering more than ever before issues such as the criteria for the diagnoses of mental illness, the vague boundaries of their operations, the clash of loyalties to patient and other parties, the paucity of reliable data on the effectiveness of their treatments, the difficulty of assessing and predicting dangerousness, and the like. No reasonable psychiatrist can avoid wrestling with the arguments proffered by these critics, and in this regard the impact of the civil-liberties movement has been favourable to the development of a socially responsible ethical sense. However, it is possible that one effect of so intense a legal involvement in psychiatric issues may have been counterproductive. To attempt to specify every aspect of the professional relationship in contractual terms leaves little room for the exercise of individual ethical judgement, and indeed may discourage its exercise. It has been observed that: 'In hell there will be nothing but law and due process will be meticulously observed.'

3. Contributing to both the previous factors for increased interest in psychiatric ethics is the fact that the treatment of the mentally ill has traditionally conjured up the image of manipulator and hapless victim; particularly so in the case of the patient who, because of his disorder, cannot provide informed consent. The relevance of informed consent for all forms of medical treatment, including the treatment of mental illness, has become well recognized in the 1980s. Controversy about their ethical permissibility has surrounded the use of all psychiatric treatments from physical manipulations of the brain—such as psychosurgery and electroconvulsive therapy—to the psychotherapies, especially behaviour-modification. In recent years there has been much questioning of the efficacy of such treatments, and their potency and dangers have been emphasized. The most drastic of these, psychosurgery, has been attacked so vigorously in the United States that a National Commission for its investigation was set up under Congressional auspices. The conclusions of the prestigious members of the Commission, incidentally, were surprisingly moderate.[13] The use of electroconvulsive therapy, too, has been decried,

its critics labelling it as hazardous and barbaric under any circumstances. The reaction was so intense that a vociferous patients' advocacy group was responsible for the passage of legislation in the state of California imposing almost impossible barriers before ECT can be used.

As a result of these controversies and criticisms, psychiatrists have had to exercise greater caution in planning treatment for their patients, and have had to be more diligent in obtaining informed consent. These developments, in the urgency of their efforts to curb ethical abuses, may ironically, have been responsible for urgent ethical problems of the opposite kind. The most pressing instance has been the emptying out of mental hospitals, especially in the US, with all the attendant evils of what has come to be known as deinstitutionalization (see Chapter 14). The difficulty in arranging for the involuntary hospitalization of severely disturbed mentally ill patients has been a particularly distressing problem, and has been the focus of a heated ethical debate (see Chapter 13).

4. The 1977 World Psychiatric Association Congress was not only momentous for the *Declaration of Hawaii*, but was also an ethical watershed in the annals of international psychiatric politics for another reason: the Soviet practice of labelling normal dissenters as mentally ill and committing them to mental hospitals was condemned by the Association. Furthermore, a commission was formed to monitor political misuse of psychiatry wherever it might occur.[14] At the previous World Congress in 1971 in Mexico City the Soviet issue had been raised, but summarily swept under the carpet. Between Mexico City and Honolulu many Western psychiatrists had moved from incredulity that such abuse could take place to a conviction that the allegations were well founded. In the process, several national psychiatric organizations reacted with resolutions condemning their Soviet counterparts, and with other interventions aimed at bringing the practices to an end.

The Honolulu Congress was also notable for the establishment of a Review Committee whose remit has been to investigate cases of the abuse of psychiatry wherever they may occur. Over two dozen cases, all from the USSR, were brought to the Committee's attention during a six-year period between 1977 and 1983. It was the increasing pressure on the Soviet Psychiatric Society which ultimately led to its withdrawal some months before the 1983 World Congress in Vienna. By then, the WPA was deeply involved (although not without a major degree of divisiveness) in an effort to restore 'ethical' psychiatry in the Soviet Union. Further pressure on Russian psychiatrists led to major changes in Soviet mental health law in early 1988, and the release of a steady stream of 'dissenter-patients' from the mid-1980s. These developments were satisfactory enough for the WPA to readmit the Soviet Society at the 1989 World Congress in Athens, although continuation of their membership was contingent on the Review

Committee's not finding any evidence of abuse by late 1990.[15] The misuse has remained a prominent feature of international psychiatric discussions. Significantly for our purposes here, it has provoked psychiatrists throughout the world to consider how readily psychiatry can be abused. (The Soviet case is discussed in detail in Chapter 24.)

5. The sacredness which psychiatrists have attached to the confidentiality they can promise their patients has increasingly come under attack and been attenuated in recent years by a number of new developments in law and psychiatric economics, especially through the demands of third-party funders. These developments have given rise to a number of significant ethical conflicts, and have made psychiatrists realize that they treat their patients in a social context (see Chapter 15).

6. Ethical aspects of psychiatric practice have been influenced in recent years by other professional disciplines besides the law; these include sociology, psychology, theology, and philosophy. For instance, after an extended silence, a significant dialogue between psychiatrist and philosopher has developed. New attitudes in the philosopher, particularly the moral philosopher, have certainly been influential. Traditionally, the philosopher may have used a form of language which proved so abstruse as to intimidate even the most eager psychiatrist. Professor Hare, a contributor to this book, recognized this poor communication by his colleagues as long ago as 1952, when he wrote: 'in a world in which problems of conduct become everyday more complex and tormenting, there is a great need for an understanding of the language in which these problems are posed and answered.'[16] His *The language of morals* endeavours to clarify the terms and concepts used by moral philosophers. Hare also emphasizes the need for moral philosophy to develop theoretical concepts which have a bearing on daily human activities, on actual concrete cases. Thus: 'The reason why actions are in a peculiar way revelatory of moral principles is that the function of moral principles is to guide conduct', and this includes the activities of a professional group like psychiatrists. The philosopher Mary Warnock highlights this movement of focus from the abstract to the concrete case in her conclusions to her book on contemporary ethics. She refers particularly to the period since 1960 in which ethics 'has become a practical subject, and therefore more urgent and more interesting'.[17] She points out that a survey of ethics during this period 'would have to show far greater awareness that what people say philosophically may affect what they do in the real world'. Contemporary figures in philosophy have put forward theoretical propositions which have a distinct relevance for day-to-day conduct. A good example is the work of the American moral philosopher John Rawls: a central assumption in his *A theory of justice*[18] is that all morality is social morality. In the present volume, Professor Hare's chapter on the philosophical basis of psychiatric ethics is written in the

same spirit as his *The language of morals*, and with a particular sensitivity to the interests and needs of the practising psychiatrist.

## Ethics: its boundaries in this book

'Ethics' has several connotations, and we need now to examine the way in which we use the term in this book.

'Ethics', derived from the Greek adjective *ēthikos*, from *ēthos* meaning 'nature' or 'disposition', is commonly used in one of two ways, which we can conveniently refer to as the philosophical and the practical. In the former case, we are concerned with a branch of philosophy, usually termed moral philosophy, whose purpose is the systematic study of human conduct with respect to the rightness and wrongness of actions and to the goodness and badness of the motives and ends of such actions. The moral philosopher attempts to show how value judgements are arrived at. Further, he tackles the question of whether ethical propositions can be proved, focusing on concepts such as 'good', 'bad', 'right', 'wrong', 'should', 'ought', 'desirable', 'justice', 'duty', 'obligation', and similar evaluative terms. A fundamental premiss of the moral philosopher is that human conduct occurs within a context of values: where people have a choice of one or another course of action and their activities are not completely proscribed, the inevitable question presents itself as to whether the particular action chosen is right or wrong, good or bad.

In tackling the questions of what constitutes ethical behaviour and how values are derived, the philosopher may offer a conceptual model or theory—this is the most general level of ethics. A number of classical models have been proposed.[19] One which has had a profound influence on moral philosophy is the *utilitarian* position of such writers as John Stuart Mill: the emphasis here is on the consequences of acts, on the balance between good and bad consequences, between benefits and harms. A person's actions should be chosen so that it produces the best result, by recognizing the needs of all those persons who will be affected by that action. The final consequence would be the greatest possible total happiness of all concerned. A competing position is the *absolutist*, or *deontological*, with its core thesis that certain acts are intrinsically wrong, regardless of their consequences, and can never be made right, and that moral judgements have universal applicability. Acts like the murder of an innocent person or the theft of another person's property, for example, are judged in the absolutist approach to be always totally wrong. Religious morality is commonly of this kind—for example, God's moral commands are viewed as absolute and must always be obeyed, or the Bible is accepted as the sole guide to moral conduct. We have already mentioned John Rawls,[18] whose central thesis is that basic morality consists of those principles chosen by the rational† person, with the important proviso that his judgements are made behind a 'veil of ignorance'—that he is unaware of the position he would have in a society in which his principles would operate. Self-interest is thus avoided by the determination of moral principles while covered behind the 'veil'.

These theories may be coherent and well-argued; but a question still remains as to how they apply to concrete, day-to-day situations. In the case of the psychiatrist, like anyone else faced with complex situations, one could argue that every situation he deals with is in one way or another unique, and that no general principles or guidelines of conduct can possibly apply. Certainly the psychiatrist must, by virtue of the nature of his work, arrive at ethical judgements in terms of real, concrete, and highly specific cases. The snag with an adherence to this 'situational' approach, however, is its exhausting and infinite quality—the psychiatrist's efforts to reach the concrete ethical position *vis-à-vis* each one of his patients, their families, colleagues, other fellow professionals, and all the other persons he must work with. Not even the most integrated individual could withstand such an onslaught of continuous decision-making.

Despite the argument of the uniqueness of each case, it seems to us that situations—many of which are discussed in this book—recur regularly in the psychiatrist's work which call for ethical judgements, and these can be studied systematically. In discussing these ethical questions, our contributors have not come up with easy, ready-made solutions, and in fact were not expected to do so, although they have in many instances offered their own views, in a tentative manner, about correct ethical conduct in difficult situations. Their chief objective is to describe the problems involved as clearly as they can, so that the reader will appreciate their nature and complexity, and, as a result be better qualified to understand how he makes his own ethical judgements. We should emphasize that even the statement of the problem sometimes is fraught with difficulty. Unfortunately the neutrality and lack of bias with which one would want the problems to be presented are not easy to attain; suppositions and assumptions lie behind the identification of the problem and the way in which it is approached.[20] None the less the project, in our opinion, is still worth pursuing.

It is tempting in a book of this kind to offer guidelines for ethical conduct. As we mentioned earlier, efforts in this direction have been made in recent years, as witnessed by the formulation of ethical codes. We feel that to succumb to such temptation would be hazardous. Neither the editors nor the contributors could possibly deceive themselves that they are in a position to prescribe immutable ethical guidelines. Ultimately, ethical

† Rawls uses 'rational' to mean 'always doing what is in one's own interest'.

conduct depends on the individual, and on his peers as a professional group, and their consent to use only those attitudes and practices which they generally agree upon as morally appropriate. Guidelines of conduct may be laid down, but they are, unlike laws and regulations, unenforceable; and, furthermore, a code can only be expressed in general terms. The psychiatrist is still left with the personal responsibility of taking ethical decisions in his daily practice which pertain to specific cases.

## 'Psychiatric ethics' in the context of general ethics

Can 'psychiatric ethics' be regarded as a specific entity, a realm distinct from other aspects of living in which ethical considerations are involved? The argument has been advanced that a separate ethics is unnecessary, not only for the psychiatrist but for the physician in general, since as a reasonable member of society he can readily adopt ethical principles which have been agreed upon by the society as a whole. Thus, the proposition has been advanced by Braceland that: 'the physician [psychiatrist included] *as a citizen* [our italics] must be an ethical man and act in accordance with the accepted standards that apply to all men'.[21] Clouser, in referring to medical ethics, has contended that: 'Medical ethics is simply ethics applied to a particular branch of our lives—roughly the area touched by medicine. And being the same old ethics that has been around for a long time, medical ethics has no special principles or methods or rules. It is the "old ethics" trying to find its way around in the new, very puzzling circumstances.'[22]

Both Braceland and Clouser's points seem valid: psychiatric ethics is, in part, the application of more or less universal principles to the moral problems of a particular professional activity. But it would seem to us that this view tends to minimize the uniqueness of these problems as the physician or psychiatrist faces them. In particular, the psychiatrist's domain is characterized by so many issues specific to the nature of his work that ethical considerations and decisions play a greater role for him than for many other professional groups. To illustrate briefly:

1. No other person apart from the psychiatrist faces the task of assessing the state of another's mind with a need to make a judgement whether to deprive a person of his liberty for the sake of his mental health. This is indeed an awesome responsibility.

2. Unlike other physicians, for whom this is a relatively rare occurrence, the psychiatrist's problems often involve a balance between individual and social responsibilities. The boundaries of the psychiatrist's work are blurred and ill-defined. He lacks satisfactory guidelines to indicate where his work starts and ends. Thus his attitude may range from limiting 'his field strictly to the suffering patient'[23] to involving himself in 'fundamental social goals'.[24]

3. There is, as yet, poor agreement on what constitutes psychiatric disorder. The debate over whether homosexuality *per se* is a diagnosable disorder, which now seems to have been settled in the negative, is a cogent example. Although contemporary diagnostic systems, such as the American Psychiatric Association's DSM III–R, have imposed a certain order on the diagnostic process, an ineradicable residue of subjectivity seems to attach itself to the formulation of psychiatric illness. Moreover, the ostensible atheoretical approach of DSM III–R has given rise to new ethical quandaries (see Chapter 7).

A perusal of the book will make it clear that the psychiatrist contributors are wrestling with problems which they face every day. These problems, of course, differ depending on the area of psychiatry considered; but certain themes are pervasive. These include: how to assess the moral costs and benefits of what they do professionally; how to maintain confidentiality and at the same time be accountable and responsible; how to come to terms with the critics of psychiatry, whether lawyers or those from among their own ranks; how to treat patients effectively while maintaining their confidence and not keeping them in the dark about what is going on; how to define the nebulous parameters of their own work while avoiding hubris or undue timidity; and how to strike a balance between the ethos of contractual equality which is becoming dominant in Western life, and a benevolent paternalism necessary to them as physicians.

As editors we hope that the second edition of *Psychiatric ethics* will help to illuminate for interested readers in the profession of psychiatry and elsewhere these themes, which permeate all areas of psychiatric practice, and in which elements of the human, the contingent, and the ambiguous take precedence over purely scientific and clinical considerations.

Finally, we wish to make a general point about this second edition of *Psychiatric ethics*. Our selection is by no means exhaustive, but we believe the topics included cover the important and common ethical issues facing the psychiatrist. Moreover, since the first edition in 1981 we have had the opportunity to witness further developments in the field. This new edition has enabled us to include additional chapters covering what seem to us important dimensions of these developments.

Two chapters tackle theoretical issues. Dyer in Chapter 5 highlights the inherent nature of a profession, as well as considering the desiderata of the psychiatric profession in particular. And Fulford in Chapter 6 presents original work on the fundamental concepts of disease and illness, which are perhaps at the heart of the psychiatrist's task. In the applied section, two areas of psychiatric practice are dealt with which are of major contemporary relevance: deinstitutionalization and the ethical aspects of psychogeriatrics. Peele in Chapter 14 examines the history of the concept of deinstitutionalization, together with an account of its manifold ethical ramifications.

And Oppenheimer in Chapter 17 reminds us that the psychiatry of the elderly warrants our careful attention, because of the complex moral dilemmas with which it confronts us.

In the first edition the section on abuse was limited to the Soviet political misuse of psychiatry to suppress dissent. We had intended to include a chapter on the unethical practices that typified Nazi psychiatry, but could not find a suitable contributor. Since then Müller-Hill, a German geneticist, has written *Murderous science*, which covers, in part, the Nazi abuse of psychiatry. His chapter on that topic for this book focuses particularly on the so-called 'euthanasia programme'. Harding contributes a chapter on Japanese abuse, in which he describes and analyses the result of a policy of state neglect of psychiatry coupled with a powerful private sector dominated by psychiatrists themselves. We are aware that psychiatry may be improperly deployed in other ways, but the three forms covered here seem the most blatant and, therefore, useful heuristically. This should not shield us from the uncomfortable fact that psychiatric abuse is prevalent universally, and presents in diverse, subtle ways.

## References

1 *American Journal of Psychiatry* **130**:1057–64, 1973.
2 Szasz, T.: The myth of mental illness. *American Psychologist* **15**:113–18, 1960.
3 Halleck, S.: *The politics of therapy.* New York, Science House, 1971, p. 13.
4 *Bibliography 1984*, Hastings, New York, Institute of Society, Ethics, and Life Sciences.
5 Reich, W. (ed.): *Encyclopaedia of bioethics.* New York, Free Press, 1978.
6 Moore, R. A.: Ethics in the practice of psychiatry—origins, functions, models and enforcement. *American Journal of Psychiatry* **135**:157–63, 1978.
7 Robinson, D. and Henry, S.: *Self-help and health. Mutual aid for modern problems.* London, Martin Robertson, 1977.
8 Szasz, T.: *The myth of mental illness.* New York, Harper and Row, 1961.
9 Szasz, T.: *Law, liberty and psychiatry.* New York, Macmillan, 1963.
10 Liefer, R.: The medical model as ideology. *International Journal of Psychiatry* **9**:13–21, 1970.
11 Laing, R. D.: *The divided self.* Harmondsworth, Penguin, 1965.
12 Robitscher, J.: *The powers of psychiatry.* Boston, Houghton-Mifflin, 1980.
13 US National Commission for the Protection of Subjects of Biomedical and Behavioural Research Involving Psychosurgery—Report and Recommendations. US Department of Health, Education, and Welfare Publication No. (OS) 77–0001 and (OS) 77–0002, March 1977.
14 Bloch, S. and Reddaway, P.: *Soviet psychiatric abuse. The shadow over world psychiatry.* London, Gollancz, 1984.
15 Bloch, S.: Athens and beyond. Soviet psychiatry and the World Psychiatric Association. *Psychiatric Bulletin* **14**:129–133, 1990.
16 Hare, R. H.: *The language of morals.* Oxford, Oxford University Press, 1952.
17 Warnock, M.: *Ethics since 1900.* Oxford, Oxford University Press, 1978.

18 Rawls, J.: *A theory of justice.* Cambridge, Mass., Harvard University Press. 1971.
19 Foot, P. (ed.): *Theories of ethics.* Oxford, Oxford University Press, 1967.
20 Montefiore, A. (ed.): *Neutrality and impartiality.* Cambridge, Cambridge University Press, 1975.
21 Braceland, F. J.: Historical perspectives of the ethical practice of psychiatry. *American Journal of Psychiatry* **126**:230–7, 1969.
22 Clouser, K. D.: Medical ethics: some uses, abuses and limitations. *New England Journal of Medicine* **293**:384–7, 1973.
23 Busse, E. W.: APA's role in influencing the evolution of a health care delivery system. *American Journal of Psychiatry* **126**:739–44, 1969.
24 Waggoner, R.: Cultural dissonance and psychiatry. *American Journal of Psychiatry* **127**:1–8, 1970.

# 2

# A historical perspective

*David Musto*

Three factors underlie the ethical questions which at all times have preoccupied those delegated to help the mentally ill: the role of the therapist, the nature of mental disease, and the cultural, religious, and even political environment in which the patient and therapist coexist. In the last decade or so these factors and the formal study of psychiatric ethics have been explicitly analysed and have become almost a new subspecialty. Before the mid-twentieth-century, however, few such formal studies existed. This lack of attention is understandable, since the profession of psychiatry developed as a medical specialty only recently, and since for much of the last century the codes discussed and adopted for general medicine appeared to have served psychiatry well. The dramatic changes in the scope of psychiatry since the Second World War, however, have brought into sharp focus ethical issues peculiar to psychiatry.

The governing factors listed above have varied widely in Western medical tradition since Hippocrates. What we call issues in psychiatric ethics during that time must represent the imposition of categories familiar to us, such as informed consent and 'right to be treated', on to a historical record for which these terms are not entirely appropriate. In reviewing the past we will be looking for ethical concepts deemed pertinent by medical or other cultural authorities when the behaviour of a person was judged to be grossly abnormal and to require treatment or limitation of freedom. Social control in a broad sense could be justified as the theme for a study of psychiatric ethics; but in this brief survey the subjects will be studied in the traditional medical context. The realization that ethical issues transcend medicine—and therefore psychiatry—constitutes a fundamental change in outlook which has marked the recent rise of interest. Restriction of the subject to the context of the history of medicine is a concession to space, not a judgement on its proper boundaries. A convenient starting-point is the Greco-Roman period.

## Greco-Roman period

It would be an error to consider the Hippocratic Oath as representing Greek or Roman medical practice. The tradition of Hippocratic thinking was akin to Pythagoreanism, a school of thought with strict moral precepts whose tenets more resembled later Christian principles than the flexible mores of Hellenistic practices, which, for example, condoned abortion and suicide.[1] The oath does include, however, some of the earliest affirmations of confidentiality and the primacy of the patient's health:

Whatever houses I may visit, I will come for the benefit of the sick, remaining free of all intentional injustice, of all mischief and in particular of sexual relations with both female and male persons, be they free or slaves.

What I may see or hear in the course of the treatment or even outside of the treatment in regard to the life of the men, which on no account one must spread abroad, I will keep to myself holding such things shameful to be spoken about.[2]

Insanity is not mentioned in the oath. In the Greek world there appears to have been little legal provision for the insane, although Roman law did provide for trusteeship of an incompetent's property and other restrictions of his rights. Mental illness as well as drunkenness were conditions that could decrease a defendant's criminal responsibility, although such decisions appear to have been made by judges without the advice of a physician or other expert on mental illness.[3]

Treatment of the insane in the ancient Western world ranged from such harsh methods, described by Celsus (first century of the Christian era), as purgation, bleeding, beatings, and cold baths to milder policies advocated by Soranus (first and second centuries), which are similar to the moral therapy espoused, although rarely practised, in the early nineteenth century: esteem for the patient, relative freedom of movement and kind treatment.

Just as a range of restraints on freedom can be identified in these early approaches to mental illness, so the causes advanced for insanity extended from divine intervention to organic or natural factors. When ethical issues are drawn from this period, the vague edges of the definition of insanity and various responses to it make firm statements about these issues difficult. Clearly, for those who were treated medically, evidence suggests that harshness of treatment or limitations of freedom were the prerogative of the physician, and that the patient and his family had little to say about either. Furthermore, the major determinant in form of therapy depended on the custodian's faith in a particular school of medicine, or perhaps in a lack of faith in any medical treatment and, instead, a dependence on religious intervention.

The marks of insanity were simple: strange, violent, suicidal, or homicidal behaviour which did not have a likely explanation from the observer's point of view. Bizarre explanations from the patient would only confirm the judgement of the family or other authorities. Treatment might be painful or harmful, but the physician administered it with a clear conscience because his theory of medicine required certain courses of action. In these instances, ethical problems may exist for us, but did not for the confident physician or the patient's faithful custodian, or, perhaps, even for the patient himself. The random manner in which those considered insane received care continued for centuries until more formal and elaborate systems evolved, first with hospitals and, much later and very recently, with the varieties of care possible when a large mental health profession exists.

## Middle Ages and Renaissance

The Middle Ages brought no medical advance to the insane; rather, the major influence on attitudes toward the mentally ill emanated from religion. For example, the Prophet Mahomet revealed that the insane are the beloved of God and especially chosen by him to declare the truth. This attitude, taken with the founding of hospitals in the Moslem world and the establishment of an enlightened medical profession, suggests that Islam was disposed towards humane care of the ill. Because of the Prophet's statement, the status of the patient was elevated to at least the same level as that of the therapist, a rare event in the history of psychiatry.[4]

Jewish tradition, as stated in the Talmud, portrayed the insane as victims of a disease, not of possession.[5] Christian religious orders provided humane though limited treatment for the deranged, but outside the monasteries Europeans had diminishing resources for care as the Roman Empire was gradually eroded. The ensuing anarchy apparently was responsible for an increase in gaolings, beatings, and torture among the insane. Compounding their misfortune, schisms among Christians led to an increase in the maltreatment of patients by equating deviant opinions with demonic possession and heresy.[6] Among competing religious factions little concern was shown for the rights of heretics whom we would now consider sane, and certainly no more concern was shown for those whose disordered fantasies and opinions were thought the product of heresy. Yet it would be unfair and misleading to suggest that European Christian attitudes toward the insane were characterized by a belief in demonic possession which had to be rooted out by the most severe methods. Toward the end of the Middle Ages, hospitals for the mentally ill were founded; humane physicians and caretakers did exist, and their numbers were to multiply in the sixteenth and seventeenth centuries.[7]

At the same time, legal care for the insane seems to have been in some specific instances balanced and thoughtful. This is the conclusion of

Richard Neugebauer,[8] who studied judicial records regarding 'natural fools' and those judged *non compos mentis* in England from the thirteenth to the seventeenth centuries; these records do not support the accepted belief that the era was cruel and dominated by demonological explanations of mental retardation and disorder. There was a growing pattern of reasonable distinctions between congenital and temporary conditions, protection of the property and interests of those judged incompetent, and a disinclination to be punitive or cruel.

In monastic hospitals the insane received good care, in keeping with the dictum of St Benedict that 'care of the sick is to be placed above and before every other duty'.[9] With suppression of the monastic orders in Protestant countries and confiscation of their property, care of patients suffered. Still, even taking into account the existence of a few hospitals and of legal protection, the Middle Ages offered only a random and unpredictable response to insanity. The ethical context in which decisions were taken was the religious tradition of the locality. This could mean emphasis on charity and understanding, or it could justify severe measures if demonic possession were suspected. It is probably reasonable to generalize that during this time a person with bizarre behaviour and beliefs was seldom classified as a 'patient', and, moreover, that no broad consensus existed for what we think of as humane treatment. The low level of institutional and public health care for all health or social problems meant that the overall quality of care for the mentally ill would be as low as that for other illnesses, such as leprosy and communicable diseases.

## The seventeenth century to the French Revolution

The two centuries preceding the French Revolution were a period of increased hospital building but no significant improvement in the care of the mentally ill. The traditional religious view of mental illness was progressively balanced by advances in anatomy and physiology which suggested that it was the product of organic change. Humane treatment, however, seems to have been related more to culturally inspired responses than to organic explanations of disordered behaviour or beliefs. An assumption that a lesion in the brain or other part of the body caused mental illness brought contrasting treatment. Powerful and destructive therapies were justified on the grounds that they were required for the correction of specific lesions, while milder treatments were advocated because of the belief that strenuous applications would impair the natural capacity of the body or mind to heal the lesion and restore health.

Mild treatment, though, appears to have been rare in the great hospitals that were built before the French Revolution, with the exception of those administered by religious orders. The rise of the sciences stimulated new explanations for the body's functions; mechanical, physical, and chemical theories challenged the Galenic tradition of four humours whose balance brought health. New theories fostered new regimens: strong medicines, bleeding, purgation, and blistering competed with methods such as isolation, beatings, and instilling fear. Faith in theory continued to outweigh empirical considerations based on the actual effects of the patient's treatment. In general, eighteenth-century therapists considered their task difficult and in need of rough procedures.

The French Revolution and, to a lesser degree, the American Revolution were movements for political equality which gave a new importance to the individual in terms of his rights in the secular order. This importance rivalled the religious tradition of immortality and equality before God. In the late eighteenth century, particularly in France, mental illness was considered the result of a wrongly ordered society: the patient was the victim of an exploitative social environment. The attitude that placed blame on society exonerated the ill person; it also suggested that care could take on a social form and promoted optimism as to the outcome—at least in the heyday of the Revolution.

Philippe Pinel, so often honoured for removing the chains from patients, was not totally original in his efforts, but he did adopt and promote more humane attitudes than his predecessors. The basis for his action in the 1790s was faith in the Revolution and one of its corollaries—the expectation that an improved society would result in fewer patients and great improvement in those already interned. He did not abolish authority over his patients—in fact, he was quite firm—but he believed that communication with them in as egalitarian a manner as possible was in keeping with the spirit of the French Republic and also beneficial to their health. Pinel was confident that few restraints were necessary if patients were treated with fundamental regard to their individuality and self-respect.[10]

In contrast, George III of Great Britain, who suffered a relapse of his mental condition in 1788, received traditional rugged care and close restraint because his physicians were determined he should receive the best care that their theories commanded: wild behaviour required a strong antidote. Even the king could not escape what we would today consider cruel treatment. Whatever anxiety the physicians felt about the king's response to their care, their consciences were untroubled. Pinel was equally at ease when he moved in the direction of more benign treatments. In both instances the physician had virtually absolute control over his patient.

Benjamin Rush, the father of American psychiatry, introduced improvements for patients under his care at the Pennsylvania Hospital in Philadelphia. As usual in the movement toward less confining treatments, reformers faced the problem of the hyperactive and threatening patient. Rush, whose own son was long a patient at the hospital, devised restraints like the 'tranquillizer chair', which prevented movement that could cause further damage to the patient, while reducing blood-flow to the brain—required by his theory of insanity. His goal was to ensure that necessary restraint and treatment created no unintended or undesirable effects.[11]

## The nineteenth century

In the nineteenth century, ethical formulations for the medical profession were promulgated in many countries. In 1803, for example, Dr Thomas Percival published a formal statement on medical ethics. Percival's immediate goal was the establishment of a code of ethics and etiquette for the Manchester Infirmary, in order to reduce controversy among the attending physicians. His comments, however, on mental patients in asylums such as existed on the Infirmary grounds, reveal the conflict between humane care and the need to preserve order. His attitude is not far different from that of Pinel or Rush when he writes:

The law justifies the *beating of a lunatic, in such a manner as the circumstances may require*. But it has been before remarked that a physician, who attends an asylum for insanity, is under an obligation of honour as well as of humanity to secure to the unhappy sufferers, committed to his charge, all the tenderness and indulgence compatible with steady and effectual government. And the strait waistcoat, with other improvements in modern practice, now preclude the necessity of coercion by corporal punishment [Percival's italics].[12]

Although he wished to be kind, he believed the physician with special knowledge of the insane could take action which to young and uninformed physicians might appear harsh. 'Certain cases of *mania*', he wrote, 'seem to require a *boldness* of *practice* which a young physician of sensibility may feel a reluctance to adopt.' When this occurs, the novice 'must not yield to timidity, but fortify his mind by the councils of his more experienced brethren of the faculty'. Yet Percival could not let his advice admit of too severe an interpretation, for he warned that 'it is more consonant to probity to err on the side of caution than of temerity'.[13] Repeatedly, these advocates of humane care faced the problem of keeping order in hospitals and regulating the admission of patients. Percival strongly favoured strict inspection of asylums for proper care and for assurance that no one was admitted without a certificate signed by a physician, surgeon, or apothecary. He emphasized the provision for writs of *habeas corpus* and other legal protection of hospital inmates. Here then are two aspects of care of the insane in which ethical problems arise: whether detention is justified, and whether care given during detention is as humane as possible.

Often the adoption of ethical codes in the nineteenth century was related to the advent of professionalism, whereby standards were set for members of a professional organization who were distinguished from physicians or laymen outside the organization. Medical etiquette was a prominent feature of these ethical codes. Procedures for consultation, details about fees, and relations with fellow physicians were regulated by the codes. Through statutory laws and third-party payment procedures, society later would begin to control aspects of practice that physicians had first governed through internal professional standards. But in the last century, especially in the United States, professionalism was not a concern of the state, and jurisdictions had few or no licensing powers. So many schools of medical practice existed that the need to distinguish among them became a matter of pride for their adherents as well as a source of economic advantage. Thus physicians established a variety of medical associations, each of which set codes of conduct and standards.

When the American Medical Association was founded in 1847 its members adopted a code of ethics based on Percival's work.[14] The American Medical Association did not become a powerful medical organization until the twentieth century, but its code of ethics is representative of mid-nineteenth-century concerns about proper clinical practice. The first section stresses the physician's high moral obligation, the need for secrecy, the requirement that a physician see a patient through to the end of his illness—whether to cure or to death—balancing hope with realistic warnings to the family. There followed a long section, entirely missing from Percival, entitled 'Obligations of Patients to Their Physicians'. The patient should choose a properly trained physician, provide all the relevant information, follow the regimen prescribed, and after recovery 'entertain a just and enduring sense of the value of the services rendered him by his physician'.[15] Later sections of the code detail courtesies of physicians to one another and the qualifications of a regular physician. The title of the last chapter is 'Of the Duties of the Profession to the Public, and the Obligations of the Public to the Profession'. The relationship of physicians to coroners, guidelines for dispensing free service, and the need to educate the public regarding quackery are stated; yet, in distinction to the detailed treatment in Percival's work, there is no discussion of medical practice within hospitals, and the only reference to insane asylums is in a list of various institutions in which medical authorities must have an interest, such as hospitals, schools, and prisons.

In 1849, two years after adoption of the American Medical Association code, Worthington Hooker, a Connecticut physician, published what is increasingly recognized as a pioneer study of medical ethics in the United States, *Physician and patient; or, a practical view of the mutual duties, relations and interests of the medical profession and the community*.[16] The titles of the chapters, 'Skill in Medicine', 'Popular Errors', 'Quackery',

'Good and Bad Practice', 'Influence of Hope in the Treatment of Disease', 'Truth in Our Intercourse with the Sick', and 'Moral Influence of Physicians' reflect his ethical concerns. Two chapters, 'Mutual Influence on Mind and Body in Disease' and 'Insanity', particularly merit our attention. Hooker, like Percival, advocated removal of the mentally ill to a retreat, and reliance upon a 'regimen, or the regulation of their occupations and amusements, bodily and mental, and very little indeed upon medicine'.[17] Hooker deplored the practice, which he admitted was widespread, of intentionally deceiving the insane, or any other patient. He recommended early treatment, and that its costs should be shared by the town and state of the patient's residence. On the subject of how best to determine whether a person is insane, Hooker approved of the French system, in which a committee of experts made the decision after an examination conducted over several days. He regretted that, in his experience, police and prison authorities too often had the final decision, and, in some instances, regarded the advice of physicians as interference. 'Such having been the opinion and practices of our courts of justice', Hooker reflected, 'it is not strange that the rights of the insane have often been trampled on'.[18] In the matter of who might commit an insane person to institutional care, he noted that in Connecticut and Massachusetts it was the civil authorities, not physicians, who made the decision. Even worse, these authorities often committed someone only after he had performed some dangerous act. 'With such defects in the provision of the law', Hooker concluded, 'it is no wonder that the community is occasionally shocked with outrageous, even fatal acts by insane persons, who through neglect have been permitted to go at large.'[19] In keeping with his desire for early treatment in cases of insanity, he suggested that those suspected of being insane be examined by a 'standing commission of lunacy ... composed of physicians who are properly qualified'.[20]

Today we witness a trend in direct opposition to a pattern whereby physicians, and particularly psychiatrists, in the United States were given wide latitude regarding commitment to mental institutions. Dr Hooker had sought to introduce expertise into decisions regarding insanity; and this is by and large what occurred in the century after his advocacy. He saw application of knowledge by professionals as increasing the rights of the committed and reducing the error during commitment procedures. It is worth noting that he did not favour waiting until an overt, dangerous act had been committed before acting on behalf of the community and the patient. He was unaware of the present-day argument that cultural bias might distort professional judgement, or that reserving entirely to medical practitioners the decision about confinement might abridge legal protection for the patient.

For several generations thereafter few issues other than the justification for commitment and the humaneness of care were raised regarding psychiatric patients. Such currently significant concerns as the ethics of behaviour-control can be dissected away from the practices and concerns of 1800, but only with difficulty. The rights of the committed patient were few, and the primitive state of what we might call the psychiatric profession of the time meant that treatment consisted chiefly in admission to a hospital and residence there until reversion to a normal state, improvement, withdrawal by relatives, or death. The chief question for those who worried about the quality of care was how to conduct a paternalistic relationship kindly, effectively, and efficiently. Personal attention to a patient was expensive, and required great devotion on the part of individual caretakers and hospital authorities. Attempts to make contact with patients through close, kind supervision, mutual respect, and a wholesome environment— 'moral therapy'—could not survive waves of pessimism about the curability of mental illness, the overloading of caretakers with patients, and the degradation of hospitals to the status of human warehouses. These conditions obtained in the mid-nineteenth-century in many countries. Attention to ethical questions suffered as the possibility of substantial reform declined.[21]

Superintendents of American institutions for the insane, who formed an organization in 1844 (later to become the American Psychiatric Association), argued especially for the right to make most decisions about their patients, from commitment to the way the hospital was organized. This body, antedating the American Medical Association, testifies to the special role these physicians had assumed within the profession. Increasingly isolated from medical practice in general, the superintendents saw themselves as experts in a field too often neglected financially, misunderstood by the community, and requiring extraordinary powers of insight and judgement. Harassed by patients' complaints of maltreatment and wrongful commitment, the superintendents were more concerned to protect themselves from legal encroachment than they were about the veracity of these accounts. To the extent that an asylum attempted moral management, to use a term of Pinel's, which was also a goal of the English reformers William and Samuel Tuke at the York Retreat, an uplifting and healthy environment was created for the patient.[22] One could hardly find fault with trying to improve the conditions of patients, the authorities believed; and if better conditions did not exist, the cause lay in inadequate financial support from governments, not with the managers of the asylums. Worry over behaviour-modification did not exist, nor did the experts wonder whether they were guided by cultural bias in designing a healthy mental environment. In fact, American psychiatrists of the time commonly found the origin of illness in disobedience or ignorance of what now could be called New England Protestant principles of conduct.[23]

An occasional dramatic error in commitment became a popular cause, stimulating the creation of new laws and procedures. Particularly note-worthy was the case of Mrs E. P. W. Packard. She was committed in 1860 by her husband, a clergyman, to an Illinois institution on the grounds that she held dangerous religious beliefs. Her husband was a strict fundamen-talist, and feared that his wife would poison the minds of their children with liberal ideas. After some years Mrs Packard was freed by the trustees; but her troubles were not over. Her husband imprisoned her in her own home, and sought to have her recommitted. Finally, in 1864, a trial was held at which she was declared sane. She then embarked on a campaign to make commitment for the expression of opinions an impossibility, 'no matter how absurd these opinions may appear to others'.[24] Events like Mrs Packard's wrongful detention seemed to give credibility to claims against the hospital superintendents, although the latter vowed that such mis-carriages were extremely rare. As one anonymous writer in the *American Journal of Insanity* explained:

There can be no clashing or division of interest between the public and the institutions. They are one and the same, and no officer of any public institution can have any possible object in receiving or retaining any sane person in an asylum.[25]

While the psychiatric profession and the mental hospitals in the United States were becoming established and stimulating a body of law and precedent regarding the care of the ill, increased experimentation with new procedures and operations raised other ethical questions within the pro-fession and among the laity. Prominent among the questioners were those severe critics of nineteenth-century medicine, the antivivisectionists.[26] Three instances of what we today might consider abuses of research in Ohio, Maryland, and Ontario led to harsh criticism from physicians in North America and Great Britain. It is noteworthy that the condemna-tion came first and strongest from peers, illustrating the alertness of pro-fessional self-regulation. One other preliminary comment might be made: these experiments were not representative of contemporary treatment. On the other hand, one should be aware that the high-minded aspirations of asylum superintendents did not necessarily reflect, in fact probably did not reflect, the reality of day-to-day existence in mental hospitals. Published reports and admonitions are not good guides to the routine practice of psychiatry.

The Ohio experiment was published in the eminent *American Journal of Medical Science* in 1874. Dr Roberts Bartholow studied the effect of electrically stimulating the exposed surface of a patient's brain through her ulcerated skull. A few days later the patient died, but Dr Bartholow denied that the experiment was related to her death.[27] However, the *British Medical Journal* criticized Bartholow's procedure and his conclusions.[28]

The editor was reaffirming Claude Bernard's comment in his *Introduction to the study of experimental medicine*:

It is our duty and our right to perform an experiment on man whenever it can save his life, cure him or gain him some personal benefit. The principle of medical and surgical morality, therefore, consists in never performing on man an experiment which might be harmful to him to any extent, even though the result might be highly advantageous to science, that is, to the health of others.[29]

In a reply,[30] Dr Bartholow tried to justify his actions, but acknowledged that the procedure was injurious to the brain; and he stated that he would not repeat such an experiment.

Reports such as that of Dr Bartholow became a refrain in the antivivisectionist literature as examples of experimenters meddling with the bodies of poor patients while observing great caution toward fee-paying patients. The antivivisectionists saw a similarity between charity patients and laboratory animals: they opposed experiments on both, and sought to arouse the public through dramatic reports.[31]

In 1897, Dr George Rohé, superintendent of a Maryland hospital for the insane, reported on his research of operating on female pelvic organs in order to relieve insanity. He based this treatment on such diagnoses as hysteroepilepsy melancholia, puerperal insanity, and mania, and claimed a recovery rate of about one-third.[32] Similar operations were reported by Dr A. T. Hobbs of the Asylum for the Insane at London, Ontario.[33]

Reproaches against Drs Rohé and Hobbs appeared in the same issue of the *British Medical Journal* which had published their papers. Dr James Russell argued that there was no scientific basis for the widespread belief that gynaecological problems lay at the root of insanity in many women.[34] 'The relation of gynaecology to psychiatry has been pretty thoroughly discussed in late years, and the general consensus of opinion gathered from alienists and neurologists alike is that ... to extol it as a great curative method in the treatment of insanity is nothing short of absurdity.'[35] The procedures closely approached criminality, since the women could not understand their possible consequences. Dr Russell even queried 120 physicians in Great Britain and in America and found, as presumably he had suspected, that few believed female organs were associated with insanity or that any operation on them would be beneficial. The operations did not meet the test of conformity with current standards of medical practice.

Dr Rohé's reply to Dr Russell's severe and sarcastic criticism was very weak; he had been misunderstood, and reasserted his claim for a cure of insanity. Dr Hobbs, 'in reply, repudiated the idea that he ever approved of operative interference unless there was actual disease'.[36] Although reports of the infamous operations had achieved publication, they did not seem to represent the practice of a substantial fraction of the profession on either side of the Atlantic. Of course, if the experimenters had not published, their questionable accomplishments might have passed unnoticed.

In looking back over the nineteenth century—keeping in mind that we are considering, rather narrowly, antecedents to the modern psychiatric profession—we see that the growth of mental hospitals and the increase in their inmates, the decline in most instances of 'moral therapy', and a deterioration in the relations between physicians and patients were all evidence of an atmosphere of pessimism about the ultimate cure of mental illness. This pessimism, in spite of advances in understanding syphilis, alcoholism, and other specific causes of mental illness, overshadowed ethical concerns, and caused them to appear unimportant. A further consequence was that patients who displayed bizarre behaviour were relegated by some caretakers to a less than fully human status. Even reformers like Benjamin Rush described such patients as animal-like and fit for being 'broken' like wild animals.[37] In the twentieth century, and especially since the Second World War, there have been powerful changes in most of these perceptions, as new concepts and sensitivities about the activities of psychiatrists have arisen.

## The twentieth century

In this century, hospital psychiatry burgeoned, with some institutions housing as many as ten thousand patients. At the same time psychiatry and other mental health professions were evolving and manifesting new optimism about therapy and the future of their disciplines. This optimism, in the face of the hundreds of thousands of patients with poor prognoses and receiving inadequate care, was based on developments in biological research and psychodynamic and social psychiatry.

Biological research moved from one success to another in medicine, reducing communicable diseases, curbing syphilis, improving surgical procedures, and ameliorating chronic diseases such as diabetes and congestive heart failure. But enthusiastic extension of this research to the field of psychiatry created ethical concerns about, for example, the introduction of prefrontal lobotomy for certain diagnoses. Other treatments for schizophrenia—electroconvulsive therapy, removal of segments of the intestine to cure 'autointoxication', and similar questionable operations— were encouraged by two features of institutional care: the need to control highly disturbed patients, and repeated frustration in attempts to find a cure for the psychoses. Confidence in a new therapy was created, paradoxically, not only by difficulty in finding any cure, but also by the belief, common in the history of medicine and science, that a line of investigation or theory successful in one area is likely to be the key to solving a problem in another area.

In the application of these new treatments in the early twentieth century paternalism was still evident. The physician decided whether to pursue an innovation and on whom to apply it; he would meet few institutional or professional obstacles. Rejection of such a paternalistic attitude is a major theme in contemporary psychiatric ethics, and is dealt with in many of the other chapters in this book. These objections are applicable not only to the rise in biological research, and to the use of drugs, surgery, and electro-shock therapy, but also to other aspects of psychiatry in the twentieth century.

The increasing importance of psychodynamic psychiatry has paralleled that of biological research. Here too, ethical issues have arisen quickly and much more explicitly than in previous centuries. Psychoanalytic psychology, particularly the work of Freud, has raised the study of ethical issues to a new level of sophistication by pointing out the many motivations which may underlie the setting and enforcement of standards for others.

In both social and biological psychiatry a central goal has been to establish norms for behaviour as well as to correct deviance. In recent years, however, the public has become suspicious of the authority of a professional élite and the standards which they have promulgated. The accuracy of expert opinion is less an issue now than the prior issue of whether experts have any right to prescribe norms of behaviour or to modify behaviour without the full consent and understanding of the patient. This attitude contrasts with the enthusiasm following the Second World War in the United States, when government psychiatrists looked forward to the full adoption of public health methods by their specialty. Early intervention would follow the pattern of testing for tuberculosis and then treating the incipient illness. The problems that unilateral psychiatric inter-vention would present in everyday life—at least from our outlook today—reveal the great changes that have taken place in just a few decades among the psychiatrists and in their attitude toward their public responsibilities.

The public health model applied to psychiatry appeared to some to be the fulfilment of a great goal—the provision of expert knowledge and treatment of mental illness for everyone, not only for those who could afford a private psychiatrist or who were forced to enter a great warehouse for mental incompetents. Here we note a profound change in the history of psychiatry: transformation of the profession from a passive role—accepting those brought to it—to an active role, seeking ways in which psychiatrists might help everyone in a community. In the United States, efforts to increase the number of psychiatrists, and the establishment of a nation-wide network of community mental health centres in the 1960s, had this new role for psychiatry in mind. Certainly there is an association between the expansion of psychiatry into new fields and the current rise in ethical concerns about the psychiatrist's proper role.

While noting the hopeful expectations and the positive therapeutic results, we cannot overlook the damage done by psychiatrists to some patients who have been excessively treated by electroshock therapy, drugs, or surgery. Some patients have been committed without adequate reason, or for any reason, and kept in institutions for many years although fit for discharge to their families or to the community. Personal catastrophes occasionally resulting from misguided psychiatric interventions have elicited new legal formulations restricting the powers of psychiatrists. Awareness of ethical issues, however, has not been limited to medicine or psychiatry.

Some of the most severe critics of psychiatry recently have arisen from within its own ranks. In his early writings the British psychiatrist R. D. Laing[38] questioned the pathological nature of schizophrenia, suggesting that it could be a 'normal' reaction to modern life and a positive experience. Other psychiatrists have followed this line of reasoning, and opposed medication or customary restrictions on the behaviour of those diagnosed as schizophrenic.

Dr Laing appears a member of the old guard compared to Thomas Szasz. Dr Szasz questions the existence of mental illness across the board, and argues that to restrict the actions of patients is unethical. For example, should a person be severely depressed and wish to take his life, Dr Szasz would oppose restraining him by force and imposing psychiatric hospitalization and treatment. Szasz is not, it should be emphasized, opposed to intervention, but only to that which is not on terms acceptable to the patient. He takes issue with coercion in the name of help, and sees psychiatrists who so impose their 'help' as policemen and gaolers, mental hospitals that confine such persons as prisons, and the insanity defence as a mechanism whereby offenders try to avoid responsibility for their acts and the courts evade their duty to punish.[39,40] In an atmosphere of suspicion about authority, and with the existence of real abuses in psychiatry and a strong activist movement in the profession, such strident criticisms from within psychiatry have had an influence greater than has been possible at any time in the past.

An interesting discussion of recent historical trends in the ethics of psychiatry has come not from a member of the psychiatric profession but from a philosopher, William J. Winslade.[41] Professor Winslade has analysed medical, philosophical, and social components of approaches to mental illness since 1870. In ethical terms, he sees a conflict today between utilitarian thinking, characterized by cost-effective treatment often relying on behavioural control by drugs, and values advocating individually tailored, possibly long-term, and expensive care.

The tragic abuse of medicine during the Second World War was an important factor in rekindling the profession's interest in ethics, and led, first, to the *Code of Nuremberg*—rules for medical research—which was subsequently incorporated into the *Declaration of Helsinki* (see Appendix). In 1948 the World Medical Association promulgated the *Declaration of Geneva*, and, a year later, the *International code of medical ethics*, which was designed to be a model for national medical codes. These two texts are modern restatements of the Hippocratic Oath. There has also been growing awareness of abuses in psychiatry, which contributed to the adoption in 1977 of the *Declaration of Hawaii* by the World Psychiatric Association. This is the first code of ethics specifically designed for psychiatrists.[42] This text was a response both to the misuse of psychiatric diagnosis and treatment in order to silence political dissidents in the USSR (see Chapter 24) and to the less dramatic but pervasive role of psychiatry in its aggressive public-health and paternalistic stances in the West. To cite a few of the *Declaration*'s statements, it calls for disclosure of diagnosis and discussion of alternative therapies with the patient, requires that detained patients should have an avenue of appeal, and calls for the seeking of patients' consent to any treatment, with third-party consent in cases of patients' incapacity.

Some national psychiatric associations have formulated their own ethical codes. The American Psychiatric Association, for example, adopted the *Principles of medical ethics* of the American Medical Association, and produced a text, the *Principles of medical ethics with annotations especially applicable to psychiatry*, in 1973.[43,44] The most relevant sections of this text concern the appropriate conduct of the psychiatrist in regard to contractual relationships in situations where he works closely with other mental health and medical colleagues; in contexts such as examinations for employment, security, and legal purposes in which the right to confidentiality must be waived; and in circumstances where the psychiatrist may feel called to draw on professional knowledge in speaking out about social issues. The American Psychiatric Association text, unlike the *Declaration of Hawaii*, does not advocate an essentially egalitarian relationship between therapist and patient; its emphasis—demonstrating its direct descent from the Hippocratic tenets—is rather on the need for the psychiatrist to merit and maintain the trust of patients and other professionals alike.

Thus in a short period thoughtful laymen and members of the psychiatric profession have moved from an almost uncritical enthusiasm for the benefits of psychiatry in the four decades since the Second World War to a more judicious attitude about what psychiatrists say they can do and what they can actually accomplish. Psychiatry is in an era of unprecedented professional development, yet finds itself in crisis in its relations with patients and the public. In this quandary the welfare of the profession depends on sound analysis of ethical questions. Should psychiatry continue to move towards a greater reliance on organic treatment, for its authority and further towards faith in a genetic basis for behaviour, powerful and broad professional control over the destinies of others may reappear—but not in the language of psychodynamics. This recurrence of psychiatry's authority is possible should hereditary determinism achieve the popular and legal respectability it once held. Ethical questions seem to lose some of their urgency when the scientific underpinning of the profession appears solid. The rise of ethical concerns in the last three decades may be due in part to the crisis in confidence through which psychiatry itself has passed. If this is the case, the growing organic basis claimed for psychiatry makes a sensitivity to ethical questions even more important for the future, when biological tests may appear to be conclusive.

## References

1 Edelstein, L.: The Hippocratic Oath, text, translation and interpretation, in *Ancient medicine*, ed. O. Temkin and C. L. Temkin. Baltimore, The Johns Hopkins Press, 1967, pp. 17–18.

2 Ibid., p. 6.

3 Rosen, G.: *Madness in society: chapters in the historical sociology of mental illness*. Chicago, University of Chicago Press, 1968, pp. 125–8.

4 Mora, G.: History of psychiatry, in *Comprehensive textbook of psychiatry*, ed. A. M. Freedman and H. I. Kaplan. Baltimore, Williams and Wilkins, 1967, p. 12. For a dissenting view, see: Mobaraky, G. H.: Islamic view of mental disorders (Letter to the editor). *American Journal of Psychiatry* **146**:561, 1989.

5 Ibid., p. 5.

6 Ackerknecht, E. H.: *A short history of psychiatry*, trans. S. Wolff. New York, Hafner, 1968, p. 17.

7 Mora, G.: History of psychiatry, in *Comprehensive textbook of psychiatry*, ed. A. M. Freedman and H. I. Kaplan. Baltimore, Williams and Wilkins, 1967, pp. 16–17.

8 Neugebauer, R.: Treatment of the mentally ill in medieval and early modern England: a reappraisal. *Journal for the History of Behavioural Science* **14**:158–69, 1978.

9 Ellenberger, H. F.: Psychiatry from ancient to modern times, in *American handbook of psychiatry*, 2nd edn, vol. 1, ed. S. Arieti. New York, Basic Books, 1974, p. 14.

10 Hunter, R. and Macalpine, I.: *Three hundred years of psychiatry 1535–1860: a history presented in selected English texts*. London, Oxford University Press, 1963, pp. 602–10.

11 Dain, N.: *Concepts of insanity in the United States, 1789–1865*. New Brunswick, NJ, Rutgers University Press, 1964, pp. 18–19, 23.

12 Percival T.: *Medical ethics (1803)*, ed. C. D. Leake. Huntington, NY, Robert E. Krieger, 1975, p. 126.

13 Ibid., p. 89.

14 Code of medical ethics adopted by the National Medical Convention in Philadelphia, June, 1847, in Hooker, W. L.: *Physician and patient; or, a practical*

*view of the mutual duties, relations and interests of the medical profession and the community (1849)*. New York, Arno Press, 1972, pp. 440–53.

15 Ibid., p. 444.

16 Hooker, W. L.: *Physician and patient; or, a practical view of the mutual duties, relations and interests of the medical profession and the community (1849)*. New York, Arno Press, 1972. See also Musto, D. F.: Worthington Hooker (1806–1867): physician and educator. *Connecticut Medicine* **48**:569–74, 1984.

17 Ibid., p. 334.

18 Ibid., p. 340.

19 Ibid., p. 342.

20 Ibid., p. 342.

21 Musto, D. F.: Therapeutic intervention and social forces: historical perspectives, in *American handbook of psychiatry*, vol. 5, ed. S. Arieti. New York, Basic Books, 1975, pp. 34–42.

22 Hunter, R. and Macalpine, I.: *Three hundred years of psychiatry 1535–1860. A history presented in selected English texts*. London, Oxford University Press, 1963, pp. 602–10, 684–90.

23 Grob, G. N.: *Mental institutions in America: social policy to 1875*. New York, The Free Press, 1973, pp. 160–1.

24 Packard, Mrs E. P. W.: *Marital power exemplified in Mrs. Packard's trial, and self-defence from the charge of insanity; or three years' imprisonment for religious belief, by the arbitrary will of a husband with an appeal to the Government to so change the laws as to protect the rights of married women*. Hartford, Connecticut, Case, Lockwood, 1866, p. 55.

25 *American Journal of Insanity* **29**:302, 1872.

26 Harvey, J.: Human experimentation in the nineteenth century. Unpublished manuscript. Harvard University, 1977. (I am indebted to Ms Harvey for calling my attention to this reference in psychosurgery.)

27 Bartholow, R.: Experimental investigations into the functions of the human brain. *American Journal of Medical Science* **67**:305–13, 1874.

28 *British Medical Journal* **i**:687, 1874.

29 Bernard, C.: *An introduction to the study of experimental medicine* (1865), trans. H. C. Greene. New York, Henry Schuman, 1949, p. 101.

30 Bartholow, R.: Experiments on the functions of the human brain. *British Medical Journal* **i**:727, 1874.

31 French, R. D.: *Antivivisection and medical science in Victorian society*. Princeton, Princeton University Press, 1975.

32 Rohé, G. E.: The etiological relation of pelvic disease in women to insanity. *British Medical Journal* **ii**:766–9, 1897.

33 Hobbs, A. T.: Surgical gynaecology in insanity. *British Medical Journal* **ii**:769–70, 1897.

34 Russell, J.: The after-effects of surgical procedure on the generative organs of females for the relief of insanity. *British Medical Journal* **ii**:770–7, 1897.

35 Ibid., p. 770.

36 Ibid., p. 774.

37 Deutsch, A.: *The mentally ill in America* (1938). New York, Columbia University Press, 1949.

38 Laing, R. D.: *The divided self* (1960). Baltimore, Penguin, 1971.

39 Szasz, T. S.: *The myth of mental illness: foundations of a theory of personal conduct* (1961). New York, Harper and Row, 1974.

40 Szasz, T. S.: *The manufacture of madness: a comparative study of the Inquisition and the mental health movement.* New York, Harper and Row, 1970.

41 Winslade, W. J.: Ethics and ethos in psychiatry: historical patterns and conceptual changes. Unpublished paper presented at the American College of Psychiatrists, Annual Meeting, San Antonio, Texas, 6 Feb. 1980.

42 Blomquist, C. D. D.: From the Oath of Hippocrates to the Declaration of Hawaii. *Ethics in Science and Medicine* **4**:139–49, 1977.

43 Moore, R. A.: Ethics in the practice of psychiatry—origins, functions, models, and enforcement. *American Journal of Psychiatry* **135**:157–63, 1978.

44 The Principles of Medical Ethics with annotations especially applicable to psychiatry. *American Journal of Psychiatry* **130**:1057–64, 1973.

# 3

# The philosophical basis of psychiatric ethics

*Richard Hare*

The editors are plainly right when they say in their introduction that 'the contemporary psychiatrist . . . is required to grapple with a broad range of ethical problems'. Some of these problems afflict other branches of medicine equally; some are, for the reasons the editors give, peculiarly pressing for the psychiatrist. On the relations in general between moral philosophy and medical ethics I have already published a paper, 'Medical Ethics: Can the Moral Philosopher Help?',[1] and this will absolve me from repeating here all the arguments for the method of thinking I there advocate. I will, however, outline the method itself, before I go on to apply it to the problems besetting psychiatrists.

In that paper I drew a contrast between two supposedly incompatible views about the right way to settle moral questions, which I dubbed the 'utilitarian' view and the 'absolutist' view. I then showed how the two views could in fact be combined into a single viable account by carefully distinguishing between two different levels of moral thinking: first, that at which we are faced with particular pressing moral problems without much time for reflection about them; and secondly, that at which we think out, in general, what our attitudes to these problems ought to be. I said that the absolutist approach was the most suited to the first kind of thinking, the utilitarian to the second.

But before I explain why this should be so, I must first outline the two approaches. Readers of the huge literature that is accumulating on medical ethics will easily recognize the two kinds of view that I have in mind. We have first those who tend to speak in terms of people's rights and the corresponding duties of other people towards them—rights and duties which are thought of as in some sense absolute. This stance is often adopted by writers on, for example, abortion. They will accordingly claim, depending on which side they take in the dispute, either that the woman concerned, or that the fetus, has certain inalienable rights which there is an absolute duty to respect. It is one of the defects of this approach that it tells us very little about how to decide *what* rights people have, or, if incompatible rights are claimed, which ought to be preserved and which overridden.

Though 'absolutist' is a convenient name for this approach, we must be careful not to confuse this use of the term with that in which it is the opposite of 'relativist'; the controversy between absolutists in this second sense and relativists has no bearing on our present topic.

The second, utilitarian, approach is the one attributed by the editors to those who 'assumed implicitly that they could perform their task without ethical difficulties by serving the best interests of their patients', and that 'inherent in the nature of the work is the psychiatrist's prime and sole interest in his patients; their optimal welfare is his *raison d'être*'. But before we assimilate this view to utilitarianism an important qualification has to be made, which, as we shall see, introduces a difficulty. A true utilitarian would, it might be said, not consider the interests of his patients solely, or even pre-eminently. For the interests of all are of equal weight for the utilitarian, and he is forbidden by his doctrine to give extra weight to those of some particular person who stands in some special relationship to him. To this question we shall return. However, in many, perhaps most, cases the interests of the patient are so paramount, and the interests of others so negligible or so equally balanced, that a utilitarian would without much hesitation make his decision solely by reference to the patient's interests. But to avoid this complication let us simply say that a utilitarian is one who thinks that when faced with a moral decision he ought to act in whichever way is best for the interests of those affected.

Here too we have to be careful in using this term. The name 'utilitarian' is used by philosophers for adherents to a wide variety of doctrines, and in common parlance has got attached to others which are not utilitarian at all in any strict sense. So it must not be assumed that any argument that has ever been brought against any view that has been called utilitarian can be brought against the view we are considering.

It is evident that psychiatrists, like most of us, think from time to time in both these ways. But it is also evident that cases can and frequently do arise in which the two methods will yield different results. For example, in a case involving treatment against the wishes of the patient, a psychiatrist might well think that the treatment was clearly in the patient's best interest and in that of everybody else concerned, and yet think that he had no right to impose it if the patient did not want it. To this question too we shall return.

Because of these apparent conflicts between the approaches, philosophers and others have suggested various more or less clumsy ways of combining them so as to avoid the conflicts. One way would be to say that the duty to do the best for the patient and others (the so-called duty of beneficence) is one duty among many, and that, as in all cases of conflicts between duties, we have to 'weigh' the relative urgency or importance of the duties in the particular case; in some cases we may decide that the duty of beneficence is the more weighty, in others the duty to respect some right. This way out is utterly unhelpful, relying as it does on a weighing process of which no explanation whatever is given.

Another equally unhelpful suggestion is that the duties in question, including that of beneficence, might be placed once for all in an order of priority, sometimes called 'lexical ordering' (from the practice of lexicographers of putting first all the words beginning with 'a', whatever other letters they contain, and then those beginning with 'b', and so on). So we should, for example, fulfil duty *a* in all cases in which it existed, whatever other duties might also be present, and so on. This suggestion is unhelpful for at least two reasons. The first is that, as before, no account is given of why the duties should have this order of priority rather than some other. The second is more subtle: will it not be the case that on some occasions duty *a* ought to have priority, on others duty *b*? In terms of the same example as before, ought we not sometimes to treat the patient against his will if the harm to which he will otherwise come is very great, but in others respect his right to refuse treatment? No lexical ordering of the duties could allow us to say this, and yet we might often want to say it. Nevertheless the idea of lexical ordering has been quite popular.

These suggestions are handicapped by their failure to distinguish between the different levels of moral thinking. It is indeed hard to see how any one-level account could solve the problem of moral conflicts; for if conflicts arise at one level, they cannot be resolved without ascending to a higher level. That we have a duty to serve the interests of the patient, and that we have a duty to respect his rights, can both perhaps be ascertained by consulting our intuitions at the bottom level. But if we ask which duty or which intuition ought to carry the day, we need some means other than intuition, some higher kind of thinking (let us call it 'critical moral thinking') to settle the question between them. And this kind of thinking has also to be brought to bear when we are asking what intuitions we ought to cultivate, or what our duties at the bottom level are (our *prima facie* duties, as philosophers call them).

An illustration of the difference between the levels, and of its relation to that between the utilitarian and absolutist approaches, may help. A simple case is that of our duty to speak the truth. A common example in the philosophical literature, which goes back to Kant, is this: a madman is seeking out a supposed enemy to murder him, and I know where the proposed victim is; do I, if I cannot get away with evasions, tell the truth to the madman? Most of us, as well as the duty to speak the truth, acknowledge a duty to preserve innocent people from murderers, and here the duties are in conflict. An absolutist will have to resolve the conflict by calling one of the duties absolute and assigning some weaker status to the other. Let us suppose that, as some absolutists have, he calls the duty to speak the truth absolute, and therefore requires us to sacrifice the life of the victim to it. A utilitarian, by contrast, is likely to say that neither duty is absolute; what we have to do is to decide what would be for the best in the particular case. In this case it will presumably do most good to all concerned, considering their interests impartially, if I tell a lie. But then it is objected that the utilitarian is making a solemn duty, that of truthfulness, of no account; he simply maximizes utility, and might as well not acknowledge any other duties.

The dispute is easily resolved once we distinguish between the two levels of moral thinking. At the intuitive level, we have these intuitions about duties, and it is a good thing that we do. A wise utilitarian, bringing up his children, would see to it that they developed a conscience which gave them a bad time if they told lies. He would do this because people with such a disposition are much more likely to do, on the whole, what is best than somebody who does cost–benefit analyses on particular occasions; he will not have enough time or information to do them properly, and will probably cook the results to suit his own convenience. Firm moral dispositions have a great utility. So the utilitarian can let the absolutist operate at the intuitive level in much the way that he proposes. But when conflicts arise, or when the question is asked, *what* intuitions we ought to have, or *what* duties we ought to acknowledge, or what would be the *content* of a sound moral education, then intuitive thinking is powerless; for if intuitions conflict or are called into question, it is no use appealing to intuitions to resolve the difficulty, since they will be equally questionable.

A utilitarian can therefore let the absolutists have their say about the intuitive level of thinking, and ask them in return to keep their fingers out of the critical level at which intuitions themselves are being appraised. That the method to be used at the critical level has to dispense with the appeal to intuitions seems on the face of it clear; that there is no other method than the utilitarian which can achieve this is more controversial, though I myself know of no other. But it is at any rate clear that *if* the utilitarian is given the monopoly of the critical level, he can readily explain what happened at the intuitive level; we form, in ourselves and others, for good utilitarian reasons, sound intuitions prescribing duties, and the disposition to feel bad if we go against them; the content of these intuitions is to be selected according to the good or bad consequences of our acquiring them; when they conflict in a particular case, we have to apply utilitarian reasoning and do the best we can in the circumstances; but when the case is clear and there is no conflict, we are likely to do the best by sticking to the intuitions.

This is not the place to give a full account of these two levels of moral thinking, the intuitive and the critical. For our present purposes it will be enough to characterize them briefly. The intuitive level, with its *prima facie* duties and principles, is the main locus of everyday moral decisions for the psychiatrist as for everybody else. Most of us, when we face a moral question, decide it on the basis of dispositions, habits of thought, moral intuitions (it makes little difference what we call them) which we have absorbed during our earlier upbringing and follow without reflection.

It is sometimes suggested that this is a bad thing, and that we ought to be more reflective in our moral thought even about these everyday decisions. It is easy to see that this is not so, however. One of the qualities we look for in a good man is a readiness to do the right thing without hesitation. A man would not, for example, have the virtue of dependability if, when the time came to fulfil some undertaking he had made, he first had to spend some time thinking about whether he ought, after all, to fulfil it. Not only do we seldom have time for such thought (especially if we are doctors); but, if we do engage in it, it is frighteningly easy to deceive ourselves into thinking that the case is a peculiar one in which our ordinary moral principles give the wrong answer, when in fact we would do better to stick to them. Our ingrained moral principles are therefore not merely time-saving rules of thumb, but necessary safeguards against special pleading. On the whole we are more likely to err by abandoning one of these principles than by observing it; for the information necessary in order to be sure that this is a case where the principle gives the wrong answer is seldom available.

Most of us get these sound general principles in the course of our normal upbringing and acquire what is called a conscience, which makes us feel uncomfortable if we break them; and this too is a good thing. However, those philosophers are mistaken who think that these moral feelings which we have are by themselves certificates of correctness in the moral judgements which they prompt. For the upbringing which led to our having them might have been misguided; if a Southerner in the old days felt bad about being friendly with blacks, because he had been brought up to believe in keeping one's distance from them, we should not regard that as a proof that he had a duty to keep his distance, but rather condemn his upbringing. In the medical and other professions the *prima facie* principles which apply specially to their members have been to some extent made articulate, if not in codes of conduct, at least in the consistent practice of disciplinary bodies like the General Medical Council in Britain and the medical licensing authorities of each state in the US. But, even more obviously in this case, it is possible to ask whether the particular practices which at any one time have this official blessing are the right ones.

That is one reason why the intuitive level of moral thinking is not self-sufficient. Another is that the *prima facie* principles, to be of much use, have to be fairly simple and general, or they could not become second nature, as they have to. This has the consequence that cases can easily arise in which the principles conflict, and thus yield no determinate answer. It is good for doctors to strive always to save life, and to strive always to relieve pain; but what if the only way to relieve pain is to kill? Or what if we can only save one life by destroying another? Such cases are the main fuel of controversy in medical ethics.

For these reasons a full account of moral thinking will include an account of the critical as well as of the intuitive level. The critical level is that at which we select the principles to be used at the intuitive level, and adjudicate between them in cases where they conflict. But how is this to be managed, and how do we know when to engage in critical moral thinking? For, as we implied above, it is sometimes even dangerous to do so.

To answer the first question I should have to survey almost the whole of moral philosophy. Good brief general introductions to ethical method are to be found in the opening chapters of P. Singer, *Practical ethics*[2] and J. C. B. Glover, *Causing death and saving lives*.[3] My own *Moral thinking: its levels, method, and point*[4] provides a full-scale account. All I can do here is to state my own view briefly, recognizing that other moral philosophers might not share it. My view is based on an analysis of the moral concepts or words, such as 'ought' and 'wrong', in order to determine clearly, first their meanings; and then, as part of these, their logical properties; and thus, as a consequence of their logical properties, the rules for arguing about questions formulated in terms of these concepts. This is really the only sound basis for an account of moral reasoning. I am perhaps unusual among moral philosophers in insisting that at the critical level no appeal should be allowed to moral intuitions. Such appeals are bound to be viciously circular; for if intuitions are in dispute, no appeal to intuitions could settle the dispute. To this, one exception can be made; some of our intuitions are not moral, but linguistic or logical, and can be shared by people with the most diverse moral views. Logical intuitions are acquired when we learn our language, not as part of our moral upbringing; they are expressed, not in moral judgements (for example, that it would be morally wrong to force the patient to submit to treatment), but in statements of logic (for example, that to say such and such would be to contradict oneself). The failure to distinguish between these two kinds of intuition is one of the main sources of confusion in moral philosophy.

It seems to me that it can be established on the basis of logical intuitions alone that whenever we make a moral judgement of the typical or central sort we are prescribing that something be done in all cases of a certain (perhaps minutely specified) kind, that is, prescribing universally for a given *type* of case. We cannot consistently claim that some particular individual has some duty, but that some other individual, however like the first in his character, circumstances, etc., might not have it. The thesis that moral judgements represent universal prescriptions can be made the basis of an account of moral reasoning which supports most of our common moral convictions (though it would be quite wrong to quote this fact in support of the account itself—for how are we to know that the moral convictions, implanted in us by our upbringing, are the ones we ought to have?). An example (which is all there is space for) will perhaps help to make clear how this can be done. We most of us accept the principle that it is wrong in general to confine people against their will. If 'wrong' expresses a negative universal prescription, or universal prohibition, this is easy to explain. For then in saying that it is wrong to do this, we are prescribing that it never be done. And the reason why we are ready to prescribe this is that we imagine ourselves in various circumstances in which other people might wish to confine us against our will, and unhesitatingly prescribe that they should not. There are some complications in the logic here which would need to be gone into in a full treatment; but it is not difficult to see intuitively that one who is prepared to prohibit involuntary confinement in all hypothetical cases in which he would be the victim will be prepared to assent to a general prohibition.

The same kind of reasoning can be used to establish exceptions to the general principle. In some cases the patient, if not confined, is likely to kill some other person. If we put ourself in the place of this other person, we find ourself ready to prescribe that the patient *should* be confined. It is a question of balancing the interests of the two parties; presuming that the interest of one in not being killed is greater than that of the other in being at liberty, we shall, if we put ourselves in the places of both in turn and respect their interests impartially, allow the confinement of the patient because this would promote the greater interest of the other person. So by this means we can build up a set of universal principles, each with the necessary exceptions written into it, to cover all contingencies.

At least, we could do this if we had complete information, superhuman powers of thought, and infinite time at our disposal. Since we are not so gifted, we have to do the best we can to arrive at the conclusions to which such a gifted being would come. That, indeed, is why it is necessary to separate moral thinking into two levels. By doing the best critical thinking of which we are capable, when we have the leisure for it, we may be able to get for ourselves a set of fairly simple, general, *prima facie* principles for use at the intuitive level, whose prescriptions for particular cases will approximate to those which would be given by a being who had those superhuman powers. This is really the best that in our human circumstances we can do.

In practical terms, what this means is that psychiatrists should, when they have the time, think about the ethics of their profession and try to decide what principles and practice would, on the whole, be for the best for those affected by their actions. In this thinking, they should consider a wide variety of particular cases, and think what ought to be done in them, for the greatest good of those affected. And they should select those principles and practices whose general acceptance would yield the closest approximation to the actions which would be done if all cases were subjected to the same leisured scrutiny. It is important to notice that cases have to be weighted for the likelihood of their occurring. In deciding whether people ought to wear seat-belts when driving, we should be more moved by the huge majority of cases in which this increases the chances of survival than by the small minority where this is not the case.

It appears that the method I have explained corresponds in general to that adopted by the contributors to this volume. I wish now to go through some of the topics mentioned by the editors at the end of their introduction, and ask how this method might be applied to them. We shall, I hope, see that the distinction between the intuitive level of thinking, at which an absolutist stance is appropriate, and the critical level, at which we should rather think in a utilitarian way, enables us to find a path through the philosophical difficulties, and at least pin-point the empirical, factual questions which we should have to answer in order to solve the practical ones.

I will start with a problem which illustrates especially well the value of the separation of levels: the problem of medical practitioners' peculiar duties to their *own* patients. As we saw, it is natural for psychiatrists to regard themselves as owing a special duty to their own patients, to safeguard their welfare—a duty which ought to override any duties they may have to the public at large. If, for example, they have as patients people who they know will be a great deal of trouble to anybody who is so unwise as to employ them, have they any duty to reveal the fact when asked for a medical certificate? Here, as before, it is obviously no use treating the duty of confidentiality to the patient and the duty of candour to the employer as duties on the same level, but ranked in order of priority; for it may depend on the case which duty should have precedence. If the patient is an airline pilot and his condition will cause him to lose control of the plane, we may think the public interest paramount; if he is a bank clerk and is merely going to turn up late for work from time to time, we may think that his condition should be concealed.

Dr Rappeport, in his excellent contribution (see Chapter 18), has many good examples of this kind of conflict between duty to one's patient and other duties. It looks at first as if a utilitarian, who is required to treat everybody's equal interests as of equal weight, can find no room in his system for special duties or loyalties to people standing in special relationships to oneself (for example, that of patient). And indeed this has often been made the basis of objections to utilitarianism. But the two-level account makes it easy to overcome them. At the critical level of moral thinking we are bound to be impartial between the interests of all those affected by actions. So at this level, we shall have to give no special edge to our own patients, but simply ask, in each case we consider, what action would produce the best results for all those affected, treated impartially. A superhuman intelligence, given complete information, might be able to provide specifications, in this way, for all cases that could possibly occur. But if this gifted person were asked to draw up some simple ethical principles for the conduct of psychiatrists, which they ought to cultivate as second nature, it is obvious that the single principle 'In every case, do what would be in the best interests of all considered impartially' would not do; for mortal psychiatrists are seldom going to know what this is. It is much more likely that the principle to do the best one can for one's own patients will figure among the principles it recommends. Why? Because if psychiatrists absorb this principle as second nature it is much more likely that the interests of all, even considered impartially, will be served than if psychiatrists think they have to do an impartial utilitarian calculation in every case. This is because the relationship between psychiatrists and their patients, based on mutual trust and confidentiality, has itself immense utility, and the destruction of this relationship is likely, except in extreme and rare instances, to do much more harm than good. So we have the paradoxical result that a utilitarian critical thinker would recommend, on utilitarian grounds, the cultivation of practices which are not themselves overtly utilitarian, but appeal to such notions as the patient's right to confidentiality.

However, this right to confidentiality is not the only right which will be entrenched in the principles of a good psychiatrist. There will be other rights there too, including the right of the public to be protected. All these rights are important; yet they will sometimes conflict. A one-level account of moral thinking based on rights is powerless to deal with such conflicts. The two rights, of the patient to confidentiality and of the public to protection, exist; but if that is all we say, we can say nothing about cases where one of these rights has to be overridden. In such cases, the psychiatrist will have to do some critical thinking; and it may have different outcomes according to the severity of the impact on the various parties' interests.

Next, let us take the right to liberty. As we saw, some sort of prohibition, in general, of forcible deprivation of liberty is likely to be part of the moral armoury of nearly everybody, because liberty is something we all value highly. For this reason, the good psychiatrist will be extremely averse to confining anybody unless there is a very strong reason. But sometimes there will be. The right of the public to protection comes in here too. So here too we have the same picture: a superhumanly well-informed critical thinker who had considered all possible cases on utilitarian lines might be able to arrive at the right answer in all of them without saying anything about rights; but if he were asked to draw up a set of principles to be imbibed by mortal psychiatrists, which would lead them in the course of their practices to the nearest approximation to his ideal solution, he would certainly place high on the list of such principles that which protects people's right to liberty. For to confine people against their will does them, normally, such enormous harm that any psychiatrist who makes light of this principle will be a public menace.

Two particular cases of this kind of problem require special consideration. The first is that of when a psychiatrist may justifiably confine people for their own good (for example, to prevent suicide). It is the case that *in general* people who kill themselves are not acting in their own best interests (as is shown by the later thoughts of most of those who have been prevented). However, it may be that some suicides do the best for themselves (for example, some who face miserable senility and have no close friends or kin). So here too the right to liberty has to be balanced against a duty to preserve the patients from great harm to themselves. Both are very important, and will be recognized as such by good psychiatrists; and this recognition can be justified on utilitarian grounds at the critical level. But at the intuitive level psychiatrists will do well to respect *both* these principles without thinking in a utilitarian way at all—until they conflict; and then they will have, perhaps at the cost of a great deal of mental anguish, to think critically and ask what, in these particular circumstances, is for the best. (See Chapter 12)

The other problem is that which arises when patients are incapable of judging for themselves what is in their own interests. This may be because they are young children, or because they suffer from some mental disability. Our ideal critical thinker would no doubt, in some of the cases he reviewed, come to the conclusion that the best interests of such people would be served if they were treated without their consent. The reason might be that patients were unable to grasp the facts of their own cases, and in particular facts about the prognoses with and without the treatment. The psychiatrist may be better able to make such prognoses. But it is terribly easy to stray across the boundary between prognosis, on which perhaps psychiatrists can claim authority, and judgements of value about possible future states of the patient, on which they cannot. Suppose that the patient, if subjected to brain surgery, will become placid and contented, but lose all his artistic flair; but that if he is not, he will remain an artist of genius, which is what he wants to be, but suffer miserably from recurrent depression, and perhaps in the end kill himself after enriching the world with some outstanding masterpieces. An exceptionally gifted psychiatrist might be better able than the patient to predict that these would be the respective outcomes of treatment and of no treatment; but that would not give him the authority to override the patient's preference for the second outcome over the first.

Looked at in terms of our two levels, the picture becomes clearer. At the intuitive level, the patients' right to decide for themselves what sort of persons they want to be will seem very important; and we can justify at the critical level the entrenchment of this right by pointing out that in the vast majority of cases patients *are* the best judges of what will in the end suit them, and also that psychiatrists are very subject to the temptation to impose their authority beyond its proper limits, that is, to stray over the boundary above mentioned. On the other hand we can also justify at the critical level the entrenchment of the duty to preserve patients from the consequences of their inability to grasp what their own future states are likely to be. In most cases there will be no conflict between these principles; but where there is, they can be resolved only by an ascent to the critical level in the particular case. However, there is danger in a too ready ascent; for it is easy to persuade oneself that there is a serious conflict between the principles, when what is really happening is a conflict between the patient's right to liberty and our own propensity to meddle.

We may next consider a group of problems about consent which are closely related to the problem we have just been considering. One of the rights on which great emphasis is properly laid is the right not to be treated without one's own informed consent. The justification, at the critical level, for the emphasis on this right is the same as before: that patients are on the whole the best judges of their own interests, and their interests are normally much more severely affected than anybody else's; so the ideal outcome from the utilitarian point of view is much more likely to be realized if this right is normally allowed to 'trump' any considerations of utility which might *seem* strong in particular cases (the 'trump' metaphor comes from R. M. Dworkin, *Taking rights seriously*[5]). But if we wish to entrench the right in this way, we have the difficulty on our hands of saying what counts as informed consent. Can people who have neither practised psychiatry, nor actually been in the state which they will get into if not treated, ever be *fully* informed about what they are letting themselves in for? If they are really pretty mad, could they not make crazy choices even if they did grasp the alternative prognoses? And would not this make their refusal of consent not fully informed? These are familiar problems. What our critical thinker will try to do is to find some principles for deciding what criteria of informed consent, if absorbed into the practice of psychiatrists, are likely to lead them in the majority of cases to do what is for the best.

An especially difficult subclass of these problems afflicts psychiatrists who have to deal with patients who are already confined in a mental institution or in prison. In either case the psychiatrist may be in a position to force treatment on patients (for example aversion therapy or psychotropic drugs); and it has sometimes been thought that this presents an ideal opportunity to do good to the patient (and also serve the public interest) against the patient's will. 'Force' need not mean 'physical force'. If the psychiatrist says to the patients that they are likely to get out much earlier if they submit to the treatment, this is not force in Aristotle's strict sense (*Nicomachean ethics* 1110 a 1) of 'that of which the origin is outside [a person], being such that in it the person who acts, or [to be more exact] is acted upon, contributes nothing'; but it is certainly duress, which Aristotle treats of in the next few sentences; the patients are faced with alternatives such that they are highly likely to do what the psychiatrist wants. It has therefore been denied that people in confinement can give meaningful consent, and it has been held, accordingly, that it is always illegitimate to use such treatments on them. But this doctrine too could lead to less than optimum results if it caused offenders to languish in prison who might, if given suitable drugs, be safely allowed out.

This could be a consequence of the failure to distinguish between our two levels, and a resulting rigidity in the application of the principle guaranteeing the right to freedom of choice to be treated or not treated. The principle is immensely important as a safeguard against abuses; if psychiatrists can break it without a qualm, they are not to be trusted with prisoners or even with patients confined in institutions. But in order to determine the limits of the principle, what is needed is not a lot of casuistry about the precise meaning of 'consent', but a set of practical rules whose general adoption will lead to the best decisions being made on the whole.

One such rule would be to insist on the separation of decisions about confinement or release from decisions about treatment. In the case of prisoners, decisions to confine would be left to judges, and decisions to release to the civil authorities; decisions about treatment would be the province of psychiatrists, who, therefore, could only say to prisoners that they might be able to improve their conditions enough to enable the authorities to release them, and not that they (the psychiatrists) would release them if they successfully underwent treatment. Certainly any mixing up of the roles of judge and doctor is likely to have bad consequences; for a decision on medical treatment requires careful observation over a period of an individual patient, which courts cannot undertake; whereas the sentence of a court aims at consistency and fairness between different offenders, and, subject to this, at the protection of the public, and the psychiatrist has neither the experience nor the expertise nor even the habits of mind required for this judicial role. Sound critical thinking would be likely to insist on such a separation of roles, and thus prevent many abuses. But whether this is so or not, the general point stands: *what* rights ought to be enshrined in *what* rules should be decided in the light of the consequences of making those rules rather than some others.

Lastly, we may consider a related problem: how are we to decide which conditions are mental diseases and which are merely deviations from the currently accepted social or political norms?[6] This is the problem raised by the political abuse of psychiatry in Russia. For example, is homosexuality a disease; and if it is, is 'revisionism'? Where do we draw the line? The term 'disease' is above all a ticket giving entry to what has been called 'the sick role'. It is an evaluative term, implying that the person with the disease ought, other things being equal, to be treated in order to remove it. If we classify homosexuality, or 'revisionism', as a disease, what we are doing is subscribing to such an evaluation. So it is no use hoping by mere conceptual analysis to settle the question of whether homosexuality is a disease. We shall call it one if we approve of the treatment of homosexuals to remove their homosexuality (if this is possible); and the same with 'revisionism'. The crucial decision, then, is whether to approve of this. And it should depend on whether the approval, and therefore practice, of treatment to remove homosexuality will on the whole be for the best for the homosexuals and others. Confining ourselves for the moment to voluntary treatment, it would seem that sound critical thinking might arrive at the following principle: if the patients want not to be homosexual and ask for treatment because they want to have sexual relations with the opposite sex, they should be given what they want; on the other hand, if they want not to be homosexual only because of the social stigmas and legal penalties attached to homosexuality, it might be better, if we could, to remove the stigmas and penalties. The reason why critical thinking would arrive at this conclusion is that in the first case the interests of the patient and others are advanced by 'cure', whereas in the second they would be better advanced by the removal of the need for it. If the situation is thus clarified, it becomes less important whether we call the condition a disease or something else.

But if *compulsory* treatment for homosexuality or 'revisionism' comes into question, the right to liberty again becomes of the first importance. Since having things done to one against one's will is something that nobody wants (this is a tautology), it is in itself an evil; it can only be justified by large countervailing gains (for example, as above, the protection of the public from dangerous mental patients). It is hard to see what these gains could be in the two cases we are now considering. In both of them the general good would be much better advanced by removing the political institutions which make 'revisionism' something that the authorities feel impelled to suppress, or by removing the habits of thought which make people want to persecute homosexuals. It will be better all round for everybody if this comes about.

Though I have not had the space to deal with all the topics raised even in the Introduction, I have perhaps done enough to indicate in general how such problems are to be handled. In all cases what we have to do is to find a set of sound principles whose general acceptance and firm implantation in the habits of thought of psychiatrists will lead them to do what is best for their patients and others. In the general run of their professional life, they need not think like utilitarians; they can cleave to principles expressed in terms of rights and duties, and may, if they do this, achieve better the aims that an omniscient utilitarian would prescribe than if they themselves did any utilitarian calculations. But if that is all they do, their thought is still defective; for, first of all, it is a matter for thought what these principles should be; and second, we have to know what to do when they conflict in a particular case. And thought about both these questions will be best directed if it has as a target the good of those affected by the application of the principles.

## References

1 Hare, R. M.: Medical ethics: can the moral philosopher help?, in *Philosophical medical ethics: its nature and significance*, ed. S. F. Spicker and H. T. Engelhardt, Boston, Reidel, 1977, p. 49.
2 Singer, P.: *Practical ethics*. Cambridge, Cambridge University Press, 1979.
3 Glover, J. C. B.: *Causing death and saving lives*. London, Penguin, 1977.
4 Hare, R. M.: *Moral thinking: its levels, method, and point*. Oxford, Oxford University Press, 1981.
5 Dworkin, R. M.: *Taking rights seriously*. Cambridge, Mass., Harvard University Press, 1977, p. xv.
6 On this question see Hare, R. M.: Health, in *Journal of Medical Ethics* 12:174–86, 1986.

# 4

# The social dimension[*]

## David Mechanic

Psychiatrists, as well as other mental health professionals, are influenced in their activities and judgement by the sociocultural context, by their personal and social biographies, by the ideologies implicit in their professional training, by the state of perspectives, theories, and scientific understanding in their disciplines, and by the economic and organizational constraints of practice settings. The practice of psychiatry involves competing roles. Although psychiatrists may select themselves into certain roles and not others, it is common for them to have multiple professional roles, with varying social and ethical requirements, but with no clear demarcation among them. Much of professional practice has important social-control functions, and mental health practitioners are in part political actors. The conflicts in psychiatry are more sharply drawn and the boundaries of appropriate activity somewhat more hazy than in other medical disciplines.

A psychiatrist plays numerous roles, including that of the scientist, the physician, and the bureaucrat. While such spheres of action overlap, it is analytically useful to separate them and examine their varying aspects and the ethical dilemmas they pose.

Freidson's work[1] has suggested the distinction between the psychiatrist as a scientist and as a physician. The goal of the physician is action, and not knowledge. The physician believes in what he is doing, and this is functional for both doctor and patient. The sceptical detachment of the scientist would only discourage the patient and erode the suggestive powers of the therapeutic encounter. While the scientist seeks to develop a coherent theory, the clinician is a pragmatist, depending heavily on subjective experience and trial and error in situations of uncertainty. While the scientist seeks to determine regularity of behaviour in relation to abstract principles, the clinician is more subjective and suspicious of the abstract. The responsibilities of clinical work make it difficult to suspend action, to remain detached, and to lack faith that one is helping patients.

The differences between the objects of science and practice suggest

[*] This chapter is adapted from David Mechanic, *Mental health and social policy*, 3rd edn. Englewood Cliffs, NJ, 1989.

different ways of proceeding in the two roles. The researcher in psychiatry must be concerned with very precise and reliable diagnosis. Only through effective distinctions among varying clinical entities can knowledge of aetiology, course, and effective treatment be acquired.[2] Although such efforts in making finer distinctions or in identifying new conditions may be uncertain and yield no benefits for the patient, they may serve the development of scientific inquiry and understanding. Such diagnostic orientations used in a clinical context, however, may be of little use, or even dysfunctional. The labelling of questionable conditions may induce anxiety in the patient, may be stigmatizing, and may divert efforts from taking constructive action on behalf of the patient. The professionalization of psychiatry in the late nineteenth century in America, and the growing assumption that mental disorders were biological in origin and required organic interventions, undermined the useful activities of social reformers who devoted attention to the social context of treatment.[3] If mental disease was an unfolding of biological propensities, why worry about the social environment? The irony, of course, was that the new conception had little to offer patients, and undermined helpful and constructive interventions.

Psychiatrists in their capacity as physicians have a social role that extends beyond their technical knowledge. The scope of their activities may be constrained by their conceptions of psychiatric activity, but they have limited control in defining the types of patients that seek their help. They have a social responsibility to do what they can to help patients who are suffering and seek assistance, and thus cannot simply be constrained by the state of established knowledge. Psychiatrists as physicians work in part on the basis of scientific knowledge and clinical experience, and in part on the basis of their social judgement of what is appropriate for the situation. As the problems faced become more uncertain, and are less resolvable through existing psychiatric expertise, the psychiatrist's social biography and values have a larger impact on decision-making.

Because psychiatry deals with deviance in feeling states and behaviour, its conceptions run parallel to societal conceptions of social behaviour, personal worth, and morality. Conceptions of behaviour can be viewed from competing vantage points, and thus they are amenable to varying professional stances. In the absence of clear evidence on aetiology or treatment, personal disturbance can be alternatively viewed as biological in nature, as a result of developmental failures, as a moral crisis, or as a consequence of socio-economic, social, or structural constraints. Remedies may be seen in terms of biological restoration, moral realignment, social conditioning, or societal change. Although all of these elements may be present in the same situation, the one that the psychiatrist emphasizes has both moral and practical implications. There is no completely neutral stance. Diagnostic and therapeutic judgements have political and social implications.[4]

In this context it is of great importance whom the therapist represents. To the extent that the therapist acts exclusively as the patient's representative, and in the patient's interest as far as this can be known, the situation is relatively simple. The patient suffers and seeks assistance, and the role of the therapist is to do whatever possible to define the options available for the patient, and to proceed in a manner they agree on. Such intervention may be at the biological, psychological, or social level, or within a medical, psychodynamic, or educational model. The definition of the endeavour, however, is in terms of the patient's interests and needs. In real situations, failure to define options is common, and the psychiatrist's values and ideologies or practice orientations may intervene, resulting in deviations from the ideal. Indeed, psychiatrists may not be conscious of their own ideologies and orientations, because they are so entrenched in their own world-view. Or they may proceed against the patient's wishes, because they assume their own greater knowledge of the patient's interests. Despite these complexities, the approach is distinctive in that actions taken are for the sake of the patient and no other.

The ethic that the physician's responsibility is to the patient and no other is itself a value, as are other norms of practice, such as confidentiality. The ethic arises from a commitment to individuals as compared to collectivities, and is not universally shared. In the People's Republic of China, for example, psychiatric practice is a public function, with primary commitment to the interests of the state and not the individual.[5] Psychiatric practice takes place openly, in consultation with family members and with community leaders. The way the patient will be handled is a public issue, and information concerning the patient's problems and management is shared with community officials and work supervisors. While the basic content of psychiatry is seen as primarily biological, the social consequences of psychiatric advice are recognized. Professional practice cannot be divorced from existing forms of social organization.

China may seem far from American psychiatric concerns, but the issues of whom the clinician represents and the proper scope of confidentiality are critical issues in the care of the mentally ill. Many families of mental patients are bitter against mental health professionals, who they feel leave them uninformed and provide them little help in dealing with the burden of a severely ill child or spouse. Most families are dissatisfied with the information they receive, feeling that communication is almost exclusively with the patient, isolating them from the treatment process.[6,7] Effective care of chronic patients often requires communication with landlords, police, employers, and others that pushes against the traditional ethic of confidentiality that defines patient–therapist relationships.

In Western societies, psychiatrists may work as agents of individual patients or as agents of collectivities or organizations, such as families, schools, industries, courts, and the armed services.[8] Under some circumstances, mental health professionals may retain autonomous roles in which they continue to act as agents for patients, but their organizational auspices make such roles more uncertain and more susceptible to encroachment.[9] Couples therapy or therapy involving parents and children inevitably involves a clash of wills and interests, and the therapist is forced to take sides, though this may be reflected only in the most subtle ways. Although such therapies may involve sufficient common interest among the parties to sustain the encounter, the therapist must walk a difficult line. Therapists in such situations often see themselves as playing an autonomous role; such a role may become more tenuous as the power of the institution employing the therapist intrudes on the relationship.

When physicians work for organizations other than the patient, their loyalties are split. Although conflict of loyalties may not be a major issue in routine everyday practice, it may at any time become problematic whenever the organization and the patient have competing needs or interests. The most dramatic examples of such forms of bureaucratic psychiatry are found in totalitarian countries, in which psychiatrists are state bureaucrats and may perform social-control functions for the state, or in the military, in which psychiatrists serve as agents of the organization. Similar pressures exist, however, whenever the psychiatrist represents some collectivity, whether it be a court, prison, school, or industrial organization. In all but the most crass cases, the role of the psychiatrist as double agent is sufficiently ambiguous that the professional can experience feelings of neutrality and of participation in the public interest. It is this comforting sense of lack of partiality that is most dangerous, because it diverts attention from the dilemmas in resolving conflicts between involved parties. The use of psychiatry to discredit political dissenters or innovators is reasonably evident, even if disputed. It is the subtle social influences on psychiatric work that are more difficult to bring into the open.

The issue of split loyalties relates to financial considerations as well as to power. Like other physicians, psychiatrists are increasingly employed by preferred-provider organizations, health-maintenance organizations, and in other capitated settings that have incentives to provide as little care as necessary. In some circumstances, physicians may substantially increase their yearly remuneration by meeting low utilization targets. The pattern of mental health services in capitated settings deviates a great deal from that in fee-for-service settings, particularly when the former involve prepaid group practice. Psychiatric bed-days are typically restricted, services are provided more by general physicians and social workers than by psychologists and psychiatrists, care is available more in group as compared with individual settings, and the intensity and costs of mental health services for patients are much lower.[10,11] It is not clear what this all means for quality, since research in this area is very underdeveloped; but it raises ethical questions for the psychiatrist nevertheless. Psychiatrists in such organizational arrangements certainly have a professional responsibility to ensure that seriously ill patients receive care appropriate to their conditions, as they do in other forms of practice. The difficulty is that because uncertainty is large almost any viewpoint can be justified. Yet there is good reason to anticipate that prepaid practice often does not provide chronic patients with the access and intensity of services they require. As prospective payment is increasingly applied to in-patient psychiatric care comparable issues of growing importance will become evident.

## Social influences on psychiatric judgement

In most instances in which psychiatric judgements are made, there are no reliable independent tests to confirm or contest them. While psychiatric diagnosis focuses on disordered thought and functioning, and not deviant behaviour *per se*,[12] judgements of disorder must be tied to social contexts and the clinician's undertaking of them based not only on clinical experience but also normal life experience. Most lay persons can recognize the bizarre symptoms associated with psychosis; it is the borderline areas that are more at issue, and at these borders it becomes more difficult to disentangle subculture, illness behaviour, and psychopathology. As the subcultural situation is further from the psychiatrist's firsthand experience, the likelihood increases that inappropriate contextual norms will be applied. To the extent that the patient comes to the therapist voluntarily and seeks relief from suffering, the lack of precision in making such contextual judgements is less of a concern than when the psychiatrist acts on behalf of some other interest. Even in the former situation, however, the prestige of the therapist reinforces his or her personal power in the encounter with the patient considerably, and may reinforce one of the alternative views of the nature of the patient's problem.

The absence of procedures or laboratory tests to establish diagnoses independent of the therapist's contextual judgement makes it relatively easy for critics to insist that psychiatrists label patients on the basis of social, ethical, or legal norms, and not on clearly established evidence of psychopathology.[13,14] Although such criticisms cannot really speak to the scientific validity of the application of a disease model to the patient's suffering or deviant behaviour,[15,2] they apply to the role of psychiatrist as clinician or bureaucrat in dealing with social problems and psychological disorder. The psychiatrist who mediates conflicts between husband and wife, between parent and child, between employer and employee, and between citizens and official agencies must inevitably mix social judgements with assessments of psychopathology. When the psychiatrist acts as an agent to excuse failures at work, to obtain special preference for housing or other benefits, to obtain disability payments, to excuse deviant behaviour, or in a wide variety of other arenas, he typically parades social judgements and personal decisions as psychiatric practice. It is therefore essential to know something about the social orientations and world-views of psychiatrists.

## Personal and social biographies

Psychiatrists have gone through a variety of selective screenings represented by their entry into medical school, into psychiatry, and into particular types of psychiatric functions, such as individual psychotherapy, hospital work, or administration. This selective process involves not only academic performance and interests, but also social background, values and ideologies, and individual aspirations. Processes of selection are also affected by the changing patterns of psychiatric practice, shifting opportunities and market conditions, and alterations in the modalities that psychiatrists use to treat patients. Various studies have shown that physicians selecting psychiatry differ from students in other specialties, such as surgery or family practice, in terms of social background, attitudes, and political orientations.[16,17] In their classic book, *Social class and mental illness*, Hollingshead and Redlich[18] reviewed the dramatic dissimilarity in the social biographies of psychiatrists in New Haven who pursued analytic-psychological orientations and those who were more directive in their approaches and depended more on organic therapies. Despite an obvious convergence in therapeutic practice, with many psychiatrists using a combination of therapies and drugs, there continues to be a distinctive selection process of mental health professionals into psychotherapy.

Therapists engaged in office-based psychotherapy are both distinctive and relatively homogeneous in their social characteristics.

Careers terminating in the private practice of psychotherapy are populated, to a very large extent, by practitioners of highly similar cultural and social backgrounds. They come from a highly circumscribed sector of the social world, representing a special combination of social marginality in ethnic, religious, political, and social-class terms.[19]

Psychotherapists coming from psychiatry, clinical psychology, and social work are more similar in social background and practice orientations to one another than to psychiatrists who are more medically inclined.[19,20] Persons who become therapists, regardless of profession, perform similar activities, have comparable work styles, share many viewpoints, and have strikingly similar developmental experiences.

The implications of similarities of development and perspective among therapists are not obvious, but very suggestive. Certainly it is reasonable to assume that therapists who are upwardly mobile, socially marginal, non-religious, divorced, and politically liberal will see social and moral issues differently from more socially integrated, conventional, and religious persons, and they will communicate quite different judgements. Because therapists' personalities and orientations are important aspects of therapy, and because psychotherapy is largely an influence process,[21] the encounter inevitably involves the transmission of values. Therapists may wish to minimize personal biases, but they cannot help but transmit what they stand for. To the extent that this is explicit to the patient, it is less of a problem than when it is masked behind a professional mystique.

Greenley and colleagues[22] provide data collected in 1973 from psychiatrists practising in Chicago, some of whom were also studied in a 1962 survey.[20] These data indicate that at least in Chicago there is a strong persistence of a dominant Freudian-analytic orientation and of office-based private practice. Although more psychiatrists report having an eclectic orientation, the enthusiasm of the early 1960s for social and community psychiatry has receded. It was noted as the orientation of only some 15 per cent of respondents in 1973. If this study was repeated today, it would probably show the growing dominance of biological psychiatry.

There is some evidence from this survey that the social characteristics of both psychiatrists and their patients are becoming more like those of the general population, although large differences exist. The growth of psychodynamic therapy in the United States can be viewed as a social movement, developing first among particular practitioners and patients facing certain existential dilemmas.[23] Psychodynamic therapies developed their roots in urban areas, with many practitioners of urban, middle-class, Jewish origins. This therapy initially attracted persons with social inclinations and characteristics similar to those of the therapists. As the movement grew, however, and therapy became more widely accepted in the culture, one would have anticipated that it would become more heterogeneous in geographic distribution and in the characteristics of both therapists and patients. The indications were that such heterogeneity was developing as psychotherapy became institutionalized, and Greenley and colleagues' Chicago data[22] illustrate this trend. Comparing cohorts of psychiatrists completing residencies in different periods from before 1950 to the time of the survey, they observe a steep decline in the proportion of those with immigrant fathers, those who were Jewish, and those who were raised in a large city. Psychiatrists in 1973, as compared with 1966, reported having more women, blacks, Catholics, and poor persons as patients, and somewhat fewer Jewish patients.

The Chicago study, as well as other data, indicates that psychiatric practice is becoming more varied and more complex.[24-26] Unfortunately very few recent data are available on the values and personal biographies of practising psychiatrists; but both national surveys by the American Psychiatric Association (APA) and other studies document changing patterns of practice. The best source of data is a national sample of psychiatrists surveyed in 1982 by the APA,[25] which can be roughly compared with earlier surveys in 1965 and 1970. Office-based practice in 1982 continued to be the primary work-setting for 58 per cent of psychiatrists, but psychiatrists were now more commonly employed in general hospitals and other settings as well. Despite these changes, individual psychotherapy continued as the dominant clinical activity, accounting for half of all clinical hours and 46 per cent of all patients seen. Half the patients now treated with individual psychotherapy also receive one or more drugs, a pattern increasingly different from the past. Approximately one-fifth of patients are seen exclusively for medication management.[25] In contrast, psychoanalysis accounted for only 6 per cent of clinical hours, and such activities as couple and family therapy, group psychotherapy, behavioural therapies, and electroconvulsive therapy constituted minor proportions of psychiatrists' time-expenditures in patient-care.

Similarly, another study comparing two surveys fifteen years apart found psychiatry to be a more diversified specialty than in the past. Psychiatrists now work in more settings and have a wider array of professional activities.[26] Moreover, individual psychiatrists are more likely to divide their time among multiple practice-settings than in the past.

Although psychiatrists earn considerably less than surgical specialists or those that perform many procedures, their earnings compare favourably with those of other cognitively oriented medical specialties, earning more on an hourly basis than these other specialties.[27] Some of the changes in the organization of psychiatric work, and the diversification of care, are probably a product of the changing financial environment and incentives of medical practice. Unfortunately, these trends seem to have increasingly made psychiatrists less accessible to public chronic mental patients, who receive their care from public institutions and community mental health centres.[28] Psychiatrists are the least likely of all specialties to accept Medicare patients, though this may substantially relate to the poor mental health coverage and limited fees allowed under Medicare regulations.[29]

In any case, the growing diversity in psychiatric practice should allow many patients greater opportunity to locate therapists and sites of care closer to their own orientations and perspectives. Thus, existing trends seem to favour increasing differentiation within psychiatry and more opportunities to work out conflicts between mental health concerns and values.

## The socio-cultural context

The socio-cultural context in which young psychiatrists develop and mature and within which they practice has a dramatic influence on their world-views, as well as on their professional activities. Varying periods of histori-cal time and specific cultural contexts provide different images of the nature of man, the boundaries of deviance, and the professional role of social and psychiatric intervention.[30] In Europe, psychiatry has remained closer to general medical practice than in the United States, where psychodynamic therapies have been viewed by young psychiatrists as more prestigious than taking care of severely disturbed or chronic patients. In the period since the Second World War psychodynamic ideas came to dominate residency programmes in psychiatry, and had a major effect on the way psychiatrists perceived their roles and practised their craft. Why the United States and not Europe was the more fertile ground for psycho-analytic ideas is a question amenable to many interpretations; neverthe-less, the fact is that it was, and this resulted in its having a dramatic influence on views of psychopathology and the treatment of patients.

During the 1960s there was a great ferment in American society, charac-terized by social activism and an ideology that government could remedy social problems through governmental programmes. This ideology had a broad sweep, and it also came to encompass conceptions of the social causes of and remedies for mental illness. Psychiatrists caught up in the ethos of the time began making grandiose claims for the potentialities of a community psychiatry. Such advocacy was not grounded in improving the programmes provided for chronic mental patients, who were increasingly being returned to their communities, but in claims for special societal expertise. In the words of one such advocate, 'The psychiatrist must truly be a political personage in the best sense of the word. He must play a role in *controlling* the environment which man has created'[31] [p. 73].

A major component of this ideology was the notion that psychiatry could engage in primary prevention to limit the occurrence of mental illness. Caplan[32] maintained that such efforts involved identifying harmful in-fluences, encouraging environmental forces that support individuals in resisting them, and increasing the resistance of the population to future illness. The programme he offered under the guise of psychiatric expertise was simply a form of social and political action. As Caplan saw it,

The mental health specialist offers consultation to legislators and administrators and collaborates with other citizens in influencing governmental agencies to change laws and regulations. Social action includes efforts to modify general attitudes and behavior of community members by communication through the educational sys-tem, the mass media and through interaction between the professional and lay communities[33] [p. 56].

Caplan cites the area of welfare legislation as one that psychiatrists ought to be involved in.

In some states, the regulation of these grants [Aid to Dependent Children] in the case of children of unmarried mothers is currently being modified to dissuade the mothers from further illegitimate pregnancies. Mental health specialists are being consulted to help the legislators and welfare authorities improve the moral atmosphere in the homes where children are being brought up and to influence their mothers to marry and provide them with stable fathers[32] [p. 59].

Clearly Caplan wished psychiatrists to become involved in matters such as morality and values, on which there were many views and differences of opinion. Caplan[33] also saw psychiatrists extending their focus to problems of personnel selection, placement, and promotion.

If he accedes to these requests, he will find that he is using his clinical skills and his knowledge of personality and human relations and needs not only to deal with persons suspected of mental disorder, but also to predict the fitness of healthy persons to deal effectively with particular situations without endangering their mental health. He will also be exercising some influence upon the nature of the population in the organization, and hopefully he will be reducing the risk of mental disorder by excluding vulnerable candidates and by preventing the fitting of round pegs into square holes[33] [p. 6].

Caplan even went as far as to speculate that a psychiatrist might 'exercise surveillance over key people in the community and . . . intervene in those cases where he identifies disturbed relationships in order to offer treatment or recommend dismissal' [p. 79]. However, he rejected this role, not because of lack of ability or knowledge on the part of psychiatrists, but because it would be a distasteful role for most psychiatrists, and because of political and social complications. That some psychiatrists do not find this role distasteful is evidenced by the thousand and more American psychiatrists who responded to an obviously biased poll by *Fact* magazine which attempted to discredit Barry Goldwater's psychological fitness to run for the presidency of the United States. A lawsuit resulted in a jury decision that Goldwater had been libelled.

Why, one might ask, do I resurrect the overblown rhetoric of the 1960s, given the widespread appreciation of the degree to which psychiatrists overextended themselves in that era? I do so because, while academic psychiatry has clearly changed, much of the interventionist and preventive ideology persists. Caplan was not a voice in the wilderness; he had substantial influence on the thinking of many practitioners and those still being trained, and the mental health field is still dominated by facile concepts of prevention. Caplan's influence may be greater in psychology and social work than in psychiatry; but these are the professionals providing many of the mental health services in our society. In addition, this kind of thinking has diffused to judges, correctional officers, and many other decision-makers in our society, and plays an important role in daily affairs.

Some of the concepts implicit in preventive psychiatry are unfortunate not only because they are grandiose, naive, and an obvious projection of political values, but also because they continue to divert attention from making many of the remedial efforts more consistent with existing knowledge and expertise. Preventive care during pregnancy and adequate post-natal care, still not fully available to the poor, are important in preventing mental retardation, prematurity, brain-damage, and a variety of other difficulties. Family-planning services and facilities for families with handicapped children are often difficult to find. The system of services in the community for chronic mental patients is at best fragmentary. By what set of values do we divert attention from these issues to pursue illusory goals? The greatest weakness of preventive psychiatry in the 1960s was the substitution of vague ideals for tangible action, and a failure to specify in any clear way how psychiatric expertise could lead to the laudable goals being advocated.

The extraordinary range of roles played by psychiatrists is reflected in the work of a Harvard psychiatrist as a consultant for the Boston Patriots football team. Among his tasks were teaching techniques 'to program the mind to achieve peak athletic performance' and 'meeting with team members before a game to help prepare them psychologically for a competition'.[34] Other functions included individual therapy, drug-use prevention efforts, helping resolve conflicts among team members, and improving relations between the coach and players. It is difficult to assess what this all adds up to. The prestigious *New England Journal of Medicine*, which publishes little on mental illness, and rations its space in the most parsimonious way, devoted more than five pages to psychiatric consultation in football.

It is essential from an ethical perspective to differentiate among varying psychiatric roles. With the psychiatrist as researcher, it is fully appropriate to examine the value of social system interventions. Caplan[32] maintained that various crises and transitional periods in the life-span, such as entering school, having a child, going to the hospital for surgery, or moving to a new environment, pose severe stresses that may burden a person's coping capacities and entail a high risk of social breakdown. He asserted that during such periods persons had a heightened desire for help, and were more responsive to it. He argued that community psychiatrists should seek out situations in which people feel vulnerable, and provide supportive help and new coping techniques. The theory argued that social breakdowns could be prevented either by intervening in the lives of people and their families during crises, or by working through various professionals, such as doctors, nurses, teachers, and administrators, who naturally come into contact with people during such crises. Among the contexts Caplan suggested for such crisis-intervention were prenatal and surgical wards, divorce courts, and colleges. The basic hypothesis, and one legitimate and worthy of detailed inquiry, is that it is possible to give people anticipatory guidance and emotional inoculation that help them cope with threatening events.

When the psychiatric role moves from investigation to practice, crisis-intervention involves major ethical dilemmas. First, although aspects of the theory are promising, it is based on a vague conceptualization to the effect that environmental trauma and the lack of coping abilities cause mental illness, a conception for which the evidence is incomplete and far from secure. Second, although such efforts may be made with laudable goals in mind, the evaluation literature attests to the fact that such programming often not only fails to achieve desired objectives, but also makes matters worse.[35] Third, there is really very little evidence that the types of trouble-shooting preventive psychiatrists advocate, although perhaps valuable in reducing distress, have any real impact on the occurrence of mental illness or are directed at those who are likely to become mentally ill if untreated. Despite these ethical concerns, the psychiatrist could justifiably engage in such programmes with interested community groups to the extent that they understand the limitations and elect to participate voluntarily. Such interventions may be viewed in the same light as any other uncertain therapy, with possible positive and possible adverse effects that must be balanced.

Preventive psychiatry intuitively seems enticing. After all, isn't it better to prevent illness than treat it after it occurs? Moreover, the proponents of prevention typically argue that it saves vast amounts of money, since treating severe illness is much more expensive than initial preventive care. But, as we have learned so well in the area of general medical care, this argument is simplistic, and often incorrect.[36,37] The success of prevention, and potential cost-savings, depend on the ability to target individuals who will become more seriously ill without treatment and the cost and effectiveness of the preventive intervention. But even when we have interventions that we believe to be efficacious, and that are not too costly, preventive efforts may still be a bad bargain unless we have the knowledge to target precisely. The number of people who become seriously mentally ill is a small proportion of the population. In contrast, the number of people who can be potential targets of preventive intervention is very large. Even a relatively inexpensive intervention spread over large numbers of people can result in large aggregate costs. But many of these people get better without formal intervention. The Epidemiological Catchment Area project estimated that 29.4 million people had a DSM III disorder[38] and many more millions have high levels of distress and dysfunction without such disorder. If we add additional vulnerable individuals, including those under high stress, those experiencing bereavement or divorce, the unemployed, and so on, we can readily identify a target population of 100 million people. Thus, an intervention costing $100, not a particularly expensive one by psychiatric standards, would in the aggregate cost $10 billion. Think of what even a small fraction of this could do for the severely mentally ill.

Preventive psychiatry is also on shaky grounds when psychiatrists are in bureaucratic positions, providing services to those neither seeking nor desiring their assistance. The imposition of such interventions in schools, divorce courts, welfare agencies, and the like, buttressed by the coercive authority of the organization, is a serious imposition on privacy and the rights of persons to lead their lives without interference. Even if the theory were powerful and its success demonstrated, involuntary application of preventive psychiatry would raise profound ethical issues.

As the optimism of the 1960s receded, preventive psychiatry lost much of its lustre, although it remains as one of many streams of psychiatric activity, and much soft thinking on the issue persists. Psychiatry in the 1980s can be more generally characterized as returning to interest in the biological bases of behaviour, and more particularly to brain processes, neurobiology, and behavioural genetics. Although psychodynamic views are highly prevalent, the field of practice is more heterogeneous than ever before, and training centres are increasingly focusing on biological research and a more rigorous approach to psychiatric diagnosis. This will, of course, affect the viewpoints and practice orientations of future psychiatrists. While these changes result in part from research advances in biological psychiatry and epidemiology, they also reflect changing conceptions of the potentialities of social reform in the society at large. Each cohort of psychiatrists is likely to retain a part of the social and value conceptions characteristic of its historical life cycle.

## Constraints of practice settings

Professional practice is influenced by the social context of practice organization and the manner in which payment for services is made. The influence of the professional's employer on professional decision-making is widely recognized, and has already been discussed. I will focus here on some practice constraints that are less widely appreciated.

In the dominant forms of psychiatric therapy in the United States, the psychiatrist is a private office-based professional contracting with patients to provide services for a fee-for-service. Although such services may be partially covered by third-party insurance, the implicit contract is between therapist and patient. Such therapy is typically organized in large time-units of 45 to 50 minutes, as often as several times a week.

Disproportionate services of this kind are purchased by the affluent or those well-covered by insurance, and the therapists view themselves as responsible to their patients, and not to some more abstract notion of need in the community. The form of payment in this situation—the fee for service per session—presumably creates an incentive on the part of the professional for long-term therapy beyond any point that such intervention would be cost-effective.

An alternative model of psychiatric work is found in such entities as health-maintenance organizations, community mental health centres, or the British National Health Service. In these contexts, the psychiatrist is theoretically responsible to a defined population who receive services from the organization. Because psychiatric services in these contexts cannot be made available to everyone who needs them, and because the use of services has implications for the economic viability of the plan, rationing decisions must be made as to who in the population most needs specialized psychiatric services and to what extent. Typically, such rationing is in part specified in the contract that patients have with the plan, such as a limitation on the number of psychiatric visits during any year. Rationing also occurs by requiring a formal referral from a primary-care physician in the plan to a consulting mental health professional. Such organizations, however, cannot sanction long-term therapy for a small number of patients at the expense of others needing services; therefore psychiatrists in such contexts are more likely to have shorter consultations, to engage in short-term psychotherapy, or to provide drug-monitoring. Although psychiatrists with such inclinations may be drawn to these types of organizations, there is little question that organizational arrangements help shape the scope and character of psychiatric services.

Similar types of constraints operate in mental hospital practice or in community care. What can be done for a patient depends on the personnel and resources available and the number of patients requiring help. Services are frequently stretched thinly or are inadequate because demand exceeds capacity. While it is typical to bemoan the fact of inadequate financing, it is unlikely that economic opportunities will ever allow psychiatrists to provide everything possible to all patients in need. Although there are no easy ways out of the ethical dilemmas posed by the need to ration, these dilemmas suggest an ethical imperative for the mental health professions. Stated simply, such professions have an obligation to evaluate their techniques and approaches in relation to their benefits and costs, in order that the resources available can be applied in the most effective way. A prudent society cannot provide public support for long-term psychoanalysis or other psychotherapies in the absence of evidence that these approaches are more efficacious than less costly alternatives.

In recent years there has been a substantial growth of private psychiatric hospitals, dedicated psychiatric, alcohol, and drug-abuse units in acute general hospitals, and a wide range of new proprietary psychiatric ventures. As reimbursement has become constrained in the general medical area, entrepreneurs view psychiatric care as a highly profitable area capitalizing on in-patient insurance coverage for mental illness available to much of the population. As a consequence of this and other factors, mental health-care expenditures as a proportion of total expenditures are rising in many employment groups. Proprietary companies now sell capitated mental health services to health-insurance plans and self-insured employers alarmed about escalating costs for mental illness. Such businesses, built around capitation, can be highly profitable, because standards of psychiatric care are unclear and highly discretionary, and it is relatively easy to shift the context of care from in-patient to out-patient settings at reduced cost. On the one hand, in-patient units have an incentive to raise occupancy rates by development of new in-patient programmes; on the other hand, capitation plans have an incentive to shift care to community contexts, and to provide less intense and less expensive services. Since standards are so uncertain, and the evidence favouring one alternative over the other is frequently lacking, the structure of the psychiatrist's employment and the incentives personally affecting professional behaviour have a large influence. It is easy for professionals to deceive themselves that behaviour in their employers' and their own interests is what is consistent with the patients' interests.

It is unlikely that ethical discussions will affect the dynamics of proprietary momentum. There are, however, a few principles that can minimize violations of ethics. In the context of budget constraints and the search for more cost-effective care it is fully appropriate to manage care more tightly, and to try to minimize care that offers little benefit. Capitated systems provide an incentive to do so; but the professional's personal remuneration should not be linked to reduced-expenditure targets. Such links clearly put the professional's and patient's interests in opposition, and can be a serious source of distrust and conflict.[39] Professionals in capitated systems, whether for-profit or not-for-profit, must maintain sufficient professional independence that they can make quality-of-care decisions without personal penalty. Some profit-oriented medical plans are alleged to fire physicians who retain such independence; but the profession must shun any organizations that do so. This is no easy issue, but the opinions of one's peers and profession can be a forceful source of social control.

More importantly, the psychiatric professions must be stronger advocates of developing effective quality-assurance systems for the mentally ill. The care provided to patients with comparable problems in varying settings must be subjected to continuing professional evaluation. It is sad that we know so little about the quality of mental health care in alternative settings.

Yet such knowledge is the central tool necessary to choose among alternative care pathways.

## A note on the care of chronically impaired patients

Deinstitutionalization and community mental health care are as much social ideologies as were earlier conceptions of the care of the mentally ill. These ideologies consist of beliefs that it is desirable that individuals, to the extent possible, live independently, assume responsibility, and show a desire to adjust in some fashion to community living. The involuntary hospitalization of patients constituted a violation of cherished beliefs about individual rights, and the abuses associated with such involuntary commitment have become widely known, making it more difficult to justify civil commitment. Perhaps less widely appreciated are the pressures now placed on patients and their families to have the patient in the community, and the growing tendency to refuse a hospital refuge to some highly impaired patients.[40]

The extent to which the community should allow such refuge, and at what point, is very much tied to economic factors and the social ethos. The issue of the extent to which coercive therapies should be used to stimulate and maintain appropriate functioning does not easily yield to a consensus, and practices vary a great deal from one context to another, depending on the values and commitments of professionals working with such patients. With the development of aversive techniques of control, 'token economies', and other forms of behaviour-modification, profound questions are raised about the limits of coercion and treatment.

In sum, every aspect of psychiatric conceptualization, research, and practice is shaped by social ideologies and assumptions. Concepts of deviance, boundaries between mental disorders and other types of problems, modes of intervention, and selection of clients all vary by time and place, by the character of social structure, and by dominant social perspectives. The biographies of mental health professionals and their practices are culturally shaped, and the economic system poses alternative opportunities and constraints. Because mental health professionals must work with models, and because such models have broad ethical implications for every aspect of their craft, there is no way of escaping the fact that psychiatric practice is as much a moral as a medical endeavour.

## References

1 Freidson, E.: *Professional dominance: the social structure of medical care*. New York, Schocken Books, 1974.
2 Mechanic, D.: *Medical sociology*, 2nd edn. New York, Free Press, 1978.

3 Grob, G. N.: *The state and the mentally ill: a history of Worcester State Hospital in Massachusetts, 1830–1920*. Chapel Hill, University of North Carolina Press, 1966.

4 Halleck, S. L.: *The politics of therapy*. New York, Science House, 1971.

5 Kleinman, A. and Mechanic, D.: Some observations of mental illness and its treatment in the People's Republic of China. *Journal of Nervous and Mental Disease* **167**:267–74, 1979.

6 Hatfield, A. (ed.): *Families of the mentally ill: meeting the challenges*. New Directions for Mental Health Services, No. 34. San Francisco, Jossey-Bass, 1987.

7 Tessler, R., Killian, L. M., and Gubman, G. D.: Stages in family response to mental illness: an ideal type. *Psychosocial Rehabilitation Journal* **10**:3–16, 1987.

8 Szasz, T. S.: *Ideology and insanity: essays on the psychiatric dehumanization of man*. New York, Doubleday (Anchor), 1970.

9 Halleck, S. L. and Miller, M. H.: The psychiatric consultation: questionable social precedents of some current practices. *American Journal of Psychiatry* **120**:164–9, 1963.

10 Wells, K. B., Manning, W. G. Jr., Duan, N. *et al.*: *Cost sharing and the demand for ambulatory mental health services* (CR-2960-HHS). Santa Monica, California, Rand Corporation, 1982.

11 Ellis, R. P. and McGuire, T. G.: Cost-sharing and patterns of mental health care utilization. *Journal of Human Resources* **21**:359–79, 1986.

12 Lewis, A.: Health as a social concept. *British Journal of Sociology* **4**:109–24, 1953.

13 Szasz, T. S.: The myth of mental illness. *American Psychologist* **15**:113–18, 1960.

14 Rosenhan, D. L.: On being sane in insane places. *Science* **179**:250–8, 1973.

15 Spitzer, R. L.: More on pseudoscience in science and the case for psychiatric diagnosis. *Archives of General Psychiatry* **33**:459–70, 1976.

16 Christie, R. and Geis, F. L.: *Studies in Machiavellianism*. New York, Academic Press, 1970.

17 Colombotos, J., Kirchner, C., and Millman, M.: Physicians view national health insurance: a national study. *Medical Care* **13**:369–96, 1975.

18 Hollingshead, A. B. and Redlich, F. C.: *Social class and mental illness: a community study*. New York, Wiley, 1958.

19 Henry, W. E., Sims, J. H., and Lee Spray, S.: *Public and private lives of psychotherapists*. San Francisco, Jossey-Bass, 1973.

20 Henry, W. E., Sims, J. H., and Lee Spray, S.: *The fifth profession: becoming a psychotherapist*. San Francisco, Jossey-Bass, 1971.

21 Frank, J. D.: *Persuasion and healing: a comparative study of psychotherapy*, rev. edn. New York, Schocken Books, 1974.

22 Greenley, J. R., Kepecs, J. C., and Henry, W. H.: A comparison of psychiatric practice in Chicago in 1962 and 1973. Unpublished MS. Department of Psychiatry, University of Wisconsin, Madison, 1979.

23 Mechanic, D.: Sociocultural and socio-psychological factors affecting personal responses to psychological disorder. *Journal of Health and Social Behaviour* **16**:393–404, 1975.

24 Redlich, F. and Kellert, S. R.: Trends in American mental health. *American Journal of Psychiatry* **135**:22–8, 1978.

25 Koran, L. M. (ed.): *The nation's psychiatrists*. Washington DC, American Psychiatric Association, 1987.

26 Fenton, W. S., Leaf, P. J., Moran, N. L., and Tischler, G. L.: Trends in psychiatric practice, 1965–1980. *American Journal of Psychiatry* **141**:346–51, 1984.

27 Astrachan, B. and Sharfstein, S. S.: The income of psychiatrists: adaptation during difficult economic times. *American Journal of Psychiatry* **143**:885–7, 1986.

28 Mechanic, D.: *Mental health and social policy*, 3rd edn. Englewood Cliffs, Prentice-Hall, 1989.

29 Mitchell, J. B. and Cromwell, J.: Medical participation by psychiatrists in private practice. *American Journal of Psychiatry* **139**:810–13, 1982.

30 Foucault, M.: *Madness and civilization: a history of insanity in the age of Reason.* New York, Pantheon, 1965.

31 Duhl, L. J. (ed.): *The urban condition: people and policy in the metropolis.* New York, Basic Books, 1963.

32 Caplan, G.: *Principles of preventive psychiatry.* New York, Basic Books, 1964.

33 Caplan, G.: Community psychiatry—introduction and overview, in *Concepts of community psychiatry: a framework for training*, ed. S. E. Goldston, pp. 3–18. Washington DC, US Government Printing Office, 1965.

34 Nicholi, A. M., jun.: Psychiatric consultation in professional football. *New England Journal of Medicine* **316**:1095–1100, 1987.

35 Robins, L. N.: Longitudinal methods in the study of normal and pathological development, in *Psychiatrie der Gegenwart*, vol. 1, 2nd edn, ed. K. P. Kisker, J. E. Meyer, C. Müller, and E. Stromgren, pp. 627–84. Heidelberg, Springer-Verlag, 1979.

36 Russell, L.: *Is prevention better than cure?* Washington DC, The Brookings Institution, 1986.

37 Russell, L.: *Evaluating preventive care: report on a workshop.* Washington DC, The Brookings Institution, 1987.

38 National Institute of Mental Health, Mental Health, United States 1985. Washington DC, DHHS Publ. (ADM) 85–1378, 1985.

39 Mechanic, D.: *From advocacy to allocation: the evolving American health care system.* New York, Free Press, 1986.

40 Morrissey, J. P., Tessler, R. C., and Farrin, L. L.: Being 'seen but not admitted': a note on some neglected aspects of state hospital deinstitutionalization. *American Journal of Orthopsychiatry* **49**:153–6, 1979.

# 5

# Psychiatry as a profession

*Allen Dyer*

Ever since university professors (the masters at the University of Paris) were allowed to incorporate in the thirteenth century, there has been ambiguity in the notion of a profession. Originally the word 'profession' meant to profess religious vows. One was 'called' to the 'discipline' the way disciples were called to their master for a vocation of service. Since the Middle Ages, however, professions have been increasingly organized into guild-like fraternities, which assure not only standards of public service, but also the economic interests of their members. So successful have professions been in looking after their own interests that, by the latter part of the twentieth century, it has been generally assumed that professions look out for themselves, while public regulatory agencies must look out for the public.

Psychiatry as a profession is caught up in our culture's attempt to rethink what is meant by a profession and how professions should be defined and regulated. Psychiatrists need to be clear about their own self-understanding as to both personal and professional goals. Should psychiatry seek to advance the standing of its guild by emphasizing its new technological prowess, or should it seek to rehabilitate its image as a profession by emphasizing the traditional ethical values of humanistic service? Are these goals compatible or exclusive?

As part of the medical profession, psychiatry faces many of the same issues of credibility faced by the rest of medicine. What defines medicine as a profession? Is it the technology which helps physicians serve their patients? Or is it fundamental ethical values which define the commitment of the physician to the patients who seek professional help?[1]

To anticipate the argument which will be developed here, I would suggest that all professions, especially medicine, and most especially psychiatry, have been increasingly drifting off course by identifying too much with their technologies rather than with their fundamental values of service. The identification with technology has appeared to make the professions more marketable, but ultimately has been costly in terms of maintaining the public trust.

There is a certain irony that attends medicine's prodigious technological success in recent decades. At a time when medicine had little to offer but sympathy, understanding, attentiveness, and a few dubious remedies, the physician was likely to be implicitly trusted. His competence or effectiveness might be questioned, but there was seldom any question that he could be trusted. For one thing relationships were one to one. The patient appealed directly to the physician for help. For the physician to survive economically it was more important to be trustworthy than to be effective. Now that the physician is more likely to be effective, economic survival can more easily be divorced from personal virtues such as trustworthiness. Furthermore, care is more likely to be offered by institutions, which are marketing the effectiveness of the technologies they offer. The physician, of course, still has a relationship with the patient, but this relationship is often very circumscribed; physician and patient may remain strangers to each other throughout their brief encounters.

In the modern institutional setting patients may legitimately question the motives of both physician and institution. Are the treatments offered consistent with what the patient wants and needs? Are the risks acceptable to the patient? Have alternatives been adequately explained? Is surgery necessary? In a terminal state would the patient want 'extra ordinary' care continued? Will the patient comply with long-term medication? Given all the options which patients and physicians now face, we routinely speak of informed consent as the basic tenet of medical ethics—as if treatment decisions were analogous to shopping for merchandise. *Caveat emptor*: Let the buyer beware. The laws and mentality of the market-place have evidently replaced the principles of trust which underlie professional ethics.

## Psychiatry as a divided profession

Psychiatry is a divided profession. It is divided in particular by competing loyalties to psychological and biological positions. I wish to state at the outset that I do not see such divisions as credible or viable. Psychiatry has no future as a divided profession. It cannot survive in the modern marketplace on the basis of a dogmatic allegiance to a physician's preferences either biological or psychological, however well-grounded in theory those preferences may be. Psychiatry's future must be based on a careful understanding of the ethical principles which have always been the basis of the professions. Technology is only useful if it is useful. This tautology emphasizes the point that technology is not an end in itself, but only serves as a means to the end of human service.

With all the challenges contemporary psychiatry faces—questions about reimbursement, complex therapies, difficult illnesses to treat, complex social problems which mimic or contribute to illness, and the stigma which attends mental illness, and sometimes those who treat it—it could be argued that it would be good for psychiatry to limit the scope of its concerns, and simply address biological problems with somatic treatments.

The rationale often given for such a limited approach is that psychiatry is part of medicine, and medicine treats biological abnormalities (not persons with biological abnormalities). This is the rationale Thomas Szasz has used in arguing that mental illness is a myth. 'Disease can only affect the body, hence there can be no such thing as mental illness.'[2] The irony in this argument is that patients—whether they are medical or psychiatric—do not perceive their ills in terms of aetiology. There is a phenomenological quality to illness. It is experienced. Patients appeal to physicians for help. If physicians do not respond, they will appeal to others: psychologists, social workers, chiropractors, nutritionists, herbalists, clergy, shamans.

It may seem at first glance to be to psychiatry's advantage to identify with medicine, even with a narrow view of what medicine is. The psychiatrist is a doctor like 'real' doctors, because psychiatry, like real medicine, treats biological illnesses. But real doctors treat patients who appeal for help. To identify medicine with physiology is to ignore the larger context of medicine. Physiology is a useful part of medicine, but a part which is amoral, has no values. To identify psychiatry with the reductionistic aspects of medicine is to buy into the same credibility problems which beset all of medicine. Can physicians be trusted to serve the best interests of each patient, or are they more interested in protecting the interests of the guild?

## Application of the anti-trust laws to the professions

I have been speaking of the professions in terms of the ethical principles which define them. Most basic of these principles (which will be elaborated in the following section) is the principle of trust. Trust as an ethical principle means the ability to rely on the integrity, ability, or character of a person. It has the religious connotation of belief and faith. It has the psychological connotation of confidence and dependency. It also has a legal meaning, with an entirely different connotation. Trust also means monopoly, a combination of firms or corporations for the purpose of reducing competition and controlling prices throughout a business or industry.

The medieval ambiguity in the notion of a profession comes to focus in the modern anti-trust laws. The codes of ethics which have articulated the trust-promoting requirements of professional life, from the Hippocratic Oath through all the revisions of most of the world's professional associations, stress the importance of members maintaining the trust of those that seek their help. The profession of these vows has until recently been seen to be something quite different from the business or corporate interests governed by the anti-trust laws or anti-monopoly laws.

In the United States the Sherman anti-trust law was passed in 1890. It stated simply that 'Any combination or conspiracy in restraint of trade is illegal.' It was left to the courts to interpret, and they held for 85 years that 'learned professions' were exempt from the anti-trust laws, which applied only to business and industry.

By 1975 it was not uncommon to refer to health care as an industry. Although patients still went to doctors, they often got their care from institutions, which increasingly were concerned with the financial aspects of the delivery of high-cost, high-tech medicine. In 1975 the United States Supreme Court ended the learned professions' exemption under the Sherman anti-trust law by handing down the *Goldfarb* decision.[3]

Goldfarb, a Washington attorney, wanted to buy a house in nearby Virginia. As an attorney he knew what most of us know—that when you buy a house you do not need the cleverest or most expensive attorney to search the title. He went shopping for the cheapest attorney, and found that they were all charging the same fee for title-searches. 'Restraint of trade,' he claimed, and took his fellow attorneys to court.

The Supreme Court agreed with him. Within milliseconds of the decision ending the learned professions' exemption, the US Federal Trade Commission, which had been waiting in the wings and expecting this result, entered suit against the American Medical Association, the Connecticut State Medical Society, and the New Haven County Medical Society, holding that they were in restraint of trade because their code of ethics prohibited advertising. Medical prices were high, the FTC contended, because doctors were prohibited from advertising, thus keeping patients from shopping for the best deals.

The Supreme Court decided for the FTC in 1982, thus inaugurating the era of advertising by physicians and other professionals. Medicine in effect was transformed from a profession into a trade. It could not have a code of ethics without getting approval from the FTC. More important than the issue of advertising, the FTC won regulatory jurisdiction over the medical profession.[4]

We might lament a significant loss in this decision, on ethical grounds. The ethics of professional advertising was not an issue in the case. The defence of the American Medical Association did not address the underlying reasons for the prohibition against professional advertising, or actually 'solicitation of patients', which is what had been proscribed. It was assumed that medicine would try to maintain a monopoly on health care, but do so in a way which was not in restraint of trade. So we are left with the question: what distinguishes a profession from a trade? If medicine is to be considered a profession, what does that mean? If psychiatry is to be considered a profession, what does that mean?

## The ethical definition of a profession

The nineteenth and (especially) the twentieth centuries have witnessed numerous occupational groups attempting to achieve the professional status occupied by the paradigm professions of medicine, law, and the clergy. Sociologists observing this cultural phenomenon have identified the formula by which such professionalization occurs. The process involves specialization, the acquisition of technical skill and expertise; but these do not suffice to establish a group as a profession. Any occupation wishing to exercise professional authority must find a technical basis for it, assert an exclusive jurisdiction, link both skill and jurisdiction to standards of training, and convince the public that its services are uniquely trustworthy.[5]

To simplify, we may say that a profession may be defined by
(a) its knowledge, techniques and expertise; or
(b) its ethics and values.

The evolution of professions usually involves a number of steps, including first becoming a full-time occupation; the establishing of the first training school, the first university school, the first local professional association, and then a national professional association; state licensing laws; and ultimately, the development of a formal code of ethics.

Established professions by these criteria include accounting, architecture, civil engineering, dentistry, law, and medicine. Developing professions would include librarianship, nursing, optometry, pharmacy, schoolteaching (often organized as a trade with trade unions), social work, and veterinary medicine. Newer professional groups are city management, town planning, and hospital administration. Doubtful contenders would be advertising and funeral direction, which, though they meet the formula, do not provide direct, recognizable personal services. There are over 140 organized allied-health professions within the United States today, all with articulated codes of ethics.

The theme of trustworthiness is a pivotal consideration in the definition of a profession. It bridges the epistemological gulf between the idea of a profession defined by its technology and a profession defined by its ethics. In order to be worthy of trust a professional must be both knowledgeable and ethical.

The codes of ethics, of course, do not assure the ethical behaviour of the members of the professional group. Professions attempt in one way or another to address the ethical standards of their members through Entry, Education, and Exit, all involving Ethics (4 Es).

(1) *Entry*: Admission standards look to the character of the individual entering the profession. In medieval England, prospective barristers were required to eat ten meals with their would-be colleagues at the inn. At

these occasions their fellows could determine if they were of suitable character to join the profession. Even emphasis on grades and board scores involves an ethical dimension, the work ethic; though hopefully admissions committees look beyond just such tangible manifestations of ability and willingness to work.

(2) *Education* does not mean merely ethics in the curriculum. The curriculum itself reflects the values of the profession. Medicine's bifurcated curriculum, basic science and clinical experience, reflects the divisions in psychiatry as a profession, and also belies deeper divisions in the field of medicine at large.

(3) *Exit* refers to professional discipline. Professions reserve the right and the responsibility of disciplining members who do not adhere to the standards of ethics specified in their codes. It is often said that professions are hesitant to police their own, and states usually have control of the license itself. However, it is also important for the profession to take discipline seriously, in order to maintain the integrity of the profession and to maintain the public trust.

Codes of ethics are more than administrative documents. They are certainly more than a list of rules by which a member of a professional group can identify and exclude would-be deviant behaviour. A code also serves to symbolize the principles by which a professional group defines itself. As such the code is a reflection of values, which are ultimately tacit and cannot be completely specified.

The Hippocratic Oath serves as a symbol that the medical profession is defined by an ideal of service. It is found wanting, perhaps anachronistic, if one looks to it as a list of rules by which one can make concrete decisions, stay out of trouble, or know what to do in a particular difficult situation. In fact any list of rules would be found wanting by such expectations. If it were possible to make clinical judgements this way, we could take a good law book and a good enough computer algorithm and never need a professional. The role of the professional is to personalize care.

The Hippocratic Oath in eight succinct statements outlines the values of the medical profession at its best over the past twenty-four centuries. It defines for the first time in history the physician as a healer specializing in caring for the sick, uninterested in and forswearing any other possibilities in the relationship with those who seek help. For the first time in history, according to anthropologist Margaret Mead, the power to heal was vested in a practitioner who was not also a shaman with the power to harm.[6] The sole purpose of the Hippocratic physician was to promote health. This was done primarily through natural means such as dietetic measures; and the physician forswore other treatments, such as cutting for the stone, leaving those treatments for those specializing in them. The Hippocratic physician swore not to perform abortions or to give deadly drugs (euthanasia), as these practices were inconsistent with the goal of healing. He forswore mischief with patients, specifically sexual misdeeds, even though prevailing cultural norms would not have required that. Significantly the Hippocratic physician swore to keep confidences. In such promises the Oath foreshadows the modern conception of a profession. The Hippocratic physician swore to teach the art only to those who agreed to keep the Oath, thus making the Oath the cornerstone of professional organization. He made these promises solemnly, swearing by Aesclepius and Apollo. Current versions of the Oath use language such as 'swear by whatever I hold sacred', which suggests the solemn and even religious quality of taking the Oath.

A recurring theme in the rhetoric of the Oath is the imperative of benefit to the patient. Although such language sounds paternalistic to the modern ear, we cannot reasonably expect our patients to be so self-sufficient as to take care of themselves. There is an obligation on the physician (and on all professionals) to refrain from self-interest, and to devote oneself to the needs of those served. This is done with a mindfulness of the autonomy of the patient and the associated goal of involving him in decision-making wherever possible, but not with the *Caveat emptor* ethic of the market-place.

Psychiatry as a profession has attended to nuances of the doctor–patient relationship in a manner which may serve as a model to all professions and all professional–client relationships. There is probably no better statement of the doctor–patient relationship than Freud's classic papers on the transference. Here we are cautioned to recognize that the patient will inevitably develop strong feelings toward the doctor, and that those feelings are more a function of the position of the physician, and are 'not to be attributed to the charms of his own person'.[7] Tempting as it may be to believe the flatterer, or frustrating as it may be to bear the brunt of a patient's anger, it is important to recognize the possibility that these feelings may be brought to the relationship. Furthermore, Freud's paper and all his psychoanalytic work require the physician to scrutinize his own conduct for clues to understand the patient's response. This psychoanalytic ethic does not just apply to psychoanalytic treatment, for such dynamics occur in all intimate relationships. The biological psychiatrist who innocently says to the ethics committee 'I didn't realize there was anything wrong with accepting her invitation to join her in the jacuzzi; I was just prescribing anti-depressants,' or 'I thought we had a special feeling for each other', should carefully review the codes of ethics, as well as the principles which underlie the written codes.

## Psychiatry's relation to other professions

If a profession is conceived of in terms of its knowledge or technical expertise, and organized to promote the economic self-interest of its members, other professions are rivals for a market share in so-called 'turf-battles'. If a profession is conceived in terms of its ethics and value of service, then other professions are allies in meeting a service need. There is often an overlap of the knowledge-base among professions with similar interests and goals.

Optometrists and ophthalmologists, for example, share a knowledge-base in eye-care. Both are capable of refracting eyes and prescribing glasses, though optometrists typically do refractions, and ophthalmologists are more likely to concentrate on surgical procedures. Both are capable of diagnosing certain diseases of the eye, though the treatment may require medical or surgical intervention which only an ophthalmologist can provide: the two professions are thus symbiotic, especially when we realize that because ophthalmologists are more likely to specialize in the more lucrative surgical procedures, patients are more likely to seek the care of optometrists for routine care and evaluation. So optometrists need ophthalmologists to treat certain diseases beyond their competence, and ophthalmologists need optometrists as a source of referrals. They are rivals in the market-place who must maintain good relationships. Even the use of drugs is an issue, since the eye can best be examined with the pupils dilated, which can be accomplished by a darkened room or by an atropine-like drug characteristically reserved for use by physicians unless state legislatures have specifically granted that privilege to optometrists as well. Furthermore, in this competitive era many states no longer require prescriptions to sell glasses, allowing them to be purchased off racks like ordinary merchandise. *Caveat emptor*: Let the buyer beware.

Such turf-battles are common among professions sharing a knowledge-base. Orthopaedic surgeons and podiatrists, osteopaths, and chiropractors. Neurologists and physical therapists. Orthopaedic surgeons and neuro-surgeons. All specialists and general practitioners. Obstetricians and midwives. Psychiatrists and a long list of psychotherapists, including psychologists, social workers, ministers, 'counsellors', and substance-abuse specialists.

Increasingly in the post-*Goldfarb* era, these turf-battles are being re-solved not by a professional appeal to public trust, but by the anti-trust courts. Psychologists, for example, recently sued the American Psycho-analytic Association, holding that it was in restraint of trade because its practice of training primarily physicians (psychiatrists) denied them access to markets they felt were legitimately theirs. The suit was settled in 1988 by a consent order allowing psychologists access to psychoanalytic training. The decision was hailed as a victory by psychologists, though in many ways it was a Pyrrhic victory, for in achieving its goals by the anti-trust route, many of the ethical tenets psychology had cherished as a profession had to be forfeited to the market mentality. The FTC has demanded that the

American Psychological Association eliminate from its code of ethics sections which prohibit fee-splitting, testimonials from clients regarding the quality of a psychologist's services or products, and, of course, advertising.[8]

Such turf-battles—including the question of psychologists' admitting privileges and the possibility of psychologists' gaining prescribing privileges—will force psychiatry to rethink both the knowledge-base and the values by which it is defined. One strategy, following the 'divided-profession' model, would be for psychiatry to jettison the practice of psychotherapy, leaving that to other professions, and retaining those aspects which are purely medical (meaning, 'biological'). In such a model, the psychiatrist's role in mental health care would be small indeed—a pusher of pills and ECT buttons and a consultant to other professionals who would serve as the primary care-providers. Indeed, in many places this is already the scenario that obtains. The psychiatrist's role is simply to medicate the more seriously ill patients so that they can talk to other professionals. Persons who are functioning adequately to make their own choices choose other professions for help.

The alternative strategy is what I prefer to call the integrative model of psychiatry, in which psychiatry's role—following the profession's ethical mandate—is to respond to appeals for help with whatever interventions best serve the patient. In other words, the service is dictated by the patient's needs, rather than by the physician's preferences.

## Psychiatry's relation to 'the rest of medicine'

When one speaks of the 'medical model' what is meant is usually a reductionist model. Medicine is often identified by its technology. So for psychiatry to identify with medicine would make it seem at first that this identification implied adherence to a reductionist biological model. The evolution of biology as a science has had an exciting history of reducing complex phenomena to more basic levels of understanding: biological life itself to the organism, then to the organ, then to the cellular, and finally to the molecular level. Each successive reduction offers a new level of detail to understanding, but adds nothing to meaning. The job of the scientist is to add new layers of understanding. The job of the clinician is to integrate that understanding with the purposes of medicine. The job of the medical scientist is to do both.

Otto Guttentag suggests that in order to keep the purpose of medicine in mind, we should speak of an 'anthropological medical model' as well as a biological medical model.[9] Such a broadening of scope helps to remind us of the purposes of biology, and for medicine helps to re-orient us to the ethic of service or patient-benefit.

When placed in the context of attempting to define a profession such considerations might seem obvious, but the bifurcations run so deep in psychiatry, in medicine, and in the Cartesian world, that we constantly slip into accepting dualities in which we don't really believe.

One such example is the recent case of *Osheroff* v. *Chestnut Lodge*. Dr Raphael Osheroff was treated for depression at Chestnut Lodge using primarily psychoanalytic treatment. He did not respond in several months, during which time he suffered losses in his family and in his business. His suit claimed that he had a right to effective treatment, namely psychopharmacological treatment, and that his losses were caused as a result of inappropriate selection of treatment.[10]

The *Osheroff* case is significant not so much because of the outcome or the precedent it might set, but because of the confusion which the adversarial process has engendered in a dichotomous situation. It does not matter for the legal decision that Dr Osheroff had already had a trial on a regimen of psychotropic medication, which had failed, or that he was ultimately treated successfully by a psychoanalyst, who used a combination of medications and psychotherapy. The legal case focused, as any legal case must do, on either/or questions, thus obscuring attempts at integrative understanding.

Psychiatry as a profession is not served by this approach. The *Osheroff* case is being discussed as if psychiatrists must choose between 'competing models of psychiatric care'. In such discussions *Osheroff* is cited as an example of the failure of psychoanalytic therapy. Psychoanalysis has promised too much, the argument goes; it has little to offer in treating the seriously mentally ill. The treatment is too long, too expensive, and not readily available.

On the other side of the coin, those who allow themselves to be caught up in this tug-of-war note that biological psychiatry also has many shortcomings, as the following account from a treatise on current controversies in malpractice litigation hauntingly suggests:

Despite the undisputed benefits wrought by the chemical revolution, biological treatments used in psychiatry today also involve many potential dangers. Counterbalancing the evidence of the efficacy of these chemical agents is evidence that they can cause side effects which harm patients as well. This fact becomes even more significant when one acknowledges that these side effects, which can be physical, emotional, or cognitive, occur even when these medications are responsibly administered by competent medical practitioners.[11]

## Towards an integrative profession

It is epistemological nonsense to accept such divisions. Given the possibility of the mind-body split, which has been the heritage of Western thought since the Enlightenment, one could attempt to reduce all mental phenomena to the physical, at the risk of the charge that modern psychiatry increasingly faces of 'losing the mind'. An alternative strategy would be to repudiate the dichotomy as specious.

Michael Polanyi has looked closely at the meaning of knowledge and suggested that the notion of strict objectivity in science, which leads to the kinds of divisions which plague psychiatry, is ultimately false and misleading. Biological sciences would be held to be more objective than psychological sciences, in part because they are more successful in their reductions. But the physical sciences, which are even more objective, are more aware of the uncertainty which follows their observations and measurements. Recognizing the uncertainty which obtains in scientific observation, and especially in the discovery of new knowledge—as opposed to the application of knowledge—has led Polanyi to remind us that knowledge is neither objective nor subjective, but rather 'personal', in so far as it relies on a tacit understanding which cannot be completely specified.

These conclusions should not be strikingly novel to the scientist working at the frontiers of knowledge, or to the clinician whose job it is to apply knowledge to the solution of human problems, and whose judgements depend on the integration of tacit experience. These conclusions may appear radical, however, to the scientist working to apply established paradigms, and struggling to be 'objective' and convincing.

In an important article entitled 'Life transcending physics and chemistry', Polanyi points out that you cannot understand a machine by reducing it to its parts. The purpose of a grandfather clock, for example, cannot be explained by giving an account of the parts which comprise it. Similarly the meaning of life cannot be explained by an analysis of its components.[12]

Psychiatry of all the professions should be prepared to understand this. The knowledge patients share of themselves is received by fellow human beings, who ideally are trained to understand not just recitations of symptoms but the meanings of symbolic communications. Nothing frustrates and angers patients more than feeling that they are not being listened to, that their stories are not being heard.

We might approach the question of what defines psychiatry by asking the question upside-down. If psychiatry is not a profession, what is it? The alternatives suggest only partial answers. Psychiatry is a science, an applied science? Psychiatry is a medical specialty? Psychiatry is a trade? Each of those partial answers begs for a more comprehensive view. Psychiatry can best be understood as a profession, seeking to apply science, but best defined by values located in a human context.

# References

1 Dyer, A. R.: *Ethics and psychiatry: toward professional definition*. Washington DC, American Psychiatric Press, 1988.

2 Szasz, T.: *The myth of mental illness*. New York, Harper and Row, 1974.

3 *Goldfarb* v. *Virginia State Bar*. 419 US 963 (US Reports), 1975.

4 *Federal Trade Commission* v. *American Medical Association*. 456 US 966 (US Reports), 1982.

5 Wilensky, H.: The professionalization of everyone? *American Journal of Sociology* **70**:137ff., 1964.

6 Margaret Mead, quoted in M. Levine: *Psychiatry and ethics*. New York, George Braziller, 1972, pp. 324–5.

7 Freud, S.: Observations on transference-love, in *Complete psychological works*, vol. XII, p. 161. London, Hogarth Press, 1958.

8 American Psychological Association: *Monitor*, March 1988, p. 1.

9 Guttentag, O.: On Defining Medicine. *The Christian Scholar*, vol. XLVI/3, Fall 1963, pp. 200–11.

10 Malcom, J. G.: *Treatment choices and informed consent*. Springfield, Ill., Charles Thomas, 1988.

11 Ibid., p. 13.

12 Polanyi, M.: Life transcending physics and chemistry. *Chemical and Engineering News*, vol. 45, pp. 54ff, 1967. Also *Personal knowledge: towards a postcritical philosophy*. London, Routledge & Kegan Paul, 1952.

# 6

# The concept of disease

*William Fulford*

There is now an extensive literature on the meanings of the key medical concepts of illness and disease.[1,2] Most authors in this literature draw directly or indirectly on the way these concepts appear in the dominant medical culture, science-based physical medicine. This approach is widespread among medical authors in particular, and thus might be called the conventional approach. The approach to be described in this chapter is in a sense the reverse of the conventional approach, in that it draws primarily on the appearances of the key medical concepts as they are employed not in physical medicine but in psychiatry. Only an outline of the main features of this approach can be given, the arguments being developed in detail elsewhere.[3] Furthermore, the approach, even in its fully worked-up form, remains in important respects tentative and preliminary. None the less, as we will see, it offers the possibility of an understanding of the medical concepts which is both more self-consistent than that provided by the conventional approach, and also potentially more fruitful practically. If it proves correct, therefore, this approach will provide a more secure foundation for psychiatric ethics.

The argument is developed in five stages, beginning and ending with psychiatric ethics. First, the place of conceptual issues in psychiatric ethics is defined. Next, the conventional interpretation of the medical concepts is considered, both in its own right and as a possible basis from which to address the conceptual issues outlined in the first stage. This shows up a number of deficiencies in the conventional approach, which then lead directly to a reverse approach, the approach from psychiatry. This is described in the next two stages of the argument, and applied to psychiatric ethics in the final section of the chapter.

## Psychiatric ethics

The medical concepts, in particular those of illness and disease, are important in relation to a wide variety of ethical problems in psychiatry. These concepts are problematic in medical ethics generally, but in psychiatric ethics they are especially so. The concept of mental illness is central, for example, to the tension between autonomy and paternalism (identified in Chapter 1 of this book as a key issue for psychiatric ethics), since it is by this that the proper scope of the authority of psychiatry as a medical discipline is defined. The concept is relevant, similarly, to a majority of the issues examined in subsequent chapters: the expanding influence of psychiatry since the Second World War, with the extension of the concept of mental illness to an ever wider range of problems, including ostensibly social and political problems, as well as those traditionally regarded as medical problems; the difficulty, made more acute by this extension of psychiatric territory, of distinguishing social and political deviance from medical deviance; the particular importance of this distinction in forensic psychiatry, in relation to 'mad versus bad' issues and questions of responsibility; and the problem in some countries of the actual abuse of psychiatry—that is the use of psychiatric treatment not for the cure of disease, nor even for the relief of suffering, but for purposes of political manipulation and control. Moreover, besides issues such as these, in which the concept of mental illness is directly implicated, are issues in which it is implicated indirectly: for example, in the distinction between therapeutic and non-therapeutic uses of drugs; in the recent upsurge of economic issues, about health-care distribution, and the responsibilities of third-party payers;[4] and in family therapy, in the issue of who is the patient, and hence in derivative ethical questions such as those of privacy and confidentiality, which depend at one remove (though of course only in part) on the notion of disorder which is adopted.

It is this wide range of difficulties that an analysis of the medical concepts must address if it is to serve as a basis for psychiatric ethics. However, the very pervasiveness of these difficulties makes it essential that their place in psychiatric ethics be carefully defined before such an analysis is embarked on. Too inflated or too restricted a view of their significance would be equally misleading. What is needed is a balance.

First a balance is needed between the medical and other concepts. The medical concepts are important in psychiatric ethics: they are important qualitatively, in that they mark out certain issues in psychiatry (such as the mad-versus-bad distinction) that are specifically medical ethical issues. But other concepts are important as well. Thus, in this book, the concept of suicide is discussed in Chapter 12, and that of research in Chapter 19. Similarly, any concept which features in ethics generally may feature in psychiatric ethics: the concept of autonomy, for instance, raises ethical issues in many other areas (law, education, politics) besides medicine. Furthermore, just below the surface of the issues raised by concepts such as these are the still more problematic concepts with which general metaphysics is concerned; causality and free will and determinism, for example, in the case of autonomy. Crucially important too, in medical as in other areas of ethics, are the general moral concepts of good, ought, right, and so on. As Hare points out in Chapter 3, improved standards of rigour in medical-ethical argument depend *inter alia* on better understanding of the meanings and implications of these terms.

A second balance that is needed is between conceptual issues in general, whether or not concerned specifically with the medical concepts, and empirical issues. In principle, there is no conflict here, of course. On the contrary, concepts without substance are empty, and substance without concepts is formless. In the present context, however, it is important to keep both sides of this equation in mind. In the past, philosophers, not least moral philosophers, have sometimes drifted too far to the concept side of the equation. Concerned too exclusively with questions of meaning, they have had little or nothing to say on the substantive issues of 'real life'. Yet in ethics at least, as Williams[5] has reminded us, if philosophy is important, so also are disciplines such as psychology, sociology, anthropology, and political science. Doctors, on the other hand, have sometimes drifted too far to the substance side of the equation. Dismissing questions of meaning as mere 'playing with words', they have tended to assume that all clinically important questions—conceptual as well as substantive, ethical as well as empirical—will be resolved by future scientific advances. Yet in psychiatric ethics at least, as we have seen, if empirical questions are important, so also are questions of meaning. All in all, then, what is needed for better clinical practice is that we avoid either extreme. As Mary Warnock, among others, has put it, we need to maintain the closest possible links between the abstract and the concrete, between theory and practice.[6]

The place of the medical concepts in psychiatric ethics is well illustrated by compulsory psychiatric treatment. Such treatment, as described in Chapter 13, is highly contentious. It raises in a most acute form the central ethical problem in psychiatry, the tension between autonomy and paternalism. Mental illness is unique in this respect. With no other condition is compulsory treatment of a fully conscious adult patient of normal intelligence thought to be justified, not for the protection of others (though there is of course provision for this), but in the patient's *own* interests. Furthermore, the difficulties here are highly practical. Leaving aside radical objections to compulsion as such, and the out-and-out abuse of compulsory treatment in some countries, it is all too often the case in everyday clinical practice that treatment decisions involving compulsion are uncertain or disputed. In such cases the difficulties may be empirical. It may be difficult to establish the risk of harm; of suicide, for example, or of danger to others. It may be difficult to establish a patient's frame of mind; whether he is, say, sad, anxious, or labouring under mistaken beliefs. But the difficulties may also be conceptual. For the grounds of compulsory treatment depend not only on the facts, but on the construction that is placed on the facts. Granted the general ethical principle that paternalistic intervention with infringement of autonomy is sometimes justified, then sadness, anxiety, and mistaken belief may all provide grounds—humanitarian or religious grounds, say—for intervening to prevent someone from killing themselves. But this is not sufficient here. The specifically *medical* grounds required for intervention in the form of compulsory psychiatric treatment, require that the patient's sadness, anxiety, or mistaken belief be construed as, or as a symptom of, illness.

Therefore, if philosophy is to contribute to better clinical practice in this area, it must be concerned with the clarification of the concept of mental illness. As in other areas of practice, it may be concerned with much else besides: with the wider ethical principles that are relevant, with logic, with the correct use of the general moral words, with the metaphysical questions raised by compulsion and so on. But clarification of the concept of mental illness is inescapably part of its brief. Nor is this a trivial part of its brief. For the properties of mental illness are subtle in the extreme. As we noted a moment ago, compulsory treatment is restricted (largely) to mental, as distinct from physical, illness; this restriction is thus a property of mental illness that any philosophical analysis of the concept must explain. Compulsory treatment is also (largely) restricted to certain varieties of mental illness, to psychotic as distinct from non-psychotic varieties; so this is a second property that must be explained. And these and other similar properties of mental illness thus amount to constraints on philosophical theory—constraints which, as we will see, crucially differentiate between the way in which the medical concepts are conventionally interpreted and the alternative interpretation to be outlined here.

## Disease—the approach from physical medicine

An important (if generally tacit) assumption in the debate about mental illness, is that the concept of physical illness, although certainly requiring analysis in its own right, is relatively transparent in meaning. This assumption is natural enough given that, compared with mental illness, there is general agreement about the application of the concept of physical illness, about which conditions are and which are not physical illnesses. Everyone, it seems, given the consistency in the use of the term, must know, or must be capable more or less readily of coming to know, what is meant by physical illness.

The influence of this assumption can be seen by comparing the arguments of Szasz,[7] an opponent of the concept of mental illness, with those of Kendell,[8] one of its supporters. For both, mental illness is the target problem: Szasz wants to 'raise the question, is there such a thing as mental illness?'; Kendell, similarly, seeks to 'decide whether mental illnesses are legitimately so-called'. Both then turn to the concept of physical illness, acknowledging the difficulties of definition, but suggesting criteria which they take to be self-evidently essential to its meaning: Szasz's criterion is 'deviation from the clearly defined norms of the structural and functional integrity of the human body'; Kendell's is 'biological disadvantage, which . . . must embrace both increased mortality and reduced fertility'. Finally, both return to mental illness. Szasz points out that for most mental illnesses there are no relevant norms of bodily structure and functioning: on the contrary, he argues, the norms of mental illness are 'ethical, legal and social'. Kendell, on the other hand, draws on epidemiological and statistical data to show that many mental illnesses are biologically disadvantageous in his sense, being associated with reduced life and/or reproductive expectations. Hence, by Szasz's criterion mental illness is a myth, whereas by Kendell's it is not.

It will be clear from this summary of their arguments that neither author's proposed criterion of physical illness is wholly satisfactory; at the very least, Szasz's is too restrictive, Kendell's is over-inclusive. However, what is important to us here is not to take sides, but rather to see that the way the debate itself, as a debate about mental illness, comes out, undermines the assumption about physical illness upon which it is based. The debate could have come out differently. Szasz and Kendell could have ended up disagreeing about the application of an agreed set of criteria for physical illness. Instead, they disagreed about the criteria themselves; and of course a wide variety of other criteria have been suggested by other authors (for a review, see Clare).[1] Hence, while it remains true that physical illness is less problematic in use than mental illness, there must be something other than transparency of meaning to explain why this should be so.

The gap here, between use and definition, is not unusual with concepts: the concept of time, for example, though far from being easily defined, is largely trouble-free in use (outside physics, at any rate). But recognizing that physical illness is a concept of this kind gives a quite different slant to the debate about mental illness. Indeed it shows the debate to be in an important sense a debate about physical illness! The ultimate practical objective of the debate is still the clinical problems associated with the concept of mental illness in everyday medical work. Equally, examples of physical illness, being generally uncontroversial, continue to provide a common starting-point for the debate. But in getting from one to the other, from examples of physical illness to the practical problems associated with the concept of mental illness, the argument, far from assuming the sense of 'physical illness' to be more or less transparent, has now actually to explain why 'physical illness' should be largely problem-free in use despite its not being transparent in meaning. Physical illness and mental illness, at the level of definition, are thus seen to be on a par, the problem-free use of the concept of physical illness being as much a matter for explanation as the problem-*laden* use of that of mental illness.

The philosopher Boorse is among those who, though concerned with the problems associated with the concept of mental illness, tackles the concept of physical illness head-on.[9] His argument, though not presented in this way, can be understood as seeking to reconcile the points of view illustrated here by Szasz and Kendell. Much of the difficulty about mental illness, he argues, goes back to a misunderstanding about the nature of health, namely that it is essentially an evaluative concept. This misunderstanding has arisen from a failure to distinguish between illness and disease, the negative terms which he appropriates to the practical and theoretical aspects of health respectively. In its practical aspects, Boorse suggests, health is indeed a value-laden concept; hence illness is too. Szasz would therefore be right, according to Boorse's argument, in pointing to ethical norms as criteria of mental illness (as distinct from disease), though wrong in denying that similar norms are also criteria of physical illness. However, at the theoretical heart of medicine, Boorse goes on, there is a body of objective knowledge which is 'continuous with theory in biology and the other basic sciences'. It is in terms of this scientific knowledge that diseases are defined, and the concept of disease is thus value-free. If Boorse is right, therefore, then Kendell is right in pointing to value-free norms as criteria of physical disease (Kendell's norms and Boorse's are in fact essentially the same); though in extending these norms to the area of mental health, Kendell (on Boorse's view) should have restricted their application to mental disease as distinct from mental illness.

Boorse's analysis of the concept of health accords well with what might be called the medical common-sense view. Most doctors would acknowledge that value-judgements come into the practice of medicine; not just ethical judgements, but also aesthetic, prudential, and legal judgements, among others. Illness, furthermore, in so far as it is a concept distinct from disease, is indeed relatively prominent in this area. It is associated naturally with the patient's experience of ill-health; it is subjective, a matter of feelings and sensations, of complaints, of symptoms. Yet all this, to the medical mind, is secondary to the area of technical knowledge in which the doctor, as a specialist, is truly expert. It is in the area of disease, defined by scientific knowledge of structure and function, that medical theory, and hence the doctor's particular skill in the diagnosis and treatment of illness, resides. Understood in this way, furthermore, Boorse's analysis provides at least a partial explanation for the relatively problem-free use of the medical concepts in physical medicine as compared with psychiatry. Boorse focuses here on the concept of illness. But even at the level of disease it can be seen that the relatively undeveloped state of the 'mental' sciences makes mental conditions, on his analysis, more likely to be problematic practically.

Yet despite its attractions, closer inspection reveals a number of objections to Boorse's analysis.[10] Some of these are technical. Illness, for example, is marked out as 'serious' disease; and while this certainly brings in the required logical element of evaluation, it conflicts with ordinary usage; for ordinarily we use both disease and illness equally readily of both serious and minor conditions. Similarly, the idea that illness should be understood as a subcategory of disease at all (i.e., the subcategory of serious diseases) has to be understood stipulatively, since it conflicts with the fact that the experience of illness ordinarily precedes knowledge of the particular disease from which one is suffering—just as historically there were ill-nesses long before the development of scientific disease-theories in terms of abnormal structure and functioning.

A more important objection for our present purpose, however, is that the main practical effect of Boorse's theory is to marginalize medical ethics. This is built right into the structure of his theory. Ethical considerations are shifted to the periphery, outside the supposed value-free theoreti-cal heart of medicine. But this marginalizing effect also comes out clearly when Boorse applies his theory to some of the practical problems with which, at the start of his paper, he says he is concerned. His solution to what he takes to be the controversial diagnosis of homosexuality, for example, amounts to no more than a solution by exclusion. Doctors, he argues in effect, should confine themselves to understanding the biology of sexuality.[11] And when he comes to 'the concept of psychosis—the key concept, it will be recalled, in relation to compulsory psychiatric treatment—his analysis gives entirely the wrong result. In this connection Boorse in fact discusses the closely related issue of responsibility in law. But his analysis leads to the counterintuitive result that psychotic disorders should be a peripheral, rather than (as they are) the central, case of loss of responsibility of this kind.[12]

It could be said that these objections to Boorse's theory are beside the point. After all, Boorse is not the first to find the concept of psychosis, though crucially important in the ethical and legal aspects of psychiatry, a tough nut to crack. While, as to ethical considerations in general, perhaps these really are peripheral in medicine. Certainly, many doctors seem to believe this to be the case. This is almost part of the medical 'common-sense' view. Then again, on the technical issues, if there are points of conflict between Boorse's analysis of the medical concepts and ordinary usage, perhaps it is ordinary usage which is wrong. Boorse himself says as much at one point, suggesting that certain features of ordinary usage are 'two thousand years out of date'.[13]

All this *could* be said were it not for the fact that there is a more fundamental objection to Boorse's theory. The marginalizing of medical ethics, and indeed (many of) the technical objections to his analysis, arise from his central contention, namely that disease can be defined without reference to values. The issues surrounding this contention are many: indeed, they include all the issues involved in the 'is–ought' debate in general ethical theory.[10] But an important observation in Boorse's case is that, although defining disease without reference to values, he continues to use it (in flat contradiction to his own definition) with clear evaluative force. For example, having defined disease in value-free terms as a 'deviation' from the normal functional organization of the species, he describes it only two lines later as a 'deficiency' in functional efficiency.[14] Similarly, a little further on, the evaluatively neutral 'environmental causes' (as an element in the elaboration of his definition of disease) becomes the value-laden 'hostile environment'. These are no mere oversights. Coming as they do at the very heart of Boorse's theory, they show that, while disease may be defined (stipulatively) in value-free terms, it cannot actually be used without value-judgements slipping back in. This feature of Boorse's theory thus suggests the possibility that disease, and hence the theoretical centre as well as the practical periphery of medicine, is essentially value-laden.

## Illness—the approach from psychiatry

The outcome of the conventional form of argument, as described earlier, leads to something of a role-reversal between physical medicine and psychiatry in their potential contributions to our understanding of the medical concepts. The conventional approach starts, as we saw, from a more or less pejorative stance towards psychiatry: mental illness/disease is perceived as the target problem, and physical illness/disease, supposedly more transparent in meaning, is thought to provide a solution. It was important to look carefully at this approach, given its prima-facie validity. But the way it comes out shows that an approach which is its exact opposite has a better chance of success. The outcome of the Szasz–Kendell version of the conventional form of argument took us part of the way to this conclusion: it showed that in an important sense physical illness/disease, rather than mental illness/disease, is the target problem. And the outcome of the Boorse version of the conventional form of argument now takes us the rest of the way. For in showing the medical concepts to be evaluative through and through, it shows the *more* overtly evaluative mental illness/disease, rather than the *less* overtly evaluative physical illness/disease, to be the more transparent in meaning; that is to say, it shows that mental illness/disease reveals, where physical illness/disease tends to conceal, the value-laden nature of the medical concepts. Hence in seeking to analyse the meanings of the medical concepts, our approach, far from starting from a pejorative stance towards psychiatry, should rather be based on the way these concepts appear in this area of medicine.

There are two principal differences between the appearances of the medical concepts in psychiatry and in physical medicine. These are implicit in what has been said already in this chapter. In psychiatry, illness, rather than disease, is the more prominent concept (hence we speak of the debate about mental *illness*): and in psychiatry the evaluative connotations of this concept are more prominent than they are in physical medicine (we have seen that the concept of mental illness is especially problematic in psychiatric ethics, and that much of the debate about this concept turns on the significance of its evaluative connotations). Correspondingly, therefore, whereas with the standard approach from physical medicine (*à la* Boorse) it is natural to treat disease, with its strongly factual connotations, as being logically primary, so with the approach from psychiatry it is natural to treat illness, with its strongly evaluative connotations, as being logically primary. And what this leads to is that whereas with the conventional approach illness emerges as an evaluative subcategory of disease, with the approach from psychiatry this relationship is reversed, disease coming out as a subcategory of the evaluative concept of illness.[15]

We will be looking at how this works in more detail in a moment. But it is important to see straight away that if the conventional theory has about it a degree of medical common sense, so too—though from a different point of view—has a reverse theory. The medical common sense of the conventional theory is as seen from the doctor's point of view. As we saw earlier, Boorse's theory, by placing the strongly factual concept of disease at the conceptual heart of medicine, rings true with doctors. This is because

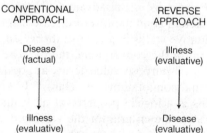

**Fig. 6.1** The conceptual relationship between illness and disease in conventional and reverse approaches to understanding the meanings of the medical concepts

The conventional approach is based on the appearances of the medical concepts in physical medicine; hence disease, defined as a factual term, is taken to be logically primary. The reverse approach suggested here is based rather on the appearances of the medical concepts in psychiatry; disease thus comes out as a subcategory of the evaluative concept of illness.

scientific knowledge of disease (of defined syndromes, of the causes of illness, and of specific treatments) has become their area of expertise. This is what matters to doctors. But what in the same way 'matters' to patients, is what was called in the last section the experience of illness: from the patient's point of view it is (normally) the experience of illness (rather than knowledge of disease) that comes first. From the patient's point of view, similarly, it is the experience of illness as a negatively evaluated condition (normally unwelcome, unpleasant, and so on) that is important. Without this, doctors would be literally out of business. Medical common sense, therefore, from the patient's as distinct from the doctor's point of view, places the evaluative concept of illness, rather than the factual concept of disease, at the conceptual heart of medicine.

To go beyond this, from a broad-brush common-sense view to the development of a detailed and comprehensive 'reverse theory' analysis of the medical concepts, is clearly beyond the scope of this chapter. In the present context, however, one particular element of such an analysis is well worth a closer look. This is the explanation that is provided by a reverse-theory analysis for the mainly factual connotations of the use of the term disease. As we will see, the reverse-theory explanation for this feature of disease avoids the contradictions inherent in the conventional theory. It also proves to be directly relevant to our understanding of the conceptual basis of psychiatric ethics.

In the conventional theory, as illustrated above, the factual connotations of disease are derived directly from its (supposed) status as a factual term. Disease, according to this approach, simply is a factual term. At first glance, then, a reverse theory, in which disease no less than illness is a value term, might be thought to be at a distinct disadvantage in this respect. However, it turns out that the factual connotations of disease can be derived just as directly from its evaluative status in a reverse theory, as they can from its status as a factual term in the conventional theory. The point is that any value term, even such all-purpose value terms as good and bad, can be used with mainly factual connotations. As Hare,[16] Urmson,[17] and others have pointed out, this is a logical property of all value terms. It comes about essentially because the criteria for the value judgements expressed by value terms are *factual* criteria. Often these criteria, in a given class of application, are highly variable, from person to person or for the same person on different occasions. But where the criteria are stable, then, as *factual* criteria, they may become attached to the meaning of the value term in question. For example, the factual criteria for 'bad' used of apples— brown skin, pulpy flesh, and so on—are relatively stable. That is to say, most people most of the time use the term 'bad' of apples with brown skins and pulpy flesh. They don't *have* to do so. 'Bad' used of apples (except where it is used as a synonym for 'decomposing') does not *mean* brown skin, pulpy flesh, and so on. In the context of cider-making, indeed, such apples are judged good. All the same, the fact that most people most of the time use 'bad' of apples with brown skin and pulpy flesh has the result that 'bad' used of apples normally implies that the apples in question have, as a matter of fact, brown skins and pulpy flesh.

Returning to the medical case, then, the same point about the logic of value terms could help to explain the relatively factual connotations of disease compared with illness. Of course, 'disease' has a wider application than 'bad' used of apples. But the basic idea is the same: namely, that in so far as it is distinct in meaning from illness, the use of disease is restricted to those conditions that are widely (by most people most of the time) negatively evaluated as illnesses.[15] It is by virtue of this idea that in a reverse theory, disease turns out to be a subcategory of illness—'illness' being used of any condition that may be negatively evaluated as illness (that is, rather than as any other kind of negatively evaluated condition, such as, say, ugliness or sin—see also below), while 'disease' is used only of those conditions that most people most of the time negatively evaluate in this way. And it is by virtue of this formulation that a reverse theory explains the factual connotations of disease while avoiding the contradictions inherent in the standard explanation. For instead of making disease a factual term, the reverse-theory formulation preserves its status as a value term, thus leaving open the possibility of its continued use with evaluative connotations. Hence, in a reverse theory, the 'slippings through' of value judgements in the use of 'disease' (as in Boorse's account), far from being an embarrassment to the theory, are actually to be expected.

A reverse theory of this kind, then, although derived from psychiatry, accounts more consistently than the conventional theory for the way the medical concepts are used in physical medicine. It also gives a more convincing explanation of the key conceptual difference between the two kinds of medicine—key in relation to psychiatric ethics—that is, of the relatively problematic uses of the medical concepts in psychiatry. This explanation rests on the same point about the logic of value terms as the explanation just given for the factual connotations of disease. On this point of logic, given that mental illness is more overtly evaluative than physical illness (and mental disease than physical disease), we should expect to find that the criteria by which the symptoms of mental illness are evaluated are more variable—from person to person and for a given person on different occasions—than the corresponding criteria for the symptoms of physical illness. And overall, this is what is found. For example, the criteria by which we evaluate anxiety, a typical symptom of mental illness, are more variable— in the sense defined here—than the corresponding criteria for, say, physical pain. Pain is at best a 'necessary evil' for almost everyone: but anxiety, though widely negatively evaluated, may be positively sought out—in horror films, for example, or through participation in dangerous sports. The difference here is a matter of psychology, not logic. We are just made this way. But given that this is the case, then for this reason alone the diagnosis of anxiety as illness will be more problematic (there will be more scope for doubt and disagreement), than the corresponding diagnosis for pain. And for this reason alone, then—rather than, as in the conventional theory, because of a supposed difference in transparency of meaning—the diagnosis of mental illness will be more problematic than the diagnosis of physical illness.

We will return to the relevance of this for psychiatric ethics in the last section. It is worth noting at this stage, though, that the reverse-theory explanation for the more problematic uses of the medical concepts in psychiatry differs crucially from that given by the conventional theory—in being neutral. The conventional-theory explanation, that mental illness is relatively obscure in meaning compared with physical illness, is all part of its pejorative stance towards psychiatry. But the corresponding reverse-theory explanation, that the more problematic uses of the medical concepts in psychiatry reflect an underlying relative variability in the criteria by which symptoms of mental illness are evaluated, puts mental illness and physical illness on an equal footing. In a reverse theory, mental illness, in being the more problematic, and physical illness, in being the less, both reflect, and reflect equally faithfully, the underlying logical properties of their respective constituent symptoms.

In general terms, then, a reverse theory provides a more satisfactory theoretical basis from which to tackle the problems of psychiatric ethics than the standard theory does. On the specifics, however, rather more is required. This is because the problems with which psychiatric ethics is concerned are mostly not so much problems of evaluation as of specifically *medical* evaluation. In the case of compulsory treatment, as we saw earlier, what is at issue, generally speaking, is not whether someone who is depressed and suicidal is in a bad condition, but whether their (admittedly) bad condition is of the specifically medical kind required to justify specifically medical means of intervention. Before returning to psychiatric ethics, then, we need to upgrade our reverse theory. We need to give account of the medical concepts as concepts expressing not just negative value judgements, but specifically medical negative value judgements. This will involve extending our analysis from illness and disease to the still more problematic concepts of function and action.

## Function and action

The relative transparency of the concept of mental illness, which helped us to see that the medical concepts are evaluative through and through, also provides an important clue to how the particular kind of value which is expressed by these concepts should be understood—namely, as arising from the experience of (a particular kind of) failure of intentional action.

Here is a thumb-nail sketch of how this part of a reverse theory works. In physical medicine, at least in hospital practice, where scientifically derived disease-theories are important, failure of function is a prominent concept. Correspondingly, therefore, in the conventional approach to the analysis of the medical concepts, failure of function (variously defined) is regarded as the root concept; that is, the concept from which disease, and in turn illness, are both derived. The theories of Szasz, Kendell, and Boorse, as described earlier, all illustrate this feature of the conventional approach. But in psychiatry the concept of *failure of action*, though not always recognizable for what it is, is, in many contexts, at least as prominent as that of failure of function. It is made explicit, for example, in many of the definitions in our official classifications: the hysterical neurotic is distinguished from the malingerer by his symptoms not being intentional (ICD-9, 300.5); the addict has 'lost control' of his use of drugs or alcohol (ICD-9, 303); and the obsessional is unable to resist senselessly repeating his actions (300.3).[18]

Hence, with a reverse approach to the analysis of the medical concepts, an approach from psychiatry, it is to be expected that failure of action rather than failure of function should be regarded as the root concept. And if it is the root concept, then this could in principle explain the particular kind of value that is expressed by the medical concepts. For intention is an inherently evaluative concept; that is to say, it is a positive evaluative concept in the sense that to claim something to be one's intention while at the same time and other things being equal denying that one evaluates it positively, is self-contradictory: like saying both that I want and (in the same sense of 'want') do not want something—a psychological, but not a logical, possibility! Therefore, *failure* of intentional action is, for the same reason, an inherently negative evaluative concept. Therefore, the experience of a particular kind of failure of intentional action could be the origin of the particular kind of negative evaluation that is expressed by the medical concepts.[19]

The difference in root concepts between the standard and a reverse theory is shown in Fig. 6.2. Obviously, as with the reverse theory of the last section, the details are all important. In the present case, moreover, the details, however carefully worked out, will certainly be more contentious. There is sufficient scope for philosophical dissent in the preceding section; as mentioned there, the logical relationship between fact and value, and in particular whether evaluative terms (such as 'illness' and 'disease') can ever be defined without reference to values, is a fundamental and continuing concern in theoretical ethics. But at least on this 'is–ought' issue there is available a body of well-rehearsed philosophical arguments upon which to

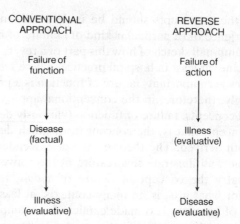

**Fig. 6.2**   The difference in 'root' concepts in conventional and reverse approaches to understanding the meanings of the medical concepts

> With the conventional approach, as developed for example by Boorse, illness is derived from disease, which in turn is derived from failure of function. With a reverse approach, by contrast, failure of action is the root concept from which illness and in turn disease are both derived.

draw (for an introduction, see G. J. Warnock).[20] The present up-graded reverse theory, on the other hand, takes us into the relatively uncharted philosophical waters of the philosophy of action, and indeed from there— with notions like 'loss of control' and 'unable to resist'—into the meta-physical deeps of determinism and freedom of the will.

Still, if the details are again beyond the scope of this chapter, it is important to see that an up-graded reverse theory, like the reverse theory of the last section, is a common-sense theory at least from the patient's point of view. The conventional theory, whatever its logical imperfections, rings true from the doctor's point of view because of the importance in medicine of scientific theories of disturbance of functioning. From the patient's point of view, though, what is important about the experience of illness is that it is incapacitating. Directly or indirectly, the symptoms of illness—pain, paralysis, dizziness, anxiety, and so on—leave us unable to do the things that we are ordinarily able to do. It is because we are unable to help ourselves that we may go to our doctor for help. It is because illness is beyond our control that its effects are not experienced as our own actions, and hence as actions for which we are responsible. The element of helplessness has been pointed out regularly by sociologists studying the ways in which illness is experienced (Lockyer).[21] And the term 'patient', as Toulmin[22] has reminded us, implies a direct contrast with 'agent'.

This is not to say that the concept of action, any more than the logical element of evaluation, is somehow at the surface of our minds every time we talk about illness and disease. On the contrary, what emerges from an up-graded reverse theory (worked out in detail) is in effect an evolutionary theory of the medical concepts. In such a theory, the properties of these concepts, in both colloquial and technical medical usage, including the elaborate development of scientific theories of disease, are all comprehensively explained by tracing their development on and from their origin in the experience of a particular kind of action-failure (specifically, failure of what is called in the theory 'ordinary' or everyday actions in the absence of perceived preventing causes).[19] In such a theory, then, this primary experience is understood to have become buried or overlain conceptually by subsequent development and elaboration of the medical concepts, much as in biological evolution ancestral bodily forms have become buried morphologically. Yet in logic, as in biology, an evolutionary theory may supply crucial insights. It is to these that we will turn in the concluding section of this chapter.

## Back to psychiatric ethics

The view of the medical concepts at which we have now arrived, although described all along as the reverse of the conventional view, is perhaps better understood simply as a more complete view. In developing this view it was appropriate to dub it 'reverse': for the approach was from psychiatry rather than physical medicine; the emphasis throughout has been on the evaluative rather than on the factual logical element in medicine; illness rather than disease turned out to be the primary concept; and now illness has been derived from failure of action rather than disease from failure of function. This whole process, however, has really been one of addition. The strategy in the conventional approach is to exclude value. The strategy here has been instead to bring it firmly into the picture, to show its central importance in the logic of medicine, and hence the importance of the concepts of illness and of failure of action.

The present approach, if correct, thus provides a more complete view of the medical concepts. It is for this reason that it can be helpful at the level of theory: in the present chapter, for example, it was our ability to draw on an aspect of the logic of evaluation that allowed us to avoid the contradiction inherent in Boorse's version of the conventional view, between his proposed value-free definition of disease and his continued use of it as a value term. More importantly for our present purpose, however, it is in providing a more complete view that the present approach offers certain practical advantages over the conventional approach, especially, as we shall now see, in relation to psychiatric ethics.

In the first place, as a more complete view, this approach makes ethics

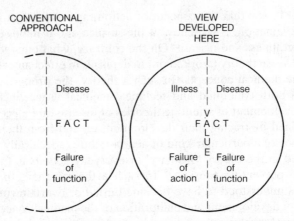

**Fig. 6.3**  A diagrammatic representation of the one-sided nature of the
conventional view of the mental concepts

> The conventional approach concentrates on only one half of the conceptual
> structure of medicine. The approach suggested in this chapter aims to complete
> the picture, adding value to fact, illness to disease, and failure of action to
> failure of function.

unavoidable. It increases the visibility of the logical element of evaluation
in medicine; and greater awareness of this element, as the editors point out
in Chapter 1, is essential if ethical standards in medicine are to be maintained and improved. In this, however, it is in principle no different from
the conventional approach, at least as presented by authors like Boorse.
Where it differs radically from the conventional approach is in showing the
logical element of evaluation to be *central* in medicine. Boorse, as we saw
earlier, regarded the theoretical heart of medicine as being value-free, and
his theory thus marginalized medical ethics, making it—at any rate as a
matter of medical theory—an optional extra. We noted also that this
corresponds broadly with the way that many doctors still view the place of
medical ethics. The present approach, on the other hand, has the opposite
effect, placing the logical element of evaluation, and with it medical ethics,
uncompromisingly at the theoretical heart of the subject.

It is important to add, though, that the present approach does not
thereby displace the factual element from the heart of medicine. In providing a more complete view, it finds a place for both. The present
approach is thus not to be understood as anti-scientific. On the contrary it
pursues efficiently the advancement of what Boorse calls a value-free
science of health. For in place of the value-excluding strategy of the conventional approach—which is essentially a strategy of denial—the present

approach offers a strategy of clarification. Some have argued that a value-free science of any subject may be an illusion.[23] But the present theory provides for the possibility of a value-free science of health by seeking to clarify the relationship between fact and value as twin and equally vital logical elements in the conceptual structure of medicine as a whole.

The view presented in this chapter thus makes science and ethics equal partners in medicine; it reconciles the 'what *can* be done' questions of medical practice with the 'what *ought* to be done' questions. And this ability to reconcile apparently disparate aspects of health care is itself a second ethically important feature of this view. For besides bringing together science and ethics, it provides a unified conceptual scheme—with the opportunities this brings for replacing conflict by co-operation, misunderstanding by communication—encompassing all the diverse disciplines involved in health care: the new view links surgery with psychoanalysis, social work with psychology, primary health care with hospital practice, and so on. More details of the approach are needed to fill out this claim.[24] However, even in the rather general form in which it has been presented in this chapter, it can be seen that it achieves at least one crucial reconciliation, that between doctor and patient. This is because the conventional approach, as we noted earlier, makes sense from the doctor's point of view, while the 'reverse' elements of the present approach— evaluation, illness, failure of action—all make equally good sense from the patient's point of view. Hence, the points of view of doctor and patient are fully reconciled once these reverse elements are brought together with those of the conventional approach to provide the more complete view suggested here.[25]

The reconciliation of the points of view of doctor and patient is significant for medical ethics—many ethical difficulties arise from doctors seeing the requirements of medical practice from a too exclusively conventional-theory point of view, and hence in an excessively scientific, mechanistic, dehumanizing way. Of course, there is nothing here, nor indeed in anything said thus far in this section, which is special to psychiatric, as distinct from general medical ethics. Indeed it is a further feature of the new view that, while it marks out a territory of specifically *medical* ethics, defined by an uncompromisingly value-based interpretation of the medical concepts, it also shows the essential unity *within* medical ethics of psychiatric and other kinds of medical-ethical difficulty.

This further feature of the present approach stems directly from the concept of mental illness being seen to be on an equal logical footing with that of physical illness. In this respect this approach coincides with the conventional views presented by supporters of the concept of mental illness, such as Kendell and Boorse. However, there is an ethically vital difference between the two approaches in their reasons for 'supporting' mental illness. With the conventional approach, mental illness is supported only to the extent that it is thought to be the *same* as the (supposedly) paradigmatic concept of physical illness. But with the present approach, the concept of mental illness is supported because it is *different* from that of physical illness: as we saw in the section before last, mental illness, in being the more overtly evaluative, and physical illness, in being the less, both faithfully reflect the properties of their respective constituent symptoms (the given psychological variability in the criteria by which the constituent symptoms of mental illness, such as anxiety, are evaluated; the corresponding stability of the criteria by which the constituent symptoms of physical illness, such as pain, are evaluated). And this is ethically vital because it shows mental illness to be of its very nature, rather than merely contingently, ethically contentious compared with physical illness. Implicit in the standard view is the hope that, with future scientific advances, psychiatry will become less difficult ethically, perhaps ending up little different from physical medicine in this respect. There are hints of this even in this book—in the suggestion, for example, that with progress in the brain sciences, the ethical problems associated with pathological aggression will be largely resolved (p. 200). But the new view shows this to be illusory. The 'facts' are always ethically relevant, of course. But without some radical change in human psychology (whereby anxiety and other similar mental symptoms come to be evaluated with the same degree of uniformity as physical symptoms such as pain), the attribution of mental illness will always (and legitimately) be more open to doubt and disagreement than the attribution of physical illness. Hence, to the important extent that ethical problems in psychiatry turn on the attribution of mental illness, psychiatry will always be ethically problematic compared with physical medicine.

The present approach, therefore, if coincident with the views of those who support the concept of mental illness, actually reinforces the concerns which have led Szasz and others to oppose it. For it shows that mental illness, if a valid concept, is none the less an ethically tricky concept. Physical illness can usually be deployed as though it were a purely scientific concept. This simplification is available because the value judgements implicit in its use are by and large uncontentious. But to deploy the concept of mental illness in the same way is to ride rough-shod over inherently different value systems. The view suggested here thus implies the need for a greater sensitivity to ethical issues in psychiatry, and more caution in the use which is made of the concept of mental illness.

Whether it is possible to go further than this raises large issues in ethical theory about the nature of ethical difficulties in general, and how such difficulties should, or whether indeed they can, be resolved. As noted at the start of this chapter, there is more to this than philosophy. But to the extent that the difficulties in psychiatric ethics are conceptual, the new view offers at least the promise of progress. We can see this if we return to the case of compulsory psychiatric treatment. In the first section of this chapter we saw that the issues raised by treatment of this kind, issues of central concern in psychiatric ethics, turn on the concept of mental illness. Yet the conventional approach was found to give an unsatisfactory account of these issues. And with the new view, in its now completed form, we can see that this could well be because this approach attempts to draw (in respect of these issues) on the wrong half of the conceptual structure of medicine. This is not an unlikely idea; after all, the issues *are* ethical, and it is likely therefore that the relevant half of the conceptual structure of medicine will be its evaluative rather than its factual half (the left-hand rather than the right-hand half of the diagram in Fig. 6.3). And if this idea is worked out in detail, what is found is an account of the key concept of psychosis in terms of failure of action rather than failure of function, an account which not only explains the unique ethical status of treatment of illnesses of this kind, but also (consistently with intuition and in contrast to the conventional approach) makes the justification of compulsory treatment stronger for psychotic than for non-psychotic mental illnesses.[26]

Overall then, the approach suggested here offers a number of attractions as a basis for psychiatric ethics: it places ethical issues in a central place in medicine, while also promoting (by way of clarification) the objective of a value-free science of health; it provides a framework for co-operation and communication between health-care disciplines, and, importantly, between doctors and patients; it defines the scope of a specifically medical ethics, of which psychiatric ethics is an integral part, quantitatively but not qualitatively different; it puts the ethically contentious concept of mental illness on an equal logical footing with the relatively uncontentious concept of physical illness; and it generates new ideas upon which to draw in tackling some of the conceptual problems of psychiatric ethics, such as those raised by compulsory treatment.

Yet the new view is no sinecure! As was emphasized at the start of this chapter, there is more to ethics than philosophy; there is sociology, psychology, anthropology, and the rest. And even to the extent that the problems of psychiatric ethics are genuinely philosophical, the difficulties are immense. The new view may indeed have something to offer by way of clarification of the medical concepts, but it takes us, as we found, into the complexities not just of ethical theory but also of the philosophy of action, and from there into general metaphysics. Mark you, the trade here will not be all one-way: if philosophy, in the form of conceptual analysis, has something to offer medicine, so too—and precisely *because* its practical problems are connected in this way with metaphysics—has medicine something to offer philosophy.[27] There is thus ample scope for a two-way partnership, a partnership between medicine and philosophy, potentially as productive as that which exists between medicine and science. But even if progress is made, the outcome for the clinician is likely to be that his task will become not easier but more difficult. At the very least, good practice will increasingly demand clear thinking about the meaning of illness as well as a sound knowledge of empirically derived theories of disease. And we should recall, finally, that even this will not be sufficient. For without the plain impulse to act ethically, better understanding of the medical concepts, no less than better knowledge of the medical facts, may be used as readily for the purposes of bad practice as of good.

## References and Notes

1 Clare, A.: The disease concept in psychiatry, in *Essentials of postgraduate psychiatry*, ed. P. Hill, R. Murray, and A. Thorley. New York, Academic Press, 1979.
2 Caplan, A. L., Engelhardt, T., and McCartney, J. J. (ed.): *Concepts of health and disease: interdisciplinary perspectives*. Reading, Mass., Addison-Wesley, 1981.
3 Fulford, K. W. M.: *Moral theory and medical practice*. Cambridge, Cambridge University Press, 1990. Besides giving a fuller account of the arguments, this book contains more clinical material than I have been able to include in this chapter.
4 Chodoff, P.: Effects of the new economic climate on psychotherapeutic practice. *American Journal of Psychiatry* **144**:1293–7, 1987.
5 Williams, B.: *Ethics and the limits of philosophy*. London, Fontana, 1985.
6 Warnock, M.: *Ethics since 1900*, 3rd edn. Oxford, Oxford University Press, 1978.
7 Szasz, T. S.: The myth of mental illness. *American Psychologist* **15**:113–18, 1960. Among the very large number of contributions to the debate about mental illness, those of T. Szasz, R. E. Kendell, and C. Boorse considered here represent particularly clear expressions of well-defined views. It will be seen by the end of this chapter that, to the extent that my own views are helpful, they build on the foundational work of these and other authors to whom I am indebted.
8 Kendell, R. E.: The concept of disease and its implications for psychiatry. *British Journal of Psychiatry* **127**:305–15, 1975.
9 Boorse, C.: On the distinction between disease and illness. *Philosophy and Public Affairs* **5**:49–68, 1975.
10 It might be thought that I overstate the extent to which doctors take medicine to be a science, and the medical concepts correspondingly value-free. However, aside from a minority of philosophically minded doctors, there is a widespread view that medicine is at heart, in its technical aspects, a science like any other. Furthermore, as Boorse's theory illustrates, it is possible to give cogent philosophical shape to this view, drawing on what I suggest in Chapter 3 of my book is a form of moral descriptivism. G. J. Warnock (reference below) gives a concise introduction to descriptivist and non-descriptivist moral theories, and to the wider philosophical debate about whether value judgements can be derived from factual statements alone (the 'is–ought' debate). The sociologist, Peter Sedgwick (*Illness—mental and otherwise*. Hastings Center Studies, 1, 3: 19–40,

1973) gave an early account of the view that disease concepts are essentially evaluative in nature.

11 By Boorse's criteria, homosexuality must be a disease, since it involves species-atypical desires which are associated with reduced fertility. But, he says, provided it is possible 'to maximise intrinsic goods such as happiness . . . it is hard to see what practical significance [this] theoretical judgement of unhealthiness would have'. In other words, according to Boorse's theory, the dispute about the status of homosexuality lies outside the scope of medical theory, for it involves an attempt 'to justify the value of health *in other terms*' [italics mine— see Boorse, 1975, section III].

12 Boorse [1975, section III] suggests that the loss of responsibility associated with mental illness might be explained by the relevant mental functions being unconscious, and hence outside our control, rather as digestive functions (such as peristalsis) are outside our control. However, as Boorse indicates, there are many problems with this account. In particular, there is not the same sharp distinction between a person and their psychological functions as there is between a person and their physiological functions. Psychotic illness, and delusional thinking in particular, is peculiarly difficult to analyse in functional terms. Yet the psychoses provide the clearest cases of loss of responsibility due to mental illness. Hence, on this important point for psychiatric ethics, Boorse's theory fails to give the (intuitively) right result.

13 Boorse, C.: What a theory of mental health should be. *Journal of Theory and Social Behaviour* **6**:61–84, 1976, p. 76.

14 See Boorse, C. (1975) (ref. 9), p. 59.

15 See Fulford, K. W. M. (1990) (ref. 3), Ch. 4. The proposed relationship between illness and disease can be visualized in terms of a Venn diagram. The universal set is made up of any condition that may be construed as an illness. This construal is according to complex criteria, one element of which (according to the theory suggested here) is a negative value judgement. But people vary in their value judgements. Hence, within the set of conditions that may be negatively evaluated as illnesses, there will be a subset of conditions that most people most of the time negatively evaluate in this way. One sense of the term 'disease', roughly corresponding with symptomatically defined diseases, is thus identified with this subset, other senses (for example, those causally defined) being derived from it. Of course, in ordinary usage the terms illness and disease, let alone different senses of disease, are not sharply differentiated in this way. An analysis of the kind proposed here seeks, however, to identify those conceptual elements which, when added together, reproduce the appearance of ordinary usage as a whole.

16 Hare, R. M.: Descriptivism. *Proceedings of the British Academy* **49**:115–34, 1963. Reprinted in Hare, R. M.: *Essays on the moral concepts*. London, Macmillan Press, 1972.

17 Urmson, J. O.: On grading. *Mind* **59**:145–69, 1950.

18 *ICD—9—Mental disorders: glossary and guide to their classification in accordance with the ninth revision of the International Classification of Diseases*. Geneva, World Health Organization, 1978. These are among the most transparent of mental illnesses in this respect. The notion of action-failure is similarly transparent in certain areas of physical medicine, for example with neurological disorders, such as paralysis, chorea, and epilepsy. It is less transparent in other

areas, mental as well as physical, for example in relation to sensations (such as pain) and emotions (such as anxiety). It is still there, however, essentially, because sensations and emotions, although not things that we do, are none the less things that we do things about (withdraw from pain, escape from anxiety). Action-failure is still less transparent in relation to what is perhaps the central symptom of mental illness, namely delusion. Yet it is here, above all, that if the analysis presented here is right, action-failure (as distinct from failure of function) becomes essential to a satisfactory understanding of the medical concepts (see Fulford, K. W. M. (1990) (ref. 3), Section III, and note 26 below).

19 Fulford, K. W. M. (1990) (ref. 3), Chs. 6 and 7. Function and action, although distinct concepts, are of course not unrelated. One aspect of this relationship is shown by the senses of 'do' in which people do things. These can be arranged in an approximate spectrum from more or less pure functioning (for example, biochemical processing) through to full-blown intentional actions. Somewhere in the middle of this spectrum there are things that, although capable of being done as full-blown intentional actions (viz with one's intentions more less consciously before one's mind), we ordinarily 'just get on and do' (J. L. Austin's phrase in A plea for excuses, in White A. R. (ed.): *The philosophy of action.* Oxford, Oxford University Press, 1968). Here in this middle ground of 'ordinary' doing, function and action may actually be equivocal: lifting my coffee cup can be construed either as me lifting my coffee cup (something that I 'ordinarily' do), or as my arm/hand functioning. The conventional approach to understanding the medical concepts concentrates on analysing them from the function side of this equivocation. My suggestion is that we may be able to achieve a richer and more self-consistent understanding of these concepts if we are prepared to explore them from its action side as well—see, for example, note 26 on the analysis of delusions. (It should be added that implicit in the equivocal relationship of function and action is the idea that function, as well as intention, is an inherently evaluative concept. In my book I argue that this is indeed so, the evaluative element in function being derived from that in intention.)

20 Warnock, G. J.: *Contemporary moral philosophy.* London, Macmillan, 1967.

21 Lockyer, D.: *Symptoms and illness: the cognitive organization of disorder.* London, Tavistock, 1981.

22 Toulmin, S.: Agent and patient in psychiatry. *International Journal of Law and Psychiatry* 3:267–78, 1980.

23 Hesse, M.: *Revolutions and reconstructions in the philosophy of science.* Brighton, Harvester, 1980.

24 Fulford, K. W. M.: (1990) (ref. 3), Ch. 11. Surgery, for example, is linked with psychoanalysis in this view of the medical concepts via the links (described in note 19 above) between function and action, concepts on the right- and left-hand sides respectively of the diagram in Fig. 6.3.

25 A specific example of where a better balance between the points of view of doctor and patient might help is in diagnosis. So long as disease concepts are assumed to be all-important there is a tendency to dismiss as a malingerer or as 'just neurotic' the patient whose illness fails to conform to an already established pathological entity. For too many doctors the identification of a specific disease, rather than the patient's experience, is still the final test of whether someone is ill.

26 Fulford, K. W. M.: (1990) (ref. 3) Ch. 10. It is with the concept of delusion that

the practical and theoretical aspects of the view of the medical concepts outlined here come together. The 'action-failure' element in this view allows an interpretation of delusion in terms of defective reasons for action rather than (the conventional) failure of cognitive functioning. The practical importance of this interpretation is that it shows why psychotic mental illness should be the *central* case of loss of responsibility (essentially because defective reasons for action represent the most fundamental failure of action). Its theoretical importance is that, as against the conventional interpretation, it is consistent with the full range of the clinical phenomenology of delusions; and this turns out to have implications beyond the logic of medicine, for general ethical theory, for the philosophy of science, and for epistemology.

27 J. L. Austin (see note 19 above) is among those who have suggested that abnormal psychology is a potentially rich resource for philosophy.

# 7

# Psychiatric diagnosis as an ethical problem

*Walter Reich*[*]

For something—a set of powers, say, or an institution, or a technology—to be capable of posing ethical problems, it must be capable of creating good or harm. In addition, it must be under the control, to a greater or lesser extent, of human will: it must be carried out, supervised, or participated in by persons who at some point possess, or believe themselves to possess, knowledge of their actions and the freedom to carry them out. Accidents of nature, such as fetal malformations or earthquakes, do not in themselves pose ethical problems, even if they cause harm, because they are not under human control. When they come under such control—for example, through the creation of a technology, such as amniocentesis or, should it ever happen, accurate earthquake prediction—that what was once an accident becomes, as a result of the possibility of human intervention, preventable or predictable, and what was once ethically neutral becomes ethically charged. If a human intervention, in some form, can, through its exercise or restraint, result in good or harm, then that intervention is, by its very nature, an ethical problem.

In psychiatry, powers, institutions, and technologies exist that, through their acts, systems, and techniques, have the potential for good as well as harm. And, as the profession's practitioners, psychiatrists believe themselves to both know their field and have the freedom to act within it. Clearly, the field, as well as those who work in it, satisfy the criteria for ethical concern.

Ever since psychiatry emerged as a separate discipline, it has been criticized for ethical abuses in every sphere of its activity. Probably, its ability summarily to cancel a person's freedom through its power to commit that person, against his will, to a psychiatric hospital has been the subject of most such criticism: psychiatrists have been accused of forcibly hospitalizing persons who have not required such hospitalizations—indeed, persons who have not even been mentally ill. Other aspects of the

[*] The opinions expressed in this chapter are the author's and are not necessarily those of any of the institutions or organizations with which he is affiliated.

profession have also been criticized on ethical grounds. Thus, institutions providing psychiatric services have often been accused of demeaning psychiatric patients. And the technologies of electroconvulsive therapy, behaviour-modification, medication, psychosurgery, and even psychotherapy have raised vexing and abiding issues regarding the control of behaviour.

But, in an important sense, all of these criticisms have missed the mark—or, to be more precise, have not gone deep enough. For, underlying all its activities—underlying all its powers, institutions, and technologies—has been one sustaining psychiatric act: diagnosis. It is the prerogative to diagnose that enables the psychiatrist to commit patients, against their wills, to psychiatric hospitals, that delineates the populations subjected to his care, and that sets in motion the methods he will use for treatment. And it is this prerogative that, therefore, should provoke perhaps the most fundamental—and the most serious—ethical examination.

Of course, the ethical problem of diagnosis has to do with its capacity for misuse. If enough is really known about mental disorders to be able to categorize them, and if such categorization does indeed represent a scientifically-based or at least pragmatically-useful professional activity, then the ethical concern must be the actual or potential misapplication of diagnostic categories to persons who do not deserve or require them—a misapplication that unnecessarily places those persons at risk for the harmful effects of psychiatric diagnosis. These effects include not only the loss of personal freedom, and not only the subjection to noxious psychiatric environments and treatments, but also the possibility of life-long labelling,[1-3] as well as a variety of legal and social disadvantages ranging from declarations of non-responsibility in family and financial affairs to, under the most extreme circumstances, such as obtained under the Nazis, the deprivation of life.[4-16]

In general, misdiagnoses may be said to originate in two ways. The first way is *purposeful*: the psychiatrist applies a standard psychiatric diagnosis to a person for whom he knows it to be inappropriate in order to achieve some end that is not, by common definition, medical. That end may vary from instance to instance. For example, the psychiatrist may be under direct and obvious pressure from a family to hospitalize a troublesome member of that family, or from political authorities to hospitalize a troublesome dissident. On the other hand, the psychiatrist may also issue a purposeful misdiagnosis at the person's own request. For example, a diagnosis resulting in hospitalization may be a protection against a worse fate, such as jail in the case of a criminal offender, the military draft in the case of a war-resister, or the birth of an unwanted child in the case of a woman seeking an abortion in a place where abortions are available only to those who can show medical need. In both types of cases of purposeful misdiagnosis, whether the misdiagnosis is unwanted by the diagnosee or wanted, harm results. In the first type, the harm is obviously to the person. In the second type, it is to the integrity of the profession. One's main concern should certainly be for the first type; but the second, largely overlooked as a sort of victimless crime, also requires attention.

But though purposeful misdiagnoses should be a serious concern, it is the other kind—misdiagnoses that result not from the wilful misapplication of psychiatric categories, but from the other, primarily *non-purposeful* causes—that deserve the greatest scrutiny. They deserve it because most diagnoses belong in this category. And they also deserve it because misdiagnoses of the first type, the purposeful, are in general clear and easily understood as unethical, while those that are non-purposeful are much more subtle and insidious, much more a part of the fabric of the field itself, and much more difficult to identify and stop.

To be sure, there is a sense in which it could be argued that this other category of misdiagnoses does not constitute a true ethical problem: after all, if they are not purposefully carried out, then they do not involve knowledge or free will on the part of the psychiatrist, and are beyond his control. But that is not quite the case. The mere fact that something is not completely purposeful does not entail that it is completely non-purposeful. This category involves, in the main, non-medical needs, pressures, and compromises that affect the diagnostic process, but that enter the psychiatrist's awareness to only a partial degree. The fact that the psychiatrist allows himself, for his own comfort, to ignore this awareness, or his responsibility to strengthen it, raises this category of misdiagnosis to the highest level of ethical concern.

Non-purposeful misdiagnoses, then, are different from *mistakes* in diagnosis. Mistakes in diagnosis result from a process in which, for want of adequate information about the patient, or lack of proper training, the psychiatrist issues a diagnosis to a person whose clinical state should be categorized differently. Rather, non-purposeful misdiagnoses result from a process in which the psychiatrist has both adequate information about the patient and proper training, but issues an incorrect diagnosis because of factors extrinsic to the patient, and does so without being aware, or fully aware, that he is doing so. Sometimes, such awareness is altogether absent: the misdiagnosis is non-purposeful in the fullest sense. Sometimes, however, awareness would be present were it not for the efforts of the psychiatrist, through the use of various techniques of denial and self-delusion, to escape the moral self-condemnation that would result from such awareness. At this most extreme end of the spectrum of non-purposefulness, the veneer of non-awareness may be so thin as to allow awareness, and therefore purposefulness, to emerge in such a manner as to make it difficult to distinguish from the purposefulness present in clear-cut cases of consciousness, fully-purposeful, misdiagnosis.

In the main, non-purposeful misdiagnosis can be traced to at least three sources. And it will be to these sources that the remainder of this discussion will be devoted.

## The inherent limitations of the diagnostic process

Certainly, the simplest source of non-purposeful misdiagnosis lies in the vulnerability of the diagnostic process to error. Over the years, it has been shown that the process can have poor or questionable reliability;[17-19] may be subject to inconsistency and change;[20] may suffer from bias;[21-25] and tends to rely on subjective criteria (such as, in the case of the diagnosis of schizophrenia, the psychiatrist's impression of the patient's 'understand-ability'[26] or 'peculiar behaviour'[27] his assessment of 'the feel of the case',[28] or his development, during the interview with the patient, of a 'praecox feeling').[29] In addition, psychiatrists may diagnose health rather than ill-ness because, as Scheff has observed, physicians as a group feel that a 'type-2 error' (accepting a hypothesis that is false) is less dangerous than a 'type-1 error' (rejecting a hypothesis that is true).[30]

Many of these limitations have been eased considerably by the introduc-tion, in recent years, of diagnostic classification systems and manuals that employ relatively objective criteria for the diagnosis of mental illnesses, particularly the third edition of the American Psychiatric Association's *Diagnostic and Statistical Manual of Mental Disorders*, which in 1987 was issued in a revised form (DSM-III-R).[31] The DSM-III-R, in particular, is constructed in a fashion that tends to reduce significantly the effects of those aspects of the diagnostic process that are influenced by subjective factors or ideologically-based theories regarding the aetiologies of mental illnesses. In the absence of clear, conclusive, and universally-accepted criteria, such as physical evidence for the presence of, say, one or another type of schizophrenia or affective disorder, such diagnostic approaches as the one taken by DSM-III (and the forthcoming DSM-IV) provide impor-tant, though by no means certain, safeguards against diagnostic error.[32-40] Nevertheless, psychiatric diagnosis, though increasingly rooted in scientific research, remains a process that is vulnerable to error; and it is the responsibility of the diagnosing psychiatrist to remember its limitations with humility, and to maintain a willingness to review his decisions and to admit his fallibility. At best, the psychiatrist is no better than his tools; and he must acknowledge their limitations as the starting-points of his own.

## The power of diagnostic theory to shape psychiatric vision

But vulnerable as the diagnostic process in psychiatry is to its own limita-tions, likely as those limitations may be to lead the psychiatrist to a misdiagnosis, and hard as he must try to guard against them, psychiatric diagnosis has yet other vulnerabilities that are even more subtle, more pervasive, and more difficult to recognize, and that, therefore, demand even greater vigilance. Again, the danger is misdiagnosis—non-purposeful but still damaging—and the ethical problem is the degree to which the psychiatrist can allow himself to ignore the forces and circumstances that lead to, and make use of, such misdiagnosis.

In large measure, diagnosis is a social act. It takes place in a social context. The psychiatrist observes behaviour and judges it against a social—often local—norm. Nor is this necessarily inappropriate. Psychiatric illnesses, particularly those characterized by psychosis, often affect persons in ways that lead them to ignore social norms and to transgress generally accepted verbal and behavioural boundaries; and such trespasses may, in fact, be the most sensitive and early indicators of possible illness. To be sure, the social basis of diagnosis is itself a problem, since the psychiatrist must know precisely where the social boundaries should be drawn, and which trespasses are the result not of illness but of some other cause—such as, for example, social activism, or artistic style, or mere eccentricity, or, for that matter, a rearing in another culture. But psychiatrists are, in the main, aware of these problems, at least dimly, having been apprised of them during training or, failing that, in the course of their ongoing practice.

Another basis for diagnostic judgement, however—one that shapes the diagnostic vision of the psychiatrist no less powerfully than the social one, but that is, nevertheless, generally unrecognized—is the diagnostic theory itself. In most countries, psychiatrists are guided by one or more theories of mental illness; and, often, those theories are associated with diagnostic systems that are their functional and practical expressions. And, depending on the specificity of the system to which he subscribes, the ways in which a psychiatrist assesses a person's behaviour, draws conclusions about it, weighs the variance between the person and the social norm—indeed, *sees* the person—may be heavily influenced by the assumptions underlying the system and the approach that system takes to recognizing and identifying mental illness. The system, after all, delineates categories of illness, and identifies the criteria by which behaviours and the persons who exhibit them deserve to be placed in those categories; and every time such a placement is made, the categories, as well as the system itself, are reified. To the psychiatrist who accepts the system as real, this occasions no concern: the reality of the system has merely found a correspondence in the reality of the patient's illness. To one who finds the categories mistaken, however, or the criteria too narrowly or too broadly defined, such reification may be simply self-deceptive and false, and may result in misdiagnoses that are as systematic as only a system can make them.

In many countries, this danger, though important, has been limited in recent years. In the United States, for example, the most recent editions of the official diagnostic manual, DSM-III and DSM-III-R (see the discussion of these above), have shifted to a descriptive, atheoretical approach to the diagnosis of mental illnesses, the aetiologies of most of which have not been established using commonly-accepted scientific methods. In the main, DSM-III and its successors define mental illnesses by describing their clinical features, which are, generally, behavioural signs or symptoms that are easily identifiable. Moreover, these editions of the DSM have classified those mental illnesses not according to aetiologies they are presumed (but have not been proved) to share, but rather according to the clinical features they share. In addition, they have listed specific diagnostic criteria for making diagnoses, the use of which increases diagnostic reliability. As a result of all this, clinicians have been more successful than in the past in agreeing on the diagnoses of mental illnesses characterized by features that are easily described and recognized, such as the psychoses; in the cases of other disorders, particularly the personality disorders, the criteria for which are more unclear, there has been less inter-judge reliability.

In other countries, the World Health Organization's International Classification of Diseases (ICD) has been widely used. The ICD (the latest version of which is the ICD-9, with ICD-10 scheduled for publication in the 1990s) provides less detail in its descriptions of mental illnesses than does DSM-III; but it, too, provides a basis for relatively good reliability in diagnosis, particularly in the diagnosis of the major mental disorders.

In one country, however, the Soviet Union, a diagnostic system has been put in place that, though in many ways highly descriptive, is, unlike DSM-III, not based on research that meets commonly-accepted scientific standards, and, in its definitions of the schizophrenic disorders, employs such broad and loose criteria that it permits the diagnosis of schizophrenia in cases in which, in the West, there would be no finding of any mental illness. As a result, Soviet psychiatrists who have used this diagnostic system have systematically tended to diagnose as ill—and genuinely to see as ill—persons who would not be diagnosed as ill anywhere else.

This Soviet diagnostic system was developed during the 1960s by Andrei V. Snezhnevsky, the founder of what has come to be called the Moscow School of Psychiatry, and, until his death in 1987, the head of the Institute of Psychiatry of the USSR Academy of Medical Sciences (renamed in 1983 the All-Union Centre for Psychiatry and Mental Health), the central psychiatric research centre in that country.

During the 1940s and 1950s, Snezhnevsky worked at and then became chairman of the Department of Psychiatry of the Central Postgraduate Medical Institute, to which the most talented academic psychiatrists in the country came to obtain their advanced degrees. Upon his ascension to the directorship of the Institute of Psychiatry in 1962, he dedicated the institute and its resources to the problem of schizophrenia, which was the focus of his central theory and of his diagnostic approach. Over the next decade, he and his staff continued to refine the system, doing clinical research designed to elaborate its details. By the early 1970s, many of his former students and trainees were in charge of the nation's academic psychiatric centres; the journal he edited, the *Korsakov Journal of Neuropathology and Psychiatry*, was the only psychiatric periodical in the USSR, and regularly carried news of his school's research and of the fine points of its diagnostic system; and the pattern of psychiatric teaching and research in centres far from Moscow felt the effect of his guidance and views, exerted through his role as an influential member of review committees for government ministries responsible for the approval of research and training grants. By the middle and late 1970s the hegemony of the Moscow School was almost complete: it was, clearly, the dominant force in Soviet psychiatry, and its system the standard Soviet approach to mental illness. This dominance continued even after Snezhnevsky's death in 1987, though it shows some signs of waning in the wake of public criticisms, in the press, of Soviet psychiatry in general and Soviet diagnostic methods in particular.[41–44]

The Moscow School's diagnostic system itself focuses on schizophrenia; but because its definition of schizophrenia is so extraordinarily broad, it takes in vast sectors of non-schizophrenic psychopathology—sectors that, grouped together, encompass almost the whole of mental illness.

The theory behind the system is based on the assumption that schizophrenia has three different forms; that these forms vary from each other not so much in their symptoms, as traditionally has been assumed in the West since Kraepelin, but in their course; and that a particular schizophrenic's course-form may be identified on the basis of a retrospective analysis of the development of his or her illness.[45–48]

A schematic rendering of the characteristics distinguishing the three course-forms is presented in Fig. 7.1. The continuous form is characterized by the development of symptoms early in life, usually by late adolescence or early adulthood, with a general worsening as life progresses. Patients falling into this category do not, as a rule, improve. The second course-form, the periodic, is characterized by periods of acute illness, interspersed with periods of remission during which the patient regains his health. The shift-like form is a mixture of the other two. As in the periodic form, there are acute attacks; but each attack leaves the patient more ill than he was prior to that attack, so that, overall, as in the continuous form, there is a general worsening of the illness during the course of the patient's life.

What is so unique—and, in the end, so problematic—about this system is the fact that two of the course-forms have subtypes ranging from mild to severe, and that in those two, the continuous and the shift-like, the mild

| Course forms | | | | | | | |
|---|---|---|---|---|---|---|---|
| Continuous | | | Periodic | Shift-like | | | |
| | | | | | Mild | Moderate | Severe |
| Sluggish (mild) | Paranoid (moderate) | Malignant (severe) | | | Mild | Moderate | Severe |
| Neuroticism; self-consciousness; introspectiveness; obsessive doubts; conflicts with parental and other authorities; 'reformism' | Paranoid; delusions; hallucinations; 'parasitic life-style' | Early onset; unremitting; overwhelming | Acute attacks; fluctuations in mood; confusion | Neurotic, with affective colouring; social contentiousness; philosophical concerns; self-absorption | Acute paranoid | Catatonia; delusions; prominent mood-changes |

Life course of the illness

Subtypes

Some characteristics

**Fig. 7.1**  Features of the Snezhnevsky course forms

subtypes are characterized by symptoms that are not psychotic. In almost all countries, psychiatrists would probably agree that persons who satisfy the Moscow School's criteria for the moderate and severe subtypes of each of these course-forms really are, by their criteria as well, schizophrenic. But they would probably disagree about the Moscow School's criteria for the mild subtypes, and would judge the persons who satisfy them to be not schizophrenic, but, rather, neurotic, suffering from a personality disorder, or even mentally well. Figure 7.1 notes the characteristics attributed by the Moscow School to persons grouped according to these subtypes.

The other feature of the system that adds to its potential danger— indeed, multiplies it—is the Moscow School's assumption that each of the course-forms represents, in essence, a separate illness, one that has its own biological basis, which is, in turn, genetically determined. This implies that a person categorized as belonging in, say, the sluggish (mild) subtype of the continuous form has the same illness as anyone else in that form, including someone belonging in the malignant (severe) subtype; and, though he has a more mildly expressed version of that illness, he has it nevertheless—and for life. Such a person may therefore be subject to many of the disadvantages, social and personal, as the person who is much more severely ill.

What is so troubling about this is clearly that the criteria given for the mild subtypes of schizophrenia apply to many persons who would be seen by most psychiatrists in the West as not schizophrenic. In fact, it could be predicted that, applied to a broad population, this system would draw into the schizophrenic fold precisely such persons—persons, that is, with neuroses, personality disorders, affective illnesses, and no mental illnesses at all. And, in fact, there is evidence that this has indeed occurred.

Some of the evidence is impressionistic. Rollins, for example, reported in her book on child psychiatry in the Soviet Union that patients with primarily neurotic or psychopathic-like symptoms were typically given diagnoses by Soviet psychiatrists in the schizophrenic range.[49] More directly, Holland has reported, after a sojourn in Moscow's Institute of Psychiatry, that Soviet patients may be diagnosed as schizophrenic even if they exhibit no signs of the illness, and that, once the diagnosis is given, even if it is further subtyped as being of the mild variety, it continues to be used on the assumption that the patient has a lifelong, genetically based condition.[50-53]

But the most telling evidence has come from the International Pilot Study of Schizophrenia (IPSS). In that study, carried out during the late 1960s and early 1970s, nine centres around the world, including Washington DC and Moscow, evaluated patients for schizophrenia and collected data about them. The centre in Moscow was Snezhnevsky's Institute of Psychiatry. As part of the study, a computer was programmed by John K. Wing to re-diagnose the patients originally diagnosed as schizophrenic at the various centres using data regarding the patients' symptoms that were gathered by the centre itself; the computer used strict criteria for its own re-diagnoses, notably those formulated by Kurt Schneider.[54] While most centres did 'well'—that is, while the computer 'agreed' with most of the diagnoses of schizophrenia rendered at those centres—two centres did poorly.

One of these, Washington, did poorly, it turns out, primarily because its diagnosticians followed the rules of their own diagnostic system, and, unlike the computer, tended not to differentiate between schizophrenia, schizophrenia-like psychoses, and paranoid psychoses; the computer gave them low marks only because it found their schizophrenics to be, by its criteria, otherwise psychotic. The agreement as to psychosis, however, was high.

The other centre that did poorly in the computer re-diagnosis exercise was Moscow's Institute of Psychiatry. But in that case, the reasons were different. A larger percentage of Moscow's diagnosed schizophrenics were reassigned by the computer not to the psychotic, but rather to the depressive and neurotic categories. Table 7.1 shows the computer classification (i.e., re-diagnosis) of patients who were originally diagnosed at the nine centres as belonging in those subtypes most likely to contain patients who would be considered by psychiatrists in many countries to be 'borderline schizophrenics', or merely 'borderline'. For eight of the centres, these subtypes were identified as 'simple' and 'latent.' For Moscow, it was 'sluggish' (the mild subtype of the Moscow School's continuous form). Although the numbers are small, the difference seems striking. The patients classified as belonging in these subtypes in eight of the centres, including Washington but not Moscow, were classified by the computer as overwhelmingly schizophrenic or as having paranoid or schizophrenia-like psychoses, while the patients classified in the mild subtype by the Moscow

**Table 7.1** IPSS computer classifications of schizophrenia subtype diagnoses

| IPSS Centre | Schizophrenia subtype diagnoses | No. of patients | Computer classifications (%) | | | | |
| --- | --- | --- | --- | --- | --- | --- | --- |
| | | | Schizophrenic similar psychoses | Paranoid psychoses | Manic psychoses | Depressive psychoses | Depressive neuroses |
| Washington | Simple<br>Latent | 4<br>2 | 50 | 33 | 17 | 0 | 0 |
| Moscow | Sluggish | 12 | 0 | 0 | 33 | 8 | 58 |
| 7 remaining centres | Simple<br>Latent | 27<br>8 | 71 | 9 | 6 | 0 | 14 |

diagnosticians, following the rules of the Moscow School, were classified by the computer as being primarily affectively ill or depressed, just as one might have predicted from an inspection of the system's broad diagnostic criteria.[55]

Finally, another confirmation of the tendency of the Moscow School's diagnostic system to overdiagnose schizophrenia has come from a Soviet psychiatrist, one working at Moscow's Serbsky Institute of Forensic Psychiatry. In an unprecedented article in a Western psychiatric journal, the psychiatrist, E. P. Kazanetz, used his own computer exercise to show that the Moscow School's system tended to overdiagnose as endogenous schizophrenics persons who were only exogenously ill—that is, it tended to diagnose as chronically ill persons whose illnesses were primarily of an acute, externally-caused type. Furthermore, Kazanetz added the observation that such overdiagnosis could be harmful to persons with acute illnesses assigned irrevocably to psychiatric registers of the chronically ill. Together with the evidence from the IPSS, Kazanetz's study reveals the degree to which an over-broad diagnostic scheme can result in over-broad diagnostic practice.[56]

What is so extraordinary about the Soviet experience, and ethically so significant, is that patients who were misdiagnosed in the IPSS and in the population studied by Kazanetz were misdiagnosed—that is, diagnosed as schizophrenic despite the fact that almost all other psychiatrists would diagnose them as belonging in less severe categories of mental illness—only because of the dictates of the official diagnostic system. Those Soviet psychiatrists really *saw* the patients as schizophrenic; or, to put it another way, *the system created a category, first on paper and then, through training, in the minds of Soviet psychiatrists, which was eventually assumed to represent a real class of patients and which was inevitably filled by real persons.* Those diagnosticians came to see schizophrenic pathology as including very mild forms, and diagnosed accordingly. Persons who should not have received those diagnoses did, to their detriment; and psychiatrists who should not have given them did, in apparent full faith. Had those psychiatrists been sensitive to the capacity of diagnostic systems to shape the way psychiatrists understand, categorize, and perceive psychopathology, they might have been able, one hopes, to avert this result.

It would be valuable to examine, in this context and briefly, the role played by the Moscow School of psychiatry's diagnostic system in the diagnosis of Soviet dissidents during the past two decades. The purposeful misdiagnosis of Soviet dissidents will be noted at the end of this essay (see also Chapter 24). A number of dissidents, however, were probably not misdiagnosed purposefully. Rather, they were misdiagnosed because their behaviour was socially odd, a kind of oddness for which there is a diagnostic niche in the Moscow School's broad definitions of schizophrenia.

For, as it happens, many of the ways in which Soviet dissidents have behaved, often in response to the governmental pressures brought to bear on them, are precisely the same, almost uncannily so, as the behaviour and characteristics said by the Moscow School to be common among mild schizophrenics, sluggish or otherwise. Table 7.2 contains a list of characteristics that were cited by Soviet psychiatrists in the case histories of certain dissidents in order to buttress their findings that those dissidents were ill. To be sure, those characteristics are typical of the ones that are often cited as signs of illness by the Moscow School's theoreticians. But they are also very typical of dissidents, particularly those who had to live the kinds of lives lived by dissidents in the Soviet Union. For example: fear, suspiciousness, and depression (hardly unexpected feelings among persons being hounded by the state); poor adaptation to the social environment (something without which you wouldn't *be* a dissident); and 'reformism' (which is another way of describing the tendency to dissent, at least before the advent of *perestroika*).

**Table 7.2**   Vulnerable styles

Overlap of common dissident styles and schizophrenic symptoms as described by the Moscow School of Psychiatry

- Originality
- Ideological formulations
- Fear and suspiciousness
- Religiosity
- Depression
- Ambivalence, guilt, internal conflicts, and behavioural disorganization
- Intensity
- Attention to detail
- Poor adaptation to the social environment
- Shift of interests
- Reformism

The result of all this has been devastating for dissidents during the past two decades, particularly before the advent of the Gorbachev era.

Dissidents were, of course, routinely arrested. Some of them were then sent, by the KGB, quite cynically, to psychiatrists, even though the KGB had no reason to think they were ill. These psychiatrists, learning of the KGB's wish that the dissidents be found mentally ill, did indeed find them ill, often giving them as a diagnosis one of the categories of mild schizophrenia. The dissidents' trials could then be held without them, they could be sent for indeterminate amounts of time to hospitals for the criminally insane, and their views could be depicted as the sick products of sick minds. Such psychiatric behaviour will be discussed later in this chapter.

But in other cases another process sometimes also occurred—a process involving different motivations but ending with the same results. In those cases, the KGB, encountering dissidents, saw before them persons who were, in a few striking ways, very different from nearly everyone else in Soviet society: in the name of goals, such as democratization or freedom of speech, that were, by all rational standards of the time, hopelessly elusive, they were willing to court inevitable and overwhelming punishment. Moreover, they were extraordinarily committed to those goals, and sometimes even chastised their interrogating officials for transgressing the Soviet constitution. Those investigators, struck by the apparent inability of these dissidents to appreciate reality, sometimes interpreted their behaviour as odd and a sign that something might not be quite right with them—that they were, perhaps, mentally ill. They then asked psychiatrists to examine these dissidents. But the psychiatrists were themselves, of course, the products of the same societies as the officials, were also struck by the same self-endangering and, by ordinary Soviet standards, apparently irrational behaviour, and were left with the same doubts about the dissidents' mental health. They knew, however, that it was precisely such behaviours that were said to be characteristic of the mild schizophrenias described by the Moscow School. And, resolving their doubts, they issued that diagnosis, beginning the process that resulted in court-ordered hospitalizations—hospitalizations on the grounds that, having committed socially dangerous crimes, and having committed those crimes as a result of mental illness, they must be socially dangerous, and therefore must be separated from society.

That this latter path to hospitalization actually took place is, I think, supported by the results of the February–March 1989 visit of the American psychiatric delegation to the Soviet Union.[57] In that visit, about half the patients who were re-diagnosed by the American psychiatrists were found not to be mentally ill by Western standards. Of these, a number had been hospitalized in 1987 or later, and others, who had been hospitalized earlier, remained in hospital in 1987 and 1988—during the period, that is, after Gorbachev's 'new thinking' on human rights had hit its stride. One could reasonably assume that, during those two years, the KGB and the psychiatrists who had so willingly served them would have been expected *not* to purposefully hospitalize dissidents they knew to be mentally well; after all, each such hospitalization could seriously undermine the effort of the Soviet Union to improve its human-rights image, an effort that was necessary if the Soviets were to achieve a number of goals in the international arena. That psychiatrists nevertheless diagnosed such people as ill suggests the possibility that, in at least some of the cases, they really thought the dissidents were ill. To be sure, some of these cases could also have been, and probably were, a result of the persistence of cynical habits among officials and psychiatrists who just couldn't change their ways; but the other explanation seems at least as compelling (and, to me, more so).[58-61]

Although the consequences of an unusually broad and vulnerable psychiatric diagnostic system have been particularly painful and destructive in the Soviet context, that context should not be considered the only one in which such damage could be wreaked. The Soviet diagnostic scheme represents an extreme spectrum system—a system that posits a spectrum of schizophrenic illness ranging in severity from the most mild to the most severe, and caused by a genetic deficit of variable clinical expression. Such diagnostic schemes are, in fact, under active consideration in the West.[62-72] To be sure, they remain under examination, and have not been introduced into formal diagnostic systems. But, given the Soviet experience, it would be valuable to weigh the potential of such systems for similar overdiagnoses; not to do so at this point would, it seems, constitute a kind of ethical trespass.

## The beauty of diagnosis as a solution to human problems

A third source of non-purposeful psychiatric misdiagnoses, and probably the most significant, is the attractiveness of the diagnostic process as a means of solving or avoiding complex human problems. With remarkable ease, diagnoses can turn the fright of chaos into the comfort of the known; the burden of doubt into the pleasure of certainty; the shame of hurting others into the pride of helping them; and the dilemma of moral judgement into the opaque clarity of medical truth. Because of their nature, functions, and meanings, diagnoses can do such things in efficient and powerful ways; and the fact that they can makes their use by psychiatrists for such ends remarkably irresistible, enormously unrecognizable, and, in the final analysis, utterly and failingly human.[73]

### Diagnosis as explanation, mitigation, and exculpation

Perhaps the most fetching beauty of diagnosis is its capacity to instantly explain: behaviour that is odd, objectionable, troublesome, or illegal can be, through the mediation of diagnosis, suddenly understood, explained, and explained away. To be sure, such behaviour may indeed be the product of diagnosable mental illness. But the capacity of a diagnosis to perform this function makes its use a temptation even in cases in which such illness does not exist, or is, at best, only marginally present.

The arena in which this diagnostic temptation has been most evident has been the law. For years, psychiatrists have been asked to testify as witnesses in cases of persons accused of various crimes. Often, both the prosecution and the defence have called upon such witnesses, who, in turn, have presented conflicting testimony about whether or not the actions carried out by the accused were a product of mental illness. While such conflicts have occasionally embarrassed the profession by suggesting that either side in a case can get psychiatric testimony in support of any diagnosis it wishes, at least they have been straightforward. Generally, the clinical questions have had to do with the presence or absence of some kind of psychosis, a group of mental conditions that can render a defendant legally not responsible for his actions; and the testimony has usually involved judgements about whether or not the defendant's behaviour and history met certain widely-accepted criteria for these, the most agreed-upon areas of psychopathology. Naturally, defendants and defence counsels have often sought findings of 'not guilty by reason of insanity', even when they have suspected or known insanity not to have played a role, because of their belief that, at least in cases of such serious crimes as murder or rape, confinement in a hospital may be shorter than the sentence that would be likely to be imposed should the defendant be found guilty and not insane. Still, some persons *do* commit crimes because they are insane: the law recognizes that insanity compromises free will, and classifies someone without free will as legally not responsible for his actions; it is the right of defendants to use that defence; and psychiatrists have a role, as a result of their expertise in recognizing such mental illness, in testifying on the substance of that defence.

The trouble is that, in recent years, attempts have been made to expand that role into realms in which psychiatrists do not have expertise. The pressure for that expansion has been the wish to explain diagnostically— and explain away legally—criminal behaviours that do not involve classical psychotic states. Instead of insanity, the clinical questions have involved issues about which psychiatry has almost no validated knowledge: questions primarily of coercion, persuasion, and influence. In a series of cases, defence lawyers have turned to psychiatrists to testify about the effects of certain environmental pressures on individual development and judgement, and on the role these factors played in the genesis of the criminal behaviour. The defence argument has usually been that these factors created a diagnosable mental condition, one that explained the behaviour and, in a legal sense, either mitigated it or totally exculpated it.

Probably the best-known case of this sort is the 1976 bank-robbery trial of Patricia Hearst, in which the defendant was said to have been incapable of criminal intent because she had undergone a process of 'coercive persuasion', a process that had affected her capacity for free will. In a sense, not only the defence, but also many observers, favoured such a diagnostic exculpation: it made it possible to understand how such an ordinary, peaceful, apolitical, and utterly American young woman could have turned so suddenly into such an extraordinary, violent, ideological, and anti-American revolutionary. The court allowed the novel defence—novel because it stepped beyond the traditional realm of insanity into the broader arena of persuasion—and a battery of psychiatrists supported it with their testimony. The jury, however, rejected it, despite its attractive advantages: diagnostic explanation, they found, was not, at least in their eyes, a basis for legal exculpation.[74-75]

The attractiveness of the diagnostic process as a means of explanation and exculpation has revealed itself in the legal arena a number of times since the Hearst trial. In each instance, the defense contended that environmental factors had influenced or determined the criminal act; and, in each instance, psychiatrists took the stand to issue their supporting diagnostic opinions. In one celebrated Florida case, for example, a young boy who was accused of having killed an old woman was defended with the explanation that his mind had been affected by television violence. As in the Hearst trial, the jury found such use of diagnosis inadequate to the task of explaining away the defendant's behaviour.

Despite these setbacks, it seems likely that the beauty of diagnosis will continue to be appreciated in the legal arena, and that psychiatrists will continue to expand the ambit of their diagnostic expertise into realms about which almost nothing certain is known. In time, it seems possible that psychiatric testimony will offer itself in support of psychological defences of all kinds—defences, for example, that attribute criminal actions to the defendant's early childhood rearing or to the pressures of his adolescent peers. While such influences undoubtedly exist, almost nothing is known about how they affect the capacity for individual judgement and the existence of free will. That some psychiatrists are willing to testify on these matters in the belief that they have such knowledge demonstrates not only the settled habit of such psychiatrists to opine on issues beyond their scientific domain, but also, it seems, the satisfaction gained from finding in the storehouse of the profession some explanation that will transform a person's criminal act into a symptomatic one, and that will turn a painful moral question into a painless medical one.

Nor should the turn to diagnosis in such cases on the part of psychiatrists occasion any wonder. It is a natural turn when an explanation for unwanted behaviour is needed, and is accomplished every day, outside the arena of the law, by non-psychiatric laymen as well. For example, journalists and other observers turn to it for simplifying explanations when political figures engage in behaviour that is inexplicable in ordinary political terms.[76-80] Still others call upon diagnostic explanations to justify forgiveness or elicit sympathy in situations ranging from breaches of airline etiquette[81] to more serious transgressions of industrial ethics[82] and literary propriety.[83] That psychiatrists similarly turn to diagnoses in the search for satisfying explanatory simplification, ones that substitute medicine for morals, is therefore not surprising; the satisfactions and advantages are the same, except that, in the hands of the psychiatrists, diagnoses achieve official status and recognition, and result in lasting effects which are not always, even in these cases, salutary.

## Diagnosis as reassurance

A second beauty of diagnosis is its power to reassure. When acts are committed whose implications are disturbing—acts that suggest vulnerabilities in ourselves, our institutions, or our communal beliefs—diagnoses often come to mind, both in the layman and in the psychiatrist, which serve to shift the frame of the behaviour from the threatening personal or social arena to a safer medical one.

In one widely publicized case, for example, this shift was effected toward its reassuring end through the co-operation of all concerned, psychiatrist and laymen alike. In 1974, Dr William T. Summerlin, a young researcher hired by the Memorial Sloan Kettering Cancer Center on the basis of his promising work in transplantation immunology, reported that he had been successful in grafting skin from genetically-unrelated animals. When other researchers were unable to confirm these astonishing results, Summerlin, in response, repeated his experiments, inking in the skins of his mice to make it appear as if the grafts had taken.

When this scientific fraud was revealed by Summerlin's research assistant, a special in-house committee was constituted to investigate the matter. The major threat posed by the Summerlin affair was the possibility that the American public might conclude that not only that researcher, but research itself, was suspect. To a community that depended on the magnificent largess of its various constituents and supporters—a largess which from US government sources alone approached at that time, more than two billion dollars a year (and is several times that figure now)—such a prospect was indeed distressing. Moreover, there were other concerns. Summerlin's story, after all, did violence to the new American dream: he was a young man from the country's heartland who had been embraced by the eastern scientific establishment only to prove himself shamefully unreliable. What of that dream? And, besides, what was to become of young Summerlin himself?

The solution to all these distressing concerns was quick in coming. First, the investigating committee issued its findings: Summerlin's 'unusual behavior involved at least a measure of self-deception, or some other aberration, which hindered him from adequately gauging the impact and eventual results of his conduct'.[84] Then, at a press conference, the cancer centre's president, Dr Lewis Thomas, a researcher and physician himself, went on to elaborate. 'The fraud in this work,' Dr Thomas informed the assembled reporters, was 'a result of mental illness'.[85]

In one stroke, all concerns were eased. Summerlin's actions were the result not of a vulnerability in research, nor of the habits of researchers, but, rather, of a fault in the man. Moreover, that fault was not moral, but, rather, medical. And, besides that, it was short-lived. At his own news conference, four days later, Summerlin volunteered that he had been suffering from an acute depression, a condition that accounted for his 'irrational act', and for which he had already begun psychiatric treatment. The psychiatrist, Summerlin explained, had prescribed rest and physical exercise, and he was already feeling much better. And so, indeed, did those who had been so distressed by the implications of Summerlin's act: the diagnosis preserved not only the good name of science, and not only the integrity of the scientific community, but also Summerlin, who could be seen now, in more reassuring terms, not as a person who would be forever morally tainted, but rather as one whose treatment would leave him clean, whole, and good, and ready to resume his professional life.

Whether Summerlin's behaviour was or was not, in fact, the result of an acute depression cannot, of course, be confirmed here; but the case is important because it illustrates the ease with which a turn to diagnosis can, at the same time, allay multiple concerns. When a psychiatrist is faced by such a case, when a means—the diagnostic process—is available that can accomplish so much, and when others are themselves inclined to think that mental illness can or should be used to explain the behaviour, it is hard to imagine that the psychiatrist will not look seriously at that option, and even find himself considering it with greater favour than ordinarily he might in other cases involving similar behaviours—which, however, in those cases pose no threat or raise no concerns.

*Diagnosis as the humane transformation of social deviance into medical illness*

Another beauty of diagnosis is its power to re-classify whole categories of socially unacceptable behaviour as the products of psychiatrically diagnosable conditions. This kind of re-classification derives, in essence, from a liberal utopian impulse: people are naturally good, and if someone acts to the detriment of society he must be ill. Hence, the social response should aim not at punishment, and not merely at control, but rather at treatment. If this approach is taken, everyone, presumably, benefits: the deviant, the 'root causes' of whose transgressions are thereby recognized and cured; society and its authorities, which are no longer in the position of exacting harsh punishments; and psychiatrists, whose redefinitions make all this possible, and who can feel themselves in the noble position of healing where others would have only hurt.

Probably the most striking examples of such re-classification may be found in connection with sexual behaviours that have traditionally been classified as socially undesirable. As a result of developments in medical technology, as well as shifts in popular views, some of these behaviours have been re-classified in psychiatric—and, therefore, diagnostic—terms. One such development, the synthesis of drugs that reduce sexual drive, has resulted in calls for their use in cases involving sexual offenders. One drug company, for example, advertised in the *British Journal of Psychiatry* that its product 'has proven to be of value in treating men who have been guilty of sexual offenses such as exhibitionism; paedophilia; indecent assault; rape; incest; voyeurism; bestiality and paederasty'. In addition, the company pointed out that other types of 'aberrant' sexual behaviours, even those not considered illegal, may also be 'controlled', including 'homosexual activities; fetishism; transvestism; compulsive masturbation; and sexual aggression in senile or mentally defective hospital patients'. In the United States, prisoners serving jail sentences for rape have gone to court demanding that they be treated with similar agents.[86] Other technological developments, those of a surgical type, have made still other 'treatment' options available, with individuals and their doctors rushing in to re-classify the aberrancy or malady in medical terms that have been tailored to fit the new treatments—and the increasing demands.

The danger here is that, despite their humanitarian goal, it is not at all clear that such re-classifications serve that end. Attributing to an exhibition-ist, or rapist, or a voyeur an underlying diagnosable psychiatric condition—hypersexualism—and then treating that condition by pharmacological or surgical means is not necessarily humane—and, in fact, has not yet been proved to work. Indeed, the surgical approach to transsexuality, a darling of the 1960s medical technology, has been shown to be seriously question-able.[87] Certainly, it is not at all clear that such redefinitions have improved the lots of the persons redefined.

Analogous attempts at re-classification have also occurred in other areas of psychiatry, with equally questionable results for both the professionals and their newly classified patients. Young offenders, for example, have been told by courts and other authorities that they would not be punished for their drug-taking or other social trespasses if they submitted to psychiatric treatment; and psychiatrists and psychiatric hospitals some-times have acquiesced in this process by making their practices, facilities, and diagnoses available to this population, usually in good faith and full belief. Instead of being recorded as criminals, such persons have been hospitalized as sociopaths or, sometimes, as persons with borderline per-sonality disorders, or even one or another form of schizophrenia—with the result that they have been labelled and treated as such, with inadvertently worse effects for the individuals than would have resulted from their original designations as deviants or criminals.

*Diagnosis as exclusion and dehumanization*

So far we have examined the beauty of diagnosis as a means of accomplishing ends that in some sense reflect the universal wish to be or do good. From time to time, we all have an urge to exculpate, to reassure, and to turn deviance into illness; diagnosis does these things, does them magically and utterly; and, in turning to it, whether as laymen or as psychiatrists, we have what we think are the diagnosee's interests at heart.

But the diagnostic process has a beauty that leads us well beyond the realm of generous human interest. We also use it because it helps us do things we otherwise could not bring ourselves to do.

The roots of this tendency are primitive, powerful, and universal. When we want to do unto others as we would not have them do unto ourselves, we find some way of turning them into others. We usually do that by labelling them, by excluding them from our own group, and by dehumanizing them—by defining their status as less than ours and, therefore, less human.

Stalin knew that, and did it on a national scale when he wanted to turn popular opinion against those who disagreed with him. Khrushchev, in his 1956 Twentieth Party Congress speech, described the process well. Stalin, he said,

> originated the concept of 'enemy of the people'. This term automatically rendered it unnecessary that the ideological errors of man or men engaged in a controversy be proven; this term made possible the usage of the most cruel repression, violating all norms of revolutionary legality, against anyone who in any way disagreed with Stalin . . . .[88]

Stalin understood that a person labelled 'an enemy of the people' would be seen by a wary and besieged population as a dangerous outsider who must be excluded from Soviet society. So seen, the outsider would be suddenly transformed into someone who is different, not truly a member of society, not truly a man—and, therefore, into someone who could and should be imprisoned, shot, or otherwise silenced, without the sympathy that ordinarily would be accorded a non-labelled fellow comrade. In her remarkable memoir of her life with Osip Mandelstam, *Hope against hope*, Nadezhda Mandelstam, the poet's widow, locates the origin of the Soviet tendency to distinguish between 'one of us' and 'not one of us' (the second group commonly being known as 'alien elements') in Lenin himself. Lenin, she points out, established that distinction during the Civil War with his 'Who whom', the phrase he used to summarize the difference between the Bolsheviks and their enemies.[89] In the same memoir she also shows how widespread was the tendency under Stalin, even among the intelligentsia, to exclude and dehumanize those officially cast out. Thus, when an acquaintance was arrested on unknown and usually arbitrary charges, people would tell each other—probably to reassure themselves that they would not be next—that 'he isn't one of us'. It was, for many, necessary 'to avoid those stricken by the plague'.[90]

Even more graphic examples of the dehumanizing power of labelling, and the universal tendency to use it, can be drawn from the context of war. In the First World War both sides had ways of turning each other into objects whose deaths would be less than tragic, somehow almost deserved. In the Second World War the Nazis pushed this strategem to the limits, using labelling to transform Jews and gypsies, and to some extent also homosexuals, and sometimes Slavs, into vermin whose extermination would be a blessing, and should certainly occasion no discomfort in the heart of a good Aryan.

And even in Vietnam the martial advantages of labelling, exclusion, and dehumanization revealed themselves. American soldiers sent there were given the task of fighting an enemy that was often indistinguishable from the general population. In Vietnam, any man, any woman, and any child was potentially lethal. And so they all became the enemy; one had to be ready to kill them. And, in order to be able to do that, one had to see them as not being in the same class as oneself. One called them 'dinks' and 'gooks'; one saw them as 'nothing but whores or thieves'.[91] These terms reflected perceptual changes that enabled American soldiers to transform the Vietnamese population into objects that could be annihilated without the danger of annihilating oneself through guilt. The power of this process was illustrated by a soldier who had to move corpses found after a battle. American corpses were bodies, while Vietnamese corpses felt, to him, like 'potato sacks'. In carrying them, he told an interviewing psychiatrist, Robert Jay Lifton, he 'didn't feel a thing'.[92]

Diagnosis is perfectly suited to label, exclude, and dehumanize in both its informal and formal usages. Informally, the terms 'crazy', 'mad', and even 'schizophrenic' often served as exclusionary labels that are used in everyday language to identify others who are annoying, discomfiting, and different. Formally applied—that is, by psychiatrists—diagnoses can make a person into someone who seems wholly other, and who *requires* exclusion. Depending on the severity of the diagnosis, he may be seen as disordered, polluted, and dangerous. In short, a diagnosis can turn him into another kind of human being, perhaps less than human, certainly not a fellow human being; and he not only has a need to be put away—he needs to be put away. Such diagnostic transformations can serve the needs of psychiatric systems under certain conditions in exactly the same way that it can serve the needs of family and social systems when their peace and tranquillity are disturbed by the symptoms of the mentally ill.

Psychiatric systems can benefit from the process of diagnostic exclusion and dehumanization because those systems subject individuals to experiences and conditions that would be difficult to impose without the advantage that such diagnostic transformation affords. Psychiatric hospitals, especially of the public variety, may be unpleasant places; and some psychiatric techniques, such as the use of drugs, electric shock, restraints, and confinement to seclusion rooms, may be experienced by patients as highly noxious. The psychiatrist knows that in hospitalizing a patient he may be, in the service of treatment, also causing him a certain degree of harm. The awareness of possible harm is compounded if the patient is an involuntary one, if the most invasive or liberty-depriving techniques are used, and if the patient responds to those conditions and techniques with the insistence that he is not sick and with a plea that they should be altered or stopped and that he should be released. At such times, the psychiatrist must harden his heart. And what enables him to do this is, among other things, the diagnosis. With it, he can see the person as a patient, one whose pleas are not simple, soulful, human importunings, but rather the routine and expected reactions of ill patients to the illnesses that have possessed them and to the treatments to which they have been subjected. With such a diagnosis, the psychiatrist can proceed, and not have to see himself as a violator of human freedom and dignity. In fact, he can see himself as helping, through the hospitalization and the use of such interventions, to transform a psychiatric case back into a human being, back into someone like himself: he can, in good conscience, allow himself to do unto the patient that which he would not have others do unto himself.

The advantage to the psychiatrist of diagnostic dehumanization is only a special instance of that disadvantage in everyday life. After all, psychiatric patients carry on the largest portions of their lives outside the psychiatric system, and place non-psychiatrists in similar, even more vexing dilemmas. The behaviours of such patients may be extremely distressing to friends, neighbours, and relatives, who, in turn, seek help for themselves by persuading the individual to consult mental health authorities, by coercing him to do so in some way, or by enlisting others, such as the police, to carry out such coercion. Sometimes, having been successful, these friends, neighbours, or relatives may recognize that their wish to be rid of the individual, and their actions to accomplish that end, were in part in the service of their own comfort; and, realizing the unpleasantness that may result to the patient because of their actions, they may feel some shame. That shame, however, can be dissipated if they remind themselves that the person is, in fact, mentally ill, that his objectionable behaviours are caused not by him but by a disease, and that their purpose in bringing him to the attention of civil and mental health authorities was related not to their own needs but to the needs of a person temporarily beset by a disease. This disease, they may reassure themselves, has obscured his usual humanity, and makes it necessary to carry out acts that, in the cases of healthy people, would constitute transgressions of their civil liberties, but that, in his case, represent only kindness, concern, and the desire to restore him to the normal community of man.

Of course, people do become psychotic, and do, in their psychoses, sometimes require interventions that we would not want inflicted upon ourselves. What is important here, though, is the capacity of diagnosis to enable persons who respect and even love such individuals to suspend their ordinary tendency to honour these individuals' stated wishes—to reverse, that is, the usual meaning of compassion, so that what the person wants is precisely the opposite of what he is given. If diagnosis enables us to do that in such cases, then it has a great capacity to do it in other cases as well, ones that involve no respect or love. For example, in cases of marginal illness, when persons annoy others by their socially unacceptable behaviour, it may become too easy to enlist the aid of diagnosis in response, so that, say, civil authorities can turn to the psychiatric system in the hope that it will aid them in removing the disturbance and in making them feel, through the issuance of a diagnosis, that they had been right in making that resort; and it may become too easy for those in the psychiatric system to acquiesce and issue a diagnosis—even when such a diagnosis may be somewhat doubtful, and even when the consequences may be unpleasant—on the basis of the self-deceptive rationale that a diagnosed person is not quite a person, and probably needs to undergo this kind of treatment, at least until it has its effect, exorcizes the disease, and brings him back to a fully human state.

## Diagnosis as self-confirming hypothesis

Perhaps the most remarkable property of diagnosis, and sometimes, for the diagnosed patient, the most enraging, is its capacity for inevitable self-confirmation. That property is used in everyday life by persons who call others 'crazy' or 'weird': once they do so, everything that the receivers of such lay diagnoses do can be attributed to, and dismissed as a result of, those or similar psychopatholizing epithets. In fact, everything they do subsequently can become a proof that the original assessment was correct.

This 'catch-22' quality of the pathological naming functions with even greater efficiency and inevitability within psychiatry itself. An actual clinical case can illustrate this well. The chief psychiatrist at a medical-school teaching hospital was asked to see a 65-year-old woman by the woman's son, a medical-school faculty member, and by her husband, a physician in a nearby community. The woman, they explained, had become 'negative' at home, disagreeable, more insistent than she previously had been about her views, and, in other ways as well, had undergone changes of personality. The chief psychiatrist, who tended to interpret behaviour and its aberrations as direct products of brain-functioning or malfunctioning, concluded that, in the case of this woman, such a malfunctioning had in fact taken place. He diagnosed an organic brain syndrome, one caused, probably, by the ageing process, and admitted her to the hospital to confirm the diagnosis.

The resident psychiatrist assigned to the case, however, could find no objective evidence of such malfunctioning. Meanwhile, the patient—finding herself in the strange circumstances of a therapeutic community, in which staff and patients were expected to aid each other in recognizing illness and in promoting health—became extremely distressed. She repeatedly insisted, to all who would hear, and in every community or group meeting, that she was not ill and should not be a patient. The response she received was consistent: she would certainly not have been admitted to the hospital had she not been ill, and the only way for her to achieve health was to acknowledge her illness. At first, she quietly tried to accept the ward routines in the hope that she would be discharged rapidly. When this failed, she complained loudly, angrily, and at length. The senior medical and nursing staff, observing her behaviour, cited it to the resident as a 'catastrophic reaction', typical of persons with her diagnosis who are challenged by tasks they can no longer master. Given fluphenazine, she quieted; and the drug-induced response was then cited as an improvement that further demonstrated the validity of the original diagnosis.

Of course the diagnosis may indeed have been correct: the resident may have been wrong and the chief right. But, given the authority structure of the ward, and the nature and effects of diagnoses, particularly those issued in such settings, it became almost inevitable that the chief's clinical pronouncement would confirm itself no matter what occurred. In the absence of objective, physically-based criteria, many psychiatric diagnoses are capable of such self-confirmation, whether they derive from a psychoanalytic orientation or, as in this case, an organic one. Indeed, even in this case, in which a psychiatric diagnosis was issued that is more susceptible to physical confirmation than most, the lack of such confirmation failed to derail the inevitable train of events. In such a climate, it becomes simply too easy to diagnose: one is rarely proved wrong, and the penchant for rapid assessment, valued so highly in general medical settings (especially academic ones) as an emblem of knowledge and expertise, has few means of objective checks in the psychiatric arena, and can result in too cavalier an issuance of diagnoses—diagnoses that, because they may be wrong, and because they have so pronounced a tendency to persist, can be highly distressing and, ultimately, damaging. Of course, this dilemma is made worse still under circumstances in which the diagnoses are issued not in the spirit of academic showmanship, or as an expression of ideological bias, but, rather, as a result of hasty or uncaring judgements. But whatever the spirit, the results to the patient are the same.

## Diagnosis as discreditation and punishment

And, finally, we come to the ultimate function of the diagnosis in everyday life, classical in every respect, as universal as the species and as old as man: diagnosis as discreditation, the attribution of a person's views, politics, actions, or conclusions to a mind gone sick: diagnosis as a weapon.

We see it everywhere. In the Middle East, for example, the Shah of Iran, before losing power, identified Libya's Colonel Qadaffi as a 'crazy fellow'.[93] In turn, Ahmed Zaki Yamani, then the Saudi oil minister, described the Shah as 'highly unstable mentally'.[94] Egypt's President Anwar Sadat diagnosed Iran's Ayatollah Ruhollah Khomeini 'a lunatic',[95] a compliment the ayatollah then passed on to President Carter.[96] In Israel, the Labour opposition had similar views about Prime Minister Begin,[97] while, on the West Bank, Ali Jabari, the Palestinian mayor of Hebron, campaigned to have the leaders of the PLO locked up in insane asylums.[98]

And elsewhere, too, and at other times. Thus Lenin, in 1919, to the poet Maxim Gorky: '. . . all of your impressions are totally sick . . . your nerves have obviously broken down . . . Just as your conversation, your letter is the sum total of sick impressions carrying you to sick conclusions. This is all a pure sick psyche . . . It is clear that you have worked yourself up into sickness . . .'.[99] The Soviet press, in 1977, on the dissident physicist Andrei Sakharov: 'pathological individualism'.[100] A West German political leader on the Carter administration's reported plan to produce a neutron bomb: 'a symbol of mental perversion'.[101] And Eldridge Cleaver's former friends on Eldridge Cleaver, after learning of his shift from black radical militant to capitalist religious conservative: 'schizophrenic'.[102]

Within psychiatry, diagnosis has also surfaced as a weapon. In 1964 American psychiatrists, polled, diagnosed a presidential candidate with whose views many of them disagreed, Barry Goldwater, as mentally ill. A decade earlier, members of the profession, supporting the Alger Hiss defence, diagnosed Hiss's accuser, Whittaker Chambers, as a psychopath, without ever having examined him. And the CIA, understanding the power of diagnosis to discredit, made plans in 1954 to use it in its covert operations.[103] Its hopes to administer LSD to those it wished to make mad—or, more to the point, to those it wished to be diagnosed by others as mad. Under the influence of the drug, these enemies of the United States would seem psychotic, with the result, presumably, that their own people, having come to that diagnostic conclusion, would reject or depose them.

But the most flagrant setting for the raw use of psychiatry to discredit—and, indeed, to intimidate and punish—has been the Soviet Union. And it is here that the category of *non-purposeful* misdiagnoses that was defined earlier in this chapter, and to which most of the chapter has been devoted, begins to merge with, and seem at times undistinguishable from, the category of *purposeful* misdiagnoses.

During the past two decades, several hundred dissidents have been arrested for political trespasses, and, as noted above, sent to psychiatrists, found mentally ill, and committed for involuntary stays at psychiatric hospitals for the criminally insane.[104–113] Of these, a number have been truly ill.[114] A number almost surely have not (as documented by the 1989 visit of the US psychiatric group).[115] To the extent that they have not, and to the extent that the diagnoses in those cases were rendered at the direct or indirect request of governmental authorities, these actions represent the worst expression of *purposeful* misdiagnoses—that is, purposeful psychiatric abuse. In many cases, however, the misdiagnoses were probably issued in full or partial sincerity;[116–119] as noted earlier in this chapter, at least some may have resulted from, or may have been made possible by, the availability or influence of the Moscow School's over-broad and over-inclusive criteria for the diagnosis of schizophrenia. Whatever the motivations behind the particular misdiagnoses may have been—whether they were issued purposefully or non-purposefully, in full awareness of their inaccuracy or in non-awareness (or only partial awareness)—the very fact that psychiatrists were asked to examine the dissidents in the first place illustrates, in a powerful way, the beauty of diagnosis in all its array—not only as a means to discredit, and not only as a means to punish, but also as a means to dehumanize, to transform social deviance into medical illness; and, in many respects, as a means to reassure and to explain.

## Comment

If we turn to diagnosis because of its non-medical beauty we are at risk, whether we are laymen or psychiatrists, of being injured by that beauty. For years people have been coming to psychiatrists to circumvent the law: they have sought diagnoses to help them get abortions or to help them evade the military draft. Psychiatrists often saw little danger in such humanitarian deeds, and responded to the requests willingly. But the danger was there, and we need only look to Russia to appreciate its extreme potential. Things went awry in that country because a powerful tool was just too attractive and too capable of misuse to be protected from it; the fear of governmental power was too great, the respect for the law too weak, the diagnostic scheme too broad, and the opportunities for self-deception on the part of both ordinary bureaucrats and well-trained psychiatrists too available. But the same attraction to diagnosis, the same appreciation of its multiple beauties, exists in the West, too; and though our laws so far have protected us from succumbing to a similar fate, the law itself has a certain weakness for diagnosis, tends to be partial to its charms, and is exquisitely susceptible to its inroads. Eventually, psychiatrists will have to understand that diagnosis plays a powerful, varied, and unrecognized role in the lives of all persons; that that role is equally powerful and no less varied and unrecognized in the lives of psychiatrists; and that all abuses of diagnoses—and, ultimately, all abuses of psychiatry—are a psychiatric problem in considerable measure because they are a *human* problem, and probably stem less from the corruption of the profession than from the needs and vulnerabilities of us all.

Naturally, psychiatrists must be expected not to misdiagnose knowingly. But in order to avert non-purposeful misdiagnoses, psychiatrists must come to appreciate the limitations of the diagnostic process itself, the capacity of diagnostic theories and schools to influence and shape psychiatric perceptions of behaviour, and the inherent beauties of diagnosis that make it so enticing to use that only the most stringent efforts on the part of the psychiatrist, and the most serious attention on the part of those who teach and train him, will keep him from yielding unknowingly to those beauties —indeed, will keep him from failing to recognize that they even exist.

# References

1 Balint, M.: *The doctor, his patient, and the illness*. New York, International Universities Press, 1957.
2 Scheff, T.: *Being mentally ill: a sociological theory*. Chicago, Aldine, 1966.
3 Levene, H. I.: Acute schizophrenia: clinical effects of the labelling process. *Archives of General Psychiatry* **25**:215–22, 1971.
4 Lifton, R. J.: *The Nazi doctors: medical killings and the psychology of genocide*. New York, Basic Books, 1968.
5 Mitscherlich, A. and Mielke, F.: *The death doctors*. London, Elek Books, 1949.
6 *Trial of Werner Heyde, Gerhard Bohne, and Hans Hefelmann*. Generalstaatsanwalt Frankfurt, Js 17/59 (GStA), 4 VU 3/61, des Landgerichts Limburg/Lahn.
7 Platen-Hallermund, A.: *Die Tötung Geisteskranker in Deutschland*. Frankfurt-on-Main, Verlag der Frankfurter Hefte, 1948.
8 Mitscherlich, A. and Mielke, F.: *Doctors of infamy: the story of the Nazi medical crimes*. New York, Henry Schumann, 1949.
9 Cocks, G.: *Psychotherapy in the Third Reich: the Göring Institute*. New York, Oxford University Press, 1985.
10 Kinter, E. W. (ed.): *The Hadamar trial: trial of Alfons Klein, Adolf Wahlmann, Heinrich Ruoff, Karl Willig, Adolf Merkle, Irmgard Huber, and Philipp Blum*. London, William Hodge, 1949.
11 Browning, C. R.: *Fateful months: essays on the emergence of the Final Solution*. New York, Holmes and Meier, 1985.
12 Ternon, Y. and Helman, S.: *Le massacre des aliénés: des théoriciens nazis aux praticiens SS*. Paris, Casterman, 1971.
13 Kogon, E.: *The theory and practice of hell*. New York, Berkley Books, 1980.

14 Hilberg, R.: *The destruction of the European Jews*. Chicago, Quadrangle, 1967.
15 International Auschwitz Committee: *Anthology*, 3 vols in 7 parts. Warsaw, 1971–4. [Articles published originally in 1961–7 in the Polish medical journal *Przeglad Lekarski*.]
16 Muller-Hegemann, D.: Psychotherapy in the German Democratic Republic, in *Psychiatry in the Communist world*, ed. A. Kiev. New York, Science House, 1968, pp. 51–70.
17 Mehlman, P.: The reliability of psychiatric diagnoses. *Journal of Abnormal and Social Psychology* **47**:577–8, 1952.
18 Overall, J.E. and Hollister, L.E.: Comparative evaluation of research diagnostic criteria for schizophrenia. *Archives of General Psychiatry* **36**:1198–1205, 1979.
19 Cantwell, D.P., Russell, A.T., Mattison, R. *et al.*: A comparison of DSM-II and DSM-III in the diagnosis of childhood psychiatric disorders. I. Agreement with expected diagnosis. *Archives of General Psychiatry* **36**:1208–13, 1979.
20 Babigian, H.M., Gardner, E.A., Miles, H.C., *et al.*: Diagnostic consistency and change in a follow-up study of 1,215 patients. *American Journal of Psychiatry* **121**:895–901, 1965.
21 Babigan, H.M., Gardner, E.A., Miles, H.C., *et al.*: ibid.
22 Pasamanick, B., Dinitz, S., and Lefton, L.: Psychiatric orientation in relation to diagnosis and treatment. *American Journal of Psychiatry* **116**:127–32, 1959.
23 Katz, M.M., Cole, J.O., and Lowery, H.A.: Studies of the diagnostic process: the influence of symptom perception, past experience, and ethnic background on diagnostic decisions. *American Journal of Psychiatry* **125**:937–47, 1969.
24 Temerlin, M.K.: Diagnostic bias in community mental health. *Community Mental Health Journal* **6**:110–17, 1970.
25 Plutchik, R., Conte, H., and Landau, H.: A comparison of symptom evaluations by psychiatrists and social workers. *Hospital and Community Psychiatry* **23**:13–14, 1972.
26 Jaspers, K.: Eifersuchtswahn: Ein Beitrag zur Frage 'Entwicklung einer Persönlichkeit oder Prozess'. *Zeitschrift für Gesamte Neurologie und Psychiatrie* **1**:567, 1910.
Fish, F.: *Schizophrenia*. Bristol, John Wright and Sons, 1962.
Astrup, C. and Odegard, O.: Continued experiments in psychiatric diagnosis. *Acta Psychiatrica Scandinavica* **46**:180–212, 1970.
27 Langfeldt, G.: Diagnosis and prognosis of schizophrenia. *Proceedings of the Royal Society of Medicine* **53**:1047–52, 1960.
28 Zigler, E. and Phillips, L.: Psychiatric diagnosis and symptomatology. *Journal of Abnormal and Social Psychology* **63**:69–75, 1961.
29 Rumke, H.C.: Signification de la phenomenologie dans l'étude clinique des délirants. *Psychopathologie Générale* **1**:125, 1950.
30 Scheff, T.: *Being mentally ill: a sociological theory*. Chicago, Aldine, 1966.
31 American Psychiatric Association: *Diagnostic and statistical manual of mental disorders*, rev. 3rd edn. Washington DC, American Psychiatric Association, 1987.
32 Baldessarnini, R.J., Finkelstein, S., and Arana, G.W.: The predictive power

of diagnostic tests and the effect of prevalence of illness. *Archives of General Psychiatry* **40**:569–73, 1983.

33 Boyd, J. H., Burke, J. D., Gruenberg, E., *et al.*: Exclusion criteria of DSM-III: a study of co-occurrence of hierarchy-free syndromes. *Archives of General Psychiatry* **41**:983–9, 1984.

34 Helzer, J. E., Brockington, I. F., and Kendell, R. E.: Predictive validity of DSM-III and Feighner definitions of schizophrenia: a comparison with Research Diagnostic Criteria and CATEGO. *Archives of General Psychiatry* **38**:791–7, 1981.

35 Hyler, S. E., Williams, J. B. W., and Spitzer, R. L.: Reliability in the DSM-III field trials: interview vs case summary. *Archives of General Psychiatry* **39**:1275–8, 1982.

36 Kass, F., Skodol, A. E., Charles, E., *et al.*: Scaled ratings of DSM-III personality disorders. *American Journal of Psychiatry* **142**:627–30, 1985.

37 Leckman, J. F., Merikangas, K. R., Pauls, D. L., *et al.*: Anxiety disorders and depression: contradictions between family study data and DSM-III conventions. *American Journal of Psychiatry* **140**:880–2, 1983.

38 Spitzer, R. L. and Fleiss, J. L.: A re-analysis of the reliability of psychiatric diagnosis. *British Journal of Psychiatry* **125**:341–7, 1974.

39 Spitzer, R. L., Endicott, J., and Robins, E.: Research diagnostic criteria: rationale and reliability. *Archives of General Psychiatry* **23**:41–55, 1978.

40 Spitzer, R. L., Endicott, J., and Robins, E.: Reliability of clinical criteria for psychiatric diagnosis, in *Psychiatric diagnosis: exploration of biological predictors*, ed. J. Akiskal and W. Webb. New York, Spectrum Publications, 1978, pp. 61–73.

41 Buyanov, M. I.: Heal thyself, medicine. *Uchitel'skaya gazeta*, 19 November 1988.

42 Churkin, A.: Interview in 'Psychiatry and Politics'. *New Times*, **No. 43**:41–3, October 1988.

43 Novikov, A., Razin, S. and Mishin, M.: Does Soviet psychiatry need a tighter rein? *Komsomolskaya pravda*, 11 November 1987, p. 4.

44 Reddaway, P.: Should world psychiatry readmit the Soviets? *The New York Review of Books*, 12 October 1989, pp. 54–8.

45 Snezhnevsky, A. V. and Vartanyan, M.: The forms of schizophrenia and their biological correlates, in *Biochemistry, schizophrenia, and affective illness*, ed. H. E. Himwich. Baltimore, William and Wilkins, 1970, pp. 1–28.

46 Snezhnevsky, A. V.: Symptom, syndrome, disease: a clinical method in psychiatry, in *The world biennial of psychiatry and psychotherapy*, ed. S. Arieti, vol. 1, 1971, pp. 151–64.

47 Snezhnevsky, A. V.: The symptomatology, clinical forms and nosology of schizophrenia, in *Modern perspectives in world psychiatry*, ed. J. G. Howells. New York, Brunner–Mazel, 1971, pp. 423–47.

48 Nadzharov, R. A.: Course forms, in *Schizophrenia*, ed. A. V. Snezhnevsky. Moscow, Meditsina, 1972, pp. 16–76.

49 Rollins, N.: *Child psychiatry in the Soviet Union*. Cambridge, Mass., Harvard University Press, 1972.

50 Holland, J. and Shakhmatova-Pavlova, I. V.: Concept and classification of schizophrenia in the Soviet Union. Unpublished, 1974.

51 Holland, J.: Draft of pilot study of joint classification of schizophrenia.

Psychiatric Research Institute USSR/Academy of Medical Sciences and NIMH/USA. Unpublished, 1975.

52  Holland, J.: 'State' hospitals in the USSR: a model of governmental psychiatric care, in *Future roles of state hospitals*, ed. J. Zusman and B. Bertsen. Toronto, Lexington Books (D. C. Heath), 1977, pp. 373–85.

53  Holland, J.: Schizophrenia in the Soviet Union, in *Annual review of research in schizophrenia*, ed. R. Cancro. New York, 1977.

54  World Health Organization: *Report of the International Pilot Study of Schizophrenia*, vol. 1. Geneva, WHO, 1973.

55  Reich, W.: The spectrum concept of schizophrenia: problems for diagnostic practice. *Archives of General Psychiatry* **32**:489–98, 1975.

56  Reich, W.: Kazanetz, schizophrenia and Soviet psychiatry. *Archives of General Psychiatry* **36**:1029–30, 1979.

57  *Report of the US Delegation to Assess Recent Changes in Soviet Psychiatry to the Assistant Secretary of State for Human Rights and Humanitarian Affairs, US Department of State*, 12 July 1989. Washington, DC, US Department of State, 1989. Reprinted as Supplement of *Schizophrenia Bulletin*, vol. 15, no. 4, 1989.

58  Reich, W.: Glasnost in psychiatry: Soviets still see dissidence as an aberration. *Los Angeles Times*, 23 September 1989, Part II, p. 8.

59  Reich, W.: The spectrum concept of schizophrenia: problems for diagnostic practice. *Archives of General Psychiatry*, **32**:489–98, 1975.

60  Reich, W.: The world of Soviet psychiatry. *The New York Times Magazine*, 30 January 1983, pp. 21–6 and 51.

61  Reich, W.: The theories and leadership of Soviet psychiatry. In *US and USSR Psychiatric Care Practices. Hearing before the Subcommittee on Health and the Environment, Committee on Energy and Commerce, House of Representatives*, 2 October 1989. Washington, DC, US Government Printing Office, 1989 Serial No. 101–82. [Note: Portions of this chapter were presented in testimony at this hearing.]

62  Rosenthal, D.: *The Genain quadruplets*. New York, Basic Books, 1963.

63  Kety, S. S., Rosenthal, D., Wender, P. H., *et al.*: The types and prevalence of mental illness in the biological adoptive families of adopted schizophrenics, in *The transmission of schizophrenia*, ed. D. Rosenthal and S. S. Kety. Oxford, Pergamon Press, 1968, pp. 345–62.

64  Rosenthal, D., Wender, P. H., Kety, S. S., *et al.*: Schizophrenic's offspring reared in adoptive homes, in *The transmission of schizophrenia*, ed. S. S. Kety, D. Rosenthal, and P. H. Wender. Oxford, Pergamon Press, 1968, pp. 377–91.

65  Rosenthal, D., Wender, P. H., and Kety, S. S., *et al.*: The adopted away offspring of schizophrenics. *American Journal of Psychiatry* **128**:302–6, 1971.

66  Wender, P. H., Rosenthal, D., Kety, S. S., *et al.*: Crossfostering: research strategy for clarifying the role of genetic and experimental factors in the etiology of schizophrenia. *Archives of General Psychiatry* **30**:121–8, 1974.

67  Kety, S. S., Rosenthal, D., Wender, P. H., *et al.*: Mental illness in the biological and adoptive families of adopted individuals who have become schizophrenic: a preliminary report based upon psychiatric interviews, in *Genetic research in psychiatry*, ed. R. Fieve, D. Rosenthal, and H. Brill. Baltimore, The Johns Hopkins University Press, 1975, pp. 147–65.

68  Fowler, R. C., Tsuang, M. T., Cadoret, R. J., *et al.*: Non-psychotic disorders

in the families of process schizophrenics. *Acta Psychiatrica Scandinavica* **51**:153–60, 1975.

69 Reich, W.: The schizophrenia spectrum: a genetic concept. *Journal of Nervous and Mental Diseases* **162**:3–12, 1976.

70 Rieder, R. O.: The schizophrenia spectrum. Presented at the 131st Annual Meeting of the American Psychiatric Association, May 8–12, 1978.

71 Kety, S. S., Rosenthal, D., Wender, P. H., *et al*.: The biologic and adoptive families of adopted individuals who became schizophrenic: prevalence of mental illness and other characteristics, in *The nature of schizophrenia*, ed. L. C. Wynne, R. L. Cromwell, and S. Matthysse. Wiley, New York, 1978, pp. 25–37.

72 Kety, S. S., Wender, P. H., and Rosenthal, D.: Genetic relationships within the schizophrenia spectrum: evidence from adoption studies, in *Critical issues in psychiatric diagnosis*, ed. R. L. Spitzer and D. F. Klein. Raven Press, New York, 1978, pp. 213–23.

73 Reich, W.: The diagnosis of everyday life. *Harper's Magazine*, February 1980.

74 Reich, W.: Brainwashing, psychiatry and the law. *The New York Times*, 29 May 1976, p. 23.

75 Reich, W.: Brainwashing, psychiatry and the law. *Psychiatry* **39**:400–3, 1976.

76 Sinclair, W.: After the upheaval: who's running what? *The Washington Post*, 21 July 1979, p. A-1. Weicker suggests Carter not run. *The Washington Post*, 22 July 1979, p. A-6.

77 Quinn, S.: Rosalynn's journey. *The Washington Post*, 25 July 1979, p. B-1.

78 Schram, M.: The troubled times of a different Billy Carter. *The Washington Post*, 25 February 1979, p. A-1.

79 Gup, T.: Brooding replaces clowning. *The Washington Post*, 25 February 1979, p. A-1.

80 Evans, R. and Novak, R.: Brother Billy: political blunders. *The Washington Post*, 2 March 1979.

81 The stewardess and the 'witch'. *Newsweek*, 30 April 1979, p. 31.

82 Berry, J. D. and Egan, J.: Alleged embezzling, maneuvering in moviedom. *The Washington Post*, 25 December 1977, p. A-1.

83 Mitgang, H.: Greene calls profile of him in *New Yorker* inaccurate. *The New York Times*, 12 May 1979.

84 Brody, J. E.: Inquiry at cancer center finds fraud in research. *The New York Times*, 25 May 1974.

85 Brody, J. E.: Scientist denies cancer research fraud. *The New York Times*, 29 May 1974.

86 Colen, D.: Drug for sex offenders called success. *The Washington Post*, 5 December 1975.

87 Myer, J. K. and Reter, D. J.: Sex reassignment: follow-up. *Archives of General Psychiatry* **36**:1010–15, 1979.

88 Khrushchev, N.: *Khrushchev remembers*, trans. and ed. S. Talbott. Boston, Little, Brown, 1970, p. 566.

89 Mandelstam, N.: *Hope against hope*. New York, Atheneum, 1970, p. 28.

90 Mandelstam, N.: *Hope against hope*. New York, Atheneum, 1970, p. 26.

91 Lifton, R. J.: *Home from the war*. New York, Simon and Schuster, 1973, p. 194.

92 Lifton, R. J.: *Home from the war*. New York, Simon and Schuster, 1973, p. 192.

93  Libya helping terrorists with arms and training. *The New York Times*, 16 July 1976.
94  Anderson, J. and Whitten, L.: Saudis suspect an Iran–US plot. *The Washington Post*, 17 September 1976.
95  *The New York Times*, 10 November 1979, p. 8.
96  Khomeini, R.: The world is not on your side. *The Washington Post*, 22 November 1979, p. A-23.
97  Farrell, W.: The furor surrounding Begin: he fights harder and doesn't budge. *The New York Times*, 25 July 1978.
98  Randal, J. C.: Role in UN session builds confidence among Palestinians. *The Washington Post*, 12 January 1979.
99  Lenin, V. I.: Letter to Gorky of 31 July 1919. *Sochineniya* (Works), 4th edn. Moscow State Political Literature Publishing House, 1951–67. Quoted in Lev Navrozov, *The education of Lev Navrozov*. New York, Harper's Magazine Press, 1975, p. 164.
100  Mrs Sakharov flies home. *The Washington Post*, 24 November 1977, p. A-39.
101  Getler, M.: Bonn party aide calls US bomb a 'perversion'. *The Washington Post*, 18 July 1977, p. A-1.
102  Allman, T. D.: The 'rebirth' of Eldridge Cleaver. *The New York Times Magazine*, 16 January 1977, p. 10.
103  Horrock, N. M.: Drug tested by C.I.A. on mental patients. *The New York Times*, 3 August 1977, p. A-1.
104  Committee on the Judiciary: *Abuse of psychiatry for political repression in the Soviet Union*. Hearing before the Subcommittee to Investigate the Administration of the Internal Security Act and Other Internal Security Laws of the Committee on the Judiciary, United States Senate, Ninety-Second Congress, Second Session. Washington, DC, US Government Printing Office, 26 December 1972.
105  Stone, I. F.: Betrayal by psychiatry. *The New York Review of Books*, 10 February 1972, pp. 7–14.
106  Chodoff, P.: Involuntary hospitalization of political dissenters in the Soviet Union. *Psychiatric Opinion*, 11:5–19, 1974. Amnesty International: *Prisoners of conscience in the USSR: their treatment and conditions*. London, Amnesty International Publications, 1975.
107  Grigorenko, P.: *The Grigorenko papers: writings by General P. G. Grigorenko and documents on his case*. London, C. Hurst; Boulder, Colorado, Westview Press, 1976.
108  Yeo, C.: The abuse of psychiatry in the USSR: the evidence. *Index on Censorship*: **Vol. 4, No. 2** (Summer 1975).
109  Bloch, S. and Reddaway, P.: *Psychiatric terror: the abuse of psychiatry in the Soviet Union*. New York, Basic Books, 1977.
110  Bloch, S. and Reddaway, P.: *Soviet psychiatric abuse: the shadow over world psychiatry*. Boulder, Colorado, Westview Press, 1985.
111  Lader, M.: *Psychiatry on trial*. Harmondsworth, Penguin, 1977.
112  Plyushch, L.: *History's carnival*, with a contribution by Tatyana Plyushch, ed. and trans. Marco Carynnyk. New York, Harcourt Brace Jovanovich, 1979.
113  Bukovsky, V.: *To build a castle: my life as a dissenter*, trans. M. Scammell. New York, Viking Press, 1979.
114  Reich, W.: Diagnosing Soviet dissenters. *Harper's Magazine*, August 1978, pp. 31–7.

115 Reich, W.: Grigorenko gets a second opinion. *The New York Times Magazine*, 13 May 1979, pp. 18ff.
116 Reich, W.: Diagnosing Soviet dissidents. *Harper's Magazine*, August 1978, pp. 31–7.
117 Reich, W.: Soviet psychiatry on trial. *Commentary*, January 1978, pp. 40–8.
118 Reich, W.: The world of Soviet psychiatry. *The New York Times Magazine*, 30 January 1983, pp. 21–6, 51.
119 Reich, W.: Glasnost in psychiatry: Soviets still see dissidence as an aberration. *Los Angeles Times*, 23 September 1989, Part II, p. 8.

# 8

# Ethical aspects of psychotherapy

*T. Byram Karasu*

Patients may forgive all the technical mistakes and none of the ethical ones.
—T.B.K.

We have evolved from an 'Age of Anxiety' to an 'Age of Ethical Crises'.[1] The psychotherapist, once left relatively undisturbed in the private confines of his office, has now been 'under siege' from within[2] and from without.[3] The 'crisis within' reflects psychiatry's own members, who extol widely different models and criteria of mental illness and its treatment, which are confusing and divisive to the field and to its future; the 'attacks from without' reflect the public confusion regarding the functions, procedures, and powers of the psychotherapist. For both patient and profession, there has occurred an increasing expectation and demand for accountability: that the patient be granted health care as a right, with greater participation in determining and assessing his treatment; and that the therapist, responding to rising social and political pressure, review the nature of his practices and their effects upon his patients. The profession's current failure to stave off challenge and criticism has been attributed to several compounding factors, including a fundamental disappointment with the limitations of science and reason in answering the problems of mankind; an anti-élitism which aims to mitigate the power of professionals as symbolic representations of the inequitable distribution of resources in society; and, most potently in the moral context *per se*, the fear of over-generalization of professional authority from scientific to ethical areas.[4]

## The interface between science and ethics

The relationship of science to ethics in psychotherapy may be considered the conceptual heart-of-the-matter. Ethics has been defined as 'the system or code of morality of a particular person, religion, group, or profession' (morals as 'relating to, dealing with, or capable of making the distinction between right and wrong in conduct'); science (which psychotherapy presumes to be) defined as 'a branch of knowledge or study concerned with establishing or systemizing facts'.[5] Theoretically, science and ethics have

been conceived of as two distinct and separate entities, almost antithetical
—science as 'descriptive' and ethics as 'prescriptive'; science relying on
'validation', ethics on 'judgement'; and science concerned solely with 'what
is', whereas ethics addresses 'what ought to be'.[6] But the lines become less
sharply drawn when the complexities of social reality are considered, as
when the psychotherapist is obliged to act as a 'double agent' to accommodate conflicts of interest not only between patient and therapist, but also
involving third parties to whom the therapist holds allegiance (for example,
family members, school, hospital, military);[7,8] and when one considers, as
the therapist straddles the ambiguous line between the science and the art of
psychotherapy, dual attitudes towards his own professional identity which
differ both in degree and quality.[9] There is still a question whether psychotherapy is a science at all, in that it deals with hermeneutics rather than
explanation, is humanistic rather than mechanistic, seeks private rather than
public knowledge—in all, is not a science but a body of knowledge with
a special status, which frees it from obligations that other sciences have.[10]

In addition, as London[11] has pointed out, while the distinction between
the principles of science and those of ethics may more readily hold for the
researcher inside his laboratory, it is less applicable to the clinician in his
daily practice. Lifton[12] especially highlighted this point in describing his
work with Vietnam veterans, which required him to combine sufficient
detachment to enable him to make psychological evaluations with involvement that expressed his own personal commitment and moral passion (in
that he had previously taken an active anti-war position). He aptly concluded, 'I believe that we [therapists] always function within this *dialectic
between ethical involvement and intellectual rigour*' [p. 386].[12]

He further recommended that 'bringing our advocacy "out front" and
articulating it makes us more, rather than less, scientific. Indeed, our scientific accuracy is likely to suffer when we hide our ethical beliefs behind the
claims of neutrality and that we are nothing but "neutral screens"' [p. 386].

With the above in mind, it is inevitable that in psychotherapy the boundaries between science and ethics are blurred. In fact, there has been a
greater recognition of the inevitable constraints upon the presumed purity
of objective treatment by the pulls of subjective commitment (unconscious
if not conscious). More specifically, the idyllic notion of psychotherapy and
the psychotherapist as 'value-free' is now widely accepted as a fallacy.[13]

This is supported by current research, which has demonstrated many
contradictions in expressed belief and reported practices in psychotherapy.[14]
One could hypothesize the existence of a 'two-tier' system—one, the ideal
or correct (i.e., value-free, non-suggestive); the other, the practical or
applied view (i.e., including direct suggestion and encouragement of
specific goals)—which interferes with a value-free frame of reference. In
brief, the application of psychotherapy represents neither pure science nor

pure ethics, but a branch of the healing profession which resides somewhere in between. Therefore it is likely that psychotherapy will only find its ethical place by locating a legitimate and unique area between the two ideological extremes—that of being an objectively applied science, and that of representing an ideology of healthy conduct.[15]

Concern with the interface between science and ethics is not new to psychotherapy. Major controversies since Freud have long pivoted upon the question of whether psychoanalysis inherently propounds particular values, especially values which may be immoral or biased. Some believe it does not do so.[16,17] Others point out its political and repressive nature by virtue of its very existence,[18,19] or, more specifically, view it as an enemy of morality and religion (see Holt's[17] refutation) or take exception to particular biases, for example its favouring of certain social classes or patient types over others[20] or its discrimination against women[21] (the issues of therapist–patient sex and sexism). Still others, while accepting that psychotherapy cannot be value-free, and even believing that in its overall goals it *should* not be,[22] see the basic issue as whether imposition of such values is 'deliberate and avowed' or 'unrecognized and unavowed'.[15]

In this regard, the ethical impact of psychoanalysis has occurred on several fronts. One major front was Freud's discovery of unconscious motivation and conflict, which posed fundamental ethical questions of psychic determinism versus free will and responsibility. But for Freud the doctrine of exceptionless psychic determinism did not preclude moral responsibility. As he put it: 'One must hold oneself responsible for the evil impulses of one's dreams.'[17] As for the therapist's ethical position, Freud foresaw the inevitable influence of therapist on his patient, and his unique power within the transference relationship both to cure and to be resisted. Classic here, of course, have been the devoted analytic attempts to maintain the purity of the therapeutic relationship through the technical neutrality of the therapist; and, when this has been inevitably violated, the full exploration and understanding of the therapist's countertransference. In addition, a legacy of analytic techniques is said necessarily to preclude the therapist's assumption of roles or his conscious manipulation and control of the patient, because this is antithetical to the development of insight.[23] Certainly Freud held an overriding ethical ideal about the conduct of psychotherapy when he wrote: 'One must not forget that the relationship between analyst and patient is based on a love of truth, that is, acknowledgement of reality, and that it precludes any kind of sham or deceit', [p. 248].[24]

## General ethical issues in psychotherapy

The following section on 'general' ethical issues in psychotherapy refers to those which are global and pervasive of its goals and to the therapist–patient relationship. Unfortunately, they often involve implicit and ubiquitous values, which, because of their complex, covert, and often intangible nature, have been those least amenable to recognition and discussion, not to speak of legislation.

## The goals of psychotherapy

*The principles of medical ethics* of the American Medical Association has set down standards of practice for physicians.[25] Although 'psychiatrists are assumed to have the same goals as all physicians', these principles have recently been revised 'with annotations especially applicable to psychiatry'.[26] The rationale was that 'there are special ethical problems in psychiatric practice that differ in coloring and degree from ethical problems in other branches of medical practice'. The format of these annotations meant no alterations in the original AMA standards; only additional qualifying statements were made.

Firstly, it may be pointed out that Section 3 of the AMA principles was the only one not annotated for psychiatry. It states that the physician (and therefore the psychiatrist equally) 'should practice a method of healing founded on a scientific basis; and he should not voluntarily associate with anyone who violates this principle' [p. 1061].[26] Further, the psychiatrist in particular is advised that 'he should neither lend endorsement of the psychiatric specialty nor refer patients to persons, groups, or treatment programs with which he is not familiar, especially if their work is based only on dogma and authority and not on scientific validation and replication' [p. 1062].[26]

Fisher and Greenberg's recent book[27] on *The scientific credibility of Freud's theories and therapy* certainly suggests that this question, despite extensive exploration, has not been decisively settled in the minds of psychiatrists themselves (although their hearts may tell them otherwise). Moreover, the proliferation of well over one hundred supposed schools of psychotherapy,[28] each presumably with its own theory of mental illness and health, therapeutic agents, overall goals, and specific practices,[29] reflects the massive nature of investigating therapeutic efficacy and the complexity of establishing 'scientific' guidelines. Given the stunning diversity of therapeutic forms now being offered to potential patients, how does one ethically equate the goals, practices, and effectiveness of a 'screaming cure' (Janov's Primal Therapy), a 'reasoning cure' (Ellis's Rational Therapy), a 'realism cure' (Glasser's Reality Therapy), a 'decision cure' (Greenwald's Direct Decision Therapy), an 'orgasm cure' (Reich's Orgone Therapy), a 'meaning cure' (Frankl's Logotherapy), and a 'profound-rest cure' (Transcendental Meditation)? Slavson,[30] for example, in assessing 'feeling therapy, nude therapy, marathon therapy, and other new remedies of the ailing psyche' concluded that 'these activities [are] untested, theoretically weak, and potentially very dangerous ...'; more specifically that 'latent or borderline psychotics with tenuous ego controls and defenses may, under the stress of such groups and the complete giving up of defenses, jump the barrier between sanity and insanity'. But the data on the efficacy of these practices are not yet available. Does the psychotherapist have an ethical responsibility to force closure on these therapies, especially if his judgement may be premature?

Such tremendous confusion in the 'state of the art' has led to a virtual 'identity crisis' for psychiatry and the psychotherapist,[31-33] highlighted negatively in the rise of the recent anti-psychiatry movement,[34] which now makes it possible for a psychiatrist to be a psychiatrist by training, accreditation, affiliation, and status, but at the same time, an anti-psychiatrist in ideology and action (all this under one ethical psychiatric roof).

At this point the goals and responsibilities of the psychotherapist are so broadly and vaguely defined that it has been said that his profession is one 'without a role-specific function',[35] and that his practice runs the gamut 'from science to social revolution'.[36] Recent observers of the field are in a quandary as to whether the purpose of psychiatry (and of the psychotherapist as one of its agents) is 'to diagnose, treat, and prevent a relatively defined number of (mental illnesses); ... to make unhappy and incompetent persons happy and competent; or to tackle poverty and civil and international strife' [p. 134].[8] While these issues are not beyond the legitimate concern of psychotherapists in their aim to improve the psychological welfare of their patients, there is a question as to whether some of these goals are beyond their competence. But at what point among these purposes is the psychiatrist no longer competent?

While broadly recognized goals include Freud's 'love and work', and variants of growth, self-realization, self-sufficiency, security, and freedom from anxiety, all of which may be noble aspirations, ethical issues are inherent in the practices which are conducted in their name. Across a spectrum of possibilities have been posed such questions as freedom to change (or not change) versus coercion, helping versus imposing the therapist's influence, and issues of 'cure' of illness versus positive growth. Thomas Szasz, probably the most prolific and vocal anti-psychiatrist, views conventional therapy by definition as 'social action, not healing', and as 'a series of religious, rhetorical, and repressive acts'.[37] At bottom is the medical model's designation of 'patient', which presupposes a restricted concept of normality and health. More radical models, on the other hand, presume to free patients from such stigma by suggesting that they may be behaving in a reasonable way in an unreasonable environment.

A fundamental ethical dilemma directly related to these various models is whether to encourage the patient to rebel against a repressive environment or to adjust to his current condition.[38] The issue has been recently highlighted in American psychiatry's definition and traditional treatment of homosexuals, for example. On a purely diagnostic level, the nomenclature of 'homosexuality' as a 'sexual deviation'[39] has been ardently challenged by gay rights caucuses; sufficient pressure was brought to bear on the American Psychiatric Association that the official designation was subsequently changed to a presumably less stigmatizing 'sexual orientation disturbance'.[40] Yet, a recent review of the literature on psychotherapy and behaviour therapy indicates that therapists still regard homosexuality as undesirable, if not pathological.[41] On a less theoretical plane, the therapist may be obliged to take a position, implicitly if not explicitly: is heterosexuality the ultimate goal for his patient, or does he wish the patient to maximize the quality of his homosexual life? The latter stance, often unpopular, was recently subject to debate when a behaviour therapist treated a man sexually attracted to boys and provided him with methods to transfer that attraction to *men*, not women![42,43] Obviously, definition of goals varies not only between therapists, but also changes with the evolution of the concept of normality.

The knotty issue of the setting of therapeutic goals by the therapist, who must achieve a balance between the needs of the individual, his family, and society, was highlighted by Malev and his co-workers[44] and Lifton.[12] In the former case, a woman, married to a permanent invalid, was torn between her loyalty to her husband and guilt lest she leave him to deteriorate, and her own personal development, which necessitated that she find a life of her own. The therapist, as the patient's advocate, may have been tempted to veer towards the latter goal for the patient in serving her best interests. He chose, as an ethical psychiatrist, not to advise her directly one way or the other, but to assist her to explore the alternatives and implications of either decision. (This might have been more complicated had he also brought in the husband for treatment.)

The dual allegiance of the therapist, not only to the patient and his family, but to others among society's representatives, was placed in bold relief in the case of psychiatrists who treated soldiers in Vietnam.[12] Lifton felt that in this situation the therapist was forced to tread a thin line between advocacy and corruption. Referral to a therapist meant to Lifton that the troubled soldier was likely to be 'helped' to return to military duty, and to resume his daily engagement in war activities (i.e., adjustment was the goal). Thus, the psychotherapist's goals became inseparable from those of the military authority. Likened to a 'catch-22', the ethical dilemma of patients and psychotherapist in the context of military commitment therefore meant that one's very sanity in seeking to escape from the environment via a psychiatric judgement of craziness rendered one eligible for the continuing madness of killing and dying.[12]

Aside from conflicting goals in psychotherapy posed by the particular interests of the individual, family, or society, Hadley and Strupp[45] found in a survey of practitioners and researchers in the field that a major aspect of the negative effects of psychotherapy was that of 'undertaking unrealistic tasks or goals'. In a compendium of such tendencies, all with profound ethical implications, were false assumptions concerning the scope and potency of therapy's goals. Misleading impressions may be given by the therapist when his need to instil hope in the patient, and the omniscience with which he is endowed (by himself and/or the patient) become intertwined. While some degree of positive expectation is said to be a requisite element for producing therapeutic effects in all psychotherapies,[46] the patient may get the erroneous impression that therapy and the therapist can solve everything. This can perpetuate unrealistic expectations and goals, which are ultimately deleterious to the patient. Such tendencies are often compounded by the therapist's failure to discuss, describe, or even acknowledge the reality of goals during treatment; or by goals which are specified, but are too broad or obscure.

Special technical problems, with ethical implications, also arise when goals set explicitly or implicitly exceed the patient's capability, fostering a false estimate of speedy progress which cannot be realized (i.e., in reality the patient requires longer treatment). Conversely, the patient may have accomplished certain goals, but the therapist then alters them, and so prolongs treatment, because he, the therapist, is unwilling to terminate (i.e., the patient in reality requires briefer treatment). Greenson[47] has aptly warned that any form or aspect of therapy that makes the patient an addict to treatment is undesirable.

The following case-illustrations highlight some of these issues, especially the ethical conflict in providing short-versus long-term goals (Case 1); and the confusion between ends and means in treatment (Case 2).

*Case 1:* How ethical is it to set limited goals when the needs of the patient may evolve as therapy progresses? Can ready-made interpretations, in the interests of time, short-change patients?

A 24-year-old woman was seen during a crisis over her one-and-a-half-year relationship with an older married man. A similar crisis had occurred two years before with another married man, and was resolved with brief treatment. Her recognition of the fact that he was not about to leave his wife and children prompted her to sever her ties with him. Two weeks following the break-up the patient was depressed and tearful, and couldn't sustain her decision; she went back to her boyfriend. In treatment, she described her suicidal ideas and her confusion regarding her love and need for him, despite her better judgement that this relationship had no future. In the ensuing 14 sessions the patient recovered from her depression, understood better her ambivalence, and learned to cope with the constraints of the relationship. Attempts were made for the patient to comprehend the unconscious nature of her conflict, unresolved attachment to her father, and her search for an inaccessible and unavailable man. Despite some intellectual recognition on the patient's part, the therapist knew well at termination that she would repeat this pattern unless a fortunate turn of events occurred in her life.

*Case 2:* The psychotherapist tends not to prescribe medication for mild to moderate insomnia, anxiety, or depression, with the presumed justification that discomfort and suffering have a potentially motivating aspect for psychological work. The ethical question is where does one draw the line? And has the patient been informed about the means and ends of treatment?

A 28-year-old professional woman with a long history of chronic depression was being treated with psychoanalytical psychotherapy twice a week. Her presenting difficulties were identified: not enjoying her work or her friends; having sexual difficulties with men; getting into highly dependent relationships. During four years of treatment in which she made good progress in working through some of the basic conflicts, she complained that her depression was not relieved. As a result of consultation, the therapist recommended a trial of medication concomitant with psychotherapy. The patient responded surprisingly well to the medication, her depression diminished, and she became socially and professionally more active. The therapist, with hindsight, realized that he might have prescribed drugs at some earlier point, which might have prevented needless suffering. But he also observed that medication, used as a crutch to provide quick or premature relief, sabotaged interest in exploring the psychological aspects of her depression.

Stone[48] describes a landmark malpractice suit in which a patient, who was also a physician, sued a private psychiatric facility for failure to treat him with psychoactive drugs, choosing instead a purely psychodynamic model of treatment. This case also includes a dispute over the appropriate diagnosis.

The private hospital contended that the patient was properly diagnosed as a narcissistic personality disorder, and that psychoanalytic therapy was the treatment of choice. The patient showed no improvement with this regimen. However, within weeks of his transfer to another hospital and the initiation of treatment with antidepressants, he made a 'dramatic' recovery. The patient's psychiatric experts asserted in deposition that 'his symptoms were obviously those of a biological depression that should have been treated biologically, as eventually was done.'[48] [p. 1386] This case was settled out of court, and the patient was awarded $250 000.

Therefore, although this action represents neither a binding decision nor a precedent, since the case has not gone to trial, it raises some serious questions, and should be duly noted by those therapists who rely exclusively on psychosocial treatment models. The 'respectable minority rule' has long been accepted in judging whether there has been negligence in the standard of care. That is, if a therapist provides a course of treatment that is followed by a 'respectable minority' of his profession, he is within the boundaries of permissible conduct.[48] This rule, which standard legal treatises universally accept at present, came into use before the biological treatment of mental disorders was shown to be efficacious. However, as our knowledge of diagnosis and treatment becomes more certain, the use of any one therapeutic model as the exclusive treatment for serious disorders will be scientifically questioned, and will be viewed as potential grounds for malpractice, as it is in the rest of medicine. Like the psychoanalytically oriented psychiatric facility in this case, psychotherapists may eventually become liable if they do not at least inform patients that alternative biological treatments are available.

In summary, the goals of psychotherapy are complex and subtle, and include professional versus personal goals, long- versus short-term, non-specific versus specific, and overt versus covert. As we shall see, it is the last contrast which is ethically the most problematic, and potentially the one most under the therapist's control.[49]

## The therapeutic relationship

Section 1 of the psychiatric annotations to the *Principles of medical ethics*[26] states that 'the doctor–patient relationship is such a vital factor in effective treatment of the patient that the preservation of optimal conditions for development of a sound working relationship between a doctor and his patient should take precedence over all considerations'. Furthermore, 'The patient may place his trust in his psychiatrist knowing that the psychiatrist's ethics and professional responsibilities preclude him from gratifying his own needs and exploiting the patient. This becomes particularly important because of the essentially private, highly personal, and sometimes intensely emotional nature of the relationship established with the psychiatrist' [p. 1061]. What are these 'optimal conditions', and what are their ethical implications in psychotherapy?

Regardless of goal, the therapeutic relationship between doctor and patient constitutes psychotherapy's strength, as well as its weakness. This duality is related to the concept of authority, which may be multiply defined.[50] In its most pure sense, it refers to an individual who is a specialist in his field, and who is therefore entitled to credit or acceptance; in another sense, it refers to power that requires submission. Different types of therapeutic relationship have been formed with various therapies,[29] or at different times in the process of the same therapy.[51] In each instance, the ethical issue of concern for the therapist is how to use his power justly:[52–54] the degree to which the therapeutic relationship is 'authoritarian' or 'egalitarian', or more specifically, to what extent the pervasive power of the 'transference' relationship, which offers the therapist a unique vehicle for exercising enormous influence over another person, is balanced by a true 'therapeutic alliance'[47] or 'therapeutic partnership'.[54] In general psychiatry, it has been pointed out that the fiduciary system, in which a patient puts his trust in the physician's ability and willingness to make crucial decisions, is being replaced by a contractual system [p. 126];[8] this trend also applies to the psychotherapies.

An egalitarian therapeutic relationship (i.e., adult-to-adult or peer-to-peer) is gaining in prominence, and is considered more humanitarian and facilitative of free exchange between patient and therapist than the traditional medical model (that is, doctor-to-patient) or the behavioural model (that is, teacher-to-student);[29] but might some aspects of this model have negative implications for the therapeutic endeavour? Myerhoff and Larson[55] have examined the major change in the image of the physician in recent times, and suggest that 'The physician ... has been traditionally depicted as a charismatic hero, a harbinger of progress, and a self-sacrificing, uniquely gifted, semi-divine figure ... Presently, this portrayal appears to be changing, and the doctor can be seen to be losing his charisma' [p. 189]. Of what importance, if any, is this change? Parsons,[56] in his analysis of the social structure and the dynamic process of medical practice, identified certain requirements of the doctor–patient relationship as necessary for successful treatment; one of the most essential was the 'social distance' between practitioner and client. A study of human organization in hospitals concluded 'we are coming to understand that faith in the doctor is a necessary element in cure, that he will not be able to exercise therapeutic leverage if we, as patients, regard him in too prosaic a light' [p. 71].[57] The authors suggested that the therapist's power to claim the patient's confidence as well as the therapist's effectiveness would be impaired by the growing familiarity between the two. Where, then, does one draw the line between the good use of power in the traditional medical model and its abuse? Where do the new boundaries of partnership end and those of 'real' familiarity and friendship begin? More importantly for the times, will there be new ethical dilemmas for the egalitarian therapeutic relationship?

Goldberg's[54] exposition of the equitable 'therapeutic partnership' suggests that not only is the nature of the therapeutic alliance (i.e., its power-distribution) critical, but so is the degree to which it is made explicit. Often within its non-explicit nature lies the ethical rub of psychotherapy. He recommends that a therapeutic contract be established with an explicitly agreed working plan (comparable to that in the medical model), the essence of which is how each agent will use his power. This should consist of agreed goals, established means to reach them, evaluation of therapy during its course, and methods of addressing dissatisfaction in the working alliance. But applying in practice what one intends in theory is not easily accomplished. In addition to the ambiguity in aims noted earlier, theory has not always been applied in new treatment modalities such as encounter-group therapy, where, despite the appearance of therapeutic virtues such as openness, autonomy, and mutuality, there is often little attention given to the participant's specific needs;[58] and treatment is often begun without inquiring about the participant's expectations.[59]

Conflict between the two models of therapeutic relationship was also highlighted in Lifton's[12] work with Vietnam veterans. Early on, most therapists felt that the essential model for the sessions was traditional therapy; Lifton held a minority view which emphasized a sustained dialogue between professional and veteran based upon a common stance of opposition to the war. This latter model did not abolish the traditional roles, but placed more emphasis upon mutuality and shared commitment. It is usually assumed that the patient knows what he wants from such a therapeutic relationship, and knows what is good for him. Lifton aptly pointed out that those in therapy were most clear about what they opposed—hierarchical distance, medical mystification, and psychological reductionism; they were presumably less clear about what they wanted and expected. Indeed, the factors they objected to may have been reminiscent of other conflicts with authority that they were grappling with in the military context. Here, the therapists—as a model of non-authoritarianism—may have contributed in a crucial way to the development of a therapeutic relationship which enabled clients to change through the process of identification.[60]

A prominent negative effect of the traditional therapeutic relationship can result from its insufficient regard for the patient's intentionality or will.[47] This may manifest itself, for example, in the therapist's fervent search for unconscious determinants, so that therapy soon becomes an end in itself; the therapist may thus assume priority over all other people in the patient's life. This may occur in an even more extreme form in some of the newer, large-group therapies, which can, in the context of group influence, encourage a belief in the godlike powers of the therapist. With or without peer pressure, the therapist's power is greatly exaggerated for reasons which have more to do with the therapist's needs than those of the patient.

The following case illustrates how close are ethical and technical aspects by examining the issue of excessive dependency and unresolved transference of patient toward therapist, and the role that the therapist may play in its maintenance.

*Case 3:* A 55-year-old woman had been in treatment for the last 17 years. She was first seen for difficulties with her husband, who neglected and frustrated her, and could not meet her dependency needs. Concerns about the prospect of separation or divorce precipitated exploration of her need for him, though chronically frustrated by his shortcomings, and most recently by his sexual inadequacy. During the last two years of treatment, her emotional dependency shifted on to the therapist, thus diluting the pressure on her husband. Although the therapist privately complained about the patient's excessive phone calls, constant advice-seeking, and magical expectations of him, he did not actively put an end to them. The therapist's rationale for continuing to treat this woman without a more identified goal of treatment was that he provided a therapeutic 'benign dependency' where she could not be harmed, and that gradual maturation would occur.

Was the patient being exploited? Dependency may be one of the most common characteristics of all patients, and allows for the early establishment of the helper–recipient relationship. In treatment other relationships develop, such as transference and a working alliance, which help to lessen that dependence, and ultimately enable the therapist to encourage independence in the patient. There are, of course, patients who need lifelong supervision even after much of the psychotherapy work is done; some of them may take the initiative and terminate treatment. But it is also possible that a therapist, because of his lack of experience, or for less benign reasons (for example, financial or psychopathological needs) perpetuates the dependency and unresolved transference of the patient. While most often seen as a technical problem in treatment, the question remains: when does a technical problem in therapy become an ethical issue as well?

## Special ethical problems of behaviour-modification

The basic ethical aspect of behaviour-modification is no different from that of other therapies, that is, the 'judicious use of power'.[52,53] However, behaviour-modification has been regarded as having some specific ethical problems, both conceptually and methodologically. These ethical issues revolve around behaviour therapy's underlying concept of man, and its alleged potential for contribution to a dehumanization or diminution of the individual—more specifically, its failure to view the patient-as-a-whole by separating the person from his problem or symptom. For many, it fosters a 'machine model of man',[52] and portrays the therapist as a technician or 'social reinforcement machine'[61] and the patient as his mechanical tool. Experimental evidence of the potency of stimulus–response patterns, and the extent to which human beings can be conditioned, have supported a view of the behaviour therapist as a possessor of extensive powers of social influence, and as an overt perpetrator of 'despotic control, brain-washing, and crass manipulation', largely irrespective of, or even against, the patient's will.[62]

In addition, behaviour therapy is said to have more profound ethical implications than other forms of psychotherapy, expressly because it 'does not expand awareness';[63] in other forms, such as individual, family, and group therapy, the therapist explicitly helps the patient to understand the meaning of his symptom. In fact, the principal merit of behaviour-modification techniques resides in their efficient and impersonal application 'without the necessity to deal with the troubling implications of what the patient's behaviour might mean' [p. 387];[63] and, because the methods work quickly, there is little time for the patient to contemplate their repercussions.

Despite these special features—often disadvantages from an ethical point of view—some observers argue that the degree to which behaviour can be altered without the intervening influence of the patient's own cognitive valuation has been greatly exaggerated.[62] As with other treatment, behaviour therapy usually cannot succeed in a person who does not wish to change. Certainly, a person's proneness to influence is ultimately an individual matter, and depends upon the type of patient. Moreover, the ethical vicissitudes of behaviour-control probably differ in the 'non-consenting patient', 'the patient under duress', and 'the voluntary patient'.[63] They are perhaps more pronounced in settings where a person is under civil or criminal commitment, and in penal institutions and state mental hospitals behaviour-modification methods have often been extensively applied in the absence of consent. Here, the most critical ethical problem may neither be the implications of behaviour therapy's concepts, nor its coercive quality, but the therapist's role as double agent, serving both the patient and the institution. Indeed, behavioral methods are regarded as 'peculiarly adaptable to meeting the needs of society' (over those of the individual).[63] More specifically, these methods may be used to increase conformity and to reinforce certain social norms, and to reduce assertiveness and deviant behaviour.

The use of specific techniques in behaviour-modification, notably aversive conditioning or negative reinforcement, raises a major ethical difficulty.[64] This is well illustrated in the case[65] of an institutionalized primary-school child who was treated for head-banging. As she was perpetually bruised, a padded football helmet was placed on her head, and her hands were tied down to her crib; nonetheless, the head-banging persisted. As an alternative plan, after all kinds of positive reinforcers had proved ineffective, the therapist slapped her sharply on the cheek and shouted 'Don't!' whenever she began to toss her head. Soon slapping was no longer necessary. Although this method had been effective, the child's parents withdrew her from the behavioural programme on learning that she had been slapped. The inevitable ethical dilemma arises: When do the ends justify the means? The obvious question of informed parental consent is equally important in this case.

The token-economy approach has also been criticized, particularly because informed consent is rarely obtained. Here, the issue may not be the type of method, but its utilization without consultation or consent. Invariably the staff make the decision about which behaviours they wish to reinforce, and the token rewards serve an essentially disciplinary function. Moreover, since the practice of token economy has traditionally relied on material incentives and 'behavioural productivity', it reflects, for some critics, an over-emphasis on the achievement ethic at the expense of a more humanistic approach.[62] The questions must be addressed: Who shall set the standards of behaviour to be rewarded or punished?—the doctors? the nurses? the patients?—and, to what extent shall these decisions be made with the consent of their recipients?

In the treatment of out-patients with neurotic symptoms, where the decision to undergo behaviour therapy is presumably voluntary, another issue emerges. In that these methods aim to abolish the symptom *per se* (in the belief that there is no underlying neurosis), does treatment merely provide superficial relief for more deeply concealed disturbance? When is the behaviour therapist obliged to refer certain patients to another form of psychotherapy, and to advise them that they need a different form of help? If he does not do so, is he deceiving the patient (as well as himself)?

In summary, although the behaviour therapist may have an advantage of technical precision over other psychotherapies; may be spared having to deal with long-term goals; can be more explicit in setting goals and applying his methods; and can thus more easily establish a mutual contract with the patient, he is no less caught up with ethical dilemmas than other psychotherapists. Moreover, he also has to grapple with additional ethical objections, arising out of his unique philosophy and techniques; namely: to his molecular (but perhaps dehumanizing) view of man and psychopathology; to his specific (but perhaps reductionistic) goals in treatment; and to his efficient and precise (but perhaps aversive, coercive, mechanical, and materialistic) methods.

## Specific ethical issues in psychotherapy

### Confidentiality and privileged communication

Confidentiality in the practice of psychiatry has been defined as 'the relationship between a physician (psychiatrist) and his patient, in which the patient may assume that his disclosures will not be passed on to others except under certain circumstances, and then only for the specific purpose of lending necessary help. This takes place within the framework of the social role of the doctor as one who treats and helps his patients, and who is ethically committed to this role' [p. 89].[65] At the same time, privileged communication is 'a right, existing only by statute, whereby a patient may bar his doctor from testifying about medical treatment and the disclosures which are an integral part of it', that is, it is 'a legal right which belongs to the patient, and not to the doctor' [p. 89].[65]

The issues of confidentiality and privilege in psychiatry have had major implications in the last decade. We need only note, for example, the disclosure, after Senator Thomas Eagleton had been nominated as Democratic candidate for Vice-President of the United States, of confidential information regarding his previous psychiatric history, including treatment for a major depressive disorder (which ultimately forced his withdrawal from public office); and the break-in to the office of the psychiatrist of Daniel Ellsberg (who had released the Pentagon Papers) to seek his medical record for possible use against him in a trial for treason. The question arises: under what circumstances are disclosures to someone other than the patient and therapist ethical? Although both of the above events received national attention, issues of confidentiality and privacy in everyday psychotherapeutic practice are more subtle, but no less crucial to the therapeutic endeavour. And, while we are concerned here with the moral rather than the legal aspects of confidentiality, the subject is often complicated by the spectre of legal sanction.

That confidentiality has long had a venerable place in the practice of medicine is seen in its inclusion in the Hippocratic Oath: 'Whatever, in connection with my professional practice or not in connection with it, I see or hear in the life of men which ought not to be spoken abroad, I will not divulge, as reckoning that all should be kept secret' [p. 154].[66] Its sanctity in psychotherapy is perhaps even more crucial, because of the inherently personal nature of the patient's communications, which cover his innermost thoughts, fantasies, and feelings. Statutes in many countries grant the relationship between psychiatrist and patient the same absolute protection as those accorded to husband and wife, and to lawyer and client.[67] Indeed, the most elaborate clause (Section 9) of the *American Psychiatric Association annotations especially applicable to psychiatry* relates to confidentiality. It declares that 'Confidentiality is essential to psychiatric treatment' [p. 1063],[26] with the additional stipulations: that the psychiatrist may reveal confidential information only with the patient's authorization or under proper legal compulsion; that he must apprise the patient of the implications of waiving the privilege of privacy; that when the psychiatrist is ordered by the court to reveal confidences entrusted to him by a patient, he may comply or may ethically hold the right to dissent within the framework of the law; and that he should disclose only that information that is immediately relevant to a given situation, and avoid offering speculation as facts. All in all, the *Annotations* call for extreme care with regard to confidential material, both written and verbal, especially in instances of consultation with other professionals; with clinical notes and records; and in case-presentations and in the distribution of teaching material. Some psychiatrists have also warned against the more insidious practice of 'gossip' among colleagues, which may inadvertently harm the patient and the therapeutic relationship.

When a therapist breaches his duty of confidentiality, he has committed an act of invasion of the patient's privacy. For example, in the case of *Doe* v. *Roe*,[68] the Supreme Court of New York found for the plaintiff, a former patient, who brought suit against her analyst to restrain her from publishing a book containing the case history of the patient and her family. The court stated that psychotherapy requires the patient to discuss personal material of the most intimate nature. Because revelation of such intimacies requires an unusual degree of trust, it ruled that a therapist who publishes such material can be sued for invasion of privacy. In addition, the 'scientific value of publication in the field of psychiatry was not established in this action' [p. 254].[69] The defendant psychiatrist was subsequently found liable by the court for the harm caused the patient by invading her privacy.

Confidentiality may, however, be breached, and privilege of communication sacrificed, if the court rules that it is more important to serve the interests of justice than those of the patient. Kermani[69] cites the case of *Schaffer* v. *Spicer*[70] as illustrative of the prevailing legal opinion. After the defendant psychiatrist had revealed confidential information to the plaintiff's husband, the patient and her husband entered into a custody battle over their child. The husband used the confidential information in support of his claim that the plaintiff was unfit to have custody of the child, after which the plaintiff sued the defendant for breach of confidentiality. The court, however, ruled that the 'defendant is protected from liability for his patient by the fact that he acted in what he thought was the best interest of the child', and that the 'patient–physician privilege must yield to the paramount right of the infant' [p. 248].[69]

Another compelling reason for a therapist to breach confidentiality is when the court demonstrates the necessity for legal disclosure of confidential information. Even in an event such as this, however, the therapist may request the right to disclose only such information as is relevant to the legal question under consideration.[71]

In recent years the confidentiality of the traditional therapist–patient relationship has been under increasing pressure, as third-party insurance and peer-review organizations have required certain information about treatment. Plaut[72] points out three forces in the escalating conflict between the right to secrecy and the right to information: increasing involvement of government in areas that were previously considered private, for example health, welfare, business-regulation, and product-control; the technological revolution in both data-collection (wire-tapping, tape-recording), and data-storage and retrieval (computerized records); and the individual's suspiciousness of authority, based on the perception that knowledge has always meant power.

In the face of these new pressures, major questions concerning confidentiality in psychotherapy are: whose agent is the psychotherapist—the patient's? the family's? society's? the law's?; what are the goals in divulging a confidence—better treatment? evaluation? consensual validation? support?; and what are the risks—will the therapeutic relationship be jeopardized? will the patient terminate treatment? Conversely, can rigid adherence to a rule of confidentiality between therapist and patient blind the therapist to certain risks and dangers to himself or to others?

In part, the issue of the therapist's allegiance is related to the type of psychotherapy he practises. Although individual therapy may be limited to traditional goals within the private framework of the patient's inner thoughts and feelings, there may be other goals whereby information communicated between therapist and patient is used to influence the patient's social milieu. A serious question that often arises is the responsibility of the therapist to the patient's family. In general, the less healthy the patient, the more important this issue becomes. With a relatively stable and independent patient, there is usually no need to contact family members, and the therapist would not encourage any communication from them. Should the latter occur, it is usually in the patient's interests that he is promptly informed of the contact, and that this is fully discussed in the therapeutic sessions. A more disturbed patient may not only need his family's support, but also involve family members with the therapist as an expression of his disturbance. In such circumstances, each communication with the family both complicates treatment and also raises ethical questions about breaches of confidentiality and whose interests the therapist serves.

In family therapy, whose purported goal is 'to treat the family as the patient',[73] the situation is usually reversed, in that an individual's confidence may be subverted in the interests of treating the married couple or family. Whether a therapist uses an individual or family approach may determine not only the goals of treatment, but the nature of the treatment of the individual within each approach. How does the therapist evaluate whether it is in the patient's best interests to be seen individually, or within the context of his family? How justifiable is it for the therapist to impose marital and family therapy if he regards the problem as stemming from the family or the marriage? The following case demonstrates the difficulties involved.

*Case 4:* A 45-year-old man with a serious obsessive-compulsive ritual which interfered with his work and social life, especially his marriage, was treated by a therapist with a family approach, who saw the man and his wife weekly in joint sessions. The man made little progress over the course of two years, although his marriage seemed less stormy. When the husband was seen alone by a consultant at the therapist's request, he confessed that he was not able to talk about his 'secret life', lest it be conveyed to his wife; nor was he able to seek the therapist for himself. It was apparent that he had unwittingly begun to identify with the therapist's viewpoint, regarding the interpersonal communication between himself and his wife as the source of his difficulties, rather than exploring intrapsychic conflicts and concerns of his own. That he should talk about personal problems to the consultant was regarded as a betrayal of his therapist, so that he was too confused and guilty to seek individual assistance.

Here, the therapist's theoretical stance of responsibility to the couple, in preference to the husband, precluded in some ways the furtherance of the best interests of the individual patient. On the other side of the coin are situations where dynamic psychotherapists so strongly believe in confidentiality and individual privacy in the dyadic relationship that they fail to divulge confidences or share information with family members which may prove vital to the welfare of the patient (see Case 5, p. 153).

Indeed, the sole exception to the rule of confidentiality between therapist and patient is the possibility of 'dangerousness' to others. This is now stipulated in the famous '*Tarasoff* decision',[74] which enunciated the maxim that 'Protective privilege ends where public peril begins'; it refers to the requirement that the therapist must warn both certain specified authorities and potential victims of possible dangerous actions by his patients. The case *Tarasoff* v. *Regents of the University of California* involved the confidential disclosure by a young patient to his therapist that he intended to kill his girlfriend. After the therapist had consulted with two psychiatrists and notified the police, the patient was detained. His release followed his denial of any violent intent. He broke off treatment in response to the therapist's breach of confidence. Two months later, he murdered his girlfriend. The therapist and his psychiatrist-supervisor were then sued by the victim's parents for failure to warn them of the peril.

The case, although unusual, places in bold relief the dilemma of the therapist in balancing the patient's right to confidentiality and society's right to protection. Many psychotherapists opposed the decision, regarding it as conceptually and practically flawed, and carrying negative implications for psychiatry.[75,76] Roth and Meisel,[75] for example, feel that the decision assumes a degree of expertise in predicting violence or danger that the psychiatrist simply does not possess; that a lowering of the threshold of dangerousness for a warning to an intended victim will result, which will compromise the patient's right to confidentiality and possibly his treatment; that the psychiatrist is not only liable if he fails to warn, but risks liability for invasion of privacy or defamation by the patient if the threat of harm does not materialize; and lastly, as happened in the *Tarasoff* case, that the patient's dangerousness will probably increase because of his sense of betrayal by the therapist and because of his premature termination of the very treatment he needs. On a more conceptual level, Gurevitz[76] argues that the *Tarasoff* decision erroneously 'defines and reinforces a social control function for psychiatry' by allying the psychotherapist 'more with the goal of protecting society than with that of healing patients' [p. 291]. It is not, Gurevitz points out, that psychiatrists reject the need to balance these functions; in fact, most psychiatrists attempt to fulfil both responsibilities.

Cases subsequent to *Tarasoff* have eased the burden on the therapist.

The court ruled in the case of *Thompson* v. *County of Alameda*[77] that, as a precondition to liability, the victim must be identifiable and the danger must be foreseeable. With the case of *Mavroudis* v. *Superior Court of San Mateo*[78] 'imminence of danger' also became necessary for the *Tarasoff* duty to exist, and with *Hedlund* v. *Superior Court of Orange County*[79] liability for harm to close relatives and associates (foreseeable bystanders) was added.[80]

No doubt because of the *Tarasoff* decision, alternative actions that can be taken by psychotherapists, short of actual warning, have been recommended. For example, because of their very strong conviction about the importance of confidentiality in the doctor–patient relationship, in no instance have Roth and Meisel[75] directly warned the potential victim without first obtaining the patient's permission. Since violence is rare, they feel it is prudent to 'rely on odds and not warn' [p. 510]. In addition, they advocate that the therapist should inform the patient of the boundaries and limits of confidentiality. If danger seems imminent, the therapist should first consider social manipulations which might reduce its likelihood, before he makes the decision to compromise confidentiality. When confronted with a potentially violent patient, options include: continued treatment of the patient; involuntary hospitalization; notification of the police; and notification of the potential victim. Each action places a different weight on the competing values of confidentiality versus protection of society. The authors cite several cases of uncompromised confidentiality with 'happy endings'.

Gross *et al.*[80] present a seven-step response-guide for clinicians to apply after hearing a patient make threats. The critical issues facing clinicians include clarity of threat, severity and actuality of danger, identifiability of potential victims, imminence of danger, and classification of potential victims. Options include family therapy, involuntary commitment to an institution, warning the victim, warning relatives of the victim, and calling the police. In any case, Gross *et al.*[80] stress that 'care must be taken to document the actions that are taken, including the rationale for the choices made. The rationale is important because therapists are held to a standard of reasonable care, not to a standard of successful performance' [p. 12].[80]

The following case, in which the therapist also maintained a strong adherence to patient confidentiality and privacy, reflects an instance not of 'public peril' (i.e., danger to others), but of the more private peril of danger to oneself.

*Case 5:* A middle-aged executive was in psychotherapy for depression following a myocardial infarction, and presented suicidal thoughts, fears of dying, sexual avoidance, and other related symptoms. He was also considering leaving his twenty-year marriage and his children, and moving elsewhere to seek a less competitive job. The patient was seen for the first time in the hospital when recovering from his MI; the patient's wife remained at his bedside during most of this time. While the psychiatrist expressed appreciation of her availability to the patient, he did not encourage further communication between himself and the wife. When the patient did not respond to weekly psychotherapy, sessions were increased to three times per week, and the patient was given antidepressant medication after consultation with a physician colleague. During three months of combined pharmacotherapy and psychotherapy, the patient's improvement was modest. During that time, his wife had phoned the therapist on a few occasions, but the therapist chose not to return the calls. Rather, the calls were discussed with the husband in the context of their marital relationship, for example, of her overinvolvement, and his dependency needs and desire to be controlled. Four months later, the therapist received a letter from the wife citing his non-response to her calls and mentioning that the patient had not been taking his medication. The therapist shared this information with the patient, who confessed that he had only taken the medication for one week, because he could not tolerate the feeling of being 'removed' that it gave him; and that he had kept the rest of the pills in case he decided to commit suicide. The patient reassured the therapist that he was not considering suicide despite the fantasy, and that he would, as the therapist requested, throw the pills away. Three weeks later, the patient committed suicide with an overdose of the medication.

Could contact with the wife have better served the therapist, and ultimately, the patient? Where does one draw the confidentiality line when the patient is a threat to himself?

In many respects, cases in which a non-hospitalized patient commits suicide are similar to those in which a patient commits a violent act towards a third party. First, they both involve the issue of prediction, and prediction in both these cases is highly uncertain. While prediction of self-harm is probably more accurate than prediction of harm to others,[81,82] studies have repeatedly demonstrated that neither can be accomplished with any degree of certainty. This is particularly true if the prediction covers more than a few days, because of the therapist's relative lack of control of the patient and his inability to make any confident assessment of his environmental situation.[83]

Second, both types of case raise the question of whether or not the therapist took adequate precautionary measures. There is no way a reliable determination can be made of how a potentially suicidal patient will respond to various treatment options. The therapist may, for example, increase the number of sessions per week and/or focus the therapy on eliminating the suicidal ideation and urges. He may prescribe medication. The therapist may also recommend hospitalization, but, unless the risk is great enough to warrant involuntary commitment, the patient cannot be forced to accept the recommendation.[83]

Ultimately, then, when an out-patient attempts suicide it must be determined whether or not the defendant was negligent in balancing the risk of suicide against the benefits of increased patient controls.

All this has led some to argue that, as with cases of potentially violent patients, the therapist has a duty to warn the parents, spouse, relatives, or other significant individuals in the patient's life of the possibility of suicide. This application of *Tarasoff* to require a warning, thereby breaching the therapist–patient confidence, was rejected by the court in a case described by Furrow.[84] In this case, in which the parents of an out-patient who had committed suicide sued the treating therapist, the court ruled that the disclosure requirement was limited to those instances 'where the risk to be prevented thereby is the danger of violent assault, and not where the risk of harm is self-inflicted or mere property damage' [pp. 44–5].[84]

Two other cases involving disclosure of confidential information are cited by Kermani.[69] In the case of *Brand* v. *Grubin*,[85] the Superior Court of New Jersey found the treating psychiatrist not negligent and not liable for his patient's suicide, even though he failed to assess adequately the patient's condition or to inform the patient's family. In another case,[86] the wife sued her husband's psychiatrist after her husband died from a drug overdose. The psychiatrist was not held liable, although the court did hold that a therapist *might* be held liable for a suicide if 'he negligently or intentionally discloses confidential communications made to him by the patient in situations where it is forseeable that the disclosure might cause the patient to harm himself and the disclosure is a factor in the decedent's decision to commit suicide' [p. 252].[19]

The above may also have ethical relevance for the therapist's position in respect of suicide and its prevention. Recently, publicized cases of so-called 'rational suicide', especially in the context of terminal illness, suggest that the psychotherapist may be faced increasingly with the need to respect decisions by patients to commit suicide. In these instances, therapist and patient alike are obliged to confront and resolve their ethical dilemmas together.

### Therapist–patient sex (and sexism)

The Hippocratic Oath includes a pledge that 'with purity and holiness I will practice my art . . . into whatever houses I enter, I will go into them for the benefit of the sick, and will abstain from every voluntary act of mischief, and further from the seduction of females or males, of freeman and slaves' [p. 236].[87] The *Annotations especially applicable to psychiatry* (of the *Principles of medical ethics*), less eloquently, but no less unequivocally, uphold this moral tradition by stating simply, 'Sexual activity with a patient is unethical' [p. 1061].[26] Indeed, it is the only activity deemed unethical between doctor and patient which is presented so unambiguously. As part of the requirement that the doctor 'conduct himself with propriety in his profession and in all the actions of his life' [p. 1061], the dictum regarding sex is stated to be especially important in the case of the psychiatrist, because his patient tends to model his behaviour after that of his therapist. Further, the necessary intensity of the therapeutic relationship may activate

sexual and other fantasies in both patient and therapist, while weakening
the objectivity required for treatment. In so far as it has earned a position
of such priority (Section 1 of the psychiatry *Annotations*), therapist–patient
sex may be considered the quintessence of the overt misuse and exploitation of the transference relationship.

Yet sexual activities, including sexual intercourse and various forms of
erotic contact between therapist and patient, have been increasingly reported in the literature; and have involved clinicians at all levels of training, from psychiatric trainee to training analyst.[88-95] This is not a new
problem for therapists, who have reported erotic transferences and their
vicissitudes since the dawn of psychotherapy. No less than Mesmer,
Breuer, Janet, Charcot, and Freud have described the emergence of strong
sexual feelings in treatment, and the inevitable problems brought about by
their presence. While sexual affairs between therapist and patient were
never sanctioned by Freud or his followers, they did occur. Often the
therapist was saved from moral indictment, as he still is, by his marriage to
his patient. But such a 'shotgun' resolution is an extreme and limited
option to deal with sexual 'acting-out'. The question remains: What are the
therapist's ethical options if he does not marry the patient?

In a recent review of legal and professional alternatives to deter, discipline,
or punish sexually active therapists,[96] four possible avenues of approach
are mentioned: criminal law (for example, a charge of rape by fraud or
coercion); civil law (for example, a malpractice suit); a medical board (for
example, revocation of licences to practise); and through a professional
association (for example, pressure to limit referrals, or threats to career
opportunities). Each in its turn has proved largely ineffectual as a system of
control in practice. In the instance of criminal law, a rape charge, as
strongly recommended by Masters and Johnson,[97] is rarely brought and
rarely sticks; most cases entail psychological, and not physical, coercion.
Both force and fraud are required, and the prevailing judicial view is that if
the patient consents, and the therapist has never claimed that sexual
activity was treatment, there has been neither force or fraud. In the
instance of civil law malpractice cases, again no legal course may be
available if the therapist has not misidentified sexual activity as treatment.
In a recently publicized incident, two factors were also held in the therapist's
favour: the patient did not press charges until one and a half years after
their relationship had begun; and she presumably did not have a normal
transference. Medical licensing boards, at least in the United States, are
not consistent from state to state, and may not have a close relationship
with psychiatric members. Lastly, professional associations have no subpoena power, and little expertise in evidentiary investigation, either to
protect the due-process rights of the therapist who is charged, or to cope
with a therapist who sues them. Davidson[41] points out that entry into

treatment may be another way for the seducing psychiatrist to escape censure, as well as serving to sabotage efforts to discipline him. Given the above failure of sanctions from without, Stone[96] concludes that ultimately 'patients must depend on the decent moral character of those entrusted to treat them' [p. 1141].

But what is deemed to constitute 'decent moral character' may change with the times, at least according to the findings of some current psychotherapists. In contrast to Masters and Johnson's position on the matter— that therapists who have sex with their patients should be charged criminally with rape, no matter who initiated the seduction—are attitudes of relative sexual permissiveness. Recent evidence suggests that the psychiatrist's value system has moved in the direction of sexual permissiveness both in terms of what is acceptable for the self and for others.[98] There is, for example, an overt endorsement of touching and so-called 'non-erotic' physical behaviour, by advocates of the human potential movement,[99,100] as these, far from being regarded as unethical or harmful, are felt to enhance the therapeutic relationship and to promote personal growth.

Attitudes towards sex between professional and patient reflect not only individual predilection, but also theoretical orientation[101] and medical specialty.[102] Kardener's[91] survey of physicians' erotic and non-erotic physical contact with patients suggests that psychiatrists had less sexual interaction than did the practitioners of some other medical specialties. Their reported rates, of erotic contact by 10 per cent of psychiatrists and sexual intercourse by 5 per cent, were lower than those for general practitioners, surgeons, and obstetrician-gynaecologists. Significant differences regarding psychotherapist–patient sex were found between 'psychodynamically oriented' and other theoretically oriented therapists. For example, whereas 86 per cent of the former group believed that erotic contact was never of benefit to the patient, this figure was significantly lower for humanistic and behavioural therapists (71 per cent and 61 per cent respectively). That there is widespread ambivalence on the subject even after the fact is seen in Taylor and Wagner's[102] review of cases of therapists who had actually had intercourse with their patients. About half reported that the experience had had negative effects on either patient or therapist, 32 per cent that it had mixed effects, and 21 per cent that it had positive effects (the authors did not question the patients). Butler[92] however found that 95 per cent of therapists who had had sex with their patients reported conflict, fear, and guilt; only 40 per cent of them sought consultation for their problem.

'Every reported malpractice case involving a psychiatrist who was shown to have had sex with a patient has resulted in a verdict against the psychiatrist' [p. 138].[84] Thus, because of the coercive position of the therapist in relation to the patient, courts and juries will undoubtedly continue to find not only therapist–patient sexual contact but also transferential exploitation in general prima-facie or presumptive evidence of general negligence.

The high levels of the court system began affirming therapist–patient sexual contact as a sound basis for malpractice in 1968, with the case of *Zipkin* v. *Freeman*,[103] in which a Missouri psychiatrist was sued by a female patient because he had 'mismanaged the patient's transference'. Mrs Zipkin began treatment with Dr Freeman in 1959 for headaches and diarrhoea, which were 'completely gone' after a few months; however, she agreed to continue a rather bizarre treatment-plan in order to get at the underlying cause of her difficulties. This treatment included joining Dr Freeman at social gatherings and skating parties, travelling with him outside the state, and investing in his business ventures. She also attended 'group therapy' swimming parties, at which some of those attending, including Dr Freeman, were nude. Mrs Zipkin's affections became completely transferred from her husband and family to her doctor, and, on his advice, she requested a divorce from her husband. As the result of her 'treatment' she gave up her friends and community commitments, and moved in with Dr Freeman. Eventually she realized that her life was a shambles, and she brought suit against him.

At the trial Dr Freeman explained that Mrs Zipkin was suffering from 'neurosis with an inferiority complex', and that whether or not the transference and countertransference had been mismanaged was not the issue. She came for psychotherapeutic treatment of her headaches and diarrhoea, and was cured.[69,104] Nevertheless, Judge Seiler, who wrote the majority opinion of the Missouri Supreme Court, stated:

Once Dr Freeman started to mishandle the transference phenomenon, with which he was plainly charged in the petition and which is overwhelmingly shown in the evidence, it was inevitable that trouble was ahead. It is pretty clear from the medical evidence that the damage would have been done to Mrs. Zipkin even if the trips outside the state were carefully chaperoned, the swimming done with suits on, and if there had been ballroom dancing instead of sexual relations [p. 761].[103]

The court thus recognized and affirmed the duty of neutrality owed by a therapist to his patient, and that a mishandling of the transference, even in the absence of sexual relations, may constitute malpractice. The court found the defendant guilty.

With regard to the culpability of therapists who have sex with their patients, many claim that they 'did not know any better'; but research shows that male psychotherapists involved with female patients tend to be in their forties and fifties, with considerable training and experience. Pope and Bouhoutsos[105] suggest that despite this evidence that they do 'know better', there are some fairly prevalent misconceptions about the ethicality of sexual conduct with a patient that could bias their judgement. The first, probably resulting from the ambiguous prohibition of therapist–patient sex 'during therapy', is that such conduct is acceptable if it occurs outside the therapeutic session, for example, at the therapist's home or a hotel. This defence has never been used successfully. The second misconception is that sexual involvement subsequent to the termination of therapy is neither unethical nor illegal. Quite a number of therapists have used this fact of therapy termination as a defence; but in no instance has a defendant been cleared on this basis.[105] No state has a regulation that specifies a time-limit when therapy ends and a social/sexual relationship can begin. The major issue at stake in determining whether malpractice has occurred is not the time-span between treatment and sexual relations, but rather the extent to which such relations are an exploitation of the therapeutic relationship.[106] In any event, the clinician will be on ethically and legally safer ground if he adheres to the motto 'once a patient, always a patient'.

*Sexism:* A related issue concerns sexism in psychotherapy. Are sexual relations with the patient—virtually always female—the tip of an iceberg of a more pervasive practice, not of sex, but of sexism in psychotherapy?[107,108] The ethics of psychotherapy in relation to patient gender has implications not only for specific abuse, such as sex between male therapist and female patient, but for other forms of sexual exploitation and discrimination. Particularly pertinent are the underlying theory, the training practices, and the nature of the doctor–patient relationships that typify many schools of therapy. Broverman and his colleagues[109] suggest that therapeutic theories have usually supported rather than questioned stereotypical assumptions about sex roles and about different standards of mental health for men and women. Thus, therapists have commonly accepted that dependency and passivity are normal qualities in women, whereas assertiveness and in-dependence are typical of men; or designated a woman's dissatisfaction with her traditional role as evidence of psychopathology.[107] Aside from the unfortunate legacy of an 'anti-feminine Freudian position',[107] women may also be harmed by a 'blame-the-mother' tradition, especially by a family therapist who regards them as potentially 'schizophrenogenic' to their children.[108] Such sex bias is often reinforced during training, in which androcentrism is unlikely to be corrected by a male supervisor[108] (female therapists are much less likely to have had supervisors of their own sex as role-models during training).[110]

The most insidious aspect of sexism in psychotherapy practice is the domination of the profession by male therapists, and the resultant tendency to replicate within the therapeutic relationship a 'one-down' position, a position in which women typically find themselves. This form of relation-ship may encourage the fantasy that an idealized relationship with a power-ful man is a more desirable solution to problems than taking autonomous action;[90,108] it may also set the stage for the kind of sexual exploitation that I discussed earlier.

The new feminist psychotherapies can provide ethical guidelines to deal with sexism in psychotherapy. The egalitarianism between therapist and patient that typifies these treatments should be replicated in all forms of psychotherapy.

## The promotion of proper ethical practice

While ethical concerns have long faced the psychiatrist (and hence the psychotherapist), codes of ethics are of recent origin—for example, that devised by the American Psychiatric Association was published only in 1974, and the World Psychiatric Association's *Declaration of Hawaii* in 1977 (see Appendix). These sorts of code have been criticized by some observers for setting arbitrary standards of professional behaviour; for the weakness of their presentation, which is likened to a description of etiquette rather than a professionally honoured document; and for the lack of moral substance in their tenets.[8,111] They are therefore felt to have serious limitations in assisting the psychotherapist to make ethical decisions in his daily practice; and they are understandably disappointing to those who confuse codes with covenants, or to those who expect to produce morally scrupulous psychotherapists.

Other observers insist that the pressing problem is not the establishment of a set of guidelines, but of enforcement.[112] The contention is that a code can always be revised to meet the professional's needs better, but that problems of peer-review will still exist: the voluntary nature of complaint investigations; conflicting roles, in which peer-review committees are required to act as investigator, prosecutor, judge, and jury; inaccurate (and insufficient) case-reporting; fear of liability by the professional reviewer; and over-concern with confidentiality, which often takes precedence over other ethical considerations, and can be used as a rationalization to resist investigation.[106] In practice, it is exceedingly difficult to know what really occurs within the therapeutic relationship. Moreover, psycho-therapists, like other professionals, are naturally reluctant to judge their colleagues; nor may they feel morally or technically equipped to do so. The ethical conduct not only of the profession, but also of the peer-review process is of concern;[113] an important criticism is that the patient has been excluded from the process, and has been poorly informed about the procedures. Consequently, it is a commonly held view that psychiatry (and psycho-therapy) is unable to police itself,[112] and that peer-review, as currently designed, is 'bound to fail'.[114] Nonetheless, positive headway has been made, and there is still hope that peer-reviews can serve some purpose.[115]

Expectations of what a code of ethics and peer-review can achieve may have been unrealistic. Perhaps their primary purpose should be education rather than control. Newman and Luft,[116] for example, have suggested that an educational peer-review system which promotes co-operation among professionals is of greater utility and is more acceptable to clinicians than a bureaucratic system of control. The difficult question still remains as to how much authority should be vested in peer-review committees.

## Conclusions and recommendations

As has been suggested throughout this chapter, ethical problems in the practice of psychotherapy are not easily soluble: the dilemmas which face the psychotherapist are varied and complex. He is virtually never a single agent. He cannot rely on codified instruments as more than broad guides to behaviour. Ultimately he must seek specific remedies to the ethical problems that inevitably arise in his practice. The following points may help the psychotherapist to exercise his ethical judgement:

(1) Greater exploration of the philosophical foundations of psychotherapeutic practice;
(2) self-awareness on the part of the therapist through, for example, constant examination and analysis of his attitudes within and outside the therapeutic relationship;
(3) active development in treatment of a 'therapeutic alliance' or partnership, in which there is equal power and participation by both parties towards mutual goals and responsibilities;
(4) greater allegiance to a code of ethics and its development, in order to better sort out ethical choices and their implications for both patient and therapist;
(5) greater responsibility on the part of the therapist for the maintenance of professional competence in himself and his peers;
(6) openness to consultation with others, and a receptiveness to outside opinions in making proper ethical decisions in treatment; and
(7) greater understanding of human nature and morality, from which timely and productive ethical alternatives can be derived.

As one author has aptly put it, 'by definition, ethical problems remain unresolved. By their unresolved quality, they provoke a continuous anxiety in the practicing psychiatrist and concomitantly a desire to search, to oppose, to think, and to research' [p. 2546].[117]

## References

1 Spiegel, R.: Editorial: on psychoanalysis, values, and ethics. *Journal of the American Academy of Psychoanalysis* **6**:271–3, 1978.

2 Osmond, H.: Psychiatry under siege: the crisis within. *Psychiatric Annals* **3**:59–81, 1973.
3 Freedman, D. and Gordon, R.: Psychiatry under siege: attacks from without. *Psychiatric Annals* **3**:10–34, 1973.
4 Michels, R.: Professional ethics and social values. *International Review of Psychoanalysis* **3**:377–84, 1976.
5 Guralnik, D. B. (ed.): *Webster's new world dictionary of the American language*. New York, World Publishing Co., 1970.
6 Fletcher, J.: Ethical aspects of genetic control. *New England Journal of Medicine* **285**:776–83, 1971.
7 Powledge, F.: The therapist as double-agent. *Psychology Today* **11**:44–7, 1977.
8 Redlich, F. and Mollica, R.: Overview: ethical issues in contemporary psychiatry. *American Journal of Psychiatry* **133**:125–6, 1976.
9 Jasnow, A.: The psychotherapist—artist and/or scientist? *Psychotherapy: Theory, Research and Practice* **15**:318–22, 1978.
10 Edelson, M.: Psychoanalysis as science: its boundary problems, special status, relations to other sciences, and formalization. *Journal of Nervous and Mental Disease* **165**:1–28, 1977.
11 London, P.: *The modes and morals of psychotherapy*. New York, Holt, Rinehart, and Winston, 1964.
12 Lifton, R. J.: Advocacy and corruption in the healing professions. *International Review of Psychoanalysis* **3**:385–98, 1976.
13 Strupp, H.: Some observations on the fallacy of value-free psychotherapy and the empty organism: comments on a case study. *Journal of Abnormal Psychology* **83**:199–201, 1974.
14 Buckley, P., Karasu, T. B., Charles, E., and Stein, S.: Theory and practice in psychotherapy: some contradictions in expressed belief and reported practice. *Journal of Nervous and Mental Disease* **167**:218–23, 1979.
15 Erickson, E.: Psychoanalysis and ethics—avowed and unavowed. *International Review of Psychoanalysis* **3**:409–15, 1976.
16 Marcuse, H.: *Eros and civilization*. Boston, Beacon Press, 1955.
17 Holt, R.: Freud's impact on modern morality. *Hastings Center Report*, April 1980, 38–45.
18 Szasz, T.: *The myth of mental illness*. New York, Hoeber–Harper, 1961.
19 Torrey, F.: *The death of psychiatry*. Radnor, PA., Chilton Book Co., 1974.
20 Hollingshead, A. and Redlich, F.: *Social class and mental illness: a community study*. New York, Wiley, 1958.
21 Horney, K.: *New ways in psychoanalysis*. New York, Norton, 1939.
22 Fromm-Reichmann, F.: *Psychoanalysis and psychotherapy*. Chicago, University of Chicago Press, 1959.
23 Greenson, R.: *The technique and practice of psychoanalysis*, Vol. 1. New York, International Universities Press, 1967.
24 Freud, S.: Analysis terminable and interminable, in *The complete psychological works of Sigmund Freud*, Vol. 23 (1937–9). London, Hogarth Press, 1964.
25 Judicial Council, American Medical Association: *Opinions and reports of the Judicial Council*. Chicago, American Medical Association, 1971.
26 The principles of medical ethics with annotations especially applicable to psychiatry. *American Journal of Psychiatry* **130**:1057–64, 1973.

27 Fisher, S. and Greenberg, R. P.: *The scientific credibility of Freud's theories and therapy*. New York, Basic Books, 1977.
28 Parloff, M.: *Twenty-five years of research in psychotherapy*. New York, Albert Einstein College of Medicine Department of Psychiatry, 17 October 1975.
29 Karasu, T. B.: Psychotherapies: an overview. *American Journal of Psychiatry* **134**:851–63, 1977.
30 Slavson, P.: *The New York Times*, 9 January 1969.
31 Brill, N.: Future of psychiatry in a changing world. *Psychosomatics* **14**:19–26, 1973.
32 Kety, S.: From rationalization to reason. *American Journal of Psychiatry* **131**: 957–63, 1974.
33 Yager, J.: A survival guide for psychiatric residents. *Archives of General Psychiatry* **30**:494–9, 1974.
34 Cerrolaza, M.: The nebulous scope of current psychiatry. *Comprehensive Psychiatry* **14**:299–309, 1973.
35 Raskin, D.: Psychiatric training in the '70s—toward a shift in emphasis. *American Journal of Psychiatry* **128**:119–20, 1972.
36 Vispo, R.: Psychiatry—paradigm of our times. *Psychiatry Quarterly* **46**:209–19, 1972.
37 Szasz, T.: *The myth of psychotherapy*. New York, Anchor/Doubleday, 1978.
38 Blatte, H.: Evaluating psychotherapies. *Hastings Center Report*, September 1973, pp. 4–6.
39 *Diagnostic and statistical manual of mental disorders*, 2nd edn (DSM II). Washington DC, American Psychiatric Association, 1968.
40 *Diagnostic and statistical manual of mental disorders*, 3rd edn (DSM III). Washington DC, American Psychiatric Association, 1978.
41 Davidson, V.: Psychiatry's problem with no names: therapist-patient sex. *American Journal of Psychoanalysis* **37**:43–50, 1977.
42 Garfield, S.: Values: an issue in psychotherapy: comments on a case study. *Journal of Abnormal Psychology* **83**: 202–3, 1974.
43 Davison, G. C. and Wilson, G. T.: Goals and strategies in behavioural treatment of homosexual pedophilia: comments on a case study. *Journal of Abnormal Psychology* **83**:196–8, 1974.
44 Malev, J. S., Kaplan, E. A., Hollender, M. H., *et al.*: For better or for worse: a problem in ethics. *International Psychiatry Clinics* **2**:603–24, 1966.
45 Hadley, S. W. and Strupp, H. H.: Contemporary views of negative effects in psychotherapy: an integrated account. *Archives of General Psychiatry* **33**:1291–1302, 1976.
46 Frank, J.: *Persuasion and healing: a comparative study of psychotherapy*. Baltimore, Johns Hopkins Press, 1961.
47 Greenson, R.: *The technique and practice of psychoanalysis*, Vol. 1. New York, International Universities Press, 1967.
48 Stone, A. A.: The new paradox of psychiatric malpractice. *New England Journal of Medicine* **311**:1384–7, 1984.
49 Zitrin, A. and Klein, H.: Can psychiatry police itself effectively? The experience of one district branch. *American Journal of Psychiatry* **133**:653–6, 1976.
50 Miller, D.: The ethics of practice in adolescent psychiatry. *American Journal of Psychiatry* **134**:420–2, 1977.

51 Karasu, T. B.: General principles of psychotherapy, in *Specialized techniques in individual psychotherapy*, ed. T. B. Karasu and L. Bellak. New York, Brunner/Mazel, 1980.

52 London, P.: *Behavior control*. New York, Harper and Row, 1969.

53 Strupp, H.: On the technology of psychotherapy, in *Psychotherapy and behavior change, 1972*, ed. I. M. Marks, A. E. Bergin, P. J. Lang, *et al.* Chicago, Aldine, 1973, pp. 3–27.

54 Goldberg, C.: *Therapeutic partnership: ethical concerns in psychotherapy*. New York, Springer, 1977.

55 Myerhoff, B. G. and Larson, W. R.: The doctor as culture hero: the routinization of charisma. *Human Organization* **24**:188–91, 1965.

56 Parsons, T.: Social structure and dynamic process: the case of modern medical practice, in *The social system*. Glencoe, Free Press, 1951, pp. 428–79.

57 Burling, T., Lentz, E. M., and Wilson, R. N.: *Give and take in hospitals: a study of human organization*. New York, Putnam, 1956.

58 Yalom, I. D.: *Encounter groups and psychiatry*. Task Force Report. Washington DC, American Psychiatric Association, 1970.

59 Goldberg, C.: *Encounter: group sensitivity training experience*. New York, Science House, 1970.

60 Offenkrantz, W. and Tobin, A.: Psychoanalytic psychotherapy. *Archives of General Psychiatry* **30**:593–606, 1974.

61 Krasner, L.: The therapist as a social reinforcement machine, in *Research in psychotherapy*, Vol. 2, ed. H. Strupp and L. Luborsky. Washington DC, American Psychological Association, 1962, pp. 61–94.

62 Bandura, A.: The ethics and social purposes of behavior modification, in *Annual review of behavior therapy, theory and practice*, Vol. 3, ed. C. M. Franks and G. T. Wilson. New York, Brunner/Mazel, 1975, pp. 13–20.

63 Halleck, S.: Legal and ethical aspects of behavior control. *American Journal of Psychiatry* **131**:381–7, 1974.

64 Goldiamond, I.: Toward a constructional approach to social problems: ethical and constitutional problems raised by applied behavior analysis, in *Annual review of behavior therapy, theory and practice*, Vol. 3, ed. C. M. Franks and G. T. Wilson. New York, Brunner/Mazel, 1975, pp. 21–63.

65 Commentary: ethical and related issues in behavior therapy, in *Annual review of behavior therapy, theory and practice*, Vol. 3, ed. C. M. Franks and G. T. Wilson. New York, Brunner/Mazel, 1975.

66 Castiglione, A.: *A history of medicine*. New York, Knopf, 1947.

67 Dubey, J.: Confidentiality as a requirement of the therapist: technical necessities for absolute privilege in psychotherapy. *American Journal of Psychiatry* **131**:1093–6, 1974.

68 *Doe* v. *Roe*, 93 Misc. 2 201, 400, N.Y.S. 2d 668, 1977.

69 Kermani, E. J.: Court rulings on psychotherapists. *American Journal of Psychotherapy* **36**:248–55, 1982.

70 *Schaffer* v. *Spicer*, 215 N.W. 2d 135, South Dakota, 1974.

71 American Psychiatric Association: *The principles of medical ethics with annotations especially applicable to psychiatry*, 1985 edn. Washington, DC, APA, 1985.

72 Plaut, E. A.: A perspective on confidentiality. *American Journal of Psychiatry* **131**:1021–4, 1974.

73 Bloch, D. A.: Family therapy, group therapy. *International Journal of Group Psychotherapy* **26**:289–99, 1976.

74 *Tarasoff* v. *The Regents of the University of California*, 118 California Reporter 129, 529, P 2d 553, 1974.

75 Roth, L. H. and Meisel, A.: Dangerousness, confidentiality, and the duty to warn. *American Journal of Psychiatry* **134**:508–11, 1977.

76 Gurevitz, H.: Tarasoff: protective privilege versus public peril. *American Journal of Psychiatry* **134**:289–92, 1977.

77 *Thompson* v. *County of Alameda*, 27 Cal 3d 741, 614 P2d 728, 167, California Reporter 70 (1980).

78 *Mavroudis* v. *Superior Court of County of San Mateo*, app 162, California Reporter 724 (1980).

79 *Hedlund* et al. v. *Superior Court of Orange County*, 34 Cal 3d 695, 669 P2d 41, 194, California Reporter 805 (1983).

80 Gross, B. H., Southhard, M. J., Lamb, H. R., and Weinberger, L. E.: Assessing dangerousness and responding appropriately: Hedlund expands the clinician's liability established by Tarasoff. *Journal of Clinical Psychiatry* **48**:9–12, 1987.

81 Halleck, S. L.: Malpractice in psychiatry. *Psychiatric Clinics of North America* **6**:567–83, 1983.

82 Leesfield, I. H.: Negligence of mental health professionals. *Trial* **23**:57–61, 1987.

83 Klein, J. I. and Glover, S. I.: Psychiatric malpractice. *International Journal of Law and Psychiatry* **6**:131–57, 1983.

84 Furrow, B. R.: *Malpractice in psychotherapy*. Lexington, MA, Lexington Books, 1980.

85 *Brand* v. *Grubin*, Superior Court of New Jersey, 329 A 2d, B2, 1974.

86 *Runyon* v. *Reid*, Supreme Court of Oklahoma, 510 P2d, 943, 1973.

87 Braceland, F. J.: Historical perspectives of the ethical practice of psychiatry. *American Journal of Psychiatry* **126**:230–7, 1969.

88 Dahlberg, C.: Sexual contact between patient and therapist. *Contemporary Psychoanalysis* **6**:107–24, 1970.

89 Truax, C. B. and Mitchell, K. M.: Research on certain therapist interpersonal skills in relation to process and outcome, in *Handbook of psychotherapy and behaviour change: an empirical analysis*, ed. A. E. Bergin and S. L. Garfield. New York, Wiley, 1971, pp. 299–344.

90 Chesler, P.: *Women and madness*. Garden City, Doubleday, 1972.

91 Kardener, S., Fuller, M., and Mensh, I.: A survey of physicians' attitudes and practices regarding erotic and non-erotic contact with patients. *American Journal of Psychiatry* **130**:1077–81, 1973.

92 Butler, S.: Sexual contact between therapists and patients. Doctoral dissertation, California School of Professional Psychology, Los Angeles, 1975.

93 Robertiello, R.: Iatrogenic psychiatric illness. *Journal of Contemporary Psychotherapy* **7**:3–8, 1975.

94 Stone, M.: Management of unethical behaviour in a psychiatric hospital staff. *American Journal of Psychotherapy* **29**:391–401, 1975.

95 Marmor, J.: Some psychodynamic aspects of the seduction of patients in psychotherapy. Presented at the 129th Annual Meeting, American Psychiatric Association, Miami Beach, Fla., May 10–14, 1976.

96 Stone, A. A.: The legal implications of sexual activity between psychiatrist and patient. *American Journal of Psychiatry* **133**:1138–41, 1976.

97 Masters, W. H. and Johnson, V. E.: Principles of the new sex therapy. *American Journal of Psychiatry* **133**:548–54, 1976.

98 Roman, M., Charles, E., and Karasu, T. B.: The value system of psychotherapists and changing mores. *Psychotherapy: Theory, Research and Practice* **15**:409–15, 1978.

99 Levy, R. B.: *I can only touch you now*. Englewood Cliffs, Prentice-Hall, 1973.

100 Pattison, J. E.: Effects of touch on self-exploration and the therapeutic relationship. *Journal of Consulting and Clinical Psychology* **40**:170–5, 1973.

101 Holroyd, J. C. and Brodsky, A. M.: Psychologists' attitudes and practices regarding erotic and non-erotic physical contact with patients. *American Psychologist* **32**:843–9, 1977.

102 Taylor, B. J. and Wagner, N. N.: Sex between therapists and clients: a review and analysis. *Professional Psychology* **7**:593–601, 1976.

103 *Zipkin* v. *Freeman*, 436 SW 2d 753, (Mo. 1968).

104 Hogan, D. B.: *The regulation of psychotherapists*, Vol. III: A review of malpractice suits in the United States. Cambridge, MA, Ballinger, 1979.

105 Pope, K. S. and Bouhoutsos, J. C.: Sexual intimacy between therapists and patients. New York, Praeger, 1986.

106 Law Firm of Onek, Klein, Farr: *Selected problems in the practice of psychiatry*. Washington DC, American Psychiatric Association, 1985.

107 Rice, J. K. and Rice, D. G.: Implications of the Women's Liberation Movement for psychotherapy. *American Journal of Psychiatry* **130**:191–6, 1973.

108 Seiden, A. M.: Overview: research on the psychology of women, II. Women in families, work, and psychotherapy. *American Journal of Psychiatry* **133**:1111–23, 1976.

109 Broverman, I. K., Broverman, D. M., Clarkson, F. E., *et al.*: Sex-role stereotypes and clinical judgements of mental health. *Journal of Consulting and Clinical Psychology* **34**:1–7, 1970.

110 Seiden, A., Benedek, E., Wolman, C., *et al.*: *Survey on women's status in psychiatric education*. A report of the APA Task Force on Women. Presented at the 127th Annual Meeting of the American Psychiatric Association, Detroit, May 6–10, 1974.

111 Jonsen, A. R. and Hellegers, A. E.: Conceptual foundations for an ethics of medical care, in *Ethics of health care*, ed. L. Tancredi. Washington DC, National Academy of Sciences, 1974, pp. 3–21.

112 Zitrin, A. and Klein, H.: Can psychiatry police itself effectively? The experience of one district branch. *American Journal of Psychiatry* **133**:653–6, 1976.

113 Sullivan, F. W.: Peer review and professional ethics. *American Journal of Psychiatry* **134**:186–8, 1977.

114 Klein, H.: Current peer review system bound to fail. *Psychiatric News*, 16 July 1975.

115 Chodoff, P. and Santora, P.: Psychiatric peer review: the DC experience, 1972–75. *American Journal of Psychiatry* **134**:121–5, 1977.

116 Newman, D. E. and Luft, L. L.: The peer review process: education versus control. *American Journal of Psychiatry* **131**:1363–6, 1974.

117 Bernaly Del Rio, V.: Psychiatric ethics, in *Comprehensive textbook of psychiatry*, ed. A. M. Freedman and H. I. Kaplan. Baltimore, Williams and Wilkins, 1967, pp. 2543–52.

# 9

# Ethical aspects of drug treatment

*Paul Brown*

## Introduction

Ethical aspects of drug treatment in psychiatry were not systematically addressed until the psychotropic drug revolution in the 1950s. The revolution began with the serendipitous discovery of chlorpromazine for schizophrenia,[1] and was soon followed by the development of potent new preparations for anxiety (chlordiazepoxide, 1957) and depression (imipramine, 1958). Lithium had been discovered in 1949, but because of fears of toxicity did not become available until the 1960s. It was widely believed that a new treatment phase had been inaugurated, with specific drug treatments for specific diagnostic conditions.

In the context of these major developments, psychiatric therapeutics rapidly evolved its own cognate scientific disciplines: evaluation of drug efficacy (clinical trials), processing of the drugs by the body (pharmacokinetics), and study of curative and unwanted effects (psychopharmacology). Paralleling the drug revolution was a dramatic global decline in the number of patients treated in psychiatric hospitals. For example, in the United States over a period of only twenty years the numbers diminished from 600 000 to the 1915 level of 100 000. This led prominent American psychiatrists to conclude confidently: 'This profound alteration in the focus of treatment of mental patients is a most convincing proof of the efficiency of antipsychotic drugs.'[2] Rhetoric, however, is no substitute for scientific evaluation. Equally eminent psychiatrists, such as Manfred Bleuler, contested such a conclusion, by pointing out the considerable placebo contribution to this 'therapeutic achievement'. He also anticipated widespread homelessness of the mentally ill, and a wholesale return of patients to custodial care. His prognosis was ultimately vindicated.[3] 'Decarceration' of the mentally ill led to widespread therapeutic neglect. The institutional settings for drug treatment were eroded without their effective replacement by community-based therapeutic frameworks. It was therefore not in

---

* This chapter owes much to the contribution by Klerman and Shechter in the first edition, and is essentially a revision and update of it; this is particularly so with the section 'Psychotropic drugs and the boundaries of mental illness'.

the least paradoxical that the drug revolution was also associated with scientific challenges and an ethical backlash.

Institutional psychiatry had already withstood a critical onslaught from sociologists,[4,5] radical psychiatrists,[6,7] and even moderate health professionals.[8] Following this, drug treatment faced a legal fusillade from patients and their advocates, and from civil-rights activists. Psychiatrists were seemingly not equipped to handle the ethical dimensions of drug treatment. Instead, they resorted to the ethical blinkers of pharmacological scientism and paternalistic control. Even had they looked to medical ethics for guidance, this would not have assisted them. Ostensibly founded on Hippocratic principles of beneficence, justice, and respect for persons,[9] it had tended to give precedence to paternalism compared to patient autonomy and social justice. For instance, the doctrine of informed consent was practised in the breach, and more often asserted the doctor's interests rather than those of the patient.

Commencing in the 1960s a spate of legal actions was brought before the American Federal Courts. At first the actions sought to uphold the right to treatment of involuntary patients;[10] but gradually the emphasis shifted to their right to refuse treatment.[11,12] Wide-ranging statutory changes followed. Already by the mid-1970s psychiatrists were becoming less defensive, and beginning to re-evaluate the ethical dimensions of drug treatment and psychiatric practice in general.[13] One of the most noteworthy aspects is applied treatment ethics. By the 1980s they were able to conduct research into the ethical basis of treatment decision-making. This research and important developments in applied treatment ethics[14] established therapeutic practice on a more ethically reflective footing.

This chapter will address a number of key ethical issues with regard to drug treatment. The consideration of risks and benefits is a prelude to a discussion of the doctor–patient relationship so far as it concerns drug prescription and informed consent. These issues will lead to a key contemporary ethical issue: doctors' duties and patients' rights. Naturally these discussions will raise more questions than provide answers; the science of drug treatment is developing so rapidly that ethical considerations are only beginning to keep pace.

## Risks and benefits of drug treatment

The psychiatrist's decision when to prescribe a drug and to which patients is based on a consideration of risks and benefits. Scientific guidelines, however, are far from clear, and in any event, treatment decisions are often influenced by value judgements and idiosyncratic biases.

*Drug risks*

The drugs used in psychiatry are potent agents, with major side-effects, and problems of toxicity and dependence. They can be particularly risky in combination with each other or with drugs used for other medical conditions. Innovative agents must pass through lengthy laboratory trials, but non-proprietary preparations avoid substantial scrutiny. There are special hazards in giving psychotropic medication to children, the mentally handicapped, the medically ill, and pregnant and nursing women.

The risks of psychiatric drug treatment become clear with the use of the phenothiazines and minor tranquillizers. When the *phenothiazines* were introduced, little was known about their potential side-effects. Although most proved troublesome, the side-effects were transitory or readily reversible with specific medications. But two in particular have proved ominously dangerous, and warrant special attention.

The Neuroleptic Malignant Syndrome is an acute medical disorder characterized by high fever, muscular rigidity, and impaired consciousness.[15] There are serious complications such as renal failure, and a mortality of up to 20 per cent. It is fortunately rare. Much commoner is the chronic and often progressive drug-induced disorder of tardive dyskinesia.[16] There is an enormous variety of presentations, but all centre on repetitive choreoathetoid movements of the lips, tongue, mouth, trunk, and limbs. Although tardive dyskinesia is commoner in older women with mood disorders, there are no absolute predictors, and it can occur in either sex and at any age. The condition usually takes up to a year to develop but can begin much earlier. It is generally precipitated by dose-reduction or drugwithdrawal, particularly when this is abrupt. The clinician must then face the uncomfortable possibility that the presence of tardive dyskinesia is masked by the very drug which is responsible for its occurrence. The treatment of tardive dyskinesia is unsatisfactory; safe, effective, and specific remedies are lacking. Prevention is the wisest course, and there have been attempts to introduce new anti-psychotic agents without this risk.[17] Given all these features it is not surprising that legal liability for tardive dyskinesia was demonstrated in 1984.[18] Obviously, tardive dyskinesia is a nightmare for patient and therapist alike.

Over the past decade, the risks of drug dependence and withdrawal with *minor tranquillizers* have increasingly come to professional and public attention.[19] It has become clear that the most vulnerable clinical group are the elderly medically ill. Dependence and withdrawal symptoms occur in up to 40 per cent of chronic users.[20,21] These symptoms, which may persist for six months or more, include insomnia (71 per cent), agitation (56 per cent), muscle twitching (49 per cent), headache (38 per cent), tremor (38 per cent), nausea (36 per cent), double vision (20 per cent), and sweating (22 per cent).[22]

In the light of these substantial problems, the medical profession was ill-prepared for critical public reaction, and patient-support groups such as 'Tranx' stepped into the breach. Consumer-protection organizations took up their cudgels, by giving these drugs negative and sensational publicity. Not surprisingly patients took fright. The prescriptive pendulum swung, as doctors became reluctant to use benzodiazepines. In the light of subsequent empirical studies this is without doubt an over-reaction; patients are being deprived of suitable medication, and are being left to the mercy of more dangerous substances—alcohol, nicotine, and barbiturates.

If psychiatric drugs such as the phenothiazines and minor tranquillizers are risky, the prescribers can be no less risk-prone[23] in their therapeutic practices. General practitioners are particularly liable to make inappropriate choices of drug and dose. This is noteworthy in the case of depression, for which condition they are apt to use minor tranquillizers alone, or antidepressants at a suboptimal dose and for inadequate duration. They are also prone to misdiagnose psychotic conditions, and by inappropriately prescribing major tranquillizers, risk precipitating tardive dyskinesia.

## Drug benefits

Psychotropic drugs are generally acclaimed by psychiatrists, and even some patient-advocates,[24] as bringing substantial benefits. They reduce symptoms and the rate of relapse, and lengthen the gap between episodes of illness. However, when the results of clinical drug trials are scrutinized, the benefits appear much more qualified. A brief consideration of antipsychotic drug trials will serve to illustrate this.

In a comprehensive survey of 100 double-blind controlled studies of major tranquillizers[2] 61 per cent of patients receiving an active drug treatment showed improvement, but only 16 per cent were in complete remission. Thirty-nine per cent were still unchanged, moderately ill, or even worse. In another survey, of 55 placebo-controlled studies of chlorpromazine, placebo proved to be as effective as the active drug in 11 trials. In fact, the combined rate of placebo-response and spontaneous remission over the whole range of mental illness, including schizophrenia and depression, variously runs between 20 per cent and 30 per cent. If we now re-examine the survey of 100 studies, we can assume that 20 per cent of the improved group can be accounted for by non-specific effects. These include patients' positive attitudes and expectations about treatment, therapists' attitudes, and the psychiatric setting. In round figures we can say that less than half (80 per cent of 61 per cent) are directly benefited by the drug at all!

The story does not stop there. If drugs are less effective than claimed, they also do not differ in any standard way in comparative efficacy. They do vary in potency and side-effects, but there is frequently little to distinguish between drugs, or between drugs and alternative biological and psychological therapies, in terms of efficacy for a given psychiatric condition.[25] One result is that prescriptive guidelines have remained obscure; whether patients receive drugs, psychotherapy or a combination of the two is often governed by value judgement or chance rather than by scientific consideration.

### Psychotropic drugs and the boundaries of mental illness

Although contemporary psychiatric nosology, embracing the core psychiatric disorders of schizophrenia, depression, and organic brain syndromes, is now well established (for example, in DSM III), there has been a contrary trend in recent years to broaden the definition of mental ill health. This has led to the risk of inappropriate medicalization, with associated abuse of drug treatment so as to achieve social control.

As was clearly noted by Klerman and Schechter in the first edition of this book, it is useful to consider the movement from mental health to mental illness along a continuum: three main areas can be distinguished (see Fig 9.1).

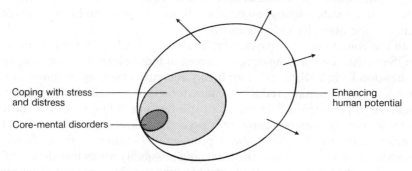

Coping with stress and distress

Enhancing human potential

Core-mental disorders

**Fig. 9.1** Boundaries between mental illness and mental health

The first includes the core mental disorders; the second, psychological problems with significant emotional distress related to stressful life events; and the third involves those seeking enhancement of human potential and personal growth. The widening of diagnostic definitions can occur within each of these three categories. The diagnosis of schizophrenia, for instance, has been malignantly applied to political dissidents (see Chapter 24), with all the attendant medication risks alluded to earlier.

Psychotropic drug-prescription has also extended to the domain of stressful life events, with their gamut of associated anxieties, tensions, and other distressing emotions. Sufferers include lonely housewives, business executives under pressure, the divorced, and the bereaved. Considerable debate prevails about whether unpleasant changes in emotional state associated with such suffering should be defined as mental illness and be treated with drugs. Brown and Harris[26] show that the most stressful life events are associated with increased psychiatric morbidity and even mortality. In these, a case can be made for brief psychotropic medication during the period of greatest risk. But clearly drugs are not appropriate for the relief of the stress and 'blues' of everyday life. There are many subtle pressures on such sufferers to seek medication, and on the doctor to prescribe, not the least from drug companies. This leads to potential ethical dilemmas. The psychiatrist's judgement to withhold medication may be met with the patient's demand for the right to prompt drug relief. As Carstairs[27] has put it 'Everyone nowadays expects to be happy. What is more, if anyone feels unhappy, he immediately thinks that something must be wrong either with him or with the state of the world, if not both.'

Not only is the public reluctant to suffer, but there may also be growing demands for psychotropic drugs to enhance human potential. These include demands for medication to promote psychological growth in psychotherapy, enhance physical prowess in competitive sport, improve concert and examination/test performance, and achieve optimal sexual satisfaction. There even exists a lobby, albeit a small one, to promote hallucinogenic drugs in the quest for enlightenment.[28]

In the context of child psychiatry, Graham (see Chapter 16) comments on the debate surrounding drug treatment in those diagnosed as having an 'Attention Deficit Disorder'. Two highly addictive drugs, methylphenidate and dextramphetamine, reduce its characteristic hyperactivity, impulsivity, and lack of persistence.[29] However, it still remains dubious whether these behavioural phenomena represent a psychiatric disorder or an expedient medical term to disguise a social problem.[30] Because of these diffuse boundaries of mental illness the leavening possibility arises that drugs will be used as chemical restraints for troublesome people where the diagnosis is in doubt. A key issue must then be addressed: whether the drug is being given for the benefit of the subject or of the staff and institution. There is ample evidence that in both psychiatric hospital and prison practice, drugs are prescribed to manage aggressive, uncooperative and rule-breaking behaviour, and even as a punitive preventive device.

'Difficult' behaviour is not a diagnosis in its own right. Rather, it is a psychological problem requiring elucidation. The snag is in deciding whether it is a feature of an underlying psychiatric illness or, say, a sign of legitimate protest. Some patients may present with aggressive behaviour as part of their psychiatric disorder, which then may warrant medication. On the other hand, staff may use tranquillization solely to tame unruly patients. This may also serve to curb the staff's own fears.[31] Clearly the responsibility of the treatment team is to make as accurate an assessment as possible of the aggression and its underlying significance, and to deal with it in the context of the therapeutic milieu with tact, understanding, and respect for patients' rights. Most psychiatrists would agree that medication is warranted in cases of extreme danger and acute emergency. The situation is more difficult to resolve when the underlying cause of the behaviour is not clearly established. It is then best to apply an approach which considers the consequences for patient, staff, and all concerned.

## Doctor–patient relationship and drug prescribing

If the substantive foundation of ethical drug prescribing is a full knowledge of risks and benefits, its procedural basis is the doctor–patient relationship, particularly mediated by the doctrine of informed consent.

### The doctor–patient relationship

Elucidation of the significance of the doctor–patient relationship was a triumph for the psychoanalytic revolution. It led to the development of dynamic psychiatry, but has had little impact on psychopharmacology. Psychiatrists with a biological orientation all too readily retreat into their traditional roles as arbiters of medical science, and subordinate the establishment of a treatment alliance to the promotion of patient-compliance. They frequently express concerns that patients might be confused, rather than enlightened, by discussion. Fears of detrimental effects from explaining side-effects, however, have proved unfounded.[32] Clinics then run the risk of becoming 'medication mills' for prescription refills and drug-depot injections. Training of these psychiatrists frequently reflects the psychopharmacological bias of their trainers, and where educational programmes neglect the psychological aspects of the doctor–patient relationship, trainees may be severely hampered.

If psychiatrists experience concerns, those of their patients are often greater. They include a fear of losing control, being damaged, or becoming addicted. Patients may not express such concerns for fear of losing their psychiatrist's interest and goodwill. On the other hand, patients may oppose or resist drug treatment. Challenges not only occur in the health conscious, the paranoid, the hypochondriac, and the help-rejecting complainer; they have also come from a new source, through heightened public awareness of the risks and dangers of psychotropic drugs. This has been fostered by the publication of articles and books, by the growth of consumerism, and by an energetic civil-rights movement.

In the context of drug treatment the psychiatrist–patient relationship is clearly fraught with difficulty. Lack of trust, inadequate communication, and manipulative or coercive tactics by therapist or patient can undermine the ethical basis of drug treatment as much as any pharmacological hazards. And yet it is this very relationship which is necessary for the optimal application of informed consent to which we now turn.

## Informed consent

Informed consent provides both an ethical and a legal definition of the therapist–patient relationship, and practical guidelines with respect to the decision to treat. It is often conceived of as a linear process, in which the therapist explains the risks and benefits of a treatment, as well as the nature and implications of therapeutic alternatives, and the patient makes a decision with regard to the options.

When so conceptualized it is all too easy for doctors to regard informed consent as a mere paper exercise, only requiring the patient to rubber-stamp his or her agreement. Two critical contextual factors should however also be taken into account: the patient's freedom and his or her competence to consent. These render medical decision-making recursive and interactive, rather than simply a one-way process.[33] For free consent to be possible, the therapist is required to discuss treatment recommendations openly. He must listen intently to the patients' questions, and try to understand their fears and objections. Where patients are ambivalent or unwilling to take drugs, the doctor must spend the necessary time to clarify the nature of their resistance. With non-urgent treatment recommendations, patients' views may have to prevail, and the therapist may need to accede to drug refusal. This is not to say that patients' beliefs about drug treatment should be accepted at face value; rather they must be assessed against objective criteria. This leads to a consideration of competence to give informed consent.

Competence is defined as the patient's ability to understand, communicate, deliberate, and make rational treatment choices.[34] Consent is generally adjudged to have occurred not when patients have merely had the risks explained, and have voluntarily accepted them, but only when they are also competent to do so. Belmaker *et al.*[35] argue that the patient's capacity to give true informed consent varies with diagnosis and therapeutic context. Many chronic patients are unreasonably willing to come off long-term medication and to try new drugs. By contrast, severe depressives are plagued by doubts, hopelessness, and pessimism, and can become more distressed by involvement in treatment decision-making. Paranoid patients frequently believe their medication and food is poisoned. In such patients there may be a serious risk of suicide or homicide, and medication can be life-saving. Medical and judicial consensus therefore exists on the necessity to waive the process of informed consent in such cases. In most incompetent patients, however, medication is not primarily an issue of survival, but rather one of preventing or stemming a relapse of a psychotic illness. When deterioration is deemed irrevocable, judicial support is once again available to enforce medication.

In the absence of firm guidelines regarding competence, and with an ever-growing civil-rights lobby, some American states have resorted to the legal doctrine of substituted judgement.[24] This requires that any treatment which the patient would have chosen, had he been able to choose, may be given. But who then should decide, and using which procedures and criteria? Suggested approaches range from judicial procedures involving independent psychiatrists, to informal review with the treating psychiatrist liaising with a legally appointed guardian.

Recent empirical research on competence to assent to medication has begun to illuminate its considerable complexity. In a noteworthy study[36] 56 state hospital patients were assessed for their degree of competence; factual knowledge was evaluated by the ability to name the medication and one of its benefits, and to be aware of tardive dyskinesia. In addition, their capacity for rational understanding was evaluated with respect to their awareness of the fact of their suffering from a mental disorder, and their recognition of the recommended drug treatment as being effective. Only 18 per cent proved to be fully competent at initial assessment. The remainder were ignorant of tardive dyskinesia, and lacked a rational understanding of the relevance of medication. Only 36 per cent of the sample were able to demonstrate factual knowledge within forty-eight hours. There was no assessment of retention, the authors suggesting that repeated testing of competence might be required.

Further studies of this kind are needed in order for the issue of competence with regard to informed consent to be properly elucidated. This in turn will facilitate optimal participation of psychiatrists in both the clinical and judicial aspects of informed consent.

## Patients' rights

Rights are the justified claims that individuals (and groups) can make on others and on society. In respect to drug treatment, Klerman and Schechter in the first edition of this volume suggested that patients' rights should include: access to treatment, necessary information, the freedom to accept or refuse treatment, and a voice in the selection of specific drugs and under what conditions to take them. Although such rights apply to all clinical contexts their assertion by involuntary patients is inevitably more difficult. Recently efforts to affirm committed patients' rights to participate in treatment decisions have intensified, particularly in the United States. Patients and civil-rights advocates are succeeding not only in focusing greater attention on the ethical issues involved, but also on testing them in the courts.

Initially, patients and their advocates campaigned for the *right to treatment.* Their aim was to apply pressure for better therapeutic conditions; in a series of court deliberations [10,37] it was found to be against due process to commit patients without adequate treatment. The focus has subsequently shifted from the right to treatment, to the *right to refuse treatment.*[11-12,38] Court actions here rested primarily on arguments that the involuntary administration of medication violates patients' bodily integrity and personal autonomy. Evidence discreditable to the psychiatric profession was adduced for a range of such violations in the context of drug treatment. They included: polypharmacy; inattention to serious side-effects, particularly tardive dyskinesia; prescribing treatment with little medical justification or for inappropriate reasons; giving medications without the patient being seen by a psychiatrist; prescription by unlicensed psychiatrists; and using drugs coercively. In summary, institutions have been portrayed as punitive, doctors as power-hungry and irresponsible, and drug treatment as a means of control.

Arising out of these legal developments, Appelbaum and Gutheil[39] argue that the fundamental issue is not the right to refuse treatment, but the right of every patient to receive 'good' treatment, to reject 'bad' treatment, and to have recourse to independent judgement. In a landmark contribution, Clayton[24] asserts that their argument fails because they do not acknowledge that what constitutes good or bad treatment depends in no small measure on the patient's values. The central issue for her is not only whether patients should be able to reject bad treatment, but also whether they can reject reasonable (on objective clinical grounds) treatment, at least in competent, non-urgent cases.

Arguing from fundamental moral principles, Clayton sets out to demolish the notion of a general entitlement of doctors to intervene in the best interests of the patient. She enlists support for this contention from the work of J. S. Mill, and from societal tolerance of those who manifestly do not act in their own best interests, cases such as smokers and hang-gliders. She further argues for the primacy of patients' rights to refuse treatment over any objective criteria as to what constitutes their best interests. In support of this she cites increasing legal authority for the position that competent adults have the right even to reject life-sustaining therapy if no important social interests are contravened. Incompetent patients, she asserts, can retain similar rights of refusal through the legal doctrine of substituted judgement.

The trend, therefore, is clearly away from the solution of conflicts of interest within the doctor–patient relationship alone, where 'informal' medical ethics may apply, to increasing legal involvement based on the principle of rights. Both medical and statutory rights are giving away to patients' rights in respect of refusal of drug treatment.

The State has an important role to fulfil in protecting its citizens; but it rarely resorts to forced medication as part of this role. Nor is it apt to deploy forced medication to protect patients intent on harming themselves. Rather, the State provides opportunities for effective and efficient drug treatment through upholding clinical decisions and by acknowledging the ethical integrity of the medical profession. This does not mean that psychiatrists have *carte blanche* to medicate. The emphasis is rather on medical duties than on rights. Doctors are no longer free (if they ever were) to ignore the patient's choices. Medication may only be enforced in cases of extreme emergency, particularly where doctors must protect themselves, other staff members, or patients and their families.

## Court actions

Public and professional debate on patients' rights regarding treatment has revolved around a series of court actions spanning the last two decades, particularly in the US. A New Jersey ruling[11] emphasized the potency and harsh side-effects of psychotropic drugs, and accorded the patient the right to exert control over their administration. The rights were to be safeguarded by an independent psychiatrist at an informal hearing, and the patient could also be represented by legal counsel.

The test case however was *Rogers* v. *Okin*[12] in 1979. Seven patients sued their psychiatrists, and called for a ban on forced medication (and seclusion) for themselves and their fellows at Boston State Hospital. The district court ruled in the patients' favour, concluding that involuntary commitment was not axiomatically a judgement of incompetence, and disagreed with the defendant's counter-argument that the State should act as *parens patriae* for the involuntarily committed. (The *parens patriae* jurisdiction originated in the power and duty of the Crown/State to protect the persons and property of those unable to do so themselves, such as minors and persons of unsound mind; a power which could subsequently be held to be practically delegated to authorized agents of the State such as psychiatrists in certain circumstances.) If a psychiatrist is of the opinion that it is necessary to enforce medication, it is the court's responsibility to judge on the patient's ability to provide informed consent, or to appoint a guardian when incompetence has been established. Gutheil[40] has subsequently attempted to demonstrate through case-examples that the guardianship approach to involuntary medication, while acceptable in theory, is unworkable in clinical practice. Roth[41] has offered an alternative remedy for the problem of how the patient's interests can be best served: he has suggested that the question of an involuntary patient's right to refuse treatment should be determined at the point when the judgement about the commitment is being considered. The commitment order could then permit the psychiatrist to treat the patient, if necessary without his consent.

The *Rogers* v. *Okin* case did not end with the 1979 ruling, and, over a period of six years, went to appeal. The Federal Court deferred to the State legislature on constitutional grounds;[42,43] but patients' rights to refuse treatment were again confirmed. In giving its judgement[44] the court took into consideration such factors as the level of intrusiveness of the treatment itself, the possibility of side-effects, the degree of emergency, the prognosis without treatment, the nature and extent of any prior judicial involvement, and the likelihood of conflicting interests. Patient-related factors, including personal preference, religious conviction, and family pressure were particularly emphasized.

The *Rogers* case was soon followed by a spate of similar court actions, in New York[36] and elsewhere in the US. Among the results have been the appointment of patient advocates, the posting of drug side-effects in wards, and the ready availability of consent forms. The effect of these changes on the traditional psychiatric institutional ethos has been striking.

## The psychiatrist's reactions

Clinical and legal conceptions of patient autonomy differ considerably. The law places a high value on the patient's stated wishes, and commonly takes them at face value or, when incompetence clearly is involved, applies the procedure of substituted judgement. Clinicians argue that the court operates on false premises. They place a higher value on *actual* intent or meaning, which is frequently regarded as different from what the patient may state at the time. Many psychiatrists therefore aver that the current emphasis on patients' civil rights fails to take into account their urgent clinical needs, and may even be in conflict with them. They point to a number of detrimental consequences.[45]

One such consequence is suboptimal patient care. There may be delays in drug treatment while doctors seek a court order to medicate.[46] Patients can indeed be neglected when staff action is legally correct but clinical decisions to offer drug treatment are withheld. As Roth states,[41] undertreatment is certainly no better than over-treatment.

Psychiatrists are also concerned about the trend away from therapeutic towards custodial functions.[47,48] For example, Leong[49] cautions against the expansion of psychiatric participation in social control, and Rodenhauser and Heller[50] draw attention to the potential role of forensic psychiatrists as law-enforcers, following a veritable pandemic of treatment-refusals. Finally, psychiatrists are worried about the erosion of their power to treat. Accustomed to having sole discretion over treatment, they see the patient's refusal as a challenge to their medical authority and the exercising of their professional expertise.

Given these kinds of complication, some psychiatrists have attempted to elucidate the basis of patient drug-refusal. Recent research shows that most cases of refusal are transient, and subsequently regarded by the patients themselves as ego-dystonic. In a couple of studies most refusers eventually gave their free consent.[51,52] Their reasons for refusal were varied, but consistent patterns did emerge. Indeed, most investigations demonstrate denial, grandiosity, psychotic perceptions, anger, ambivalence, negativism, and conflict with their family or with the treatment team. Refusals on account of side-effects are remarkably uncommon.[53,54]

In a most illuminating study, Schwartz and his colleagues[55] sought to investigate patients' attitudes to treatment after involuntary medication by interviewing 24 refusers. Initially, a third exhibited psychotically-based denial, and felt that they had no need for medication. At discharge however, 70 per cent felt that their refusal had been correctly overridden, and that they would wish to be treated against their will again if it proved to be necessary. The other patients resisted at every stage in the process, were mostly suffering from manic-depressive illness, and showed denial of psychotic proportions. The authors concluded that: '. . . the decision to refuse psychotropic medication is a manifestation of the patient's illness and does not reflect autonomous functioning or consistent beliefs about mental illness or its treatment. Consequently treatment refusal should be considered primarily a psychotherapeutic issue and in most cases, should be subject to clinical rather than judicial review'.

Even with these substantial research findings the patient's right to drug refusal remains much emphasized. Perhaps, as Gutheil suggests,[40] the legal view has become too dominant, and: 'The way is paved for patients to "rot with their rights on"'. Rather than taking this type of adversarial stand, it seems preferable for psychiatrists to adapt constructively to these legal developments. At the clinical level this means elucidating drug refusal, and where at all possible grappling directly with it. Psychiatrists can also collaborate with patient-advocates in developing safeguards both within and without the clinical arena. Ziegenfuss[56] even recommends the reorganization of psychiatric services in order to accommodate patients' rights. This would include improving general management and the design of clinical programmes, and a thorough implementation of ethical procedures. Through a process of mutual support, neither patient nor professional would then be victimized by 'the system'.

Finally, it must be reiterated that rights are always associated with duties; this applies to doctors and patients alike. Osinga[57] draws attention, in a useful way, to the patient's duty to collaborate, from which can be derived a preparedness to co-operate with the professional.

## Drug costs and social justice

Ethically-based drug treatment does not only consist of balancing risks and benefits and weighing up patients' rights. Powerful market forces operate in regulating the access to and the availability of drug treatment, and severely restrict the application of the principles of fairness and non-discrimination, that is to say, of justice.

Two decades ago, Muller[58] lamented the over-medicated society. Drugs were promoted to deal with all the ills of living—50 per cent of psycho-tropic drug prescriptions were of minor tranquillizers, resulting in substantial dependence and abuse. Szasz[6] regarded this as the doctor's evasion of moral responsibility, and Muller[58] as economic exploitation by doctors, pharmacies, and drug companies. Illich[59] combined these factors under the rubric of the 'medicalization of life'.

By the 1980s the economic tide had turned. Psychiatric consumerism continues, but the relative public fisc for mental health is dwindling. In the community sector, the main problem has become access to care, and allocation of increasingly scarce resources to the underserved—the poor, the elderly, prisoners, and refugees. Deinstitutionalization was initially hailed as a triumph for drug treatment and social enlightenment (see Chapter 14). It undoubtedly has been for some psychiatric patients; but for most it has been associated with homelessness and poverty. Patients are frequently deprived of access to hospital, pharmacies, and drug treatment. There is no poor psychiatric lobby, and patients have no political power. Further, although the legal safeguards of patients are in place, actual service provision is woefully inadequate.

The trend to privatization has brought its own ethical dilemmas.[60] With a limit on mental health resources, treatment providers seek the least costly and shortest route. In consequence there is less out-patient service-provision, reflected in fewer visits and reduced long-term care. Privatization encourages cost-control and patients' sharing the financial risk with the provider. For psychiatrists, this leads to the dilemma of acting as double agent, when they have to serve both the patient's interests and those of the payment system. The economics of the market-place encourage minimalist ethics.

## Conclusion

At a fundamental level, psychiatry is beginning to develop an ethical basis for drug treatment. This is founded on a balanced consideration of psychopharmacological factors, moral principles, and fiduciary interests. More specifically, psychiatrists are taking a variety of initiatives. For instance, continuing medical education and peer-review programmes have been instituted to ensure that practitioners stay abreast of the psychiatric literature, and are able to assess developments in drug treatment.[33,61–63]

The profession is promoting intra-institutional and peer review. These are now well established for psychopharmacology research, and are also being extended to routine clinical practice. While psychiatrists proceed along these lines, there is a debate on the pros and cons of intra-versus extra-institutional review. Clayton[24] has drawn attention to the inadequacy of the former. She claims that although the courts can be slow and costly, they, together with lay review bodies, are more likely to pay due regard to all competing interests.

Formulary systems in institutional psychiatric settings enhance patient welfare through effective and economic drug-usage. Van Voort[64] comprehensively discusses the ethics of drug-review in terms of four dimensions: tight versus loose regulation, who should regulate, how review bodies and psychiatrists should interact, and how review data should be handled. With these in mind, he recommends monitoring by psychiatrists, pharmacists, administrators, patient-advocates, and other involved parties. This seems a commendable process of dialogue and consultation.

These kinds of procedures are timely and desirable. It is to be hoped that psychiatrists will commit themselves to such pursuits, thereby enhancing the ethical foundations of drug treatment.

# References

1 Delay, J. and Deniker, P.: Le traitement des psychoses par une méthode neurolytique derivée de l'hibernothérapie, in *Congrès des Médecins Alienistes et Neurologistes de France. Luxembourg* **50**:497, 1952.
2 Davis, J. M., Barter, J. T., and Kane, J. M.: Antipsychotic drugs, in *Comprehensive textbook of psychiatry*, ed. H. I. Kaplan and B. J. Sadock. Baltimore, Williams & Wilkins, 1989.
3 Roth, L. H.: Four studies of mental health commitment. *American Journal of Psychiatry* **146**:135–7, 1989.
4 Goffman, E.: *Asylums: essays on the social situation of mental patients and other inmates*. Chicago, Aldine, 1962.
5 Scheff, T. J.: *Being mentally ill: a sociological theory*. Chicago, Aldine, 1966.
6 Szasz, T. S.: *The myth of mental illness*. New York, Harper, 1961.
7 Laing, R. D.: *The politics of experience*. New York, Pantheon, 1967.
8 Joint commission on mental illness and health: *Action for mental health*. New York, Basic, 1961.
9 Thompson, I. E.: Fundamental ethical principles in health care. *British Medical Journal* **295**:1461–5, 1987.
10 *Wyatt* v. *Stickney*: 325 F. Supp. 781 (M.D.Ala.) 1971.
11 *Rennie* v. *Klein*: 720 F 2d. 266 (3d Cir) 1983.
12 *Rogers* v. *Okin*: 478 F. Supp. 1342 (D. Mass.) 1979.
13 Redlich, F. and Mollica, R. F.: Overview: ethical issues in contemporary psychiatry. *American Journal of Psychiatry* **133**:125–36, 1976.
14 Clements, C. D. and Ciccone, J. R.: Applied clinical ethics or universal principles. *Hospital and Community Psychiatry* **36**:121–23, 1985.
15 Pearlman, C. A.: Neuroleptic malignant syndrome: a review of the literature. *Journal of Clinical Psychopharmacology* **6**:257, 1986.

16 Jeste, D. V., Wisniewski, A. W., and Wyatt, R. J.: Neuroleptic-associated tardive syndromes. *Psychiatric Clinics of North America* **9**:183, 1986.

17 Kane, J., Honigfeld, G., Singer, J., and Meltzer, H.: Clozapine for the treatment of resistant schizophrenia. *Archives of General Psychiatry* **49**:789, 1988.

18 Wettson, R. M. and Appelbaum, P. S.: Legal liability for tardive dyskinesia. *Hospital and Community Psychiatry* **35**:992–4, 1984.

19 Hallstrom, C.: Use and abuse of benzodiazepines. *British Journal of Hospital Medicine* **41**:115, 1989.

20 Tyrer, P.: Prescribing psychotropic drugs in general practice. *British Medical Journal* **296**:588, 1988.

21 Higgitt, A. C., Lader, M. H., and Fonagy, P.: Clinical management of benzo-diazepine dependence. *British Medical Journal* **291**:688–90, 1985.

22 Gorman, J. M. and Davis, J. M.: Antianxiety drugs, in *Comprehensive textbook of psychiatry*, 5th edn. ed. H. I. Kaplan and B. J. Sadock. Baltimore, Williams & Wilkins, 1989.

23 Schwartz, H. K.: Legal and ethical pitfalls in family practice. *Psychiatry* **35**:103–8, 1987.

24 Clayton, E. W.: From *Rogers* to *Rivers*: the rights of the mentally ill to refuse medication. *American Journal of Law and Medicine* **13**:7–52, 1987.

25 Klerman, G. L., Dimascio, A., Weissman, M. M., Prusoff, B. A., and Paykel, E. S.: Treatment of depression by drugs and psychotherapy. *American Journal of Psychiatry* **131**:186–91, 1974.

26 Brown, G. W. and Harris, T.: *Social Origins of Depression*. London, Tavistock, 1978.

27 Carstairs, G. M.: A land of lotus eaters? *American Journal of Psychiatry* **125**:1576–80, 1969.

28 Clark, W. H.: Ethics and L.S.D. *Journal of Psychoactive Drugs* **17**:229–34, 1985.

29 Wender, P.: *Minimal brain dysfunction in children*. New York, Wiley, 1971.

30 Bosco, J. J. and Robbins, S. S. (eds.): *The hyperactive child and stimulant drugs*. Chicago, Chicago University Press, 1976.

31 Main, T. F.: The ailment. *British Journal of Medical Psychology* **30**:129–45, 1957.

32 Munetz, M. R. and Roth, L. H.: Informing patients about tardive dyskinesia. *Archives of General Psychiatry* **42**:866–71, 1985.

33 Sider, R. C. and Clements, C.: Psychiatry's contribution to medical ethics education. *American Journal of Psychiatry* **139**:498–501, 1982.

34 Winslade, W. J.: Ethics in psychiatry, in *Comprehensive textbook of psychiatry*, 5th edn, ed. H. I. Kaplan and B. J. Sadock. Baltimore, Williams & Wilkins, 1989.

35 Belmaker, R. H., Klein, E., and Dick, E: Ethics and psychopharmacologic research, in *Pharmacology: impact on clinical psychiatry*, ed. D. Morgan. St. Louis, Ishiyaku Euro America, 1985.

36 Beck, J. C.: Determining competency to assent to neuroleptic drug treatment. *Hospital and Community Psychiatry* **39**:1106–8, 1988.

37 *O'Connor* v. *Donaldson*: 422 US 563, 1975.

38 *Rivers* v. *Katz*: 495 NE2d 337 (NY), 1986.

39 Appelbaum, P. S. and Gutheil, T. G.: The right to refuse treatment: the real

issue is quality of care. *Bulletin of the American Academy of Psychiatry and the Law* **9**:199–202, 1981.

40 Gutheil, T. G.: In search of true freedom: drug refusal, involuntary medication and rotting with your rights on. *American Journal of Psychiatry* **137**:577–80, 1980.

41 Roth, L.: Mental health commitment: the state of the debate, 1980. *Hospital and Community Psychiatry* **31**:385–96, 1980.

42 *Mills* v. *Rogers*: 457 US 291.

43 *Rogers* v. *Okin*: 738 F 2d. 1 (1st Cir.), 1984.

44 *Rogers* v. *Commissioner of Department of Mental Health*: 458 NE 2d. 308 (Mass.), 1983.

45 Appelbaum, P. S.: The right to refuse treatment with antipsychotic medications: retrospect and prospect. *American Journal of Psychiatry* **145**:413–19, 1988.

46 Appelbaum, P. S. and Hoge, S. K.: The right to refuse treatment: what the research reveals. *Behavioral Sciences and the Law* **4**:279–92, 1986.

47 Brooks, A. D.: Law and antipsychotic medications. *Behavioral Sciences and the Law* **4**:247–63, 1986.

48 Sidley, N. T.: The right of involuntary patients in mental institutions to refuse drug treatment. *Journal of Psychiatry and the Law* **12**:231–55, 1984.

49 Leong, G. B.: The expansion of psychiatric participation in social control. *Hospital and Community Psychiatry* **40**:240–42, 1989.

50 Rodenhauser, P. and Heller, A.: Management of forensic psychiatric patients who refuse medication—2 scenarios. *Journal of Forensic Sciences* **29**:237–44, 1984.

51 Kalman, T. P.: An overview of patient satisfaction with psychiatric treatment. *Hospital and Community Psychiatry* **34**:48–53, 1983.

52 Keisling, R.: Characteristics and outcome of patients who refuse medication. *Hospital and Community Psychiatry* **34**:847–8, 1983.

53 Marder, S. R., Mebane, A., Chien, C., *et al.*: A comparison of patients who refuse and consent to neuroleptic treatment. *American Journal of Psychiatry* **140**:470–2, 1983.

54 Marder, S. R., Swann, E., Winslade, W. J., *et al.*: A study of medication refusal by involuntary psychiatric patients. *Hospital and Community Psychiatry* **35**:724–6, 1984.

55 Schwartz, H. I., Vingiano, W., and Bezirganian Pérez, C.: Autonomy and the right to refuse treatment: patient's attitudes after involuntary medication. *Hospital and Community Psychiatry* **39**:1049–54, 1988.

56 Ziegenfuss, J. T.: Conflict between patients' and patients' needs: an organisational systems problem. *Hospital and Community Psychiatry* **37**:1086–8, 1986.

57 Osinga, M.: But the patient has responsibilities as well. *Australasian Journal of the Medical Defence Union* **38–39**, Summer 1989.

58 Muller, C.: The overmedicated society: forces in the market place for medical care. *Science* **176**:488–92, 1972.

59 Illich, I.: *Medical nemesis: the expropriation of health*. New York, Pantheon, 1976.

60 Webb, W. L.: Ethical issues in modern mental health delivery. *Hospital and Community Psychiatry* **38**:917, 1987.

61 Appelbaum, P. S. and Reiser, S. J.: Ethics rounds: a model for teaching ethics in the psychiatric setting. *Hospital and Community Psychiatry* **32**:555–60, 1981.

62 Bloch, S.: Teaching of psychiatric ethics. *British Journal of Psychiatry* **136**:300–1, 1980.
63 Sider, R. C.: The ethics of therapeutic modality choice. *American Journal of Psychiatry* **141**:390–4, 1984.
64 Van Voort, W. B.: Ethics of nonformulary review in psychiatry. *Hospital and Community Psychiatry* **39**:1253–5, 1988.

# 10

# Ethical aspects of the physical manipulation of the brain

*Harold Merskey*

In this chapter, I base my discussion of ethical issues in the physical manipulation of the brain upon some current attitudes which can be summarized in a banal way as follows:

(1) Physicians advise and do not impose their advice except in special circumstances. Thus the treatment of individuals to save their lives or relieve their own distress is normally highly ethical but it may be unethical to impose any such treatment (even though legally allowed).

(2) Children and others in a condition which precludes them from deciding rationally may have decisions taken for them by people (usually their next of kin) who have appropriate concern for their interests and welfare.

(3) Physicians may ethically give some treatments to those people who come under Rule (2) but the types of treatment which may be given require careful scrutiny and the status and motives of the other person who makes the decision require careful assessment.

(4) Ethical actions may or may not be sanctioned by law. Physicians normally do not consider themselves bound to pursue ethical treatments for the patient's benefit if they are forbidden to do so by law. (But a difficult situation arises, for example, with physicians who wish to treat injured persons in secret when police forces or other security agencies are in pursuit.)

(5) Coercive treatments for the benefit of a third party are unethical. (To say 'You must have this behaviour modification or drug or lobotomy which you do not want because otherwise we expect you to murder your mother' is not a medically ethical approach.)

(6) The treatment of individuals against their wishes to change them for the sake of the needs of society or a political system is even more repugnant to ethical physicians than the previous conditions.

(7) Patients may consent to treatment which benefits either themselves or others but there are peculiar difficulties in confirming the presence of 'free consent' in some circumstances.

These rules partly reflect ethical considerations and partly reflect practical problems. The latter as will shortly be seen are capable of solution.

## Clinical cost–benefit ratios

There are three major types of physical manipulation of the brain, namely, electroconvulsive therapy (ECT); surgical ablation by scalpel or other technique which deliberately damages tissue; and the insertion of recording or stimulating electrodes, which is an advanced form of surgery. Each of these types of procedure has been attacked on many grounds and often ignorantly. The purpose of this discussion is to sketch the reasonable basis for their use, if any, in terms of medical ethics. In all cases much of the controversy turns upon the usefulness or otherwise of the procedure and the morbidity due to it. Those are necessary aspects for any physician to consider in regard to any treatment. They do not determine the ethical justification for the use of a treatment. The decision about whether a treatment is justified must always pass the test of a clinical judgement that the chance of benefit outweighs the hazards. If the chance of benefit is held to outweigh the risk of suffering or loss from the morbidity and mortality of the treatment the recommendation is ordinarily that the treatment be given. As every clinician knows these matters are often difficult to put in quantitative terms. If radical mastectomy for carcinoma of the breast gives, say, an 80 per cent chance of five-year survival (with a 10 per cent chance otherwise), and less than a 1 per cent chance of immediate operative death the calculation is fairly simple even though the operation also gives a near 100 per cent guarantee of some days of pain and discomfort to say the least. It is harder to decide how a thalamotomy for chronic pain with perhaps a 70 per cent chance of significant relief for 12 months can be evaluated in relation to a 20–30 per cent chance of some exacerbation of the pain and a 5 per cent chance of stroke or aphasia (which may also improve or partly remit). Nevertheless, carcinoma of the breast continued to be treated by radical mastectomy so long as odds of the order quoted existed and no other treatment offered better prospects, whilst thalamotomy has largely or wholly been discarded for pain (and not at all because it was an operation on the brain).

Thus procedures are assessed or remain in vogue on the basis of informed knowledge of what they can do for patients. If ECT is attacked on grounds of seeming barbaric because it incidentally causes convulsions that is an irrational view by comparison with the acceptance of surgery in which a breast may be mutilated or a larynx removed. Each procedure can be done for the benefit of the patient and, in the light of the information provided to him, he may ordinarily choose if the disadvantages are more or less than the advantages.

## Refusal of general surgery

If the non-psychotic adult does not choose to have some general surgical operation, despite his knowledge of the risks, an operation is not pursued. One important practical reason is that patients who undergo operations without some degree of acceptance often do badly. The patient who fears his operation excessively is dreaded by the surgeon. Clinical lore holds that such patients suffer serious complications and often die. The attitude of the patient thus becomes a factor in the cost–benefit equation. If it were not so, surgeons might be tempted to press necessary operations upon patients more vigorously. Practical wisdom reinforces the ethical position of not doing things to patients who refuse consent.

The wisdom of not operating on the strongly unwilling individual applies to psychotic patients also. If they refuse some general surgical operation there is usually no more chance of their doing well with it than if they are sane. Children, however, are treated differently. Johnnie, aged 7, may protest he does not want an urgent appendectomy. He may be forcibly anaesthetized against his strongest expressed wishes and physical resistance, the operation is done and he recovers nicely. It would take an unusual person, medical or lay, to maintain he should have been allowed to refuse although death was otherwise likely.

We can conclude that practical wisdom limits the frequency with which extra-cerebral operations are undertaken against the patient's wishes. Nevertheless, in some patients, who cannot decide for themselves, namely children, practice and feeling both hold that it is right to disregard the patient's wishes and wrong to accede to them where life or perhaps disability is at risk. Even John Stuart Mill so often quoted by those who argue against compulsory treatment, has the following to say about the right of the individual to take actions which might be harmful to his physical or moral health:

It is, perhaps, hardly necessary to say that this doctrine is meant to apply only to human beings in the full maturity of their faculties. We are not speaking of children, or of young persons below the age which the law may fix as that of manhood or womanhood. Those who are still in a state to require being taken care of by others must be protected against their own actions as well as against external injury.[1]

## The unique status of the brain

When procedures are considered which affect the brain an important fresh consideration arises. Even if the patient can consent we have to ask if it is right to alter, probably irreversibly, the structure of the organ on which the patient's volition and power to decide about treatment is based. If he cannot consent or refuses to agree to treatment is it justified at all to override his wishes in such a way that one may physically abolish the structural elements of his brain which have enabled him to sustain his objection? In either case, with or without consent, would we be in the position of chopping off the hands not of a thief but of a man who has created a work of art which we do not like, or perhaps an idol of which we disapprove?

Many psychiatrists past the age of 55 have no difficulty with one aspect of the question which is easily answered for them on the basis of a particular experience. Although the operation of frontal leucotomy was probably over-used, and sometimes crudely practised, there was a time when ECT was sometimes not sufficient to cure all cases of severe endogenous depression and antidepressant drugs were not available. During those years from approximately 1945 to 1959 a number of patients in chronic misery from prolonged depressive illness and the endogenous (or unipolar) type accepted leucotomy. In well-selected cases the cost–benefit ratio was such that in the view of patients, family, and physician the operation was usually held to have been a substantial success. Formal reports testify that the procedure, and especially some of its later modifications had a worthwhile cost–benefit ratio.[2–8]

Men and women who were ill had accepted that their structurally normal brains could be cut into, and had recovered, resuming happy and effective lives. Before operation the mood of many of them was appalling and their judgement of life and events was often made irrational by that mood. They had still perhaps enough command of their thoughts to be able to make a valid decision about whether they would have an operation, and the consequences were beneficial for many of them. Yet the brain was the organ of decision as well as the site of operation. In principle and in practice there should be no difficulty with the proposition that it is acceptable to operate on the brain to relieve emotional discomfort provided that the patient is able to make a valid decision about the risks and advantages and provided of course that those risks are small enough and advantages large enough.

A more specific argument could also be offered. The part of the brain subjected to treatment may not be involved in decision-making. Hence that portion is open to operation on the same terms as a limb or abdominal viscus. I find this argument unattractive however because profound disturbances of mood usually affect judgement and it may be specious to say that the site of operation does not have a function in the process of making decisions. It is better to rely on the presence of feelings and of reasoning which validate consent.

Similar considerations apply to the use of ECT for depressive illness which has not responded to medication and which is of the type known to be likely to respond to treatment. If the patient is willing, there is no ethical problem about giving it. Hazards to life are minimal, any impairment of brain function is minimal or temporary, it is doubtful if any recognizable structural disturbance results from well-conducted courses of treatment (up to 15 ECT in a course), and therapeutic results are frequently dramatic.

This situation, however, represents the optimal circumstances from physical manipulation of the brain. The anticipated cost–benefit ratio is highly favourable, the risk to life is low, significant personality change is not an issue, the patients are suffering intensely, and they can reasonably expect good results and minimal disadvantages. More difficult problems arise with patients who refuse treatment, with patients whose illness may pervert their judgement, with patients whose treatment may be recommended for the sake of others because of their aggressive or other unacceptable behaviour, and with patients who are constrained by circumstances such as imprisonment so that their consent or agreement to treatment may be felt to be forced upon them in some way by conditions which others impose. Some of these major problems require consideration with respect to each type of physical manipulation of the brain.

## Electroconvulsive therapy

The status of ECT has been assessed in the valuable report of the American Psychiatric Association Task Force on the subject.[9] ECT is now mainly used for severe depression in which suicide is a major risk.[10,11] Occasional other firm indications include some forms of schizophrenia[9] and mania.[9] The risk to life is very small,[12] as little as 1 in 28 000 treatments in one survey.[13] In five other reports the death-rate ranged from nil to 0.8 per cent of patients treated.[9] The treatment is both scientifically proved for depression and highly regarded clinically. Compared with drugs ECT is the more effective treatment for depression, particularly psychotic depression.[14,15,9] ECT compared with mock ECT is highly effective according to one report.[16] A double-blind controlled trial which did not show a good result from ECT in depression[17] has been criticized as inadequate[18] and also as allowing a possible favourable interpretation.[19] Others have favoured ECT moderately[20] or markedly.[21] Another blind trial[22] favoured ECT against placebo, although the treatment was complicated by the use of active medication in some of the subgroups. Costello,[23] who notes the failure of trials to be methodologically perfect, recognizes that ECT produces unique effects on memory which might not be mimicked by placebo so that a truly blind controlled trial may be impossible to achieve.

Controlled trials are perhaps not necessary if the long-known work of Cronholm and Ottoson[24] is accepted. They showed a quantitative relationship between the amount of epileptic discharge produced and the remission of depression. This is probably the strongest evidence available for the significance and effectiveness of the actual convulsion. More recently a consistent relationship has been shown between the dose–response ratio with ECT and the overall results.[25] This has long been observed by practising psychiatrists gauging the response to treatments and looking for the typical stepwise improvement in the successful case.

The main complication of ECT is a temporary impairment of memory. Objective tests of memory indicate that after a conventional course of treatment (six to twelve applications, either bilateral or unilateral) ECT produces no detectable permanent loss of memory for the one or two years preceding treatment and for a still earlier period in the patient's life.[9] Memory is lost for some events around the time of treatment. New learning is not detectably affected six to nine months after ECT.[26] Prospective work over seven months comparing patients having ECT and those not having it showed no relative impairment in the ECT group on an extensive battery of psychological tests.[27] However, two-thirds of patients who have had ECT, especially bilateral ECT, do tend to complain of greater memory difficulties prospectively. There is thus a suspicion that bilateral ECT may produce some, not currently demonstrable, memory impairment. Extended courses of 250 bilateral ECT have been shown to be associated with long-term memory impairment.[9] Three retrospective reports[9] found impairment on tests of memory and cognitive function but as the American Psychiatric Assocation Task Force report indicates, there are alternative possible explanations in terms of the patient's diagnosis or treatment which might have been factors in causing the memory damage. It seems reasonable to assume that after six months ECT will rarely cause more than mild memory difficulty, but that the risk will increase with successive treatments, particularly bilateral ones. Brain damage is known to result from anoxia, which may cause gliosis. There are no convincing reports of these phenomena after ECT which can be dissociated from the occurrence of anoxia due to more primitive methods of treatment than are currently available.

Attempts have been made to forbid or curtail the use of ECT, most notably in Alabama, where in state hospitals no less than three specialists and five others have been required to approve the treatment for a patient.[28] In California the law specifies that before ECT can be given to a voluntary patient, even in a private office, informed consent must be obtained from the patient according to a standard written consent form which shall be supplemented by the physician with appropriate information pertaining to the particular patient being treated. The information to be given includes 'significant risks ... especially noting the degree and duration of memory loss (including its irreversibility)' and that 'there exists a division of opinion as to the efficacy of the proposed treatment ....'[29] Thus 'informed consent', as specified by the law, has to include a scientifically unproved criticism of the treatment and a misleading allegation about its efficacy which disparages the available scientific information. ECT may not be given in California to minors (under the age of 12) and only in emergency, as a life-saving procedure and after three child psychiatrists have approved it, to those between 12 and 16 years. It requires a court hearing as well as the consent of the appropriate relative or guardian to give ECT to a patient of any sort who is not competent to give consent. Winslade *et al.*[30] comment on this to the effect that interposing laws between physicians and patients results in delays or denial of service while failing to resolve critical legal issues involving competence and consent.

Such political activity over a highly successful treatment owes little to knowledge of clinical practice and is also an interference with a patient's free choice of treatment. To some extent such measures are stimulated by claims that ECT is over-used for inappropriate conditions and to punish recalcitrant patients. Oddly enough they seem to have owed little if anything to the worst example of professional misuse of ECT, the practice of 'de-patterning' through multiple treatments, advocated by Cameron[31] but quickly ignored or rejected by almost all other psychiatrists.[32] These are matters for technical decision and competent professional practice and not for arbitrary legislative interference. The currency which such wild law-making gains is to some extent due to irresponsible journalism. Psychiatry is a common subject for the news media and physical manipulation of the brain of any sort is a dramatic and appealing topic. In contrast with these political activities and legislative interference it can be noted again that ECT has a very favourable cost–benefit ratio as demonstrated by the studies reported. When given unilaterally it involves only a very small risk of long-term memory impairment which for the great majority of people is of minimum importance compared with the suffering and hazards of depression.

Whether ECT should be given to patients against their will is a more troublesome issue. The problem was common but is now infrequent; yet occassionally it still arises with patients who have a severe (usually acute) depressive illness which is not adequately relieved by medication or other measures. A few such patients object strongly to having ECT. Some may have had it and developed fear of it even though it is beneficial. Some of these may yield to sympathetic persuasion. Others remain adamant. There may be a very serious risk of suicide or other self-damage, the distress of the patient is often severe or his or her judgement disordered. This situation can be compared with forcible appendectomy in children. The patient stands to gain far more than he will lose and cannot decide rationally for himself. The physician has an ethical commitment to attempt to relieve suffering and to prevent suicide. On the few occasions on which I have known it to be done the patient has continued to accept both ECT and a relationship with the physician long after the compulsory status has lapsed, the patient's family are grateful, and there is no recrimination. It seems right to do so, and a legal system which fails to provide the patient with the opportunity to have his suffering relieved by such an effective available measure could be regarded as lacking in humane concern.

The American Psychiatric Association Task Force Report[9] allows the possibility of treatment in circumstances where the patient is incompetent but objects to treatment, and indicates that in some jurisdictions a court procedure may be required. It emphasizes rightly that the guiding principle should be good overall medical management with a minimum of delay and no unnecessary restrictions on the exercise of good clinical judgement. Edwards and Flaherty[33] in New South Wales, Australia, clearly imply that ECT may be given despite a patient's refusal but subject to review procedures.

The practical qualifications in this context are important. The diagnosis and alternative avenues of treatment should be double checked by independent physicians. Perhaps the patient does not respond because there is a dementia or physical illness underlying the depression and the treatment is less appropriate than might be thought. The agreement of the nearest relative is essential, not only on legal grounds as in some jurisdictions but also on ethical grounds. If those who are likely to be most concerned for the patient cannot also approve the treatment there should be doubts as to its justification. The physician should also be satisfied that even if he has the support of the patient's family that support is given out of love and not, as may happen, out of antagonism. We should be sure also that he is not himself responding out of irritation or frustration or other illegitimate motives. But granted that these conditions have been met and that the physician is supported by the law of the jurisdiction in which he practises it is humane and appropriate to insist on effective treatment being provided. Not to give it could be regarded as negligence.

In my view the decision to give treatment against a patient's wishes should always be validated or confirmed at least by a fully independent professional opinion.

The position adopted in this discussion is paternalistic. However, the paternalism is shared with colleagues, and just as to have good parents is valuable for children so to have good fatherly (or motherly) physicians can be valuable to psychotic patients. It is not necessary to reject paternalism totally because it is sometimes confused with authoritarianism. Some readers, particularly in the United States, may feel that a contractual relationship which relies on an ethic of mutual equality offers a better position than the above. My personal view is that the patient has more to gain from a 'scrupulous' and responsible fiduciary approach in which the professional does not take personal advantage of his inevitably greater knowledge of the illness and its treatment. Since physicians are expected anyhow to observe fiduciary self-restraint it seems mistaken to suppose that they are not influential in the outcome of the patient's decision.

Apart from depressive illness ECT is rarely needed today in psychiatry. A few excited manic or catatonic schizophrenic patients may require it briefly and the considerations which apply are essentially the same as those which relate to acute severe depression in which the patient directly refuses treatment and protests at being given an anaesthetic for the purpose. More often the question of consent is a paper issue. The patient will not sign a form, or is not competent to do so, but accepts preparation for treatment, fasts as required before the anaesthetic, knows that he or she will receive electricity to the brain, and receives the anaesthetic injection before treatment without complaint. As with depression, the doctor who will not proceed to give ECT after all the above qualifications are satisfied could be regarded as negligent morally, even if not legally.

## Definition of psychosurgery

The main neurosurgical procedures which have been advocated for psychiatric illness are leucotomy and amygdalotomy, the former for the control of depression as already discussed, the latter for control of aggressive behaviour whether against the self or others. Occasionally, in Germany, operations on the hypothalamus have also been proposed for certain sexual offenders.

Neurosurgical operations undertaken on putatively healthy tissue to relieve psychiatric symptoms are generally called psychosurgery. The definition requires some care. A recent World Health Organization booklet[34] defines psychosurgery as 'the selective surgical removal or destruction ... of nerve pathways with a view to influencing behaviour'. Bridges and Bartlett[7] point out that this definition is incorrect because most modern psychosurgery is concerned with the treatment of severe intractable affective illnesses without any intended effect on behaviour at all, although of course behaviour may alter where it is directly influenced by the illness. Unfortunately, the United States Department of Health Education and Welfare has taken the same view as the WHO booklet and has defined psychosurgery as: (1) surgery on the normal brain tissue of an individual not suffering from physical disease for the purpose of changing or controlling behaviour or (2) surgery on diseased brain tissue of an individual if the sole object of the surgery is to control change or affect behavioural disturbances.[35] As Bridges and Bartlett state[7] 'a better definition of contemporary psychosurgery is: the surgical treatment of certain psychiatric illnesses by means of localized lesions placed in specific cerebral sites'. This matter is important as will be seen since the incorrect definition has served as a basis for unreasonable conclusions which are likely to affect the availability within the United States of certain valuable operations.

## Operations for disturbed affect

Psychosurgery as we know it began with an operation on the frontal lobes proposed by Egas Moniz, a neurologist, and undertaken by a surgeon, Almeida Lima on 12 November 1935.[36] However Burckhardt,[37] the medical superintendent of a small Swiss mental hospital, actually undertook operations on the intact brain in 1890, removing areas of cerebral cortex from six patients.[4] Freeman and Watts[38] pioneered the work in the English-speaking world operating on their first case in 1936, and thousands of patients were leucotomized in the 1940s and 1950s. At the start of that time, according to Dax:[4]

Two aspects have to be mentioned to put the popularity of the operation in perspective. First, patients were much more disturbed than we know them now and the nursing staff was fewer in numbers. Barbiturates were fairly new and sodium amylobarbitone was greeted as the new wonder drug ... Padded rooms were in frequent use, incontinence of urine and faeces was rife and many patients wore strong canvas clothing. Some were extremely violent and tube feeding was frequent. Depressives on suicide caution cards were stripped of their possessions, spoon fed and marched from one room to another. There was sentinel walking, echolalia, flexibilitas cerea and frequent stupor, with constant danger from the catatonics.

Personality changes from the operation were of course recognized.

The results of leucotomy and its modifications are today somewhat thoughtlessly despised. We should note however that it was introduced against a background of relevant neurophysiological and psychological information and the representative results obtained in England between 1942 and 1954 in 10 365 patients[3] showed that even with chronic schizophrenia and the old standard operation, 41 per cent approximately, were 'at least greatly improved' and only 3 per cent had marked deleterious changes of personality; 2 per cent were worse, mortality related to the procedure was 4 per cent, and the incidence of chronic epilepsy was 1 per cent. The availability of antidepressants and phenothiazines together with ECT and improvements also in the environmental and psychological management of patients made leucotomy redundant for most patients. Nevertheless it was established as an effective treatment, particularly for affective illness. However, more sophisticated techniques have produced good results for anxiety (94 per cent), obsessional symptoms (49 per cent), and depression (79 per cent) in the few patients who still require operation, without submitting them to high rates of morbidity. For example, with stereotactic procedures, operative mortality has been reduced to 0.2 per cent, chronic epilepsy to 0.6 per cent, postoperative intellectual impairment to 0.6 per cent, and marked personality change to 0.5 per cent.[39] These good results are confirmed in reports from independent and reliable studies.[5,6]

An even more advantageous technique was developed and practised by Crow and his colleagues, where the implantation of indwelling electrodes was accompanied by stimulation and subsequent ablation of successive small amounts of cortex so that any bad effects on personality could be almost totally prevented.[8]

The number of operations done in Britain is not large. Between 1974 to 1976 the rate was 3.4 per million population aged over 15, or 431 operations.[40] In the 240 patients operated on in the three most active units 21 (8 per cent) were for repeated violence whilst 85 per cent were for mood disorders. Thus the bulk of psychosurgery was undertaken for illnesses in which the patients' symptoms were primarily subjective and consent was quite likely to be informed and valid.

An enquiry in the United States[41] found that about 400 procedures, meeting the definition of psychosurgery which the Department of Health Education and Welfare has adopted, were being performed annually in the United States. No significant psychological deficits were attributable to the psychosurgery in the patients evaluated and the treatment was efficacious in more than half of the cases studied. The data presented did not indicate that the procedure had been used for social control (as had been alleged) or that the procedure had been applied disproportionately to minority or disadvantaged populations (as had been noisily claimed). Indeed from correspondence with the most active psychosurgeons in the United States, it was found that out of a combined total of 600 patients, one was Black, two were Oriental Americans, and six were Hispanic Americans. Seven operations were reported to have been performed on children since 1970 and three prisoners underwent psychosurgery in 1972. Most psychosurgery patients were middle-class individuals referred to neurosurgeons by psychiatrists and were about equally divided between males and females. The National Commission for the Protection of Human Subjects of Biomedical and Behavioural Research in the United States found that psychosurgical treatment constituted a minuscule proportion (estimated to be less than 0.001 per cent) of psychiatric treatment in general.

Hussain *et al.*[42] have shown, even very recently, in a follow-up of all cases from a defined urban population, that psychosurgery still provides valuable results for a selected population, particularly in those with depression, agoraphobia, obsessional neurosis, and certain aspects of schizophrenia.

From the evidence reviewed it appears that at least some forms of psychosurgery are accepted procedures in the sense that many different physicians refer patients for these treatments at the hands of particular surgeons, recognize appropriate indications for the referral, and are able to anticipate the probable outcome with considerable accuracy. Thus in their opinion the treatment is 'accepted' on normal clinical grounds. It is therefore surprising that the United States National Commission cited came to the conclusion that 'the procedure' did not constitute 'accepted practice', seeming to confound indiscriminately a variety of different operations. The conclusion seems to have more to do with the political and social atmosphere in which the Commission worked than with the merits of the case, even though the Commission was regarded as having produced a surprisingly favourable report in respect of psychosurgery.

This is not to say that some psychosurgical procedures are not experimental—but rather that certain operations are indeed as well proved as many other valid medical or surgical procedures. Stereotactic subcaudate tractotomy[2] and varieties of limbic tractotomy[4] and Crow's procedure[8] surely constitute accepted forms of treatment, as probably do a number of other modified leucotomy operations.

## Operations for pain

Although cerebral operations have been carried out to alleviate pain and have been briefly mentioned they do not currently present an issue because they are almost never indicated and because, so far as I know, they were always done with consent. Pain may be due either to physical lesions or to an emotional state.[43–45] It is accordingly defined as 'an unpleasant sensory and emotional experience which we primarily associate with tissue damage and describe in terms of tissue damage'.[46] Whatever the cause the experience is subjectively the same, an unpleasant one in the body. Leucotomy for pain when done in the presence of an appropriate psychiatric illness such as depression was successful. However in the last 25 years in regular work with patients with pain, I have only seen one who seemed to require an operation for pain and depression and he had a stereotactic subcaudate operation. This modified version of leucotomy was used primarily because he was depressed. When depression was not the main cause, leucotomy for pain only worked if the lesion was so large as to damage the personality.[41,47]

Thalamic and mesencephalic operations have also been undertaken for pain but were largely unsatisfactory.[48] These were for patients presumed to have, usually, peripheral lesions causing pain. Hypophysectomy is currently undertaken with benefit for pain from carcinoma,[49] but no one talks of this organ as sacrosanct. Thus operations for pain can either be assimilated to the argument concerning those for affective disorder or are not in significant use. However should a new operation be discovered for pain due to peripheral lesions, or central lesions, it is hard to imagine anyone saying that they should not be done. This suggests that the wrong sort of distinction is made between psychiatric illness and physical illness, viz. that it is all right to operate on the brain for a physical illness arising elsewhere in the body, but not for a psychological disturbance. This seems unfair not only to the patient who has pain for psychological reasons but also to all those patients who might benefit psychiatrically from brain surgery.

## Operations for aggression

The human brain, as much as the animal, has highly developed anatomical and physiological systems which subserve self-protective defensive and aggressive responses and are accompanied by emotional changes. It may also, like some animal brains, provide for cool predatory aggression.[50] Most human aggression is affect-laden. When it is not it is probably unpredictable by anybody other than the aggressor. Much human aggression also can be clearly linked to environmental triggers, to cultural patterns, to childhood experiences, and to a variety of social and psychological factors. Even so, the prediction of aggressive behaviour is extremely difficult and for clinical purposes often very unreliable, despite the fact that better prediction would be of enormous value for judges in passing sentence and in connection with offenders seeking parole. Nevertheless there are a few individuals who engage in violent repeated aggressive behaviour against themselves or others. As a result of animal work and from operations on patients who had temporal lobe lesions (often with epilepsy) it became evident that aggressive behaviour might be modified by means of surgical lesions, particularly in the region of the amygdala. Such stereotactic operations have been undertaken in retarded patients,[51] on children who are overactive and self-damaging,[52] and on violent offenders.[53-55] As the earlier discussion indicated the number of operations in this group is small in Britain and the United States and the operations are comparably few in the rest of the English-speaking world. Several hundred operations on children in India apparently required consent not only from the children's parents but from grandparents as well.

The results of such operations have been reviewed by Kiloh.[51,55] Some apparently striking successes have been obtained,[51,56] although the results are not nearly as good overall as those for the latest development of leucotomy. Nevertheless, Kiloh points out that these stereotactic procedures appear to be relatively safe and free from undesirable sequelae. The success rate is 50–75 per cent at 2 years or more and the successful cases become more effective and indeed happier human beings. Perhaps, given time, the results might become as good as those for the modern developments of leucotomy, but the opportunities for steady development of the technique in suitable patients are increasingly circumscribed because of public concern expressed by a variety of groups. The United States Department of Health Education and Welfare[35] points out that the National Commission for the Protection of Human Subjects of Biomedical and Behavioural Research was called into being after 'widespread expression of public and congressional concern ... including allegations that these procedures were ... being used for "social control" of dissidents and violence prone individuals and ... were performed disproportionately on members of minority populations'. In the event the results already quoted indicate a truly enormous disproportion between the outcry and the facts. It is doubtful that any operation was done for 'social control' and minorities were under-represented, as already described. The main issues which remain are whether the social considerations form an invalid part of some decision to operate, and whether operations may be done without consent.

The first of these questions relates mainly to psychosurgery for violence. The other two relate both to surgery for mood states and to that for violence.

## Social definition of disease

For those who like it, as well as for those who do not approve, it is still a fact that the attribution of the word 'disease' to a set of circumstances is determined in many cases by social factors. Fabrega[57] has described how social behaviour is used as a criterion of disease in different societies. Conventionally doctors give disease labels to 'conditions' about which they are consulted. Those 'conditions' may be organic changes or disabilities (for example, pneumonia), psychotic disorders with or without organic causes (delirium, mania), and neurotic and behavioural disorders (phobic anxiety, enuresis, sociopathic personality). Some conditions such as mania or depression may be 'spontaneous' or induced by organic change (steroid treatment, influenza, depression with dementia). The same phenomenology in mania or depression may have an overt organic cause or none. Sociopathic behaviour may perhaps be 'constitutional'-XYY linked, induced by social conditions or childhood ill-treatment or a consequence of epidemic encephalitis or head injury. Without arguing the details of these particular instances it seems to me and perhaps to most psychiatrists that disease patterns are determined at least in part by social expectations combined with biological knowledge, and that biological knowledge is not the sole criterion. More precise definitions of disease (or health) have long eluded agreement. Physicians see themselves as trained to recognize 'diseases' or 'conditions'. If a physician has something to offer in the treatment or care of a 'condition' he is normally willing to provide his professional services. These may be along the lines of drug or other physical treatment, psychological treatment, and even manipulation of the environment. For example, patients with peptic ulcer or conversion hysteria alike might receive a recommendation for discharge from the armed services, and so on.

All this need not stop the physician from limiting his functions to those which are 'medical' and refusing to be involved primarily as an agent to deal with social issues.[58] The physician who adheres to the traditional role will help a patient to get better social conditions but will not *qua* physician seek automatically to change the conditions. In some cases (cholera due to contaminated water) his view of a social arrangement will be deservedly accepted. In others (the advisability of conscription or imprisonment in general) he is wise if he is content only to exercise the role of an ordinary citizen.

This being said, let us consider the situation of the physician and of the patients who are recommended for treatment of disorders of thought, mood, or behaviour. The disorder may be recognizable to the physician as a syndrome with or without biological cause. There is no reason why he may not offer to treat it if that is what the patient asks. If it is not what the patient asks, the doctor may then determine if the failure to ask arises from a failure of reason. If so he might treat the patient who does not ask, but does not oppose, provided that the proper representatives of the patient (family, guardian, etc.) request him to do so and do not have a disproportionately selfish interest in the treatment. (The wife of a depressed man once asked me if leucotomy would help the impotence from which he had suffered even before depression supervened.)

If the patient is clearly opposed to treatment then the physician will only rarely if ever undertake it. Those special circumstances where this might happen in relation to the brain will be discussed shortly. At this point it is sufficient to have indicated that I take the following position: our notion of illness is partly biological and partly social; treatment by physicians is on the 'medical model'; we may recognize and sometimes act in relationship to social causes but only within the limits of our agreed function as physicians, which is to diagnose and promote cure where we can, and to advise on how individuals and society may take the responsibility for prevention and control. It is from this standpoint that I consider the ethics of psychosurgery.

## Brain surgery with consent

Relevant considerations for physicians include as always the cost–benefit ratio. Another consideration is more 'ethical' in nature: whether it is right to destroy putatively normal brain tissue in order to relieve emotional distress. Edgar[59] points out that there is no objection to operating on the brain as such, e.g. to remove a tumour. He argues that in the face of evidence that a person's aberrant behaviour resulted from a tumour we would not reject operation because it might be at a brain site related to personality or the 'will'. Thus we are prepared to operate on the brain in circumstances where there is also evidence of structural change and we accept possible effects from this upon personality. If individuals who are able to give free and valid consent wish to accept a surgical procedure which offers worthwhile benefit in the absence of overt pathology there is no reason why they should not do so, and it curtails their freedom if we refuse permission. General surgery also is not confined to abnormal tissue. Legs may be shortened, ears or noses reshaped (although healthy). Normal organs are removed—as in adrenalectomy for carcinoma or hypophy-sectomy for severe pain.[49] Also, operations have been performed on putatively normal brain tissue in order to relieve pain attributed to organic disturbances elsewhere in the body.[48] Although it is sometimes technically difficult to do useful surgery on the substance of the brain there should be no objection to brain surgery for psychological disorder solely because the brain controls thought, feeling, judgement, and personality. Logically it is the most appropriate site of intervention in a consenting individual. But it will be very necessary to consider in due course what constitutes consent or valid agreement.

The relevance of brain pathology is a practical issue. Mark and Ervin[56] and Mark and Neville[60] rejected psychosurgery for aggression except in patients with brain lesions. They seem to accept in principle that psycho-surgery for aggression might be allowed without physical pathology but they rule it out in the short run. Physical pathology may be one source of evidence that intervention at a particular site is 'good medicine', particularly if (a) the patient's brain is damaged in a particular way, (b) most people who have such damage behave aberrantly as does the patient, and (c) this operation has worked to change that behaviour in other patients.[56] However, to limit brain operations for psychological illness to cases which only have brain pathology would make for a number of difficulties.

If a patient is distressed and regretful over his aggressive behaviour why should he not have the opportunity to receive surgical help, assuming it to be effective, just as much as a man with phobias or a woman with chronic pain due to an emotional disorder or to a lesion outside the brain? There are also problems in defining pathology broadly and yet perhaps it should be so defined. While EEG abnormality is less easily related to disease than histological change it could have valid associations with pathophysiological disturbances in the temporal lobes. Except in the dementias, relevant chemical abnormality cannot be shown by present techniques in any specific brain area in life but may well be significant. Micro-anatomical differences will not be found before surgery.

Brain pathology alone is too restrictive and uncertain as a criterion in consenting patients. Hostile public attitudes to psychosurgery have presumably contributed to a reduction in the opportunities for it to be provided. In Ontario a detained patient, even if competent, cannot consent to psychosurgery (Mental Health Act 1980, revised 1987, Section 35). If he did so, it would be difficult to arrange, since no one seems to be undertaking it in the province or elsewhere in Canada.

In Britain, unfortunately, the attempt to control medical decisions has also extended to leucotomy, to the detriment of work at a highly respected specialist centre with exceptional experience. The Mental Health Act 1983, Section 57, empowers a Mental Health Act Commission, under a non-medical chairman, to supervise psychosurgery. The patient, his general practitioner, his regular psychiatrist, and the specialist to whom he is referred may all concur in a decision for surgery. A separate medical commissioner and two lay persons are required also to determine the validity of the patient's consent, but carry no responsibility for the further care of the patient. If he wants such help the patient has to accept an intrusion of a person who has no therapeutic role, and his request may still be denied by this 'independent medical commissioner'. Patients considering treatment of this type have to make difficult decisions in which discretion and careful weighting of feelings are required from their advisers. A committee procedure and legal process are likely to help less than they hinder. Suicide followed one such refusal.[61-65] It is difficult to regard these arrangements as anything but a violation of the patient's rights, brought on by a combination of anti-psychiatry and bumbling officialdom. The numbers affected are few, but the violation of principle remains troublesome.

## Brain surgery without consent

If it is humane and proper to undertake appropriate surgery to change the mood or behaviour in individuals who can make an appropriate judgement and therefore give valid consent would it not also be humane and morally unobjectionable to operate for the same purposes on individuals who cannot give consent because they are too disordered to be able to approve the situation? In principle the answer appears to be yes. Special precautions are of course required in such circumstances. It should first be abundantly clear that the patient really is not decided or able to decide about the matter. Any hint of reluctance, perhaps expressed in behaviour like eating a meal before an anaesthetic is due, or failing to co-operate with preliminary procedures, should be taken as an indication that consent is refused even though the patient does not explicitly put the matter into words. The decision should also obviously be made by more than one person, and should be subject to review and special supervision. As usual, it would require the approval of the next of kin. Perhaps too it should be agreed upon by some independent non-medical professionals. I do not think such people would be in a better position to judge than experienced physicians. But the need to present a case before intelligent disinterested parties should provide a helpful safeguard. In particular, those parties should establish that dependence upon the doctor's goodwill is not the patient's reason for consent. Some of these conditions are essential, some of them optional. Given that enough of them were satisfied it should be acceptable to treat with brain surgery those patients who do not consent but who do not explicitly or implicitly refuse. If neither the patient's indifference nor his consent can be established then the case has to be seen as one in which consent is refused.

In my view it is unacceptable to perform leucotomy or other brain surgery on patients who are specifically or implicitly unwilling. This differs from the view offered on ECT. The first reason is the minimal or absent risk of permanent detrimental physical brain changes with ECT compared with the potential risk of such changes with surgery. It is unacceptable to enforce even such infrequent hazards as those of some brain surgery upon unwilling patients in the present context. The second reason is more fundamental. Even if there were no deleterious changes possible with surgery or if the manipulation were not a physical one, it seems wrong to impose potentially permanent changes in a man's mental state against his wishes. In case this should seem to be at variance with my willingness to recommend occasional ECT to patients who refuse it, I would point out that the effects of ECT are essentially temporary and may be required as emergency even life-saving treatment. Although psychosurgery may also be life-saving it is inconceivable that its effects could usually be classed only as temporary (even though they are sometimes not sufficiently sustained to be therapeutically worth while). Thirdly, while the giving of ECT compulsorily also violates a man's mental state against his wishes it is done in conditions which give him later opportunities to protest at what was done. It does not carry any risk of permanently changing his original personality and basis of judgement or take away his opportunity later to seek redress for unfair treatment.

It may be the case that legal and social systems do sanction interventions on men's minds which change them permanently. All reformatories, correctional institutions, and penal establishments usually have some such aims for unwilling participants but they are not founded upon medical considerations. If we are considering procedures which depend on medical expertise the refusal of consent is a fundamental objection to all procedures which aim at irreversible personality change. If this position is accepted it should safeguard against the appalling possibility that procedures of psychosurgery would be used on unwilling political prisoners.

There remains an important issue to do with consent, namely that of men or women under legal constraints in prison or comparable institutions. Mark and Neville[60] argue strongly that no one in prison or prison-like conditions should receive psychosurgery. Against this view a hypothetical case may be postulated of a criminal who develops a depressive illness for which in freedom he would have a neurosurgical procedure. Provided that the conditions of his imprisonment and the length of his sentence have no bearing on the treatment recommended, which could, say, be a modified leucotomy, the question of whether he should have an operation should be decided on the same basis as for a free individual. However, psychosurgical operations suggested for prisoners sometimes do not satisfy these requirements. They are in any case few in number. It is likely that there is a ratio of a score of articles on the topic to every operated prison case. But what these operations tend to do is offer a treatment for aggressive behaviour; treatment which may change the personality as well as simply reduce the frequency of aggressive antisocial actions. Let us assume for the moment that such treatments are effective. The question then arises whether it is right to offer them to men in detention, and on what conditions. Some patients engage in self-mutilation and other harmful activities against their own persons; some of them may be glad to accept an operation which relieves them of this behaviour. If in frustration one day we are engaged in banging our head against a wall we may welcome some assistance which relieves us of the inclination to do so. Operation in those cases may be as valid and as justified as for depressive illness.

Still other patients might feel a deep regret at behaviour which they do not manage to control but which is harmful to others—say repeated assaults or fighting. One such man sought treatment for his aggressive outbursts by attending a hospital out-patient department. An oral phenothiazine was included in his treatment and was partly helpful, but supposing that surgery gave the best chance of success and that the risks were acceptable, would it have been justified to operate on his brain? A conditional yes seems the correct answer. If so, perhaps the treatment should be available also for prisoners with the same motives and wishes. Again the right answer appears to be in the affirmative. However, prisoners present great difficulties.

At this point let us consider only established procedures with known benefits and hazards. The problem is whether the prisoner is giving his consent not because he wants to change his behaviour and avoid harming others in future but because he wishes to alter the terms of his sentence. It can be presumed that a man who is at the end of a long sentence or only has a short sentence of less than 12 months will not be unduly influenced by the hope of early release. A prisoner with a longer sentence might well assent to operation for just that reason, that he wishes to shorten the sentence. While his consent might not be called free it might be valid in his own interests. But we are reluctant to accept that an external constraint should be influential in such a decision. In the one case the decision may be correct. But since constraints from the civil authority can be varied then a variety of new constraints might appear (perhaps with a new revolutionary government?) and psychiatrists would be asking surgeons to take on new cases because of new political changes. The thought is anathema. It is even not too far-fetched to imagine a society where imprisoned psychiatrists might be invited to accept some intracerebral lesion which would change their responses so that they would become more accepting of the tenets of the government of the day. Some of our colleagues have been tortured in Argentina, or vanished without a trace. Doctors Gluzman and Koryagin suffered in the Soviet prison system because of their adherence to medical ethics (see Chapter 24). Less resolute physicians (and who can say he would be a hero like one of these two?) might prefer the option of surgical treatment. It seems hard to assent to any brain operations under conditions of constraint.

In the United States a famous court action was brought to prevent psychosurgery on a prisoner.[66] The man in prison for 18 years for murder (followed by necrophilia), had satisfied an 'Informed Consent' Review Committee consisting of a law professor, a priest, and an accountant that he wanted the operation. Ironically the attorney who brought the case 'Kaimowitz representing himself and certain individual members of the Medical Committee for Human Rights on behalf of John Doe', had never consulted the prisoner. The lawyer appointed by the court to represent the man thought that he desperately wanted the operation,[67] but proved to the court's satisfaction that the man was held unconstitutionally as a prisoner. Despite the fact that the prisoner was therefore freed, the hearing continued on the question as to whether a prisoner could give free informed consent to psychosurgery and it was held that he could not. It has been argued[68] that this conclusion violates the right to treatment, so that it seems unlikely that the Kaimowitz case represents a definite conclusion in United States law.

The issue may be hard for American lawyers or judges. It also presents a problem in practical ethics for doctors. It seems that physicians, lawyer, priest, and accountant all believed, probably correctly, that the prisoner wanted the operation. But after he was released, he changed his mind. Burt's account[67] gives clear reason to think that the circumstances of imprisonment and medical surveillance at least contributed to the prisoner's consent without any attempt being made by physicians to press the prisoner to agree.

In the light of this finding it can be argued that no prisoner's consent should be accepted for psychosurgery related to the type of behaviour which has caused his imprisonment. That however might be called double jeopardy. It seems desirable to insist that the attempt should be made to avoid prisoners accepting operation with a view to facilitating release. In the case in question that condition was not apparently fulfilled.

Some arrangements might however be proposed which would allow long-term non-political prisoners (very strictly defined) to obtain treatment for repetitive violence or chronic maladjustment. One necessary condition could be that the prisoner is clearly aware that no immediate change in his sentence is to be expected. Only long-term evidence of change over, say, a minimum of three years, would be acceptable evidence leading to a reduction of the sentence. Such change should be equally helpful to him if it occurred in the absence of operation. It would be up to him to decide whether he wanted the procedure to facilitate his own efforts. Secondly, a substantial independent review of the proposal would be required for each case, involving at least three expert psychiatrists and including preferably one from outside the country, and a substantial lay review body as well, drawn similarly from beyond the institution. A hearing in open court could also be required. The consent of the prisoner and his relations would be obligatory and the review personnel would be specially required to assess if the individual's consent was reasonable and consistently held and was not dependent on the hope of release. With such safeguards very few operations might be done, but it is conceivable that they would be worthwhile for the patients. Prisoners too should have 'the right to treatment'. It is of course unthinkable that anyone who did not give consent should have psychosurgery.

On the basis that minors, prisoners, and civilly committed mental patients should not be denied the benefits of treatment the United States National Commission accepted that psychosurgery should be allowed for them provided their rights were rigorously guarded.[35] The American Psychiatric Association largely supported the Commission's report but opposed psychosurgery on children because of insufficient data and approved it only for prisoners if its indications were unrelated to criminal behaviour. The United States Department of Health Education and Welfare[41] decided not to fund psychosurgery research or treatment by any of the institutions which it supports, for any of these three groups. This action going against the recommendations of both the National Commission and the American Psychiatric Association seems to be like the Commission's conclusion that psychosurgery was not 'an accepted procedure' in that it is perhaps related more to considerations of public noise than to the facts or merits of the matter.

In regard to children and the mentally incompetent I suggest that stringent procedures, similar to some of those outlined for prisoners, might be used to establish that: (1) the procedure offered worthwhile benefit and appeared to be in the patient's interest, and (2) consent was not refused implicitly.

To sum up this discussion I have argued that psychosurgery should never be forced but it might be done with non-competent individuals or prisoners subject to stringent safeguards, some of which have been considered.

## Depth electrical stimulation

Electrical stimulation offers similar problems to the longer-established forms of surgery, and one additional problem. The similar problems arise because electrical stimulation is not without risk of permanent harm. Any electrode or sheaf of inserted electrodes might rupture a vessel. Indwelling electrodes, further, can give rise to a fibrotic reaction—particularly when used for repeated electrical stimulation. These risks require assessment in relation to any electrical stimulation procedures; those of a haemorrhage are perhaps minimal but those of fibrotic reactions may be greater than is currently anticipated. It is known that implanted electrodes used for dorsal column stimulation for the treatment of chronic pain have given rise to fibrotic reactions. Intra-cerebral electrodes, no matter how sophisticated, might do something like this, or promote some other form of continuing damage to cells. Nevertheless both Heath[69] and Crow[8] appear satisfied that this technology is minimally damaging, and it is not intended for permanent implantation. At present only occasional operations with indwelling electrodes in the brain have been done for pain[70] and they do not appear to be very successful.[71] They have been used for chronic pain from peripheral lesions. As with the unsuccessful thalamic operations it is hard to imagine moral objections being raised to these treatments in the event of their being successful.

The additional problem is that indwelling electrodes may provide the possibility of pleasurable self-stimulation. This is not often the case but if it were, someone would be sure to want to stop it. At the present time there are patients who have been given batteries which they can turn on and off and which deliver stimulation by the implanted electrodes. When this is done with animals which are taught to do certain acts, for example lever-pressing, to initiate self-stimulation the animals may work tremendously hard to stimulate themselves, and do little else.[72] Some neglect food, water, and natural functions. For a further account see Valenstein,[73] who indicates that such phenomena are rare and difficult to reproduce in both animals and man consistently.

Apart from these practical considerations there is a theoretical issue. Medicine has so far aimed mostly at correcting abnormalities, not at obtaining a subjective Elysium. Self-stimulation which achieves the latter would be socially objectionable. Should we take heed of such a consideration? Perhaps not in principle if we accept the individual's right to self-determination. Again, in practice the operation would probably not get far since it would be biologically disadvantageous, leading to failure of reproduction as well as death. There appear sufficient reasons for physicians not to wish to support the achievement of super-normality by self-stimulation.

There are hypothetical situations in which surgery and especially self-stimulation could make people function more actively and with greater success. Perhaps intelligence could be improved. Mark and Neville[60] point out that this makes medical men authorities on what constitutes the good life. A case could be argued for that conclusion without suggesting that we are the sole authorities. But the profession is certainly neither ready nor prepared to assume such a role.

The dangerous attraction of electrical stimulation of the brain is that in the short term it offers possibilities of scientific investigation of the brain in patients with psychoses and perhaps some others by means of recordings taken from the electrodes which are used for stimulation. We would clearly like to know more about the patterns of activity in different parts of the human brain in all sorts of psychiatric conditions—and even non-medical circumstances. This motive is not a legitimate guide to the ethical management of patients. The justifiable attraction of electrical stimulation of the brain is that firstly, it offers much improved chances of precision in placing lesions, and secondly, it allows graded ablation of tissue. After stimulation in a given part, tissue between the electrodes may be destroyed by increasing the current used. Only small amounts of tissue need be destroyed at one time. Careful, painstaking steps can be taken to secure relief without personality change. Such advantages are enormously attractive. Despite the problems outlined, this is presumably the optimum way to conduct psychosurgical ablations.

## Surgical innovation

In the discussion so far reference has been made to operations where established knowledge is fairly extensive and to hypothetical situations where such extensive knowledge was postulated. Most controversy attaches to innovations in treatment. This is a difficult subject in any branch of medicine. Is the first patient to have a particular operation being treated ethically? If not, how can any operation be developed? Medicine is not alone with this problem. Everyone with a legal difficulty deserves an experienced barrister. If so, how can a new barrister be morally justified in getting experience?

It is clear that new procedures should not ordinarily be introduced on those who cannot give valid consent. This might be qualified to the extent that the new procedure is reasonably supposed to be less risky than any other established treatment. A coronary patient may be able to give valid consent for a new type of graft if it is explained to him. But can any psychiatric patient needing treatment for his mood, thoughts, or behaviour give valid consent to an unproved treatment? The answer is uncertain but it is equally uncertain whether a patient with advanced carcinoma can make a free valid judgement on some last-chance new procedure. Some, for example Mark and Neville,[60] recommend the criterion of physical pathology. In the development of techniques this is plainly sound. If we start from a base where verification of the facts is relatively easy, we have more chance of finding beneficial new procedures with least risk to patients.

However neither psychiatric nor carcinoma patients should be excluded from the possibility of being helped by an unproved treatment which has reasonable scientific justification. Innovations which carry hazards should therefore be allowed with due precaution for both of these groups. Innovations in treatment are now subject to increasing control with special review mechanisms. It seems best to argue that they may occur in consenting free patients without physical disease, that the control procedures will be maintained and that they will not be done in prisons or on patients who are not competent in the usual sense: but if an innovation were suggested which could only help prisoners or the incompetent this conclusion might need to be revised.

## Some practical issues

The theoretical issues have been considered so far, with reference to practical problems as required. We need next to discuss briefly some practical points. In all the procedures examined the outstanding precondition is that they should be capable of yielding the patient worthwhile benefit at minimal risk and that the benefit should be significantly greater than that from alternative less traumatic procedures. By this criterion ECT is outstandingly attractive. Its morbidity rate is much less than that of antidepressant drugs (with perhaps one exception, flupenthixol, which is not yet approved as such in North America). It causes some transient memory disturbance, very few fatalities, and little else in the way of trouble. In contrast, antidepressant drugs almost invariably cause discomfort (dry mouth, constipation, blurred vision), quite often cause hypotensive faint feelings, and can provoke a variety of significant illnesses such as prolapsed haemorrhoids from constipation, epileptic fits, retention of urine, and, theoretically, glaucoma. The cardiotoxic effects of the antidepressants probably also cause fatalities several times more frequently than does ECT.

Although leucotomy-like procedures are rarely performed in North

America and Britain, the modified versions have high standing, as has been described, because of their lack of morbidity and for their therapeutic success.[2,5,8] They still have a proper place in psychiatric treatment.

Among the major psychosurgical procedures amygdalotomy or amygdalectomy and hypothalamic operations[74,75] are less well-established. This is not only because of opposition to treating behaviour rather than distress, it is also because knowledge of their benefits and risks has been available for a much shorter time and the technology of investigation (criteria for selection of patients and for assessment of results, etc.) is still embryonic. There is further an inherent difficulty in assessing aggression compared with depression or obsessional neurosis or schizophrenia because the manifestations of aggression are frequently intermittent. Some patients are continuously assaultive of themselves or others. But major assaults are liable to be committed by individuals who have 'over-controlled hostility'.[76,77] Discussions in the literature[78] indicate that the prediction of dangerousness is handicapped by the infrequency with which dangerous behaviour occurs. Cocozza and Steadman[78] with a particular population developed a score which correctly predicted dangerous behaviour by eleven patients and no dangerous behaviour by three who did behave dangerously. Twenty-five were predicted by the score as dangerous and did not prove to be so. Thus the score produced statistically significant results (P <0.001) which were however clinically insufficient. The best conclusion we can draw is that operations for aggression should be developed first for those who are frequently assaultive, so that a time-span of one or two years will help to indicate significant improvement.

The difficulty in prediction also provides a further reason why operative intervention on prisoners should be avoided if possible in circumstances which would make the results of operation a condition for release. Psychiatrists normally operate on the principle that the patient who is interested in cure will be as frank with them as he is able. This does not hold for some aggressive prisoners. Psychiatric skill is reasonably good for the management of psychotic patients and neurotics. It is poor with deceivers and we need not be ashamed of this since we do not or should not purport to be detectives. We are another type of investigator. Assessing patients who might say they are cured by operation so as to promote their own release is fraught with difficulty. Nevertheless in principle it seems to be wrong to deny to prisoners the benefits of worthwhile operations, especially since not all of them present the above problems. Sufficient safeguards ought therefore to be sought to allow the performance of some psychosurgery on prisoners who consent. A novel safeguard would be one which follows from the Detroit case,[66,67] and that would be to call for a legal review of a prisoner's sentence, before psychosurgery, such that any neglected opportunity for him to challenge his incarceration could first be pursued.

# Conclusions

The conclusions in this chapter can be stated briefly. ECT is a valuable treatment which on occasion may be given even to incompetent patients who object. Stereotactic types of leucotomy are of proved value but only rarely indicated; neurosurgical operations for aggression have some potential but need more evaluation; it is reasonable to operate on brain tissue which is not the site of known gross disease; it is not reasonable or ethical to undertake neurosurgery against the patient's wishes; prisoners may have appropriate treatment of any type for illnesses unrelated to their crime; operations on violent prisoners may only be considered with stringent precautions. Brain stimulation by implanted electrodes is a form of brain surgery and subject to the same considerations as psychosurgery; it has some advantages and no great practical disadvantages compared with other brain surgery.

# References

1 Mill, J. S.: *On liberty* (1859), London, Watts and Company, 1929.
2 Knight, G. C.: Further observations from an experience of 660 cases of stereotactic tractotomy. *Postgraduate Medical Journal* **49**:845–54, 1973.
3 Tooth, G. C. and Newton, M. P.: *Leucotomy in England and Wales 1942–1954.* Reports on Medical Subjects, No. 104. London, Her Majesty's Stationery Office, 1961.
4 Dax, E. C.: The history of prefrontal leucotomy, in *Psychosurgery and society*, ed. J. S. Smith and L. G. Kiloh. Oxford, Pergamon, 1977, pp. 19–24.
5 Mitchell-Heggs, N., Kelly, D., and Richardson, A.: Stereotactic limbic leucotomy—a follow-up at sixteen months. *British Journal of Psychiatry* **128**:226–40, 1976.
6 Goktepe, E. O., Young, L. B., and Bridges, P. K.: A further review of the results of stereotactic subcaudate tractotomy. *British Journal of Psychiatry* **126**:270–80, 1975.
7 Bridges, P. K. and Bartlett, J. R.: Psychosurgery: yesterday and today. *British Journal of Psychiatry* **131**:249–60, 1977.
8 Crow, H.: The treatment of anxiety and obsessionality with chronically implanted electrodes, in *Psychosurgery and society*, ed. J. S. Smith and L. G. Kiloh. Oxford, Pergamon, 1977, pp. 71–3.
9 American Psychiatric Association: Electroconvulsive therapy. Task Force Report No. 14, Washington DC, 1978.
10 Guze, S. and Robins, E.: Suicide and primary affective disorders. *British Journal of Psychiatry* **117**:437–8, 1970.
11 Huston, P. E. and Locher, L. M.: Involutional psychosis: course when untreated and when treated with ECT. *Archives of Neurology and Psychiatry* **59**:385–94, 1948.
12 Beresford, H. R.: Legal issues relating to electroconvulsive therapy. *Archives of General Psychiatry* **25**:100–2, 1971.

13 Barker, J. C. and Baker, A. A.: Deaths associated with electroplexy. *Journal of Mental Science* **105**:339–48, 1959.
14 Bruce, E. M., Crone, N., Fitzpatrick, G., *et al.*: A comparative trial of ECT and Tofranil. *American Journal of Psychiatry* **117**, 76, 1960.
15 Medical Research Council: Clinical trial of the treatment of depressive illness. *British Medical Journal* **5439**:881–6, 1965.
16 Sainz, A: Clarification of the action of successful treatments in the depressions. *Diseases of the Nervous System* **20**:53–7, 1959.
17 Lambourn, J. and Gill, D.: A controlled comparison of simulated and real ECT. *British Journal of Psychiatry* **133**:514–19, 1978.
18 Ottosson, J. O.: Simulated and real ECT. *British Journal of Psychiatry* **134**:314, 1979.
19 Watt, J. A. G.: Simulated and real ECT. *British Journal of Psychiatry* **134**:314, 1979.
20 Johnstone, E. C., Deakin, J. F. W., Lawler, P., *et al.*: The Northwick Park ECT trial. *Lancet* **ii**:1317–20, 1980.
21 Brandon, S., Cowley, P., McDonald, C., Neville, P., Palmer, R. and Wellstood-Eason, S.: Electroconvulsive therapy: results in depressive illness from the Leicestershire trial. *British Medical Journal* **288**:22–5, 1984.
22 Wilson, I. C., Vernon, J. T., Guin, T., *et al.*: A controlled study of treatments of depression. *Journal of Neuropsychiatry* **4**:331–7, 1963.
23 Costello, C. G.: Electroconvulsive therapy: is further investigation necessary? *Canadian Psychiatric Association Journal* **21**:761–7, 1976.
24 Cronholm, B. and Ottosson, J. O.: Experimental studies of the therapeutic action of electroconvulsive therapy in endogenous depression. *Acta psychiatrica et neurologica Scandinavica* **35**:(Suppl. 145) 69–97, 1960.
25 Price, T. R. P., MacKenzie, T. B., Tucker, G. J., and Culver, C.: The dose response ratio in electroconvulsive therapy. *Archives of General Psychiatry* **35**: 1131–6, 1978.
26 Squire, L. R. and Chace, P. M.: Memory functions six to nine months after electroconvulsive therapy. *Archives of General Psychiatry* **32**:1557–64, 1975.
27 Weeks, D., Freeman, C. P. L. and Kendall, R. D.: ECT III. Enduring cognitive deficits? *British Journal of Psychiatry* **137**:26–37, 1980.
28 *Wyatt* v. *Hardin*, No. 3195–N (M.D. Ala. 28 Feb. 1975, modified 1 July 1975): 1. *Mental Disability Law Reporter* **55**, 1976.
29 California Welfare and Institutions Code, 1979. SS. 5325.1, 5434.2, 5326.7, 5326.8.
30 Winslade, W. J., Liston, E. H., Ross, J. W. and Weber, K. D.: Medical, judicial and statutory regulation of ECT in United States. *American Journal of Psychiatry* **141** (11): 1349–55, 1984.
31 Cameron, D. E.: Production of differential amnesia as a factor in the treatment of schizophrenia. *Comprehensive Psychiatry* **1**:26–34, 1960.
32 Gillmor, D.: *I swear by Apollo.* Montreal, Eden Press, 1960.
33 Edwards, G. A. and Flaherty, B.: Electroconvulsive therapy: a new era of controversy. *Australia and New Zealand Journal of Psychiatry* **12**:161–4, 1978.
34 World Health Organization: *Health aspects of human rights.* Geneva, WHO, 1976.
35 *Determination of Secretary regarding recommendation on psychosurgery of the*

National Commission for the Protection of Human Subjects of Biomedical and Behavioural Research. Federal Register, 15 Nov. 1978. Part VI, pp. 53241–4.

36 Moniz, E.: Les premières tentatives opératoires dans le traitement de certains psychoses. Encéphale 31:1, 1936.

37 Burckhardt, G.: Ueber Rindenexcisionen, als Beittag zur operativen Therapie der Psychosen. Allgemeine Zeitschrift für Psychiatrié 47:463–548, 1891.

38 Freeman, W. and Watts, J. W.: Psychosurgery. Thomas, Springfield Ill., 1942.

39 Smith, J. S.: The treatment of anxiety, depression and obsessionality, in Psychosurgery and society, ed. J. S. Smith and L. G. Kiloh. Oxford, Pergamon, 1977.

40 Barraclough, B. M. and Mitchell-Heggs, N. A.: Use of neurosurgery for psychological disorders in the British Isles during 1974–1976. British Medical Journal iv:1591–3, 1978.

41 US National Commission for the Protection of Subjects of Biomedical and Behavioural Research involving Psychosurgery: Report and Recommendations with Appendix. Bethesda, MD: US Department of Health, Education and Welfare, Publication No. (OS)77-0001 and (OS)77-0002, 14 March 1977.

42 Hussain, E. S., Freeman, H., and Jones, R. A. C.: A cohort study of psychosurgery cases from a defined population. Journal of Neurology, Neurosurgery, and Psychiatry 51:345–52, 1988.

43 Beecher, H. K.: Measurement of subjective responses. New York, Oxford University Press, 1959.

44 Merskey, H. and Spear, F. G.: Pain: psychological and psychiatric aspects. London, Baillière-Tindall and Cassell, 1967.

45 Sternbach, R. A.: Pain: a psychophysiological analysis. New York, Academic Press, 1968.

46 Subcommittee on Taxonomy of the International Association for the Study of Pain: Definitions of pain terms. Pain, Suppl. 3, 1979.

47 Elithorn, A., Glithero, E., and Slater, E.: Leucotomy for pain. Journal of Neurology, Neurosurgery, and Psychiatry 21:249–61, 1958.

48 Cassinari, V. and Pagni, C. A.: Central pain: a neurosurgical survey. Cambridge, Mass., Harvard University Press, 1979.

49 Moricca, G.: Pituitary neuroadenolysis in the treatment of intractable pain, in Persistent pain: modern methods of treatment, ed. S. Lipton. London, Academic Press, 1977.

50 Sheard, M. H.: Neurobiology of aggressive behaviour, in Aggression, mental illness and mental retardation: psychobiological approaches, ed. D. Zarfas and B. Goldberg. University of Western Ontario, London, Ontario, pp. 76–93, 1978.

51 Kiloh, L. G., Gye, R. S., Rushworth, R. G., Bell, D. S., and White, R. T.: Stereotactic amygdalotomy for aggressive behaviour. Journal of Neurology, Neurosurgery, and Psychiatry 37:437, 1974.

52 Balasubramaniam, V. and Kanaka, T. S.: Amygdalotomy and hypothalamotomy in a comparative study. Confinia neurologica 37:195, 1975.

53 Narabayashi, H., Nagao, T., Saito, Y., et al.: Stereotaxic amygdalotomy for behaviour disorders. Archives of Neurology 9:1, 1963.

54 Heimburger, R. F., Whitlock, C. C., and Kalsbeck, J. E.: Stereotaxic amygdalotomy for epilepsy and aggressive behaviour. Journal of the American Medical Association 198:741–5, 1966.

55 Kiloh, L. G.: The treatment of anger and aggression, in *Symposium on psycho-surgery and society*, ed. J. S. Smith and L. G. Kiloh. Oxford, Pergamon, 1977.

56 Mark, V. H. and Ervin, F. R.: *Violence and the brain*. New York, Harper and Row, 1970.

57 Fabrega, H., jun.: *Disease and social behaviour: an interdisciplinary perspective*. Cambridge, Mass, MIT Press, 1974.

58 Merskey, H.: A variable meaning for the concept of disease. *Journal of Medicine and Philosophy* **11** (3): 215–32, 1986.

59 Edgar, H.: Regulating psychosurgery: issues of public policy and law, in *Operating on the mind: the psychosurgery conflict*, ed. W. M. Gaylin, J. S. Meister and R. D. Neville. New York, Basic Books, 1975.

60 Mark, V. H. and Neville, R.: Brain surgery in aggressive epileptics: social and ethical implications. *Journal of the American Medical Association* **227**:765–72, 1973.

61 Bridges, P. K.: Psychosurgery and the Mental Health Act Commission. *Bulletin of the Royal College of Psychiatrists* **8**:146–8, 1984.

62 Bridges, P. K.: Addendum to 'Psychosurgery and the Mental Health Act Commission'. *Bulletin of the Royal College of Psychiatrists* **8**:172, 1984.

63 Lord Colville: The Mental Health Act and second opinions. *Bulletin of the Royal College of Psychiatrists* **9**:2–3, 1985.

64 Thompson, C.: An open letter to Lord Colville. *Bulletin of the Royal College of Psychiatrists* **9**:100, 1985.

65 Bridges, P. K.: The Mental Health Act Commission and second opinions. *Bulletin of the Royal College of Psychiatrists* **9**:120, 1985.

66 *Kaimowitz* v. *Department of Mental Health*. Cir. Ct Wayne City, Mich., Civil, No. 73–19434 AW, 10 July 1973.

67 Burt, R. A.: Why we should keep prisoners from the doctors. *Hastings Center Report* **5**:25–34, 1975.

68 Greenblatt, S. J.: *New York Law School Law Review* **22**:961–80, 1976–7.

69 Heath, R. G., John, S. B., and Fontana, C. J.: Stereotaxic implantation of electrodes in the human brain: a method for long-term study and treatment. *IEE Transactions on Biomedical Engineering* Vol. bme 23:296–304, 1976.

70 Hosobughi, Y., Adams, J. E. and Linchitz, R.: Pain relief by electrical stimulation of the central gray matter in humans and its reversal by Naloxone. *Science* (New York) **197**:183–6, 1977.

71 Gybels, J.: *Electrical stimulation of the central gray for pain relief in humans*. Pain Abstract 1:170, 2nd World Congress on Pain. Montreal, International Association for the Study of Pain, 1978.

72 Delgado, J. M. R.: *Physical control of the mind: toward a psychocivilized society*. New York, Harper and Row, 1969.

73 Valenstein, E. S.: *Brain control*. New York, Wiley, 1973.

74 Sano, K.: Sedative neurosurgery, with special reference to posteromedial hypothalamotomy. *Neurologia medico-chirurgica* 4:112, 1962.

75 Sano, K.: Sedative stereoencephalotomy: fornicotomy, upper mesencephalic reticulotomy. *Progress in Brain Research* 21:350, 1966.

76 Megargee, E. I.: A critical review of theories of violence, in *Crimes of violence*, ed. D. J. Mulvihill, M. M. Tumin, and L. A. Curtis. Washington DC, US Government Printing Office, 1969.

77 Quinsey, V. L., Pruesse, M., and Fernley, R.: A follow-up of patients found

'unfit to stand trial' or 'not guilty' because of insanity. *Canadian Psychiatric Association Journal* **20**:461–7, 1975.

78 Cocozza, J. J. and Steadman, H. J.: Some refinements in the prediction of dangerous behaviour. *American Journal of Psychiatry* **131**:1012–14, 1974.

# 11

# Ethical aspects of sexuality and sex therapy

*John Bancroft*

In general, the purpose of ethical guidelines for the psychiatrist is threefold: (1) to protect the patient from exploitation, incompetence, and pressures to conform; (2) to uphold the rights of that patient, his entitlement to make decisions about his own life and to have access to information that is important to his welfare; and (3) to foster, by the psychiatrist's own behaviour, desirable social attitudes and action.

The first two objectives, protection of the patient and the promotion of his rights, often coincide, but they also conflict with one another, and present some of the most difficult ethical dilemmas that we have to face. These are circumstances when, in respecting the patient's rights, we may be acting against his interests or well-being. As members of a caring profession, we have to take that dilemma seriously. Fortunately such a dilemma is seldom involved in sex therapy, though there are a few examples that I will consider. Problems do arise for the sex therapist when dealing with the sex offender, when there may be conflict between the interests of the offender and those of society.

In considering the third objective, the fostering of desirable social attitudes, we are acknowledging that our responsibilities as psychiatrists extend beyond our patients to the societies in which we live. Such influence as we may have stems not only from our explicit public statements, but also from our day-to-day work. Public attitudes and social policy concerning many forms of behaviour have been extensively influenced by medical opinion, often it seems disadvantageously. For example, the medical condemnation of various kinds of non-procreative sex in the eighteenth and nineteenth centuries has been well documented.[1] More recently, in the 1950s, the evidence of the British Medical Association to the Wolfenden Committee on prostitution and homosexuality involved a strong assertion of values that were quite unjustified by any rational medical appraisal.[2]

Since the first edition of this book, social attitudes to sexuality have been in a state of upheaval as a result of two major developments, in both of which the medical profession finds itself inextricably involved. One is the world-wide epidemic of HIV infection and AIDS; the other is the extraordinary increase in awareness of the extent that children are sexually abused within their families.

The AIDS issues has resurrected old ethical problems, particularly the role of the medical profession in reinforcing negative attitudes to homosexuality and other forms of nonconformist sexual behaviour, and the ostracizing of victims of infectious disease. But we are also confronted with new and exceptionally difficult ethical dilemmas concerning confidentiality and informed consent for serological testing. For the most part these issues are beyond the scope of this chapter, which is primarily concerned with the treatment of sexual problems. However, the reappraisal of sexual attitudes that is under way does impinge on several aspects of this chapter, and the surfacing of child sexual abuse as an issue does have more direct implications for sex therapy which will be discussed.

The ethical issues will be considered in this chapter under a number of headings. These include the sexuality of the patient–therapist relationship; the influence of the therapist on the patient; informed consent and the appropriateness of treatment; problems of confidentiality; and the professional qualifications of the sex therapist.

Three types of clinical situation will recur and require separate consideration. The first is treatment of sexual dysfunction and general problems in sexual relationships. Numerically, this is the most important, the large majority of patients seeking sex therapy coming into this category. Typically these are individuals or couples who complain of loss of interest or enjoyment in their sexual relationship or impairment of more specific sexual responses, such as erection, ejaculation, or orgasm. The second is the treatment of deviant or stigmatized sexual behaviour, and the third, a particular form of the second, the treatment of the sexual offender.

## The sexuality of the patient–therapist relationship

This is not an issue confined to sex therapy. Any medically qualified clinician or nurse has to recognize that the involvement of nudity and physical contact in their dealing with patients has sexual implications that are not present in other types of professional relationship. Sexual feelings may arise in either the patient or the doctor. But in sex therapy there is not only the explicit focus on sex but also the need to increase comfort with sexual matters and to give permission to overcome sexual inhibitions. Hence sexual feelings that arise in the relationship may have therapeutic potential. Prolonged discussion of the patient's sexual history and current feelings inevitably introduces a degree of vicarious sexuality, even without a physical examination. Thus this issue has special significance for all sex therapists whether medically qualified or not.

As a result of the taboo against a sexual relationship between doctors and patients, any such relationship, even when occurring outside the professional context and when quite unrelated to sexual problems, may be regarded as grounds for withdrawal of professional status. Most doctors accept this without question; and yet it does happen that doctors engage in sexual activity with their patients on the grounds that it is therapeutic to do so. A number of anonymous surveys of mental health professionals have been consistent in finding that 5 to 10 per cent of male and 1 to 2 per cent of female therapists admit to having had sex with a patient.[2]

The professional taboo has been likened to the taboo against incest.[3] Elsewhere, I have argued that the incest taboo may serve a useful function by permitting a degree of sexuality in the parent–child relationship which facilitates sexual development, while at the same time protecting from the destructive effects that a fuller sexual relationship might bring.[4] In a similar way, the security derived from the taboo in the doctor–patient relationship may allow sexual feelings to be used constructively in therapy either implicitly or explicitly. This includes the sexual attraction the therapist may feel towards the patient. Pope *et al.*[2] found that only 5 per cent of male and 24 per cent of female therapists had never felt sexually attracted to a patient. Such feelings are important not only in what they tell the therapist about the patient, but also in the ways that they may influence the therapist's behaviour, unwittingly and with potential harm unless they are recognized.[5]

Certainly the argument that is most commonly put forward to support the professional taboo is that the special relationship that is required for effective professional help, which perhaps combines caring and detachment, is incompatible with an overtly sexual relationship with its potential for emotional involvement and self-interest on the part of the professional. In particular, the requirement for the patient to lower his or her defences for the purpose of treatment produces a vulnerability that makes exploitation especially reprehensible.[6] It has been pointed out that such ostensibly therapeutic sexual interaction almost always involves a male therapist and a young female patient, and that there is little evidence of the therapist's providing such help for the fat or ugly who might receive from it more benefit to their self-esteem. Although it should not be assumed that every case of such patient–therapist sexuality is harmful, there is now well-documented evidence of a syndrome of traumatization, anger, and distrust in women patients with such experiences.[2,7,8]

If I declare my support for this taboo, I must admit to some uncertainty as to where to draw the line. Should you ever touch your patient except for obviously clinical purposes? An arm around the shoulder or a hug to comfort distress might be construed as sexual, and professionals are often advised to avoid even these basically caring gestures, if only to safeguard themselves from the occasional histrionic manipulative patient. I would find such limitations to my therapeutic relationships unacceptable, and am prepared to take the risk, providing that I am quite clear of my own motives. Other professionals may hold different views.

This issue is of particular relevance to health workers in institutions where they provide day-to-day contact and support for their patients or clients. Sexual exploitation of institutionalized patients by staff is common,[9] yet it would be undesirable to foster institutional atmospheres in which no bodily contact occurs. And there are special situations where physically or mentally handicapped individuals may need some instruction in sexual matters, such as how to masturbate. To avoid such interaction may be to deny such individuals an important source of pleasure in their restricted lives. Yet to help in this way involves treading a precarious path between genuine help and what might be regarded by many as sexual abuse. There is undoubtedly a need for more guidance and training in these highly sensitive issues for institution staff as well as the helping professions.

Some doctors, anxious to avoid inducing any sexual feelings during their genital examination, use a purposely brusque and mildly unpleasant examination technique. Whether intended or not, this conveys a negative message about sex. Others, by contrast, feel that the occurrence during physical examination of sexual responses which do not lead to overt sexual interaction not only reinforces the sexual security of the professional relationship, but may provide information of therapeutic value. In Britain sex therapists trained in the Balint approach rely a great deal on the *emotional* reactions of the female patient to vaginal examination. Tunnadine[10] calls it 'the moment of truth'. This method involves female therapists treating female patients, but that does not exclude sexuality of either a homosexual or a parent–child kind. Within the safety of the professional relationship such experience can lead to crucial permission—as Tunnadine puts it—with a shift from the fantasy: 'this part is bad, prohibited, still belonging to mother who has not handed over permission for a sexual life'—to the fact of a motherly woman saying: 'go ahead—it is yours to explore, use, love with, just like lips or hands: a decent, beautiful organ of pleasure'.[10]

Concentration by this group of workers on the treatment of female problems has in part stemmed from their difficulty in finding an equivalent of the vaginal examination for the male patient. In the male, examination may not have the same potential for 'permission giving'. But it can nevertheless facilitate a special openness between the male doctor and the male patient if used appropriately. But are such factors relevant when the doctor and patient are of the opposite sex? The relevance is clear when the sexual problems stem from the patient's relationship with the opposite-sex parent, although the therapeutic use of such factors may require considerable skill. Also, a therapist of the opposite sex may effectively desensitize the patient to sexual fears of the opposite sex within such a 'safe' relationship. A case can therefore be made for allowing and exploiting the sexuality of the physical examination when it occurs within the security of a professional relationship and when the purpose of the physical examination is not *explicitly sexual*.

What of direct sexual stimulation during such an examination? Hartman and Fithian[11] use what they call a 'sexological examination'. During examination of the female patient, both the male and female therapists take turns in stimulating the vagina. The woman is encouraged to regard any positive or erotic feelings that are elicited as acceptable. At a later stage, the male partner is called in to the room and encouraged to examine his wife and stimulate her vagina in a similar fashion. Their sexological examination of the male partner by contrast does not involve any attempt to stimulate and is much briefer. The reason for this discrepancy is not given. Hoch[12] reported a comparable approach in which the female patient is sexually stimulated by a male therapist during the course of a vaginal examination and in front of her husband. In both these cases, this form of examination is seen as therapeutically valuable. A modification which comes midway between the sexological examination and a 'simple' sexual relationship between therapist and patient has been euphemistically called 'body work therapy'.[13] Here sexual touching of the patient by the therapist or vice versa is encouraged and the patient's emotional reactions to the experience discussed at the time. Although one can recognize the obvious educational potential of this approach, the question that its proponents have not succeeded in answering is the effect that such precedures have on the therapist–patient relationship. Is the rationale of the therapy accepted at face value by the patient, or does the relationship in the patient's eyes transform into a sexual game? It is far from clear that possible negative effects on the therapeutic relationship are outweighed by the assumed advantages.

The sexuality of the therapeutic relationship is perhaps most explicit as a result of physical contact, but as mentioned earlier, there are other manifestations. Both verbal and non-verbal behaviour of either therapist or patient may be seductive or sexual in meaning. The therapist may be influenced in his choice of questioning or advice by the vicarious sexuality that ensues. The patient's responses may be influenced in a similar way. Acceptance or rejection of a patient for therapy, or the allotment of time in therapy may be similarly affected. While there would be agreement that such tendencies on the part of the therapist should be both recognized and controlled, there are aspects of the structure of sex therapy which have a relevance not always acknowledged.

First, whether the sex of the therapist is the same or different from that of the patient is a therapeutic variable which ideally should be chosen to

meet the needs of the case. The potential sexuality of the relationship may
be desirable in one case, to be avoided in another. In practice, there is
often limited choice in this respect. Secondly, the therapist may work
either with an individual patient or with a couple. In the latter case, the
sexual potential for the therapeutic relationship is reduced but not eliminated. Any sexuality that arises between the therapist and one of the patient
couple may have an adverse effect on that couple's relationship. This
provides one of the justifications for co-therapy—using two therapists, one
male and one female. The above problem can then be minimized, particularly if the principal responsibility for relating to each member of the
couple is taken by the same-sex therapist.

Most of the points that have been raised so far have concerned heterosexuality in the patient–therapist relationship, but the homosexual parallel
in each case should also be considered.

One of the most controversial issues in sex therapy is the use of surrogate
partners. Here the therapist provides someone *other than himself* to become sexually involved with the patient. The advantages that are claimed
are due to the surrogate being concerned and sympathetic as well as
knowledgeable about sexual problems; in other words, all the advantages
of having sex with your therapist without the disadvantages. One objection
often raised is that such a procedure is indistinguishable from prostitution.
This does not solve the problem, as the ethical status of prostitution itself is
far from clear. The similarity is beyond dispute and in fact therapists do
sometimes use sensitive, caring prostitutes for this purpose. Such practice
is by no means of recent origin.[14] But usually the women involved as
surrogates in no way regard themselves as prostitutes. Their motives are of
interest and not readily apparent. Masters and Johnson[15] reported that 9 of
the 13 female surrogates in their research studies justified their participation on the grounds of having had personal experience in helping a family
member with sexual problems and wanting to extend that help to others.
Only three openly declared that their motives were sexual.

Masters and Johnson discontinued the use of surrogates after a few years
because of their concern about the ethical issues. In Britain the main
advocate of surrogate-therapy has been Cole,[16] who has used surrogates,
predominantly female but a few male, since 1970. He gives some details of
34 women and 9 men who have acted in this way. They ranged in age from
the early 20s to the late 40s in the women and the late 50s in the men.
Almost half were currently married. Most approached his clinic offering
themselves for this work on their own initiative. They were selected on the
basis of three principal criteria: they needed to be sufficiently intelligent to
understand the basic ideas behind sex therapy; they should be relatively
uninhibited sexually, so as to be able to engage in a full sexual repertoire;
and they should be free of the resentment that the sexes often harbour

against each other. Otherwise a range of personalities and appearances was sought, to allow the therapist flexibility in assigning surrogates appropriately, a process which according to Cole is of considerable therapeutic importance. Cole[16] gives details of the efficacy of this approach in 390 men and 35 women. As with many other innovative treatment approaches, he reports results, after 15 years or so of experience, which are much more modest than his early claims.[17] It is also noteworthy that he has been unable to follow up these patients, except for a group of 42, most of whom volunteered evidence of their progress. While follow-up in more conventional sex therapy is notoriously difficult, it is a relevant comment about this particular form of therapy that Cole regards follow-up enquiry to be unacceptable in the majority of cases, particularly in those who may have succeeded in progressing to a new sexual relationship. Nevertheless, Cole makes a persuasive case for at least the initial efficacy of surrogate therapy in a proportion of cases, particularly with such problems as heterophobia and secondary erectile failure.

The ethical acceptability of surrogate therapy is a complex matter. If the sexual distress of an individual can be overcome by a person who is motivated to help, what is the objection? Objections will vary from those in which such behaviour is considered immoral because it is a form of adultery, regardless of its outcome, to those which are concerned with the nature of the change in sexuality which results. Is the success of such treatment based on the quality of the sexual performance or of the sexual relationship with the surrogate? Do changes in that particular relationship generalize to other relationships? These concerns highlight one of the most basic controversies amongst sex therapists—is treatment aimed at sexual function or at the sexual relationship? Those who stress the former may be more inclined to accept surrogate therapy as a useful option. Those who favour the latter may reject this approach on the grounds that it either divorces sex from the relationship, leads to complications resulting from the relationship with the surrogate that does develop, or causes confusion about the role of sexuality in loving and intimate relationships.

This controversy is receiving fresh impetus with the vigorous debate accompanying the AIDS epidemic. The entirely proper emphasis on 'safe sex' by those concerned with the spread of the HIV virus, with the encouragement to use condoms because of a lack of knowledge or trust in our partner's previous or current behaviour, is causing many to ponder the nature of sexual relationships. In any case the AIDS issue must loom large in surrogate-therapy circles. Cole[16] stresses the need for extra vigilance about sexually transmitted disease as a result of AIDS. But it will undoubtedly be a challenge to the efficacy of this approach for it to be effective with the additional requirements of 'safe sex'. Much of sex therapy is about establishing emotional security in sexual relationships. The security of the condom is of a different kind.

Cole has, I believe, been sincere in his pursuit of this highly controversial treatment method. After entering the field with the air of the rebel against sexual orthodoxy, there is a more resigned feel, in his recent writing, that surrogate therapy is not going to be accepted. He points out that, with the law not recognizing motives, therapists making use of surrogates are vulnerable to prosecution in the United Kingdom under three sections of the Sexual Offences Act 1956: procuring, living on immoral earnings of a prostitute, and keeping a brothel. He reports that so far no legal proceedings have been taken under this Act against *bona fide* professional sex therapists using surrogates. But he points out that this is due to the exercise of discretion by the police. He nevertheless sees fear of such prosecution as the reason why many therapists will not use surrogates. In the United States, Malamuth *et al.*[18] found that 28 per cent of the professionals they questioned had at some time used surrogates, whereas 87 per cent said they would only now do so if they were certain about the legality of the practice.

An aspect of surrogacy which has arisen in the United States, is the extent to which it has become professionalized. As was discussed earlier, there are strong reasons for ensuring that the patient is not exploited sexually by the therapist. The concept of the surrogate partner may avoid or minimize such exploitation if, in spite of the money involved, the surrogate is not seen as being in a professional relationship with the patient. On the West Coast of the United States, where surrogate therapy is widely practised, the surrogate has emerged as a form of helping professional.[19] The International Professional Surrogate Association (IPSA) now provides training programmes, legal advice, and ethical guidelines. The distinction between surrogate partner and therapist has become blurred. This is the main reason put forward by Masters and Johnson[20] for ceasing to use surrogates.

## The influence of the therapist on the patient

For a number of reasons, the therapist is usually in a position to influence his patient. The patient, because of his presenting problem and his need to lower his psychological defences, is often in a psychologically vulnerable state. The therapist, as a member of a helping profession, will often be seen by him as having status and kudos. The esteem accorded to the therapist by the patient is likely to be enhanced by his understandable need to have faith or to put trust in the therapist. From this position of relative power, the therapist has to consider to what extent he is imposing his own values on the patient (see Chapter 21).

But there is a wider influence that also has to be considered. The therapist, because of his status, may influence a much broader range of opinion not only by what he says in the form of public statements, but also as a consequence of the types of treatment he is known to use. There may be considerable misunderstanding of his motives or opinions for which he cannot be held directly responsible; but it is his responsibility to recognize these wider influences so that he can modify them or amplify them according to his ethical principles. I will consider some specific examples below.

The doctor, working in a medical setting, is used to taking an advisory role with his patients. He is the expert on illness, and the 'sick' patient, if sensible, will put himself into the doctor's hands and do what he says. This is one aspect of the 'medical model' and there is no doubt that, in many instances of severe illness, it is appropriate.[21] But such circumstances rarely prevail in the treatment of sexual problems. It is true that there are many medical factors which impinge on sexual function, and medical advice on their management will be needed. But the bulk of treatment should be seen as crucially different, as more of an educational process where the therapist helps the patient or couple to learn new ways of relating sexually. Although considerable psychotherapeutic skill may be required to help a patient to overcome the resistance to specific change, the primary purpose is still the change to new ways of behaving. Not only is the onus of change on the patients but they have to be clear that such change is what they seek. The treatment thus involves 'the negotiation of a contract', whereby patient and therapist reach agreement about goals of treatment and methods of reaching them. To use the concept of transactional analysis, the relationship between therapist and patient is of an 'adult–adult' type, rather than 'parent–child' or 'doctor–sick patient'. I have argued elsewhere[22] that this type of relationship is necessary for effective treatment of sexual problems, whereas the more dependent relationship which characterizes the medical setting is less conducive to the type of learning that is required. If that is so, the ethical implications of therapist influence are twofold. First, by wielding such influence, the therapist may unwittingly undermine the appropriate therapist–patient relationship and hence the efficacy of treatment. Secondly, and most obviously, the therapist is in a position to impose his own values or beliefs on the patient because of his influential position.

Given this potential for influence, is it *necessarily* wrong for therapists to impose their own values? In the past, the medical profession has acted as the guardian of sexual morality to an extent second only to the Church. The usual justification stems from the confusion of health and morality, exemplified in the Mental Hygiene movement of the 1920s. There is no doubt that sexual values have been powerfully influenced by medical opinion. In the eighteenth and nineteenth centuries, warnings from doctors of the dire medical consequences of non-procreative sex—coitus interruptus or masturbation or homosexuality—added a particularly heavy load to sexual guilt that is still very much in evidence.[23] Members of the medical profession may be less naïve about compounding medical advice with morality nowadays, but more subtle versions undoubtedly continue. There is a dilemma here. Are physicians to avoid using their position of influence to encourage attitudes that they believe are for the public good? Given this position, it is difficult for the medical profession to avoid criticism. They will be attacked for bolstering values which are regarded as unacceptable by the critic or they will be attacked for failing to encourage values that the critic upholds.

Whether a doctor is capable of remaining neutral is a matter of some doubt. The ethical requirement is perhaps that he should be clear when he is not doing so, that he should avoid the deceit of justifying his own morality on quasi-medical grounds, and that by the same token he should be active in countering similar deceit stemming from his medical colleagues. Before encouraging a patient to adopt values or attitudes that the therapist holds as important, he should consider carefully whether this would create distressing conflict with the patient's cultural or religious mores. Let us consider some specific examples.

One of the most debated issues of this kind is the treatment of homosexuality. In virtually all Western societies, homosexuality carries social stigma. This may range from outright hostility and ostracism to tolerance, rather than acceptance, of abnormality or more commonly of 'sickness'. Although there are many homosexuals who lead perfectly satisfactory and happy lives in spite of this, there are many others who at some stage experience unhappiness and depression that seems to be directly related to their homosexual life-style.[24] The extent to which their distress is a consequence of social stigma is not measurable but is likely to be substantial. When a person seeks professional help for distress of this kind, there are, in simple terms, two obvious goals: one, to learn to adapt more happily within a homosexual role, the other, to explore an alternative such as heterosexuality, asexuality, or bisexuality. What are the ethical issues facing the therapist in this situation? If he has a genuinely open mind about homosexuality, the problem is relatively straightforward. If, for instance, he feels quite comfortable helping people to adjust either to a homosexual or a heterosexual role, he can proclaim his neutrality and set about helping his patient to find the goal and life-style that suits him best. If the therapist has more definite views—for example he believes that life as a homosexual is never satisfactory or acceptable and that an asexual or heterosexual alternative should be sought, or by contrast, he believes that someone with homosexual preference should *always* accept those preferences and not try to change them, he is faced with an ethical dilemma. In either case, he is in danger of pressing the patient to conform to his, the therapist's, own values. And yet he may feel strongly that pressure is justified.

For some years there has been a broad consensus among the helping professions that homosexuality is not an illness and is not something that requires treatment to 'cure' or change it, however disadvantaged the homosexual may be in our society. There have been many who have taken the view that any attempt to help someone with homosexual preferences to establish heterosexual feelings or relationships is ethically unacceptable (see for example Davison[25]). Twenty years ago this was a topical issue; it was then by no means unusual for homosexually-oriented men (seldom women) to seek help of this kind. More recently it has become much less frequent, reflecting, I believe, changing social attitudes to homosexuality. Unfortunately, with the AIDS epidemic and the dramatic increase in anti-homosexual prejudice, we must expect some reversal of this seemingly desirable trend. In any case, this issue raises some ethical points of more general relevance, and therefore continues to warrant our attention. I have debated this matter in more detail elsewhere,[26] but I will briefly outline the three principal issues at stake, and consider how each may be affected by the current climate of opinion.

The first concerns the effect of such treatment on social attitudes to homosexuality. Any treatment aimed at helping homosexuals to be non-homosexual is regarded as reinforcing negative social attitudes to homo-sexuality and giving medical support to the notion that homosexuality is bad. Undoubtedly there is some truth in this idea. Greater tolerance of homosexuality in a social group is often attained only by an increase in the number who regard it as a 'sickness' rather than a 'sin'. The knowledge that there is a 'cure' for the 'sickness' encourages that tendency. Hence, it is argued, all such treatment should be avoided. And yet, what about the needs of the individual who seeks help? Can one justifiably deny him help because of the effects that help may have on society in general? Placing the needs of society before those of the patient seems to threaten a most basic principle of the caring professions. But does it have to be an either–or situation? Much depends on the aims of any specific treatment. If the aim is unequivocally to suppress or eliminate homosexual interest, the above argument carries weight. Clinical evidence has shown that such treatment is unlikely to succeed in this aim, providing a second powerful reason for its unacceptability. If, on the other hand, the goals of treatment are to extend the individual's scope for sexual relationships to include the heterosexual the argument fails. It may be said, to sustain the argument, that therapists never help heterosexuals to establish homosexual relationships. This may be true, principally because such an objective is seldom, if ever, sought; no doubt because heterosexuality *per se* is not stigmatized. It is not unusual, on the other hand, for a therapist to encourage an individual to acknow-ledge and accept homosexual feelings which he, the therapist, believes to be present when that individual is striving unsuccessfully to maintain a heterosexual identity.

Opinion may remain divided on this issue, but I have no doubt that it is possible to help an individual to explore alternative sexual roles without reinforcing anti-homosexual feelings. A good example of a balanced approach was shown in the book on homosexuality[27] by Masters and Johnson, in which they described two types of treatment, one aimed at improving homosexual relationships, the other at establishing heterosexual relationships in people with previous homosexual feelings. While their patients may not have been representative of homosexuals in general, they nevertheless sought help. Unfortunately, even a balanced and basically positive report on homosexuality such as that by Masters and Johnson can be taken out of context and used to support a totally opposite point of view. In a public debate that occurred soon after the book was published, following prosecution of a British politician with previous homosexual experience, one commentator cited a report of therapeutic success as evidence that homosexuality is always 'learnt'; hence, it was justified to take steps to prevent it by fostering anti-homosexual values. Such gross misuse of clinical research data can hardly be taken as justification for condemning Masters and Johnson's efforts at treatment, though it certainly helps one to understand how opposition to their approach arises. Attitudes to the treatment of homosexuality have been confounded by this type of statement for some time. Since the late nineteenth century, when the 'sinfulness' of homosexuality was being challenged by people with more humanitarian beliefs, evidence of treatability has been used by the opposing camp to demonstrate that homosexuality is acquired rather than innate and hence, for some curious reason, sinful.[1]

It is easy to see how, at the present time, with growing anti-homosexual feelings amongst sections of the public and press, recourse will be had to the 'illness' model. It will be seen by many as preferable to outright rejection of the homosexual 'cause', though probably no more humanitarian in its effects. The medical profession has a particular responsibility to avoid reinforcing such views. When seeking to influence sexual behaviour to lessen the dangers of the AIDS epidemic, it is important to distinguish between certain types of homosexual behaviour and the status of 'being homosexual', in the same way as one would normally distinguish between certain form of heterosexual behaviour and the status of 'being heterosexual'.

The second issue concerning the treatment of homosexuality is that the patient who seeks help does so because of social pressure. His apparent 'free will' is an illusion. The implication of this point of view is that one cannot freely choose to conform. If taken seriously, this argument would throw doubt on the 'free choice' of most forms of psychiatric treatment. Obviously in the capacity of professional advisers we have a responsibility to give as much relevant information as we can to someone who is confronted by such a choice. But to assume that a person is unable to make the most appropriate decision for himself is to take on a responsibility which raises other much more difficult ethical issues.

This problem again has renewed relevance in the AIDS era. Whereas ten years ago one could recognize some definite improvements in the social reaction to the homosexual, now the homosexual man is confronted with a frightening prospect. Even if he is committed to an 'exclusive' relationship, he will have little confidence in finding a partner with no risk of exposure to HIV at some stage in his sexual career. Should the opportunity to explore the possibility of a heterosexual life-style be denied him?

The third issue derives from the idea that homosexuality is the natural state for the homosexual. An attempt to conform or encouraging someone to conform to an unnatural state, such as heterosexuality, would therefore be regarded as unacceptable. 'Unnaturalness' (i.e. recourse to 'natural law') is often used to justify the moral unacceptability of homosexuality itself,[28] and not surprisingly a similar argument is sometimes used to oppose attempts to change from homosexuality to heterosexuality. If such an argument were to have any rational basis, it would require sufficient knowledge of the origins of homosexual and heterosexual preferences to allow us to recognize which was the innate or constitutional preference in any particular individual. In fact, we have little understanding of why either homosexual or heterosexual preferences develop, and the reasons are likely to be many and various.[29]

There is also growing uncertainty about the stability or immutability of sexual preferences. For some time it has been widely believed, particularly by those in the Gay community, that sexual orientation is not only fixed but established early; bisexuality has been treated with scepticism if not hostility. Such a reaction at a time when the Gay subculture was struggling to assert itself and to encourage the belief that a Gay identity is valid and worth while, is understandable. To be confronted with the idea that one might enjoy both homosexual and heterosexual relationships whilst attempting to cope with the heterosexual world's rejection of one's Gay identity would be less than welcome. During the past decade, as the Gay world has started to establish itself and Gay militancy has passed its peak, attitudes to bisexuality have started to change. Bisexuality amongst women has perhaps always been less of a contentious issue, and has been further reinforced by the women's movement, with its alliances between lesbian and straight women united in their distrust of men.[30] But more recently there have been signs of greater acceptability of bisexuality amongst men (see for example Klein[31]). This is relevant to the therapist, who may, as a result, think more positively about helping an individual to explore hetero-sexual as well as homosexual relationships. But whereas we might see this change as a healthy move away from a socially reinforced dichotomy of sexual identities, it has been endowed by the AIDS epidemic with a bitter irony. Perhaps the last thing that the heterosexual world now wants is for male homosexuals to become bisexual.

While opinions about homosexuality still vary, attitudes to sexual contact between adults and children are almost universally negative. In the past, most of the professional attention in this respect was directed at extra-family sexual abuse, in particular the sexual proclivities of the paedophiliac, whose sexual preference is for children. Intra-family abuse, in the form of incest, was recognized but received comparatively little attention. In the past ten years we have seen a major shift of emphasis, so that now intra-family sexual abuse appears to be almost widespread. Certainly sex therapists are encountering a dramatic increase in the number of adults, mainly women, who reveal such episodes from their childhood. It is a matter of some discomfort for many sex therapists to contemplate the inevitable conclusion that in the past, before altered public awareness made it easier for victims to reveal their secrets, they must have worked with many individuals in sex therapy without uncovering this potentially crucial information.

The determinants of social attitudes to adult–child sexual interaction are complex and unclear. When the paedophiliac outside the family was the main object of attention, unqualified hostility to any form of child sexual abuse was not only almost universal but often extreme, and in many individual cases, out of proportion to the harm that the abuse itself may have caused to the child. The picture that is now emerging suggests that intra-family sexual abuse is not only more common but substantially more damaging in its effects. It is as though the universal revulsion towards 'adult–child' sexuality has been a 'reaction formation' stemming from a suppressed awareness of the extent of intra-family sexuality and the deep anxiety that it engenders.

In many respects, sex therapists are now faced with a new challenge in working out the best way of helping the adult whose sexual problems may be related to such childhood experiences. This whole development confronts us with an ethical issue of some fundamental importance. Has the earlier tendency for victims of childhood sexual abuse to keep their secrets resulted from their expectation that, in any case, they would not be believed? And if so, what part has psychotherapy played in reinforcing this expectation? Masson[32] in a compelling book examines the early days of Freudian psychoanalysis and asks why Freud's early belief in the aetiological importance of intra-family sexual abuse gave way to his later view that such abuse represented fantasy of a wish-fulfilling kind? Much of the structure of psychoanalytic theory was built on this revised view. Masson gives evidence of an upsurge of awareness of child sexual abuse in the 1880s in France, which, according to his account, was followed by a process of social denial, as if the reality was too horrendous to contemplate. He proposes a similar explanation for the change in Freud's position. Are we now living through another period of reawakened awareness of intra-family sexual abuse? And what will be the consequences this time? The crucial point from Masson's analysis which is relevant to our topic is that, as a result of Freud's revised theory, generations of psychoanalytic patients have been told or led to believe that their experiences of sexual abuse as children were wish-fulfilling figments of their imagination. For someone who has experienced such childhood trauma, it is difficult to think of any way in which a professional could aggravate the trauma more than by this process of invalidation. This therefore provides us with a particularly disturbing example of a therapeutic process which may have more general relevance; the imposition by the therapist of an interpretation of the patient's experience which, while satisfying the theoretical needs and hence justifying the therapeutic method of the therapist, also harms the patient. How often, and in how many different types of psychological treatment, does this type of harm result?

At the present time, as the prevailing reaction to this disturbing increase in awareness, it is now frequently regarded as unacceptable to doubt in any way the truth of an individual's account of childhood abuse. That state of affairs is likely to produce its own problems as time goes on.

Another clinical example from sex therapy evokes an ethical dilemma which is more insidious, perhaps because it is less contentious. This concerns the individual who presents with low sexual interest or drive. Usually this is seen as a problem because of its incompatibility with the greater sexual interest of the partner. The therapist may seek a cause for this 'disability' or recommend treatment, with the implication that diminished sexual interest is wrong or pathological. A parallel may be drawn with low intelligence. Obviously there are circumstances when an individual's intelligence becomes impaired, even occasionally undeveloped, because of a pathological process which deserves attention. But usually, if problems in a relationship stem from a difference in intellectual capacity, help is given to the couple to come to terms with the difference rather than to try to reduce it. But not so with low sex drive; sex therapists often justify intervention on the grounds that low drive is a consequence of active psychological inhibition. Doubtless that is sometimes the case, but some therapists have difficulty in accepting that a person's low sexual interest may be intrinsic. In such circumstances, we encourage conformity to a norm of sexual activity.

A comparable and perhaps more contentious issue concerns female orgasm. While it is relatively unusual for an adult man to be non-orgasmic, it is far from rare among women. There seems little doubt that many women have become orgasmic with help, realizing the potential that had lain dormant. But a corollary of this has been the growing expectation that every woman should be orgasmic; yet there is no evidence or even likelihood that this is possible. The issue has become confounded by its political implications. An orgasm has become a 'woman's right' of the kind which has often been denied by the self-centred sexual chauvinism of men. A male therapist may now expect feminist censure if he suggests to a woman that she may not have the capacity for orgasm. Obviously it is no more justified to make that assumption than it is to make the opposite, but it is difficult to avoid the process of reinforcing 'norms' and the consequent pressure to conform to them. This is one area in which the therapeutic activities of sex therapists have unwittingly influenced public opinion by generating new expectations. How does one strike the correct balance between encouraging women to realize their sexual potential and creating dissatisfaction with their individual limitations?

Another relevant ethical issue concerns the conflict between the goals of therapy and the cultural or religious norms of the patient. Many sex therapists emphasize the importance of mutual self-assertion and self-protection in the sexual relationship, stressing the need for equality both in the give-and-take of sexual pleasure and in the relationship more generally. In the context of white, Anglo-Saxon, Protestant, or Jewish middle-class culture, from which these therapeutic approaches originate, such principles make sense. But to what extent should they be encouraged in couples from different cultural or religious backgrounds? For the Muslim this may present conflict with Islamic expectations of the sexual roles of men and women. In many societies, particularly those more obviously 'macho-oriented', the sex therapist's principles may conflict with the cultural criteria of masculinity or femininity. By advocating his principles, the therapist may create disharmony within the couple's social environment. When do the advantages of the therapist's 'model relationship' outweigh the social dissonance that it may produce? This also, once again, takes us into the realm of sexual politics. The amount of conflict produced tends to vary with the degree of cultural or religious support for the subordination of women. I have to admit to a degree of missionary zeal in this respect. I firmly believe in the social and interpersonal value of equality in sexual relationships as described above, yet I am conscious of the conflict that it may produce in some of my patients. Usually my zeal is overpowered by entrenched social influence. The therapist should not get the extent of his 'power' out of proportion. But the ethical dilemma is there, and it is accentuated by the increasing tendency for women to reject traditional social norms, and hence to be receptive of therapy goals, while their partners prefer the status quo. In such cases, therapy may only reinforce tension that had already developed in the relationship because of the changing expectations of women. It is pertinent to ask when it is helpful to increase tensions in this way.

## Informed consent and the acceptability of treatment methods

Having considered the potential influence of the therapist on his patient, what other ethical issues arise in the negotiation of treatment for sexual problems? The need for goals that are acceptable both to patient and therapist has already been stressed. But what about the acceptability of the treatment method itself?

Most forms of sex therapy present no particular problems in this respect, relying on the active co-operation of the patient or couple to carry out 'homework assignments' in the privacy of their own home—tasks which are within their control to do or not to do. Nevertheless, it is desirable from every point of view to give a clear account of what will be involved, such as the type of homework assignment, content of the counselling sessions, and frequency and duration of treatment. When this is done a proportion of patients or couples decline the offer of treatment, either explicitly or by default, and this emphasizes the importance of *informed* consent. If informed consent is not sought, patients may enter a form of therapy which they do not understand or like but from which they cannot ecape without loss of face. Such a situation is commonplace in many psychiatric clinics, particularly within the British Health Service, where the patient does not pay for treatment. Treatment proceeds from one session to the next with no clear objective or plan having been stated and no clear opportunities for the patient to say 'yes, I do want to give this a try' or 'no, I don't'. Initial assessment merges imperceptibly into ill-defined treatment; the patient complies or is seen to be uncooperative or 'poorly motivated'.

Most sex therapists recognize the desirability of establishing a clear 'contract' with the patient at the outset. This not only requires him to make a responsible decision whether to accept this particular offer of help, but is also therapeutically beneficial if treatment is accepted. The patient may reject the offer not because he is 'poorly motivated' but because he does not like or trust the therapist or does not feel comfortable with the style of treatment proposed.

There are specific components of treatment that present problems and there may be a need to correct patients' false expectations. They may, for example, incorrectly and apprehensively believe that therapy will require them to 'perform sexually' in front of the therapist. The need for a physical examination and the particular form it takes can create difficulties. Some therapists may be inflexible in following certain procedures, such as having the partner present or involved at this examination. Failure to prepare the patient or couple for this procedure may result in alienation or rejection of treatment. Obviously it is not possible or even desirable for every eventuality to be agreed upon at the outset—but if the therapist is sensitive to possible rejection of a new idea and allows proper and unprejudiced discussion during the course of therapy, these difficulties can often be avoided. A common problem is the unacceptability of masturbation techniques for some patients. When these techniques are rejected by the patients they may be led to feel that they are unreasonably old-fashioned or uncooperative. This can have a destructive effect on treatment and also affect the patient's self-esteem, a further example of the abuse of patients by the theoretical approach, as discussed earlier.

A form of treatment which has caused particular concern is aversion therapy. In the 1950s and 1960s it was used quite commonly for the treatment of various forms of deviant sexuality including homosexuality. The inefficacy of treatment methods aimed at eliminating existing behaviours rather than establishing new ones has already been mentioned and in the light of clinical experience, as well as theoretical reappraisal, aversive techniques are now seen to have a much more limited role. They may be useful, however, in helping the patient who is in danger of committing a sexual offence to increase his self-control, particularly if combined with other more positive methods of treatment.[1,29] But can the use of noxious stimuli such as electric shock or induced nausea ever be justified on ethical grounds? Much of the criticism of these techniques involves a comparison with 'brain washing'. I have closely examined this assumption elsewhere[1] and pointed out that the similarity between 'thought reform' techniques and aversion therapy, *as generally used*, is negligible, not only because of the differences in noxiousness and duration involved, but also because of the need, in the case of thought reform, for total control of the individual's environment. In the absence of such 'total manipulation', there is little chance of altering a person's reactions or beliefs unless such changes are sought by him. Hence providing that aversive techniques are only used in a setting where the patient is able to reject or withdraw from treatment, the ethical problem is not one of *Clockwork Orange* control.

Obviously there are ethical considerations in the type of noxious stimuli used. They should be safe and no more unpleasant than they need to be for the purpose. Their intensity should be chosen to suit the tolerance of the individual patient and he should still have control over the level of intensity used. There have been several reports of methods which do not follow these principles and they have consequently received just criticism.[33] But if we ensure the fully informed consent of the patient in the use of safe and tolerable aversive stimuli, do we satisfy ethical requirements? Does aversive treatment differ from other painful forms of treatment such as surgery or dentistry? In my view, the remaining ethical issue involves, once again, the nature of the patient–therapist relationship. At best, an aversive technique should be seen as one particular form of help incorporated into a more broadly-based approach. It should not be seen as a complete or sufficient treatment method in its own right. Of crucial relevance is the effect that the aversive procedure has on this relationship. Two consequences are likely: the patient may feel anger towards the therapist, and he may feel humiliated by the experience.

From my earlier experiences with aversion therapy[1] I concluded that ethical safeguards lay in the maintenance of or striving for the same kind of mutually respecting 'adult–adult' relationship between patient and therapist that we discussed earlier. The patient's anger should be understood and dealt with appropriately; any likelihood of humiliation should be countered, in what ever way possible, by the therapist. Following such principles would preclude certain types of 'aversion' therapy which rely not on aversive stimuli such as electric shock but on systematic criticism and humiliation of the patient—so-called 'shame therapy'.[34] Happily the indications for aversive techniques are now so limited that they are seldom used. But the principles involved may have more general relevance.

The use of aversive techniques to facilitate self-control over unwanted sexual behaviour brings me to the next ethical issue—consent to treatment by the sexual offender, which is not only informed but also free from coercion. It is not unusual for an offender, say a sexual abuser of children, to be referred by the court for treatment, such treatment to be given as a condition of sentence. How can one establish, at a stage when the sentence has not been passed, what the offender himself wants, other than his understandable desire to placate the court? With psychological methods of treatment, particularly counselling or psychotherapy, the issue is less crucial because treatment is not likely to be effective unless the offender wants it to be. Nevertheless, he may find himself 'trapped' in therapy because of his sentence. The use of aversive techniques in these circumstances is clearly a cause for concern, and even more critical is the prescribing of drugs such as the anti-androgen cyproterone acetate, oestrogens, or benperidol to control sexual drive. Once sentence, which includes the condition for treatment, has been passed, control for what is done passes from the court, with its public safeguards, to the doctor, with probably no external scrutiny at all. The crucial distinction arises between 'therapy', which is usually regarded as in the interest of the recipient, and 'social control', where the aim is primarily to protect society. The use of a penal procedure like imprisonment is straightforward in that it comes unequivocally into the second category and is only administered with the public safeguards of the legal system. But when 'social control' becomes confused with medical treatment, those safeguards disappear and ethical problems ensue because of the possibility that the offender's interests are dealt with at the same time as those of society. The use of drugs to suppress libido in sexual offenders creates a precedent which, with the development of drugs to control other drives such as aggression, may have much wider and more fundamental ethical significance.

Clearly a case can be made for the use of libido-suppressing drugs both to the benefit of the individual and as a means of 'social control'. There may be individuals who have not as yet tangled with the law but who are in danger of doing so and who seek medical help. Drugs may then be useful and the problem of informed consent does not differ substantially from that with other types of drug therapy. There will also be those who following conviction are regarded as a serious threat to public safety and for whom the use of drugs as an alternative 'social' control' to imprisonment may be justified; can 'consent free from coercion', normally required before administering medical treatment, ever be obtained with sufficient confidence when the alternative is another method of penal control? In these cases I would argue that treatment should be administered by the court in the same way as any other penal measure and not be labelled euphemistically as medical treatment. Currently, there is no legal machinery for such administration. This is a complex and important ethical issue which remains unresolved.

There are other forms of 'treatment' for sexual offenders which deserve separate consideration because of their irreversible nature and potentially far-reaching effects. Both surgical castration and various forms of psychosurgery (see Chapter 10) have been used, and the ethical question is whether they should be used under any circumstances. Castration is much less commonly used today, partly because it has been shown to be relatively ineffective or at best its effects unpredictable.[35] The value of psychosurgery is not clear from the available evidence, but as with castration it has been strongly criticized on both scientific and ethical grounds.[36] Given the generalized effects that both procedures may have on personality, I would require solid evidence of predictable outcome in each case before I could begin to justify their use. It is difficult to see how such evidence could be obtained.

## The management of the transsexual patient

Transsexualism as a clinical problem poses ethical issues that are perhaps unique, and require separate consideration. Transsexuals believe themselves to be, or seek to become, members of the sex opposite to that of their own bodies. The causes for this condition are not understood and even professionals concerned to help these people find it a puzzle. Because of transsexuals' overriding desire to live and be accepted as members of their psychological sex, they seek medical help to change their bodies to conform with their psychological gender identity. Such sex reassignment may require, apart from an adjustment in behaviour, in the case of a male to female transsexual, electrolysis of facial hair, oestrogenic hormones to feminize the skin and body fat, mammoplasty, penectomy, orchidectomy, and vaginoplasty. For the female to male transsexual, androgenic hormones to increase body and facial hair and muscle bulk, mastectomy, hysterectomy, oophorectomy, and possibly phalloplasty may be sought (as yet the advantages of phalloplasty are very uncertain because of problems of surgical technique). An enormous amount of medical help is likely to be required in the long-term process of sex reassignment, which, at best, is always difficult.

The first ethical issue concerns the basic acceptability of the procedure, especially as it involves surgical alteration of the anatomy. It may be regarded as immoral because it is seen to tamper with nature.[37] Some surgeons have been reluctant to involve themselves, or have been discouraged by their legal advisers from doing so, for fear that they may be prosecuted under the archaic mayhem statutes. These derive from feudal England and were intended to deter men from evading military service by having some part of their body removed (usually fingers or toes). The surgeon responsible for the maiming was liable. Holloway[38] however was able to find only one case in the legal literature in which a surgeon had been convicted under such a statute and this was not for sex reassignment surgery.

Graham[39] has more recently reviewed the legal aspects and his conclusions lend support to the idea that responsibly taken decisions about sex reassignment with properly informed consent are unlikely to be successfully prosecuted as illegal. He points out, however, the variation in legal opinion on this matter particularly in the United States where the law relevant to mayhem varies from state to state. And he gives examples of legal opinion that genuinely informed consent for such surgery may be impossible for the transsexual seeking reassignment.

These uncertainties have not applied to those cases, such as adreno-genital syndrome or Klinefelter's syndrome, where there is an identifiable physical cause for the incongruity between psychological and physical gender. A further objection has come from some psychiatrists, who view transsexualism as a form of psychosis and sex re-assignment surgery as a totally unacceptable collusion with the patient's delusional system. The mental state of the transsexual is indeed important in deciding whether he is able to give 'informed consent'. It is usually not possible to justify a diagnosis of psychosis or any other particular psychiatric condition.[40] Transsexuals often have personality problems, perhaps particularly the male-to-female,[41] but this is often an understandable consequence of prolonged gender-identity confusion, and is as likely to be a justification for sex reassignment as a contra-indication.

Transsexualism has been described as an iatrogenic condition; before the first surgical reassignment there was not the demand for such treatment that now exists. It is perhaps not surprising that before such a procedure is regarded as feasible it is not often requested. In fact, many people with gender-identity confusion may resolve much of their confusion once they learn that such a change is possible, even if the prospect is remote. There certainly seems little doubt that apart from the specific request for surgery, the other manifestations of transsexualism have been well-known for centuries.[42]

As the medical profession has become more familiar with this condition, there has been a greater preparedness to seek solutions to the transsexual's problems. With recognition that a proportion of transsexuals are clearly better off after reassignment surgery than they were before, a number of centres around the world have provided this type of treatment. The professional in such a centre faces a further ethical problem: the conflict between the rights of the patient and the doctor's responsibility for his patient's welfare. The relationship between transsexual patient and doctor is to a considerable extent a game in which the patient has no doubts about his or her wishes and whose primary purpose is to persuade the doctor to accede to them. The doctor in return is conscious of the possibility of an unfavourable outcome—that by no means all transsexuals fare well following surgery. Failure is of two principal types. First, the patient's expectations of the benefits of surgery may be unrealistic, looking for resolution of most of his problems. In fact, the problem of 'passing' or being socially accepted successfully in the new sex will not be affected by genital surgery except indirectly through an increase in self-confidence. Commonly the patient discovers that life is still difficult and he may return for more surgery. The second kind of failure is in surgical technique. Vaginoplasty and phalloplasty pose considerable technical challenges to the surgeon and frequently go wrong. Postoperative complications may be prolonged or serious.

The doctor when confronted with a patient seemingly determined to pursue sex reassignment, naturally wishes to establish that the patient will cope with, and benefit from, this major change. Hence, more or less all specialist centres now require a period of one and a half to two years of 'real-life testing' in the new role before irreversible surgery is carried out.

The Harry Benjamin International Gender Dysphoria Association has published standards of care for hormonal and surgical reassignment, reflecting the opinions of most experts in the field.[43] They stress the importance of a conservative approach in which irreversible decisions involving surgery should only be taken after a period of time in which the transsexual demonstrates his or her ability to cope effectively with the chosen gender role. They also advocate the involvement in the decision-making of clinicians whose training and experience is in the assessment and management of psychological and sexual problems. Unfortunately there are still surgeons who will operate on transsexuals without such safeguards, providing that they can be paid for the surgery. Such clinical practice must be regarded as ethically suspect. The management of the transsexual remains an unusually difficult area from the ethical point of view, and while there is little doubt that many of these individuals live happier and more fulfilled lives after full sex reassignment (and this author continues to recommend patients for surgery after careful selection), it is an aspect of clinical care which should be kept under constant review.

## Confidentiality (see Chapter 15)

In most forms of psychiatric treatment information obtained from patients is of a highly confidential nature. This is particularly so where sexual problems are concerned. Special consideration has therefore to be given to the method of keeping records and to the type of information recorded. The use of special files, distinguishable and separate from general medical files, is probably mandatory.

Psychiatrists are usually trained to take a detailed history which is systematic and far-ranging. They are less well trained to select crucial information in a particular case, and usually follow the principle that the more information one has, the less likely it is that some important factor will be overlooked. The acquisition of large amounts of confidential and intimate information may also enhance their 'charisma' in the patient's eyes. We need to question seriously the amount of information we obtain (and especially record) in the management of sexual problems. There are two implications. The first is related to the therapeutic consequences: the vulnerability produced in the patient by a one-way exchange of information may reinforce a tendency to take a passive role in therapy rather than the active 'adult' role that is needed. The second implication is more directly ethical. Is the therapist justified in obtaining information which is not clearly relevant to the patient's treatment? In the newer, more behavioural forms of sex therapy, specific behavioural tasks, usually small steps towards the goals of treatment, are set by the therapist. If the patient or couple can carry these out satisfactorily then the next tasks are assigned and so on. Only when difficulty is encountered in achieving the tasks is it necessary to look for explanations, and relevant background information may then be sought. A couple can go through a course of such therapy with little problem and consequently with the therapist knowing very little about their past lives.[29] Obviously a certain amount of information has to be obtained at the outset in order to arrive at a reasonable contract for treatment. Yet many therapists consider that they have failed in their professional duty if they do not find out about important past events. The need to justify requests for confidential information remains an important ethical issue in sex therapy as well as other kinds of psychiatric treatment.

When working with couples, particular problems of confidentiality may arise when one partner gives the therapist information that is to be concealed from the other. With information about past events, it is usually appropriate to accept the patient's request for continued confidentiality. When the confidence concerns a continuing or current aspect of the patient's life, this may pose problems for the therapist. The most obvious example is when one partner reveals an on-going extramarital relationship and expects the therapist to keep the information from the spouse. This may impose a considerable handicap on therapy and can be considered unacceptable on those grounds. My own policy in these circumstances is to indicate that I am only prepared to work with a couple if they commit themselves to their relationship, at least for the duration of treatment. I explain that the basis of my approach is to facilitate an open, self-assertive, and self-protective relationship, and that to attempt that with the therapist and one partner concealing highly relevant information from the other makes a mockery of that approach. There is however a need for caution. The spouse with current extramarital activity may not anticipate this response from the therapist. Having made the revelation, the withdrawal of the therapist from a treatment contract may place the patient in a difficult position with his spouse. It may therefore be appropriate, when such circumstances are suspect, to make a general comment about therapeutic policy before the patient has revealed anything specific.

Our entry into the AIDS era is also presenting the sex therapist with formidable problems when dealing with couples of which one partner is HIV-positive and does not wish the other to know. This problem, which of course has arisen in the past with other forms of sexually transmitted disease, is by no means confined to the sex therapist. But there are special difficulties when both partners are equally involved in the therapeutic transaction, and when the therapy is predicated on the fundamental importance of mutual trust in sexual relationships.

## Professional qualifications

A continuing concern among sex therapists is the maintenance of satisfactory standards of training and clinical practice. It is not unusual for people who have no professional training of any kind, and whose qualifications are based on their own sexual experiences to designate themselves as expert sex therapists. It may be argued that the maintenance of professional standards is not an ethical issue, however desirable it is to foster competent practice. On the other hand, the point is often made that professional bodies establish and enforce ethical guidelines. Individual therapists working outside such organizations have no such guidance or constraints. This point has even been used to justify the exclusion of all non-medical professionals (such as clinical psychologists) from involvement in sex therapy, on the grounds that only medical doctors have a 'Hippocratic Oath', which bars them from sexual contact with their patients and a disciplinary body to enforce it. (The fact that most doctors on qualifying don't take any such oath is perhaps irrelevant). This issue is a complex one, and I shall only deal with it briefly. Much of the problem stems from the difficulty in defining what are the requirements for a good sex therapist. In matters of unequivocal pathology, it is relatively easy to justify the need for medical training.

In the past few years there has been a dramatic increase in our awareness of the role of physical factors in the causation of sexual dysfunction, mainly erectile problems in men.[29] Clearly there is now a need, in many cases of erectile dysfunction, for access to the appropriate medical skills in investigating the aetiological significance of such factors. But whether or not physical factors are found to be relevant, the mainstay of management remains psychological. Apart from the educational and communication-improving aspects, which are central to much of sex therapy, 'permission' is often required to approach love-making in different ways, which previously the couple would have considered 'abnormal' or unacceptable, in order to adapt to the limitations imposed by physical disease or the ageing process. There is therefore no escaping the need for the sexual counsellor with the appropriately sensitive and informed approach. A medical training is not required for that role. Indeed, some hold the view that medical training creates barriers to such counselling skills. There is therefore a requirement for good clinical practice that sex therapists, who are not medically qualified, should have good working relationships with medical colleagues who can carry out appropriate physical assessment. The converse is not only true but of particular importance at the present time. The recent vogue amongst surgeons for the investigation of erectile dysfunction with intracavernosal injections of smooth muscle-relaxing drugs has led to a growing use of self-injection of such drugs as a form of treatment. Increasingly patients are being referred to surgeons and started on such self-injection regimens with a minimum of assessment of the psychological aspects of the problem or the psychological reactions of the man and his partner to this type of treatment. This presents us with one of the principal ethical concerns in the management of sexual problems at the present time. It is too early to appraise the full significance of this development, but if it continues unmodified I predict considerable problems both clinically and medico-legally. To a lesser extent, and for somewhat longer, there have been comparable concerns about the use of surgical prostheses for erectile failure. There are undoubtedly cases where such use is beneficial. But it is not unusual for surgical treatment of this kind to be recommended without adequate assessment of the psychological aspects of the case. The solution, once again, is for surgeons working in this field, who undoubtedly have a valuable part to play, to work closely with colleagues whose expertise is in the psychological assessment and management of sexual problems. Increasingly we are confronted by the need, for both ethical and clinical reasons, for interdisciplinary sexual problem clinics. Regrettably they are still rare, and in general are given low priority within the National Health Service in the United Kingdom. This issue is of even greater importance in the private sector, where often of necessity clinicians work in relative isolation.

In my view, the field of sexual problems has the particular advantage that a simple educational approach can be used in the first instance, often with good effect and frequently sufficient in itself. In cases where this is not enough, additional help and skills can be introduced at a later stage without disadvantage. The borderlines between sex education, simple counselling, and more complex therapy are ill-defined.

It may be agreed, nevertheless, that with the various ethical complexities that have been considered in this chapter, there is a strong need for a special or 'professional' status for the sex therapist. If so, we must seek ethically acceptable ways of meeting that need.

## References

1 Bancroft, J.: *Deviant sexual behaviour: modification and assessment.* Oxford, Oxford University Press, 1974.
2 Pope, K. S., Keith-Spiegel, P., and Tabachnik, B. G.: Sexual attraction to clients: the human therapist and the (sometimes) inhuman training system. *American Psychologist* **41**:147–158, 1986.
3 Kardener, S. H.: Sex and the physician–patient relationship. *American Journal of Psychiatry* **131**, 1134–6, 1974.
4 Bancroft, J.: Commentary on 'incest' by Noble, M. and Mason, J. R. *Journal of Medical Ethics* **4**:69–70, 1978.
5 Schover, L. R. and Jensen, S. B.: *Sexuality and chronic illness: a comprehensive approach.* New York, Guilford, 1988.
6 Marmor, J. The ethics of sex therapy, in *Ethical issues in sex therapy and research*, ed. W. H. Masters, V. E. Johnson, and R. C. Kolodny. Boston, Little Brown, 1977.
7 Apfel, R. J. and Simon, B.: Patient–therapist sexual contact: II. Problems of subsequent psychotherapy. *Psychotherapy and Psychosomatics* **43**:63–8, 1985.
8 Feldman-Summers, S. and Jones, G.: Psychological impacts of sexual contact between therapists or other health care practitioners and their clients. *Journal of Consulting and Clinical Psychology.* **52**:1054–61, 1984.
9 Edelwich, J. and Brodsky, A.: *Sexual dilemmas for the helping professional.* New York, Brunner-Mazel, 1982.
10 Tunnadine, L. P. D.: *Contraception and sexual life; a therapeutic approach.* London, Tavistock, 1970.
11 Hartman, W. E. and Fithian, M. A.: *Treatment of sexual dysfunction.* California, Centre for Marital and Sexual Studies, 1972.

12 Hoch, Z.: The sensory arm of the female orgasmic reflex. Paper read at 5th Annual Meeting of International Academy of Sex Research, Prague, August, 1979.

13 Williams, M. H.: Individual sex therapy, in *Handbook of sex therapy*, ed. J. LoPiccolo, and L. LoPiccolo. Plenum, New York, 1978.

14 Schrenck-Notzing, A. von: *The use of hypnosis in psychopathic sexuality with special reference to contrary sexual instruct*, trans. C. L. Chaddock, 1956. The Institute of Research on Hypnosis Publication Society and Juhan Press, 1895.

15 Masters, W. and Johnson, V. F.: *Human sexual inadequacy*. Boston, Little Brown, 1970.

16 Cole, M.: Sex therapy for individuals, in *Sex therapy in Britain*, ed. M. Cole and W. Dryden. Open University Press, Milton Keynes, 1988, pp. 272–99.

17 Cole, M.: Human sex behaviour and sex therapy, in *Sexual problems*, ed. J. Jacobson. London, Elek, 1975.

18 Malamuth, N., Wanderer, Z. W., Sayner, R. B. and Duknell, D.: Utilisation of surrogate partners: a survey of health professionals. *Journal of Behaviour Therapy and Experimental Psychiatry* 7:149–50, 1976.

19 Jacobs, M. Thompson, L. A., and Truxaw, P.: The use of sexual surrogates in counselling. *Counselling Psychologist* 5:73–7, 1975.

20 Masters, W. H., Johnson, V. S., and Kolodny, R.: *Ethical issues in sex therapy and research*. Boston, Little Brown, 1977.

21 Bancroft, J.: Crisis intervention, in *An introduction to the psychotherapies*. 2nd edn, ed. S. Bloch. Oxford, Oxford University Press, 1986.

22 Bancroft, J.: Sex therapy, in *An introduction to the psychotherapies*. 2nd edn, ed. S. Bloch. Oxford, Oxford University Press, 1986.

23 Bullough, V. L.: Homosexuality and the medical model. *Journal of Homosexuality* 1:99–110, 1974.

24 Bell, A. P. and Weinberg, M. S.: *Homosexualities. A study of diversity among men and women*. London, Mitchell Beezley, 1978.

25 Davison, G. C.: Homosexuality: the ethical challenge. *Journal of Consulting and Clinical Psychology* 44:157–62, 1976.

26 Bancroft, J.: Homosexuality and the medical profession: a behaviourist's view. *Journal of Medical Ethics* 1:176–80, 1975.

27 Masters, W. H. and Johnston, V. E.: *Homosexuality in perspective*. Boston, Little Brown, 1979.

28 Boswell, J.: *Christianity, social tolerance and homosexuality*. Chicago, Chicago University Press, 1980.

29 Bancroft, J.: *Human sexuality and its problems*, 2nd edn, Churchill Livingstone, Edinburgh, 1989.

30 Blumstein, P. W. and Schwartz, P.: Bisexuality in women. *Archives of Sexual Behavior* 5:171–82, 1976.

31 Klein, F.: The need to view sexual orientation as a multivariable, dynamic process. In *Homosexuality/heterosexuality; the Kinsey Scale and current research*, 2nd Kinsey Symposium, ed. D. McWhirter and J. M. Reinisch. New York, Oxford University Press, 1990.

32 Masson, J. F.: *The assault on truth: Freud's suppression of the seduction theory*. New York, Farrar, Straus & Giroux, 1984.

33 Campbell, D., Sanderson, R. E., and Laverty, S. G.: Characteristics of conditioned response in human subjects during extinction trials following a single

traumatic conditioning trial. *Journal of Abnormal and Social Psychology* **68**:627–39, 1963.

34 Serber, M.: Shame aversion therapy. *Behaviour Therapy and Experimental Psychiatry* **1**:219–21, 1974.

35 Heim, N. and Hursch, C. J.: Castration for sex offenders: treatment or punishment? a review and critique of recent European literature. *Archives of Sexual Behavior.* **8**:281–304, 1979.

36 Rieber, I. and Sigusch V.: Psychosurgery in sex offenders and sexual deviants in West Germany. *Archives of Sexual Behavior* **8**:523–28, 1979.

37 Green, R.: Attitudes towards transsexualism and sex re-assignment procedures, in *Transsexualism and sex reassignment*, ed. R. Green, and J. Money. Baltimore, Johns Hopkins Press, 1969.

38 Holloway, J. P.: Transsexuals: legal considerations. *Archives of Sexual Behavior* **3**:33–50, 1974.

39 Graham, D.: Legal aspects; should the law be changed? In *Transsexualism and sex reassignment*, ed. W. A. W. Walters and M. W. Ross. Oxford, Oxford University Press, 1986, pp. 135–43.

40 Hoenig, J. and Kenner, J. C.: The nosological position of transsexualism. *Archives of Sexual Behavior* **3**:273–88, 1974.

41 Walinder, J.: *Transsexualism: a study of 43 cases.* Gotenburg, Scandinavian University Books, 1967.

42 Bullough, V. L.: Transsexualism in history. *Archives of Sexual Behavior* **4**:561–72, 1975.

43 Walker, P. A., Berger, J. C., Green, R., Laub, D. R., Reynolds, C. L., and Wollman, L.: Standards of care: the hormonal and surgical sex reassignment of gender dysphoric persons. *Archives of Sexual Behavior* **43**:79–90, 1985.

# 12

# The ethics of suicide

*David Heyd and Sidney Bloch*

## I. The special status of the problem of suicide

Suicide presents perhaps the most dramatic and demanding clinical situation psychiatrists have to face. At the annual rate of 5000 successful suicides in England and 20 000–30 000 in the United States, and with an increase in the 15–35 year age-group since 1975,[1] no psychiatrist can deny the gravity of the problem. And as the number of attempted (unsuccessful) suicides is roughly 8 to 10 times the number of fatal suicides, there is but little chance that any psychiatrist is spared the direct and personal experience of treating suicidal patients and their families. While the widespread incidence makes suicide impossible to ignore, its very nature makes it difficult to confront—psychologically, therapeutically, and ethically.

Suicide differs in at least four important respects from other clinical circumstances that involve ethical dilemmas. First, most medical and psychiatric problems are concerned with the adjustment of the right means to a given end that is basically shared by doctor and patient; suicide however focuses on the end itself, about which the two parties may hold polarly opposite views. Suicide is not only a *functional* problem to which therapeutic techniques are applied but also an *existential* one—in both the literal and the philosophical sense of the word. The question is not how to achieve a better, more fruitful life, but whether to live at all. The fact that the starting-point in the treatment of the potentially suicidal person is seen in such radically divergent terms by doctor and patient makes suicide a particularly difficult case: the psychiatrist's task extends beyond technically assisting his patient in attaining his own desired goals; he is required to persuade the patient to change his most basic desires and attitude to life.

Secondly, the conflict between the psychiatrist's values and his patient's goals is deeper than a particular and incidental disagreement. The value of life as an end in itself is not only shared by the great majority of people, but also considered as possibly the most important ethical value. Accordingly, the very phenomenon of suicide is generally regarded as a threat or even as an insult to our deepest convictions about the 'sanctity of life'. To some extent this intolerance of the idea of the cessation of life is manifest in our attitude to death in general, which we find hard to face directly, but it is especially acute in the case of suicide, which expresses a *voluntary* and irreverent repudiation of the value of life.

Thirdly, it is difficult for us to rid ourselves of this sense of insult or threat, because the dilemma of suicide is logically and ethically puzzling. As we shall see in the next section, there are unsolvable problems in supplying a rational justification for the value of life and for the alleged moral duty to go on living. Our belief in the obvious value of life is further offended by the relative failure in preventing suicide, either by means of psychiatric treatment or through some form of social engineering. It seems that whatever we do, the rate of suicide in a particular society will remain fairly constant.[2] And the optimism raised by successful prevention in individual cases is partly offset by the alarming number of people under psychiatric and other medical care who nevertheless succeed in taking their own lives. Psychiatry does not seem (yet) to fare better than the more traditional menacing attempts of moralists, theologians, and legislators at stopping people from killing themselves. Suicide is disturbingly ubiquitous and universal—across cultures and ages.

Finally, it is a well-known fact that the suicide rate among physicians including psychiatrists is substantially higher than that in the general population.[3] This special proneness places the psychiatrist in a vulnerable position when he treats a suicidal patient. In other spheres of treatment (of both mental and physical illness) the doctor can more readily remain detached. But the possibility of suicide is considered by almost every human being at some stage of his life and this makes it harder for the doctor to take a balanced and objective view of his suicidal patient. As a result there is the danger of an unsympathetic or unduly paternalistic attitude replacing rational evaluation and humane understanding of the patient's situation.

So, unlike many kinds of psychological dysfunction, suicide is not a *state* which may gradually improve (or deteriorate) with the application of particular forms of treatment. It is rather a radical *event* taking place at a specific moment, often totally unpredictable and always irreversible. Furthermore, the act of suicide is motivated by what seems to us to be an unnatural drive or choice, with results which none of us can easily imagine or experience.

Beyond those very concrete problems facing the clinician, there are certain methodological difficulties which the student and theorist of suicide cannot ignore. Although suicide could be thought to be an easily definable concept, closer examination reveals a wide range of definitions and a plethora of partially synonymous terms ('suicide', 'self-killing', 'self-murder', 'self-poisoning', 'attempted suicide', 'para-suicide', etc.). Not being a case of malfunctioning, suicide cannot be defined in terms of a normal or standard state or behaviour. The fact that the business of suicide is the denial of some value, a normative choice, and not just a physical act of terminating biological life, makes the definition of suicide *value-laden*, that is to say not purely descriptive. The language of suicide reflects this characteristic: for example, the lack of any specific Biblical term for self-killing, the emotive phrase 'self-murder' used by Augustine, the attempt to neutralize the value-laden concept by using a scientific term ('intentionally caused self-destruction'), or the more modern clinical and restricted jargon 'self-poisoning'. 'Suicide' itself is a relatively new (seventeenth-century) term whose function was to replace the more incriminatory 'self-homicide'.[4]

On the other hand, ethical analysis, let alone moral judgement, cannot ignore the scientific theories about the nature of suicide, that is to say the *descriptive* studies of psychiatry, psychology, and sociology. Both the way suicide is conceptualized and defined and our approach to the moral question of the right to intervene will depend heavily on these descriptive studies, especially on the questions whether suicide constitutes a mental illness or a rational choice, and whether it is an expression of a pure intention to die or a 'cry for help'. Furthermore, the analysis of the element of voluntariness—one of the conditions of suicide according to many definitions—partly depends on our general theory of mind and human behaviour, including in particular the criteria for distinguishing between an impulsive response to a certain stimulus under conditions of stress and a rational choice based on systematic consideration of alternative courses of action.

The awareness of this inevitably 'circular' nature of all definitions and theories of suicide (the interdependence of descriptive and normative factors) is of both theoretical and day-to-day clinical importance. This interdependence will become especially clear when some major views concerning suicide in the history of Western thought are studied (in section III) and the contemporary clinical scene is discussed (in section IV). In the philosophical discussion (in section II) we will suggest that the difficulties in refuting the 'rationality' of suicide are considerable, but nevertheless leave room for a significant measure of morally justifiable intervention. The ethical basis of such an intervention policy is spelled out in more detail in the final part of the chapter (section V). We hope that our philosophical and historical analysis, by broadening the clinical and ethical perspective, will highlight certain principles in the light of which the psychiatrist's own approach can be critically tested.

## II. The philosophical point of view: the value of life

That life has value, or indeed is the most valuable thing we have, is usually taken for granted. Being such an obvious 'good', it requires no theoretical justification. Being so naturally held by human beings as a primary value, it needs no inculcation. The principle of the sanctity of life is invoked (either in theoretical discussion or in moral upbringing) only when the value of *other* people's lives is at stake, as in the context of the prohibition of murder, abortion, involuntary euthanasia, and killing in war. In these cases elaborate argument and reasoning are usually called for. But in the case of one's *own* life, the very questioning of its value is taken by many people as a sign of crisis, or even of 'illness' and abnormality.

Yet, the persistent occurrence of suicide (which apparently is a specifically human phenomenon) constitutes a challenge to the obviousness of life's value. On the one hand, it proves that the basic drive to preserve one's life is not always powerful enough to override other drives and wishes. On the other hand, it casts doubt on the possibility of rationally justifying the value of life because it forces us to admit that most people go on living not as a result of a rational choice or well-grounded conclusion of philosophical reasoning. This may not be a disturbing conclusion as long as we are not confronted by a person's explicit preference for death over life. Besides the tragedy of the person's death itself, the absence of rational justification is perhaps the main cause of the shattering impression suicide leaves on us. It also explains the effort, typical of many cultures, to conceal and suppress the occurrence of suicide, either by linguistic euphemism, or by explaining the resulting death as an 'accident', or by other cover-up methods and taboos. In a more Existentialistic vein we can say that the tragedy of suicide is not only the victim's but also that of the survivors, since the act lays bare the absurdity and meaninglessness of life.[5] As Camus put it: 'There is but one truly serious philosophical problem and that is suicide. Judging whether life is or is not worth living amounts to answering the fundamental question of philosophy.'[6] This philosophical hypothesis is psychologically substantiated by the feeling of emptiness and despair experienced by many people who have survived an unsuccessful attempt on their lives.

The main source of philosophical difficulty in justifying the value of life lies in the symmetry between the two choices of life and death. The prolongation of life does not mean the shortening of death, and cutting life short does not imply having more of the other state (death).[7] Therefore, even if we could assign 'values' to life and death they would be typically incommensurable. How can we compare the state of conscious experience of an identifiable subject with the complete loss of consciousness and personal identity? We are reminded of the famous Epicurean argument: we should never fear death or regard it as an evil, because as long as we live it is not with us, and when we die we are not there to suffer it. We can show how a certain kind of existence and experience is preferable to another kind of existence or experience, but we have no scale of values, no 'parameter', by which we could choose between existence and non-existence.

This intellectual perplexity is reflected in the psychological difficulty of conceiving one's own death. Indeed, Freud was convinced that we can never imagine ourselves dead, and that if we try, we always remain there as spectators.[8] This is evident to psychiatrists dealing with suicidal patients, who often have fantasies of retaining some form of identity and experience after their deaths (e.g. enjoying the relief from pain, or the revenge on those whom the act was meant to punish).

A possible attempt to avoid the puzzling logical asymmetry of the respective values of life and death consists in shifting the emphasis from life *as such* to the *good life*. It is often argued that what carries value is the good or meaningful life—pleasant, happy, honourable, virtuous, and so forth—not sheer biological life. Thus, assuming any scale of values of the types just mentioned, not only can we compare the value of different lives, but we can also declare certain lives (especially our own in certain circumstances) as not worth living at all. This line of argument underlies the more 'rational' cases of suicide: King Saul kills himself to avoid shame; the terminally ill patient opts for voluntary euthanasia in order to avoid pain; Socrates refuses to escape from prison and drinks the poison to avoid the immoral life of an outlaw; Captain Oates sees no value in his life if it risks that of his companions; and the religious martyr dies in order to avoid the violation of divine commands. In all these examples, considerations of the quality of life rather than the comparative value of life versus death lead to the suicidal conclusion.

It should however be noted that the logical problem of the incommensurability of the values of life and death is thus circumvented only at the price of introducing other controversial values of a moral or theological nature. Ascribing value to life rather than to life of a certain quality has the advantage of universality and independence of subjective belief. Moreover, the proponents of the quality-of-life theory have to concede that life as such is a necessary condition to the meaningful or worthwhile life, and therefore has some secondary and indirect value. These remarks are highly relevant to our practical approach to suicidal behaviour because they have far-reaching ethical implications. As we shall see in section V, there are good reasons to prevent a person from committing suicide even if he sincerely believes at a certain moment that his life has lost all meaning and value. These reasons appeal to the value of life itself, from which a new meaning might be created. In other words, even if philosophically speaking only the good or meaningful life is intrinsically valuable, life should be morally respected and enhanced as the only way or opportunity to attain that meaningfulness.

This last point suggests that there is a significant difference between the point of view of the person considering suicide and that of the psychiatrist, relative, or any bystander. For the subject himself the question is that of the meaning of life, the subjective assessment of its value *for him*. For those who judge his decision to take his life, the question is whether it is right or wrong to do so, rational or irrational, permissible or prohibited. Thus far we have considered suicide mainly from the point of view of the agent. We have examined the abstract notions relating to the value of life and the grounds for its continuation or termination. On this level suicide has no specifically moral meaning because morality is concerned with the rules and guiding principles of 'the game of life', whereas suicide is a decision to opt out of the game altogether. From the point of view of the agent, the decision to die lies beyond the reach of moral arguments. But the point of view of others is the moral and ethical one on which we should focus—by considering, albeit schematically, the major ethical approaches to suicide in the history of Western thought and then by examining the moral dilemma of those who may be in a position of responsibility in the face of a person's intent to kill himself.

### III. Major ethical approaches towards suicide in Western thought

The Biblical approach to suicide is usually mentioned only as a curious exception and indeed there is no specific term for intentional self-destruction. Throughout the Old Testament there are only five cases of self-killing—Saul, his slave, Samson, Achitofel, and Zimri—and in the stories relating their fate any moral condemnation (or praise) of the act is conspicuously absent. Death by one's own hand is described as a natural concomitant to another well-grounded and legitimate intention such as avoiding torture by the enemy, loyalty to the King, and wreaking revenge. In the same factual and morally neutral manner the New Testament describes Judas hanging himself (only with Augustine is Judas's suicide condemned as doubling his sin).

Suicide played a more prominent role in Greek and Roman culture. Under certain conditions it was approved and even praised. Aristotle,[9] however, claims unambiguously that killing oneself is 'contrary to the right rule of life' and unjust to the State; the State consequently is justified in taking punitive measures against the suicidal person and his family. Aristotle seems to appreciate the difference that we mentioned earlier—between the subjective point of view which is morally neutral (since suicide is voluntary, it cannot be considered according to Aristotle as 'unjust to oneself') and the objective moral judgement of others (if there is an injustice, it must be to the State). A similar extension of the meaning of suicide beyond the subjective can be traced in Socrates'[10] prohibition on taking one's own life. Again, as with Aristotle, it is argued that self-annihilation may be viewed as unjust towards some 'person' other than the agent (thus making it a *moral* wrong), but it is the gods rather than the State who are wronged by the taking of life. For a person is not the owner but only the custodian of life given to him by the gods.

The Romans, however, considered the question of suicide mainly from the agent's point of view, and concluded that it was not subject to moral censure. In Seneca's words, 'mere living is not a good, but living well. Accordingly, the wise man will live as long as he ought, not as long as he can.'[11] Trouble, lack of peace of mind, or a bad turn of fortune are for Seneca sufficient reasons for suicide. Like other Stoics he also values the ultimate exercise of freedom which characterizes our choice of one of the 'many exits' from life. Dying is typically described as a liberating event. In this kind of freedom, says Pliny, we are superior even to the gods. And indeed the incidence of suicide in Imperial Rome was widespread, with no legal sanction against it.

The rise of Christianity as a persecuted religion of a minority group led to many acts of suicide which were justified as martyrdom. The Church responded to the almost epidemic rate of self-destruction by banning it formally in the sixth century. St Augustine[12] presented the theological argument against suicide by interpreting the sixth commandment prohibiting murder as applicable to self-killing no less than to the killing of others. Countering the thesis that suicide was a legitimate way of avoiding sin, Augustine states that suicide is itself the gravest sin. Suicide should be thus considered as wrong under all circumstances with the exception of the definite command of God (as in Samson's case). The most systematic argument against suicide in medieval Christianity is that of Thomas Aquinas (thirteenth century). Thomas[13] presents three reasons:

1. Suicide is a violation of the natural law according to which 'everything naturally keeps itself in being' and which prescribes self-love.
2. It is a violation of the moral law, being an injury to the community of which the suicide is a part.
3. It is a violation of the divine law, which subjects man to God's power and leaves to God the right to take life.

The first reason is self-regarding; the second and third are other-regarding and typically moral in nature. The second reason is a utilitarian one and accordingly conditioned by the assumption that suicide indeed has bad consequences for society. The first and third reasons are absolutist or deontological, that is to say derived from general rules in an unconditioned and an *a priori* manner. Suicide is declared as a triple sin—against oneself, society, and God.

This severe condemnation of suicide had a long-range effect on European attitudes. A more tolerant and balanced view of suicide gradually emerged from the time of the Renaissance (for example, in Montaigne and later in the poet John Donne). An explicitly liberal position regarding suicide can be found in the writings of the eighteenth-century philosopher, Montesquieu.[14] Montesquieu sharply criticizes the anti-suicide laws in Europe as cruel and unjust. No person is obliged to work for society when he has become weary of life, since the relation between the individual and society is based on reciprocity, and the laws of the State have authority only on those who decide to go on living. On the theological level Montesquieu also denies that the separation of body and soul disturbs the order of Providence in the Universe, and thus rebuts the attempts to base the opposition to suicide on 'cosmic' arguments of divine order. The first bold and systematic challenge to Thomas's reasoning came only after half a millennium. In a posthumously published essay, the Scottish philosopher David Hume[15] critically considers the three reasons against suicide, although in reverse order to that of Thomas:

1. If God is omnipotent and governs the world down to the minutest detail, then the act of suicide must also be seen as conforming to his laws and will, and not as an encroachment upon his power. And if suicide is a disturbance of the natural order of the universe, so must be any act of saving life from natural destruction, and this is absurd.
2. Suicide does no harm to society because death absolves man from all his social duties, which are reciprocal and binding only as long as the individual benefits from society. Indeed, sometimes an act of suicide may reduce the burden borne by society and hence be even laudable.
3. Suicide is not necessarily against the agent's interests. Misery, sickness, and misfortune can make life not worth living. The fact that people commit suicide despite the 'natural horror of death' proves that in some cases it is not unnatural.

Kant,[16] however, tried at about the same time to support the absolute moral prohibition of suicide using rational, non-utilitarian, and non-theological arguments. Kant does not appeal to the unnaturalness of the act but to its inherent inconsistency: we cannot attempt to improve our lot—escaping pain, misery, and despair—by destroying ourselves altogether; suicide is an egoistic act and therefore is paradoxical and logically self-defeating. We have a duty to ourselves to choose life rather than death. Kant shows by means of his Categorical Imperative that the maxim 'from self-love I make it my principle to shorten my life if its continuance threatens more evil than it promises pleasure' can never become a 'universal law of nature'. This is due to the fact that the function of the feeling of self-love is 'the furtherance of life', and it would contradict itself if it led to its destruction. This philosophical argument is especially interesting in the light of modern psychological studies of suicide which note the two incompatible goals often manifest in suicide—the wish to die and the wish to improve one's life.

Both Hume and Kant, although holding opposite ethical views on suicide, reflect the modern tendency, starting from the Renaissance, to discuss it on a purely moral level, and not as a religious sin. This change allowed on the one hand the introduction of State laws in which suicide and attempted suicide came to be regarded as crimes, and on the other hand also paved the way for a growing interest in the scientific study of suicidal behaviour and hence a more tolerant approach in moral judgement. In a seventeenth-century study, Robert Burton suggests a clear causal link between depression ('melancholy') and suicide, and interestingly regards it as a mitigating factor in our moral judgement of those persons who are 'mad, beside themselves for the time . . . deprived of reason, judgement'.[17] This attempt at a scientific understanding of suicide was crowned in 1897 by the famous study of the French sociologist Emil Durkheim. This is a purely descriptive account of a social phenomenon which assiduously avoids value judgement either by way of assumption or conclusion. Although Durkheim uses the terms 'altruistic' and 'egoistic' to characterize suicides of different types, he definitely does not mean to praise or condone the first and to condemn the second. He is merely analysing the motives of the agent and his relation to the social environment.[18] If there are any normative implications, they consist of a criticism of society and its institutions rather than any blame of the individual, who is regarded as a victim of a poorly integrated society.

The development of psychiatry and clinical psychology in general and psychoanalysis in particular contributed to the process of 'de-moralization' of contemporary attitudes to suicide even to a greater extent than sociology and epidemiology have done. In the light of his belief in the strong life instinct and self-love, Freud found the phenomenon of suicide puzzling. In the earlier stages of his theory he solved 'the riddle' by claiming that thoughts of suicide are 'murderous impulses against others' turned back upon the self—treating the self as an object of aggression and hostility. This theory of introjected aggression was later supplemented by the concept of 'the death instinct' displayed by the superego against the ego; if ego defences break down under the thrust of super-ego attacks, the patient is liable to commit suicide.[19-21] Beyond that theoretical interest of attempting to explain the psychodynamics of suicide, modern psychiatry has sought to develop the most effective treatment of potential suicides and methods to prevent actual attempts. Modern psychiatry is also concerned with the care of survivors of unsuccessful suicide attempts and with the bereaved families of successful cases.

Historically, this is a radical shift in the approach to suicide. Instead of a *post hoc* judgement—whether it is theological, moral, or legal—there is an effort to diagnose and prevent: rather than trying to discourage suicide by means of threat (of worldly or divine punishment), there is an attempt to eradicate the causes of suicide. Treating has replaced preaching! Like many other phenomena in our culture (madness is a good example) suicide has undergone a deep process of medicalization. This process has, as we shall see in section V, significant ethical implications, and it is by no means universally agreed that the medicalization of suicide has created a more enlightened and humane moral approach. At this stage it will suffice to point out that in both psychological and sociological attitudes to suicide, the subject is regarded as a victim of external forces or as a patient; he is thus absolved from any moral responsibility for the act. It seems that society can avoid having to make moral judgements about suicide only at the cost of eliminating all moral meaning from the act.

Our more 'liberal' view of suicide in the contemporary era is not only a function of the rise of scientific and medical interest in it. Our whole attitude to the value of life and to the valuable life has changed. With the weakening of religious belief and values there is a growing scepticism about the possibility of justifying the value of life and about the traditional criteria of the valuable life. For example, an increasing proportion of couples are dubious about the morality of bringing children into the world. According to the Existentialists the meaning of life, and indeed the value of life itself, are derived from a purely subjective choice rather than from any objective facts and norms. As with many other issues in current ethics, more value is placed on individual autonomy than in previous times, and as—according to many people—a woman has a right over her body in the case of abortion, and a citizen has a right to emigrate from his country, so must we ascribe to everyone the right to opt out of life.

Of course this liberal view of autonomy is not easily applied to concrete cases in the clinic and is incompatible with views held by the vast majority of psychiatrists. Moreover, the search for scientifically valid causes of suicide, which has replaced the moral judgement of the act, paradoxically leaves us in a more ignorant and hence psychologically vulnerable state. For it is certainly easier for society to declare an act of suicide as moral cowardice, virtuous heroism, mortal sin, or even demonic intervention than to face it as a social or psychological problem whose cause is still largely unclear. It is therefore not surprising that the law's view of suicide has changed only very slowly; for example the criminal offence of suicide was abolished in Britain as recently as 1961.

## IV. Clinical aspects

As we suggested in the last section, the clinical and scientific view of suicide is in itself a link in the history of the social evaluation of that ever-present phenomenon. The attempt to strip the concept of its moral overtones is best reflected in modern definitions of suicide, which are a necessary starting-point to any consideration of its clinical aspects. According to Durkheim:

The term suicide is applied to all cases of death resulting directly from a positive or negative act of the victim himself, which he knows will produce this result.[22]

This broad definition covers cases that we do not ordinarily label 'suicide' such as religious martyrdom, self-sacrifice of soldiers in war, hunger-strikes and self-immolation as a political protest (for example, Jan Palach in Czechoslovakia), and even smoking. Durkheim's definition requires only the agent's *knowledge* of his resulting death and only an indirect causal link with his action. Indeed, no specific decision to kill oneself is regarded as a necessary condition. Yet, we usually describe as suicide only causes involving an *intention* or a *wish* to die, carried out *actively* by the agent as the result of a specific *decision*. This is a much more narrow and restrictive definition of the concept. Beauchamp's[23] definition may be particularly useful in the clinico-ethical context. A person commits suicide if: (a) that person intentionally brings about his or her own death; (b) others do not coerce him or her to do the action; and (c) death is caused by conditions arranged by the person for the purpose of bringing about his or her own death.

But philosophers since the Middle Ages have known only too well how difficult it is to assess the intention behind an overt act. As in the Roman Catholic doctrine of the Double Effect, an intentional act may have two effects—one intended, the other unintended, though foreseen. For example, a termination of pregnancy may result both in saving the woman's life and in the death of the fetus: only the first outcome is actually desired, whereas the second is seen as a necessary and undesirable means or a concomitant result. But we should be careful in applying this distinction between directly intended result and reluctant acceptance of secondary effects, because on the one hand direct intentions may lie hidden beyond the persons' level of conscious awareness and on the other hand intentions which he explicitly claims as primary may not necessarily be so. For example, there may be a 'suicidal' intention behind at least some cases of heavy smoking or drinking, dangerous sports like mountaineering and motor-racing, duelling, and heroic altruistic actions. And no less clear for the psychiatrist is the well-recognized observation that explicit expression of suicidal intention is, in many cases, really a cry for help, a desperate wish to gain sympathy, a desire to take revenge, or a hope to be relieved from pain, and so forth. Thus the distinction between direct and oblique intention is not a subtle academic exercise but of utmost importance to the clinician, who assumes a parallel distinction between the conscious and the unconscious, between overt expression of intention and covert motivating forces. It determines both whether a given case should be classified as 'suicide', and the ethical criteria for the right or even the duty of the psychiatrist to intervene.

Most people are naturally inclined to label as suicide: active rather than passive acts of self-destruction; the egoistically rather than the altruistically motivated; the consciously rather than the subconsciously intended; and the action leading to certain death rather than the risky action of gambling with life. However, the active–passive distinction has been criticized as morally and psychologically irrelevant.[24] Durkheim's inclusion of both egoistic and altruistic forms of suicide seems valid from a psychiatric point of view, at least in some cases; the unconsciously intended death may be more effective in causing death than a consciously-expressed suicidal intention; finally, as Stengel has forcefully claimed, the 'suicidal attempt' is no less meaningful a form of suicidal behaviour than the cause of completed suicide, although there are reasons to distinguish between the two.[25] Theoretical and clinical studies therefore cast doubt on the common tendency to view as suicide only the first sort of case in each of the above-mentioned pairs. Yet, it is again interesting to note that our moral intuition about the right to intervene in a potentially suicidal act is still based on that natural tendency rather than on more sophisticated philosophical and clinical views of suicide: we do not usually feel morally bound to intervene in the case of a patient who refuses to comply with essential treatment (passive suicide), or in an extravagant and 'irrational' act of heroism or hunger-strike (altruistic suicide), in the heavy drinker's life-threatening habit (unconscious suicide), or in a game of Russian Roulette ('probable' suicide).

The crucial issue in a clinical context is the relation between suicide and mental illness: is suicide itself a psychiatric disorder? Is it caused by mental illness? Is it always associated with mental illness? We should not be surprised that answers to these questions are inconclusive and agreement among those who have studied them limited. There are serious theoretical difficulties in defining both the concepts of mental illness and suicide, and there are major obstacles to empirical research in the form of unreliable sources of information and the different sorts of data and methodology used in psychological autopsies (reports of failed suicides, of surviving relatives, of doctors, of coroners, etc.). Then, of course, suicide is directly linked with other factors such as age, sex, marital status, place of residence, physical condition, family history, social class, and even with 'cosmological' factors such as time of the day or season. Methodologically we should be aware that if we take as our data cases of suicide in a particularly suicide-prone group (elderly men living on their own in big cities), we might end up with different results regarding the weight of mental illness in suicide than if we studied another population in a different social context.

Despite the methodological complexities, the available data are persuasive. Barraclough and his colleagues[26] in their impressively thorough examination of suicide in England found that of 100 cases studied 93 were judged to be mentally ill by a panel of three psychiatrists, each of whom independently reviewed all the available evidence on each case. A similar level of psychiatric disorder (94 per cent) was found in a noted American study of 134 successful suicides.[27–28]

In the British study the majority of patients (64 per cent) were diagnosed as suffering from a primary depressive illness; the next sizeable group were cases of alcoholism (15 per cent). The strong link between suicide and depression has now been found by several investigators. In follow-up studies of patients diagnosed as manic-depressive or endogenous depressive, there is a consistent finding that about 15 per cent of them will die by suicide. In one comprehensive review[29] of 30 follow-up studies of patients with various forms of depression, including neurotic depression, Miles obtained the same average figure of 15 per cent.

Other findings pertinent to the association between mental illness and suicide are that: successful suicide is frequently preceded by one or more attempts at suicide; the risk of suicide is high in patients in the period immediately following their discharge from hospital; suicide occurs among patients who have been admitted to a psychiatric hospital; most suicides give direct or indirect warning signals before realizing their plan; and a substantial proportion of suicides consult a physician, their family doctor, or a psychiatrist in the weeks preceding their death—to a far greater extent than the normal population.

All these data support the assertion[30] that suicide-proneness can be effectively diagnosed, and even predicted with some degree of accuracy in individual cases. This is an important matter in the ethics of suicide prevention because it is a well-known principle that we ought to do only what we can do: intervene only when we know we can both identify those who intend to kill themselves and stand a good chance of preventing them from doing so.

Prevention can assume various forms. The family doctor can play a vital role by being sensitive to early signs of serious depression; the Samaritans and other lay organizations claim to have reduced the suicide-rate in Britain;[31] effective treatment in psychiatric hospital, and no less important, efficient care following discharge appear to be basic means of reducing the suicide-rate. However, it still remains an open question whether these various measures can succeed in preventing suicide in the long run and on a large scale, or whether the basic cause, and hence also cure, of suicide lies on a social rather than psychological level.[32–33]

If we believe that the ability to prevent suicide has been demonstrated and an important association between suicide and mental illness confirmed, are there still moral grounds for intervention in cases of potential suicide? Suicide prevention may obviously require involuntary hospitalization and forced drug or electro-convulsive treatment, particularly in the case of psychotically-disturbed depressives; it also involves the serious risk of erroneously imposing treatment on a person who is not in fact contemplating suicide, or on someone who wishes to die but is definitely not mentally ill. The justification to intervene is considerably more complicated if the clinical observations mentioned above are rejected *en bloc*. Thomas Szasz, for example, is known for his strident attack on the conventional psychiatric approach to suicide when he states: 'Successful suicide is generally an expression of an individual's desire for greater autonomy—in particular for self-control over his own death'.[34] He proceeds to argue that intervention in suicidal behaviour is always wrong: it is tantamount to a curtailment of a person's freedom and a reflection of the psychiatrist as coercive paternalist. On the other hand, Szasz is not against the psychiatrist's involvement in the situation where a patient *seeks help* for 'being suicidal'. He also seems to be ambivalent about the mental health professional's ultimate duty in the case of a person showing suicidal behaviour when he indicates that the professional ought: '. . . perhaps, to try to persuade him or her to accept help'[35] (see also Narveson[36]).

The vast majority of psychiatrists would not subscribe to the views of Szasz, even those expressed more recently, which are less dogmatic, but instead operate on the premise that their role is to save the life of a person whose suicidal thoughts are in all likelihood the product of psychological disturbance. But as we shall see in the following section, it is by no means obvious whether intervention is justified, even if we assume that suicide is virtually always an indication of mental illness; or that intervention is always wrong, even if suicide is considered as a rational and voluntary act of a 'healthy' person.

## V. The ethics of psychiatric intervention and suicide prevention

For psychiatrists the ethics of suicide primarily centres around the moral justification and limits of an intervention policy; this involves both the general prevention of potential suicidal acts and the life-saving measures applied to a person who has actually made an attempt on his life.

The ethical dilemma of whether to intervene in a suicidal act is intensified by the fact that whatever we do, a price must be paid. This dilemma is presented schematically in Table 12.1.

In the light of this scheme of the ethical dilemma of whether to intervene, let us consider three actual clinical cases.

*Case A.* A 65-year-old widower has insisted on learning the truth about his prognosis from his physician. Two years have passed since his first symptoms led to the discovery of cancer of the colon. Now, with widespread secondaries, he is fully

**Table 12.1**

| Intervention | Non-intervention |
| --- | --- |
| Taking the *patient*'s decision as irrational, impulsive, distorted by mental illness. | Taking the *patient*'s decision as authentic, deliberate, clear-headed, and rational. |
| On the assumption that his decision is reversible, certain steps, which are also reversible, are taken to prolong his life. | On the assumption that his decision is irreversible, no steps are taken, thus irreversibly letting him commit suicide. |
| Paternalism: forcing the patient to act rationally as an expression of care for his real interests. | Respect for the *patient*'s autonomy and liberty to kill himself as to take any other decision, even if it seems irrational to us. |
| Care for the patient's family, who usually ask for intervention. | Taking the *patient*'s side rather than that of his family. Priority of his freedom over the family's interests. |
| *The price*: forcing him to act against his will, prolongation of his mental and physical misery, serious loss of liberty. | *The price*: missed opportunities, the infinite loss involved in death, possibility of the most 'tragic mistake'. |
| *Underlying assumption*: the instinctive drive to save other people's lives plus the professional duty and practice of doctors to do so. | *Underlying assumption*: 'nothing in life is as much under the direct jurisdiction of each individual as are his own person and life' (Schopenhauer) |

aware that the prognosis is grave. He has but a few weeks or months left to life. Throughout his life he has been an advocate of voluntary euthanasia, and concludes now, that he does not wish to battle futilely against his impending death; he would rather die 'with dignity' and in his full senses than in excruciating pain which calls for massive doses of narcotic drugs. He is also steadfast in his conviction that it would be grossly unfair to saddle his only daughter with his problems. He knows that he can no longer fend for himself and that his only options are to be hospitalized or to move in with his daughter's family. Both prospects are completely unacceptable to him. He has always been proud of his self-reliance, and will not easily forgo it now. He talks candidly about his wish to die—through his own hand. His only 'need' is to collect a sufficient number of hypnotic pills to enable him to die in what he avows to be a decent fashion.

*Case B.* A 35-year-old married woman and mother of three small children has been feeling utter despair since the tragic death in a domestic fire of her youngest child some eight months earlier. During this period, her feeling of loss has increased to the point where she now believes that she must join the 'the kiddy in heaven'. She has always been a devout Roman Catholic, now more so than ever. Her belief is strong that the deceased child needs her whilst the three living children can be cared for by her husband and relatives. She is convinced that she is to blame for the tragedy—she should not have left the child unattended. There is absolutely no point in continuing to live her life as at present when 'Paul needs me elsewhere'. She tried to hang herself on the day of consultation but her husband, close to breaking point because of his wife's insistence on being reunited with Paul, managed to intercede. He has no doubt that she will kill herself unless some help can be provided. On the other hand, as a devout Catholic himself, he can appreciate his wife's wish to 'join Paul in heaven'.

*Case C.* A 40-year-old housewife and mother of three teenage children presents with apathy, withdrawal, and self-neglect over some weeks. During this time she has lost interest in her family and friends, wakes at about 2 a.m. each morning and cannot return to sleep, and has lost one stone in weight. She has developed the unshakeable belief that she is worthless, has let her husband and children down, and deserves to die. She feels quite helpless and sees no future for herself. She suffered a similar episode three years previously for which she was treated as an inpatient with antidepressant medication. She made a good recovery then and had felt content and cheerful until the onset of her present state.

*Case D.* A 60-year-old retired teacher and mother of two children feels physically unwell and is diagnosed as suffering from the side-effects of long-term treatment with lithium. During the course of her admission to a general hospital to investigate the physical problem, she shows features of depressed mood; these become so severe as to require her transfer to a psychiatric unit. There, her pessimism, anergia, insomnia, and more particularly her intense suicidal thoughts, lead to a decision to apply electroconvulsive therapy (ECT). She responds reasonably well but the improvement is short-lived. ECT is resumed, again with the evidently good result. Periods of home leave follow, with the anticipation that recovery is almost complete and full discharge imminent. By this time she has spent six months in a hospital. The depression soon recurs, this time more severely and also more frustratingly to herself, her family, and the ward staff. There seems to be a doubt developing as to whether the condition is treatable. A third course of ECT is instituted, in conjunction with antidepressant medication. And, because the patient is constantly preoccupied with ways of 'ending it all', her status of voluntary admission is converted into a compulsory one. Not only is this drastic step taken, but also the practice of 'constant observation', even to the point of supervising her toiletries. There is immense concern about the patient's safety following her disappearance for thirty-six hours. Found by the police on a golf course, she explains how she is 'longing for death' and feels 'utterly desperate'. Yet another course of ECT treatment begins, although the staff feel confused about their action in persevering when after some nine months it is fairly obvious that their patient is determined to die. They feel all the more bewildered in the face of her repeated requests for them to advise her on how she can best accomplish her wish, and her spurning of her family's concern.

Two months later sees a mounting desperation in all the protagonists, culminating in the patient's attempt to asphyxiate herself. Saved from death, she repeatedly expresses the wish to die, but also joins in ward activities and even exhibits a dry humour. Exactly one week later she is discovered in the bathroom with a plastic bag over her head. A determined effort to resuscitate her proves to no avail. The one-year saga is at an end, save for the profound feelings of the bereaved family and of the medical and nursing staff.

One final point needs to be made. The patient had been successfully treated for bouts of depression 32, 26, and 20 years previously, and in the intervening periods had led a reasonably contented life in her various roles of wife, mother, and teacher.

Case A can be confidently classified as an example of voluntary euthanasia and can hardly be labelled as 'irrational'. Most doctors would respect the patient's wish 'to die in dignity', although they might find it psychologically (and legally) difficult to co-operate actively in his suicide. No psychiatrist would consider forced hospitalization for such a person. In terms of our scheme, we can assume that the patient's decision to die is deliberate, authentic, and, in all likelihood, irreversible. The family might well be relieved rather than distressed by his act. Forcing him to continue to live means the prolongation of despair, pain, and loss of dignity.

Case C is a common occurrence in clinical practice and characterizes a large class of suicides caused by depression. Virtually all psychiatrists would suspect that her wish to die is not rational and sincere, but that her thinking has been distorted by certain reversible causes. Previous treatment proved helpful, and it can be assumed that therapy for the present state might be equally effective. Unlike the widower of case A, whose liberty is to all intents and purposes lost until his natural death if life is forced on him, the deprivation of liberty through involuntary hospitalization in the treatment of the depressed woman will be temporary and in all likelihood reasonably short. There is much hope of applying therapy which will relieve her of the sense of helplessness and enable her to see that her interests, and those of her family, are better served by her continuing to live.

It is case B which is puzzling and difficult to decide about. Her wish to die can be labelled as irrational only on the grounds of our rejection of her deep religious convictions. Her suicidal wish is not irrational in the sense of being impulsive, lacking deliberation, ambiguous, or distorted by mental illness. Even her close relatives, who stand to 'lose' from her decision, are basically sympathetic to her reasoning. On the other hand, the psychologically sensitive observer would no doubt be tempted to ascribe her desperate decision to her intense grief over the death of her child, and conclude that her despair can be relieved, at least partially, with psychiatric treatment. How far should the psychiatrist intervene in such a case? Note that case B is typical of many suicides, not in the specific circumstances but in that blend of basically sound reasoning (at least from the agent's point of view) and non-rational motives; it is a complex which resists disentanglement. The area in the spectrum of cases lying between type-A and type-C cases is unfortunately 'grey' and ethically indeterminate; and no ready-made recipe for solving the dilemma of intervention can be offered. A methodological remark may however prove useful.

There is an asymmetry between the two horns of the dilemma of intervention, because of the irreversibility of the act of suicide, and correspondingly of the decision not to intervene. This source of asymmetry—being temporal in nature—is not often considered by philosophers, who tend to discuss the ethics of suicide on an abstract, theoretical level. But it is of crucial importance in the practical clinical context, such as case D. The irreversibility of non-intervention places a particularly heavy burden of moral responsibility on the psychiatrist. By contrast, a decision to intervene can always be reversed, if subsequently shown to be mistaken. The psychiatrist's responsibility for an irreversible act is even more serious because the decision is often taken under conditions of uncertainty: is the suicidal intention final, is it authentic, is it rational, will the person be grateful if saved?

Case D is particularly difficult in this context, for unlike cases A and C, the issue is not the rationality and authenticity of the suicidal person's *choice*, but rather the chances of success of the therapeutic intervention. In other words, the moral dilemma is not whether to force treatment on someone who does not want it now, but whether to force treatment on someone who is untreatable. It seems that if the suicidal condition is indeed incurable, the only point in hospitalizing the patient is to compel her to live.

On the basis of our remarks in section II regarding the dependence of the value of life on the idea of a valuable life, we can raise serious doubts as to the legitimacy of such compulsion. However, the question whether a certain condition is really untreatable is basically a matter of professional diagnosis rather than of moral judgement. And as all diagnosis is prone to mistakes, the psychiatrist tends to ward off responsibility by continuing to apply treatment despite his belief in its inefficacy. Although this strategy is psychologically understandable, it should be remembered that there is a vast difference between a heroic medical effort to save the life of a 'hopeless' case (such as a victim of a serious accident) and the struggle against an 'untreatable' patient with a mental illness set on a suicidal course. The slightest chance of a 'miraculous' cure in the first case justifies the policy of 'never giving up'. A similarly slight chance in the second case cannot justify the violation of autonomy and privacy of the patient and the creation of so much pain as that involved in enforced treatment.

However, in cases such as A, B, and C this direct responsibility over a potentially irreversible decision under conditions of uncertainty suggests a 'policy of postponement'. In our view, we are justified in asking or even forcing potential suicides to reconsider their attitude, to give themselves a second chance, or to defer a final decision lest there be a change in circumstances. This postponement policy is logically sounder than one of non-intervention because the intervention itself is a reversible act. If further study of the case shows that suicide is indeed 'rational' and authentic, or every effort at treatment fails to alter the person's frame of mind, or the person persists in his wish to kill himself regardless of change of circumstances—then there is always the option of letting him carry out his intentions. Although there is no good reason to argue that paternalistic regard for the person's interests, and those of his family, is in principle more important than respect for his autonomy and liberty, it seems that the reversibility of the decision to intervene makes the violation of autonomy less weighty. Only in extreme cases such as, for example, a paraplegic who can be technically prevented from killing himself indefinitely, can we question the moral legitimacy of such an act of prevention. The freedom to terminate one's own life, or at least the capacity to do so, remains one of the most basic consolations to human beings. Beyond those temporary measures we may take to save life, ultimately we must remind ourselves of the need to respect this fundamental freedom.

Throughout this section the focus has been on the question of the moral justification of *preventing* suicide. Although our remit does not extend to the subject of euthanasia (see Rachels[37] for a clear account of this topic), the controversial issue of the psychiatrist's potential role in assisting or at least abetting a patient to commit suicide requires our consideration. The circumstances of Case D certainly point to the potential relevance of the issue; and the case of Elizabeth Bouvia demonstrates its actual complexity.[38]

Ms Bouvia, a twenty-six-year-old woman with incapacitating cerebral palsy, declared herself as a suicidal patient upon her voluntary admission to the psychiatric service of a Californian county general hospital in September 1983. She both refused nourishment and sought a court order preventing the staff from force-feeding her or discharging her. Her wish to die was the result of a belief that her future prospects were utterly hopeless.

The Court ruled in favour of the hospital upon the grounds that while Ms Bouvia was competent in arriving at her decision, the requirement of the common good overrode respect for her autonomy. Concluding that: '. . . society's interest in preserving life and the medical profession's obligation to do so outweighed her right to self-determination', the judge referred to the 'devastating' effects that assisting suicide would have on other patients and others afflicted with handicaps.

Most commentaries on the case have concurred with the Court's decision (as do the authors) although their arguments have differed. For example, Bursztajn et al.[39] have adopted an approach based on empirical grounds, namely that 'physical illness alone, *per se*, is rarely a cause of suicidality'. Rather, it is the associated swirl of emotional feelings, especially depression, which clouds the patient's judgement. Intervention, in the form of a 'therapeutic cooling-off period' (and of at least six months duration) provides an opportunity for the alleviation or amelioration of the state of depression. This position is similar in many respects to our own policy of postponement. But Bursztajn and his colleagues also contended that the autonomous patient is a myth, and that a patient, like Ms Bouvia, who presents to the hospital in a distressed state is likely to be calling for professional assistance because of an ambivalence about her decision to die.

Alan Stone[40] has criticized this analysis, claiming that the patient's mental state is irrelevant. Following the Bursztajn line of argument, the Court should have found Bouvia incompetent and forced her doctors to intervene on that basis. What is central for Stone is that hospitals and doctors are not duty-bound to passively abet the suicide of a patient, competent or incompetent, who is not terminally ill; and, conversely, patients have no right to compel their doctors to participate, even passively, in their suicide. He would wish to dispel a double myth by adding to the original myth of the autonomous patient the one of the 'omniscient and omnipotent psychiatrist'.

A third approach is based on an argument concerning the common or public good, and probably comes closest to the gist of the Court's decision in the Bouvia case. Kane[41] has asserted that her plea could not be based merely on an appeal to the right to self-determination. Even if a person should have the freedom to commit suicide, '. . . it does not follow that the civic community has the responsibility to assist anyone in that act of suicide'. Kane asked rhetorically about the freedom of the doctors, nurses, and hospital staff, if the judge had ordered their collaboration in Ms Bouvia's suicide. Almost certainly, most of them would have been forced to violate their codes of ethics and to act against their consciences. We end up in the dilemma of having to respect the liberty of both the patient and the professional staff. Even if personnel could have been found to voluntarily assist in the suicide, their collaboration would still have had detrimental effects on the broader community, including the rest of the professional staff, other patients, and society as a whole. In the final analysis, Kane argues for the primacy of the common good, which must override private interests.

All these positions have no doubt been associated with the long-standing acceptance by legal jurisdictions that to aid, abet, or counsel suicide is an offence. Thus, the medical profession is legally bound to act in a highly specific fashion. But the advent in the Netherlands from the mid-1970s of a series of guidelines (although they are not enshrined in law) dealing with the active euthanasia of terminally ill patients is challenging our customary notions. Although these guidelines are confined to terminally ill patients who are afflicted with intolerable pain and other physical symptoms, and who freely, voluntarily, competently, and repeatedly request that their lives be ended because of their suffering, they do facilitate the assisting of a form of suicide. We would assert however that these clinical circumstances differ in many fundamental respects from those obtaining in the psychiatric context dealt with in this chapter, and the arguments advanced against the assistance of a 'psychiatric suicide' are likely to prevail.

In turning to the question of suicide within a psychiatric framework, we may conclude by saying the following—that it is better to err on the side of preserving life than on the side of letting it be lost. Although philosophical considerations may show that there is no logically valid argument for the preference of life over death and that our basis for life is completely irrational, we should always remember that the potential suicide may, deep in his heart, share that irrational preference with us.

## References

1 Platt, S.: Suicide trends in 24 European countries 1972–1984, in *Current Issues in Suicidology*, ed. J. Moller, A. Schmidtke, and R. Wetz. Berlin, Springer, 1987.

2 Durkheim, E.: *Suicide*. London, Routledge and Kegan Paul, 1952, pp. 46–9.

3 Roy, A.: Suicide in doctors. *Psychiatric Clinics of North America* **8**: 377–87, 1985.

4 Daube, D.: The linguistics of suicide. *Philosophy and Public Affairs* **1**: 415–17, 1972.

5 Yalom, I.: *Existential psychotherapy*. New York, Basic Books, 1981.

6 Camus, A.: *The myth of Sisyphus*. Harmondsworth, Penguin, 1975, pp. 11–12.

7 Nagel, T.: Death, in *Moral problems*, ed. J. Rachels. New York, Harper & Row, 1975, p. 403.

8 Freud, S.: *Thoughts on war and death*. Standard edition, **14**: 289–90.

9 Aristotle: *Ethica Nicomachea*. London, Oxford University Press, 1925, 1138a.

10 Plato: Phaedo, in *The dialogues of Plato*. Oxford, Clarendon Press, 1953, Vol. 1, 62b–c.

11 Seneca: Epistle 70, in *Epistulae morales*, Loeb edn. London, Heinemann, 1925, Vol. II.

12 Augustine: *The city of God*. Harmondsworth, Penguin, 1972, Book I, Chapters 17–27.

13 Thomas Aquinas: *Summa Theologica*. New York, Benziger, 1947, II, ii, Q. 64, Art. 5.

14 Montesquieu, Baron de.: *Persian letters*, No. 76. Harmondsworth, Penguin, 1973

15 Hume, D.: On suicide. In *Essays*, ed. T. H. Green and T. H. Grose. London, Longman, 1882, Vol. 4, pp. 406–14.
16 Kant, I.: Groundwork of the metaphysic of morals, in *The moral law*, ed. J. Paton. London, Hutchinson, 1948, p. 89. Cf. *Lectures on ethics*. New York, Harper & Row, 1963, pp. 148–54.
17 Burton, R.: *Anatomy of melancholy*. London, The Nonesuch Press, 1925, pp. 224–6.
18 Durkheim, E.: *Suicide*. London, Routledge & Kegan Paul, 1952, Chapter 1.
19 Freud, S.: *Mourning and melancholia*. Standard edition, 14:239–60, 1957.
20 Freud, S.: *Beyond the pleasure principle*. Standard edition, 18:1–64, 1955.
21 Freud, S.: *The Ego and Id*. Standard edition, 19:1–66, 1961.
22 Durkheim, E.: *Suicide*. London, Routledge & Kegan Paul, 1952, p. 44.
23 Quoted in Rachels, J.: *The end of life*. Oxford, Oxford University Press, 1986, p. 81.
24 Glover, J.: *Causing death and saving life*. Harmondsworth, Penguin, 1977, pp. 176–81.
25 Stengel, E.: *Suicide and attempted suicide*. Harmondsworth, Penguin, 1964, pp. 82–3.
26 Barraclough, B., Bunch, L., Nelson, B., and Sainsbury, B.: A hundred cases of suicide: clinical aspects. *British Journal of Psychiatry* 125:355–73, 1974.
27 Robins, E., Murphy, G. E., Wilkinson, R. H., *et al.*: Some clinical considerations in the prevention of suicide based on a study of 134 successful suicides. *American Journal of Public Health* 49:888–98, 1959.
28 Robins, E.: *The final months: a study of the lives of 134 persons who committed suicide*. New York, Oxford University Press, 1981.
29 Miles, C. P.: Conditions predisposing to suicide: a review. *Journal of Nervous and Mental Disease* 16:231–46, 1977.
30 Sainsbury, P.: Depression and suicide prevention. Paper read at the 10th Anniversary of The Belgian Group for the Study and Prevention of Suicide, 1980.
31 Bagley, C.: Social policy and the prevention of suicidal behaviour. *British Journal of Social Work* 3:473–95, 1973.
32 Jennings, C., Barraclough, B., and Moss, J. R.: Have the Samaritans lowered the suicide rate? A controlled study. *Psychological Medicine* 8, 413–22, 1978.
33 Dew, M. A., Bromet, E. J., Brent, D., and Greenhouse, J. B.: A quantitative literature review of the effectiveness of suicide prevention centers. *Journal of Consulting and Clinical Psychology* 55:239–44, 1987.
34 Szasz, T.: The ethics of suicide. *The Antioch Review* 31:7–17, 1971.
35 Szasz, T. S.: The case against suicide prevention. *American Psychologist* 41:806–12, 1986.
36 Narveson, J.: Moral philosophy and suicide. *Canadian Journal of Psychiatry* 31:104–7, 1986.
37 Rachels, J.: *The end of life*. Oxford, Oxford University Press, 1986.
38 *Bouvia* v. *County of Riverside*. No. 159780, Supreme Court, Riverside County, CA, Tr. 1238–1250, 16 December 1983.
39 Bursztajn, H., Gutheil, T. G., Warren, M. J., and Brodsky, A.: Depression, self-love, time and the 'right' to suicide. *General Hospital Psychiatry* 8:91–5, 1986.
40 Stone, A.: Response to the article 'Depression, self-love, time and the "right" to suicide', by Bursztajn, H. *et al*. *General Hospital Psychiatry* 8:97–9, 1986.
41 Kane, F. I.: Keeping Elizabeth Bouvia alive for the public good. *Hastings Center Report* 15: 5–8, 1985.

# 13

# The ethics of involuntary commitment to mental health treatment

*Robert Miller*

The previous edition of this volume contained a chapter on the ethics of involuntary hospitalization. In this update, I have revised the title and broadened the focus of the chapter to reflect the fact that involuntary commitment is no longer limited exclusively to treatment in in-patient settings. Because of the increasing use of the criminal justice system as an alternative to civil commitment, I have also included criminal commitments in addition to civil procedures in the discussion. Although I have used the term psychiatrists to refer to clinicians responsible for the evaluation and treatment of involuntarily committed civil patients, it should be understood that many of the responsibilities and ethical dilemmas to be discussed increasingly apply to non-medical mental health professionals as well.

To the extent that a profession controls its own practice, it is comparably free to establish ethical standards for that practice, based only on what its members feel would advance the profession's goals for its members and for its clients. Until the 1960s, organized medicine, including psychiatry, was largely free from external influence and regulation, and occupied a morally and economically powerful position in society. It was therefore relatively free to concentrate its ethical deliberations on patient welfare, without consideration of outside interference. In the last three decades, however, a variety of factors have led to the loss of a significant amount of the autonomy of psychiatry as well as of medicine as a whole. As a result, psychiatry has also lost a considerable amount of freedom to determine its own standards of practice independent of external forces, and has become increasingly reactive to those forces in the reshaping of its ethical codes. As I shall argue throughout this chapter, ethical concerns should dictate that it is no longer sufficient for clinicians to practice their clinical specialties in a vacuum while remaining ignorant of, and therefore reactive to, the external political, legal, and social forces which increasingly shape their practices. It is necessary for psychiatrists to adopt proactive stances with respect to courts and legislatures in order to further their ethical goals.

It should also be noted that while current legal procedures result in a number of problems for clinicians working with involuntarily committed patients, not all of those problems are chiefly ethical in nature. In this chapter, I will attempt to focus on the ethical aspects of involuntary commitment. As many of the issues are not explicitly addressed in formal statements of ethical principles from various sources, I will of necessity draw on my own clinical experience and on my subjective interpretation of the ethical dilemmas inherent in working with involuntary patients. In the process, more questions will of necessity be raised than answered; the goal of this chapter is to raise clinicians' consciousness to new conflicts posed by recent changes in commitment procedures, and to provide frameworks within which to analyse and resolve them in the real world of clinical practice, where clinicians do not have the luxury of philosophical discourse, but must make decisions with significant ethical ramifications on a daily basis.

In order to discuss the ethical dilemmas associated with involuntary commitment, it is first necessary to examine the factors which have increasingly become important in setting external parameters for its imposition and implementation.

## The impact of attorneys and advocates

Perhaps the major factor in the growing challenge to psychiatric autonomy has been the rise of the mental health bar.[1] Since the civil rights movement which began in the 1960s in the United States (and which has also increasingly affected the practice of involuntary hospitalization in other countries as well, as will be discussed below) lawyers, judges, advocates, and legislatures have had a growing impact on all aspects of psychiatric practice, but particularly on situations involving coerced treatment. The research studies in the United States have convincingly demonstrated that changes in substantive or procedural criteria for commitment which were designed to restrict involuntary hospitalization have had little impact in the absence of active representation of patients by knowledgeable attorneys.[2]

## Moral right versus legal right

Many of the conceptual differences between clinical and legal professionals have been discussed in the literature.[3] For the purposes of this analysis, the most significant include (1) the legal focus on liberty interests (defined as freedom from external restraints) as contrasted with the clinical focus on treatment needs and the internal restraints imposed by the mental disorder itself; (2) the legal emphasis on procedural rights as contrasted with the clinical emphasis on outcome; and (3) the criminal justice representation model, which requires concentration on the rights of individual clients without regard to the rights of others who might be affected by the individual's behaviour, as contrasted with the interest of clinicians (particularly those who work in in-patient settings where patients have less opportunity to avoid each other or staff) in the rights of all patients and staff in a given facility.

Clinicians have frequently, and accurately, been characterized as paternalistic in their approach to patients, both by themselves and by their critics.[4] Unfortunately, paternalism has come to have a pejorative connotation because of the history of abuses in psychiatric facilities which were justified in its name. Paternalism (and the *parens patriae* rationale for involuntary hospitalization which was based on it) has become suspect, equated by critics with unjustified deprivation of liberty under an unsupervised, clinically-dominated power structure. (The *parens patriae* jurisdiction originated in the power and duty of the Crown/State to protect the persons and property of those unable to do so for themselves, such as minors and persons of unsound mind; a power which could be subsequently held to have been delegated to authorized agents of the Crown/State, such as psychiatrists, in the case of the mentally ill in certain circumstances.) This *post hoc ergo propter hoc* fallacy has led many clinicians, particularly those working in in-patient facilities, to become defensive about their paternalistic motives, and to denounce them, publicly, while often continuing to subscribe to them privately.

Kaplan[5] has put forth one reason for the paternalistic tradition in medicine which is directly relevant to our discussion. Drawing on Strauss's historical analysis,[6] he points out that the Greek philosophers conceived of moral worth in terms of rationality. Under this system, the highest moral duty was to assist others to achieve their potentials for rational thinking and action. As with the political system based on these principles, the duty of the wise man was to lead others along the path of rationality, and the duty of the less wise to follow that lead. It is no coincidence that the ethical principles which still form the basis for medical practice were also established at this time. Physicians possessed wisdom concerning health, and patients had a moral duty to follow their advice.

Physicians, including psychiatrists, are still socialized, implicitly if no longer explicitly, under the belief that it is their duty not only to offer the best clinical advice possible, but also to ensure that the patient follows it. This concept becomes particularly significant in psychiatry, in which the patient's rationality itself is often affected by illness. Thus it is easy to understand how psychiatrists interpret the right to treatment as the right of the treater to impose needed treatment on the patient,[7] and why many psychiatrists reject the concept of a right to refuse treatment, which prevents them from fulfilling their moral responsibility to treat patients whose rationality has been impaired through illness, and (even worse) makes them responsible for incarcerating patients without providing the necessary treatment. In the subsequent sections of this chapter, this moral duty will be considered in the discussion of the various ethical dilemmas posed by the involuntary treatment of patients.

## The prediction of dangerousness

The dangerousness criteria for involuntary hospitalization which have been established in virtually all jurisdictions in the United States have led to a number of ethical dilemmas for psychiatrists. The threshold dilemma, of course, is that of the ethics of predicting future dangerousness, required by all police power statutes. While the prediction of 'imminent' dangerousness at the entrance to the commitment system, particularly in the emergency detention provisions of most state statutes, may be reasonable,[8] although difficult to study,[9] the longer-term predictions of behaviour in different contexts required for extension of commitment beyond an initial observation period have been shown to be so inaccurate that the official policy of the American Psychiatric Association is that psychiatrists are incapable of making them.[10] The *Annotations* to the American Psychiatric Association's ethical guidelines state that 'A psychiatrist who regularly practices outside his/her area of professional competence should be considered unethical'[11] (Section 4[1]). It is certainly arguable that the routine prediction of long-term dangerousness, even if genuinely believed to be accurate by the clinician,[12] might constitute a breach of ethical conduct. While such predictions have been the subject of vociferous criticism from clinicians when made in the context of capital-punishment sentencing hearings,[13] there is little conceptual difference between such opinions and those rendered in re-hearings for involuntarily hospitalized patients.

This is not to say that psychiatrists have *no* expertise in predicting dangerousness; rather it is to argue that such predictions should be offered only if the data on which they are based are first presented, and the conclusions qualified by statements concerning what is known about their validity. To the extent that psychiatrists continue to offer such predictions, the profession is under an ethical obligation to pursue methodologically sound research to enhance our predictive capacity and to provide more precise data concerning the accuracy of those predictions.

On the other hand, the dangerousness criteria for commitment place clinicians in a very difficult ethical position in several ways. First, clinicians who wish to secure hospitalization for patients who are perceived to need it clinically, but who decline to accept it voluntarily, must make allegations of future dangerousness in order to obtain the authority to provide the needed treatment. The fact that predictions of dangerousness are rarely challenged in commitment hearings in most jurisdictions[14] simply facilitates their routinization. As Treffert[15] has said in the context of hearings to determine competency to refuse treatment, rights are converted into 'rites', phrases uttered for their symbolic value, but often devoid of substance. Clinicians find themselves between the Scylla of 'fudging' on their predictions of dangerousness and the Charybdis of abandoning those in need of treatment. If psychiatrists were to be honest about the current state of predictability of dangerousness, particularly future dangerousness in unknown contexts, the result would probably be a short-term decrease in the hospitalization of patients who need it on clinical grounds. But as long as clinicians continue to distort the process of predicting dangerousness in order to secure commitments, it is less likely that the social and political pressure necessary to effect changes in the commitment statutes toward more clinically-based criteria will occur.

Second, to the extent that dangerousness criteria are effective in determining the characteristics of in-patient populations (and there is evidence that, despite the perfunctory nature of most commitment hearings, there has been a significant shift toward more dangerous patients)[16] the character of those populations has changed toward a population which is both demonstrably more dangerous and also less likely to suffer from mental disorders which can be effectively treated with current techniques. As will be discussed below, a major factor in the decision to hospitalize dangerous but untreatable patients is the threat of liability for acts committed by such patients,[17] thus placing clinicians in the dilemma of choosing between possible harm to third parties (and liability for themselves) and placing persons for whom treatment is unlikely to be effective in preventive detention, at the further cost of withholding increasingly scarce clinical resources from patients who could benefit from them.

A related dilemma is posed by chronic patients who deteriorate in the community sufficiently to merit initial involuntary hospitalization, and who reconstitute sufficiently in the period prior to the formal hearing (generally 3–14 days after admission) to appear to no longer satisfy the commitment criteria, but not enough to be able to remain safely in the community after release. Such patients typify the 'revolving door' population of the repeatedly-admitted chronically mentally ill, who may respond well to treatment in the structured environment of a hospital, but do not get the chance under such circumstances. In response to the frustration of watching such patients come and go, some clinicians have decided to withhold treatment from such patients prior to the hearing, in order that the court can appreciate the patient's mental status without treatment, and thus provide the patient with sufficient time in the hospital that improvement can be maintained after release. Some states provide for commitment (particularly to out-patient treatment) based on the establishment of a likelihood that, without the structure and treatment provided by the commitment, patients would deteriorate to a condition which would satisfy the existing criteria for involuntary hospitalization. Clinicians should therefore be familiar with such statutory provisions if they exist in their jurisdictions, and work to effect their inclusion if they are not.

*Case 1:* Ms A was a 45-year-old single chronically schizophrenic woman who lived by herself; she received a small disability payment, but was unable to manage it effectively. She never bathed or cleaned her house because of her beliefs that hygiene was unnecessary, and she lived off food stored in her refrigerator despite the fact that her power had been cut off for six months because she did not pay her bills. At the time of initial hospitalization, her malnutrition was significant, but not life-threatening. She was bathed against her will (her head had to be shaved because her hair was so matted), clothed, and fed. She refused treatment with medication, denying that anything was wrong with her. By the time of her judicial commitment hearing ten days after admission, she appeared normal, although she continued to deny the need for treatment or change in her life-style. She was released at the hearing without conditions, because of no demonstrable imminent danger to herself.

Morse[18] has argued against involuntary hospitalization in part on the basis that there are too few mental health professionals to provide adequate treatment for those who seek it voluntarily, and thus utilitarian principles alone would argue that those who resist hospitalization or treatment should not be forced to accept it. On superficial analysis, such a course appears to present fewer ethical problems than does the incarceration and coerced treatment of unwilling persons; but, on further reflection, it becomes apparent that selection of patients based on their willingness to participate voluntarily in treatment raises other significant ethical concerns, by replacing clinical judgement with consumer desires. Morse's proposal might be appropriate if voluntariness were randomly distributed along the continuum of severity of mental disorder; but, as has been demonstrated by the experience of community mental health centres,[19] service-delivery systems based on patient self-selection tend to select for less severely disordered patients rather than for those most in need of the scarce resources available.

In addition, there are data which indicate that the majority of patients who refuse treatment do so because of denial of illness,[20] and that after treatment has had the opportunity to become effective, most involuntary patients report that hospitalization has been beneficial, although their disorders prevented them from appreciating it at the time they were committed.[21] Thus abolition of procedures for involuntary hospitalization and/or treatment would be tantamount to abandonment of this severely ill population of patients.

## Informed consent

The legal doctrine of informed consent has become a major factor in involuntary treatment over the past two decades. Most familiar in this context is the central place that consent has assumed in the 'right to refuse treatment' controversy. Although it has received far less attention in the legal literature, consent is also a significant problem in the area of voluntary admissions to hospitals, as well as in out-patient treatment.

Current clinical as well as legal philosophy supports voluntary treatment whenever possible, as part of the evolution of health-service delivery from a fiduciary to a contractual system. Despite the criticisms of those such as Szasz,[22] who argues that, because of the (implicit or explicit) threat of commitment should the patient refuse the services offered, voluntary admission is 'medical fraud', voluntary acceptance of treatment, including hospitalization, is perceived at least as the lesser of two evils. The major problem with this policy is its underlying assumption that patients are capable of giving such consent, which requires (a) the provision of sufficient information to enable a decision to be made; (b) the patient's capacity to comprehend the information and to use it in a rational decision-making process; and (c) lack of any coercion. Unfortunately, the studies which have been done all indicate that few patients are in fact capable of meaningful understanding of that information, particularly at the time of admission.[23]

*Case 2:* Ms B was a 45-year-old woman who was brought to the hospital for admission by her family. She had a long history of debilitating mental illness, and had been hospitalized on seven previous occasions, each time with significant remission of her psychosis after medication was resumed. Her family described another relapse, with social withdrawal, apparent paranoid delusions, refusal to eat, and intermittent outbursts of aggressive behaviour toward her family. In the admission office, Ms B remained unresponsive to all questions and declined to sign the request for voluntary admission, although she did not resist coming to the hospital. The admitting psychiatrist felt that she would benefit from hospitalization and treatment, and instructed her family to initiate civil commitment procedures, as Ms B did not appear to be competent to sign herself in voluntarily.

The fact that patients are frequently unable to comprehend or to retain information necessary for valid consent to hospitalization or treatment does not relieve clinicians of the ethical responsibility to persist in their efforts to provide that information when patients are capable of understanding it. While mental patients, by virtue of their disorders, may be more likely than other medical patients to deny the presence of illness, or to distort information presented to them, they are also more likely to have experienced prior treatment, particularly with anti-psychotic medication, and may in some cases be more capable than other medical patients of understanding the real risks and benefits of treatment.

Given this fact, clinicians are faced with an ethical (as well as a potential legal) dilemma when patients come (or, as is more frequently the case, are brought) for treatment, appear to the clinician to need the treatment sought, but are incapable of demonstrating sufficient understanding to satisfy even the most superficial requirements for informed consent. Prior to the advent of formal requirements for informed consent, such patients were considered to be 'assenters', a category intermediate between con-senters and refusers, and were treated as consenters for purposes of admission and treatment; but the advocates of affirmative informed consent have argued that assenters should be considered refusers unless they are capable of giving informed consent, and in fact do so after being provided with sufficient information upon which to base their decisions.

Despite the drawbacks resulting from more formal requirements for informed consent, there have been clear benefits as well. Before the late 1960s, when clinicians in the United States had the unquestioned authority to treat patients as they deemed clinically appropriate, time pressures (particularly in the public mental hospitals to which the great majority of involuntary patients were committed) mitigated against substantive efforts to involve patients actively in their treatment plans. Accreditation require-ments,[24] as well as patients' rights rules, now require clinicians to make such attempts, and most studies demonstrate that most civilly committed patients will in fact give their consent to appropriate treatment if it is adequately explained to them, and if they are given some realistic choices. Many 'refusals' of medication have turned out on closer inspection not to be blanket treatment-refusals, but rather patients' choices for particular anti-psychotic medications, frequently based on their personal experience, which differed from their psychiatrists' own idiosyncratic preferences.[25] Although no data are yet available, it is logical to assume that patients whose preferences are accepted by their treaters will be more likely to continue treatment after their commitments expire.

Another advantage of explicit requirements for informed consent is the provision of an external mechanism for review of clinical decisions in difficult cases, such as those involved for patients with severe psychoses and early signs of tardive dyskinesia. Such decisions not only pose ethical dilemmas for clinicians, but increasingly place them at risk for legal liability no matter which choice they make. By bringing the issue before an external decision-maker (judicial or clinical), the treating clinician can obtain explicit guidance in how to proceed, as well as protection from subsequent liability for making the 'wrong' choice.

Since patients at risk for this currently untreatable side-effect of psycho-tropic medication are usually suffering from severe mental disorders, their ability to give informed consent to treatment is always suspect. But while most such patients have been treated with psychotropic medications before, and thus generally have extensive personal experience with the risks and benefits of such treatment, few have such experience with tardive dyskinesia, and are rarely capable of understanding the full impact of developing it. Even psychiatrists who have become comfortable with making vicarious judgements in favour of treatment are often uncomfortable with the responsibility (and the potential liability) of making such decisions when tardive dyskinesia has been diagnosed. The procedures established for review of treatment decisions can also provide a mechanism for assisting treating clinicians in making these difficult decisions. While this same function can be provided by clinical consultation, available psychiatric resources in most public hospitals have often precluded such an approach unless mandated by a court or legislature.

*Case 3:* Mr C was a 22-year-old mentally retarded schizophrenic patient who had been institutionalized much of his life in a facility for the developmentally disabled because of impulsive and unpredictable violent behaviour. His delusions and hallucinations were adequately controlled on moderate doses of anti-psychotic medication, but his violence was controlled only with high doses (60 mg of haloperidol plus 2000 mg of chlorpromazine per day); other medications prescribed to counter aggressive behaviour had proven ineffective. Without such treatment, Mr C spent much of his time in seclusion, because of the serious danger he posed to other patients and staff. The state statutes at that time did not require informed consent in order to treat committed patients. The attorney who headed the facility's human rights committee had himself appointed as Mr C's guardian, and instituted a lawsuit against the facility alleging inadequate treatment. After a careful evaluation, the consulting psychiatrist found no evidence of tardive dyskinesia, but recommended that Mr C's guardian be presented with the realistic alternatives (frequent seclusion versus treatment which had a high probability of leading to tardive dyskinesia) and required to choose between them.

## Disclosure of information

As a result of the increased emphasis on patient autonomy and informed consent, another problem has developed recently, involving the nature of the information which must be given to patients concerning their rights while being treated at a mental health facility. For example, twenty jurisdictions in the United States provide patients facing involuntary hospitalization with the right to remain silent, although only ten require that the patient be informed of that right at the time of admission.[26] Many clinicians fear that such requirements will encourage patients to withhold information necessary for their treatment, although the only study of the implementation of this right found no such effects,[26] and there is actually some evidence that provision of such warnings may have the paradoxical effect of causing some patients to disclose more information than they would have without the warnings.[26,27]

With the proliferation of external requirements to share previously confidential information with others, such as is the case with third-party reimbursement, requirements to provide information to courts in child custody and psychic trauma cases, obligations to assess proactively patients' abilities to operate motor vehicles, requirements to report sexual or physical child-abuse,[28] requirements to report sexual abuse by previous therapists,[29] and the more general duty to protect third parties from patients' dangerous behaviour, clinicians are faced with an increasing problem of what to tell patients about the disposition of information they give during therapy. There is evidence that many patients would drop out of therapy or not seek it in the first place if they were aware of the potential consequences of divulging information which is essential to effective treatment.[30]

In some situations, legal requirements for disclosure are explicit, such as the previously-mentioned statutory requirements to inform patients facing civil commitment that they have the right to remain silent, and in pre-trial or post-conviction evaluations of criminal defendants;[31] but there are few, if any, statutes or court decisions which explicitly prescribe requirements for disclosure of information in other situations, in which the need for disclosure can rarely be anticipated at the initiation of the psychiatrist–patient relationship. The American Psychiatric Association's *Principles of medical ethics*[11] (Section 4, no. 2) states that 'the continuing duty of the psychiatrist to protect the patient includes fully apprising him/her of the connotations of waiving the privilege of privacy'; but this principle was formulated in an era in which clinicians had both the responsibility *and* the authority to decide what information to divulge and under what circumstances, based only on their clinical judgements. They no longer have that privilege, and statutes and ethical codes provide little guidance as to when or how to warn patients of possible future disclosures of information.

There are also few data available concerning the incidence of disclosure of information in actual practice, even in criminal evaluations in which it would appear to be legally mandated. Miller and Weinstock[28] surveyed sex-offender treatment-programmes in all 51 jurisdictions in the United States, and found that there were few state policies concerning warnings to patients, even though most had been criminally convicted. A number of respondents (particularly those working in correctional facilities) reported that they felt that their primary responsibilities were to the government rather than to their patients. Many said that they gave blanket warnings to their patients at the time of admission that there was no guarantee of confidentiality with respect to possible disclosure to courts of information derived from therapy.

*Case 4:* Mr D had been found not guilty by reason of insanity of assaulting his parole officer, and committed to a forensic hospital. After a six-month hospitalization, he obtained a court order requiring his treating psychiatrist to evaluate him for conditional release; the criterion for release was that he should be able to live in the community without posing danger to others. The psychiatrist informed Mr D at the beginning of the interview of the purpose of the evaluation and the criterion for release, and told him that the report would go directly to the judge who ordered the evaluation. Despite this warning, when Mr D was asked what he intended to do after release, he immediately said that he would find the parole officer and kill him. That information was included in the report, and resulted in a denial of Mr D's release. For two years after the hearing Mr D would scream curses and threats whenever he saw the psychiatrist, even after transfer to another ward. His feeling of betrayal extended to other clinicians for much of that period, and significantly interfered with the development of a therapeutic relationship.

## The right to treatment

The concept of a right to treatment has been the repository of a variety of agendas since Morton Birnbaum coined the term in the United States in the 1960s.[32] Birnbaum conceived of the right as an obligation of government to provide effective mental health services to all citizens; but the US courts have not recognized the right on a constitutional basis, although several have ruled that involuntarily committed patients have a right to treatment as compensation (*quid pro quo*) for loss of freedom.[33] As previously mentioned, the interpretation of this right varies considerably, from the legal position that the patient's right is that of being offered appropriate treatment, to the moral rights position that patients have a right to be treated effectively, even against their expressed wishes, if they are so impaired by their disorders that they require involuntary commitment.[7,15]

It makes little difference how the right is interpreted, however, if clinicians are not provided with adequate resources to provide the treatment in question. Although there has been relatively little in the literature concerning rights of treatment staff, Rachlin[34] has argued that they at least should have the right to the resources necessary to carry out their responsibilities. Perhaps the major ethical dilemma faced by clinicians who work in public civil and forensic mental hospitals, to which the majority of involuntary patients are still committed, is whether to accept the substandard resources (particularly staff time) available as compared with what is found in other types of psychiatric practice, or to leave for another setting. Solomon[35] in his 1958 presidential address to the American Psychiatric Association called for psychiatrists to stop working in public mental hospitals, and a growing number of psychiatrists have followed his advice.[36] To compound the shortages of psychiatrists, restrictive immigration laws designed to diminish the 'brain drain' from Third World countries, and stricter accreditation standards at the state and national level, have limited the numbers of foreign medical graduates practising in the United States; such immigrants had previously comprised the majority of physicians practising in public mental hospitals. The problem with Solomon's solution, of course, is that if the most principled psychiatrists abandoned the public sector, it would simply compound the problem of lack of resources.

## The right to refuse treatment

Depriving people of their freedom, whether by hospitalizing them against their will, by forcing them to report to an out-patient facility for treatment, or by forcing them to accept a particular form of treatment (such as medication), invariably poses significant ethical dilemmas. Although intrusions on individual autonomy are common in US society, when they are due to the exercise of governmental authority they must be justified either by the state's police power to protect others from a person's actions, or by its *parens patriae* power to protect people from their own actions. The overriding of people's autonomy with respect to their own bodies, and therefore their rights to determine what medical procedures will be applied to them, has been justified on both grounds: under police power when the treatment in question is necessary to reduce present or future danger to others, and under the *parens patriae* power when the proposed treatment appears to be in the person's best interest, but is rejected because of reasoning impaired by the very mental disorder for which treatment is indicated. The problems posed by people who refuse non-psychiatric medical treatment because of a mental disorder are not conceptually distinguishable from those posed by psychiatric treatment, but are generally dealt with through different legal procedures.

Although at this point fewer than half the jurisdictions in the United States have court decisions or statutes which explicitly recognize a right to refuse treatment,[37] it is to be expected that most jurisdictions will be forced to grapple with the issues over the next decade. The trend seems clear: every court which has examined the issue of refusal of psychiatric treatment has concluded that there is a constitutionally-mandated, but qualified, right to refuse. All have recognized that medication may be administered against their will or without their consent to patients in emergency situations, usually defined as those involving imminent danger of physical harm to the patient or to others, although variations exist in the definitions of the severity and/or imminence of the threatened harm required to invoke the emergency exception.

The major differences which exist lie in the procedures established to determine if refusals should be sustained or overturned in non-emergency situations. To date, all such decisions require for overriding refusal a finding that the patient is incompetent to make informed treatment decisions; but the majority of courts have ratified independent clinical review, while others have mandated judicial review.[38] There are also some differences in the procedures required for the review process itself, such as whether representation by counsel is required.

For clinicians who initiate external review of patient treatment-refusal in order to be able to provide appropriate treatment for patients under their care, it is not the nature of the review process (clinical or judicial) which poses ethical problems, although it certainly poses logistical and other problems. The dilemmas lie in the areas of the choices available to clinicians whose patients refuse treatment. In many states clinicians have the option of utilizing seclusion and restraint as an alternative to forced medication in emergency situations; in either case, the intervention can be utilized only as long as the emergency itself exists, and therefore cannot be used to justify ongoing involuntary treatment of the disorder underlying the behaviour which created the emergency. Such use of medication, if strictly interpreted, is in effect chemical restraint, rather than treatment of a mental disorder, and raises significant ethical problems by creating staff pressure on psychiatrists to subject patients to the side-effects (if not the long-term risks) of psychotropic medication without their major therapeutic benefits.

The emergency use of medication is not, however, applicable in the case of severely ill patients, who need effective treatment as much as do their aggressive counterparts. Such patients pose fewer management problems to line staff and to other patients, and thus create less pressure for immediate attention from psychiatrists, particularly in public hospitals with significantly lower psychiatrist–patient ratios. Ethical problems occur when allocation of resources is determined on a 'squeaky wheel' basis rather than on individual clinical need; and the significant increase in psychiatrist time needed for the hearing process, particularly in states with requirements for judicial review, is often a major determinant in decisions as to which patients' refusals should be appealed.

*Case 5:* Mr E was a 32-year-old chronic schizophrenic with many prior hospitalizations, frequently after having been arrested for assault on police officers. At the time of his most recent hospitalization, for treatment to competency to stand trial, he was not aggressive, but was severely disorganized in his thinking and regressed in his behaviour. As on previous admissions, he denied that he was ill, and refused medication which had been effective on all previous admissions, but which he stopped taking as soon as he was released from the hospital. A petition for a hearing on his refusal was sent immediately, but was misplaced in court, resulting in a five-week delay in the hearing. During that time, Mr E spent his time mumbling incoherently and smearing faeces and urine over himself and his room. He had to be secluded to prevent him from smearing other patients, but could not be medicated compulsorily because his behaviour did not satisfy the statutory criteria for emergency treatment. He was found incompetent to refuse treatment at the hearing, was started immediately on medication, was restored to competency to proceed, and was discharged from the hospital within a week.

For those few patients who are determined after a review process to be competent to refuse treatment (reported to be between 0 per cent and 33 per cent of refusing patients, with most studies reporting fewer than 10 per cent), and for all refusing patients prior to hearings on their competency to refuse, psychiatrists are in the position of chiefly providing preventive detention for the benefit of society. Although non-psychiatrists have argued (successfully in many courts) that other forms of treatment, such as individual, group, or milieu therapy, may be as effective as medication in psychotic patients,[39] in practice most patients who are sufficiently psychotic to require hospitalization are not capable of benefiting from such treatment until their psychoses are controlled with medication. Because of the frustration associated with serving as gaolers for treatment-refusing patients, pressures exist for psychiatrists to utilize very low thresholds for incompetency to make treatment-decisions, either at initial commitment hearings or in subsequent proceedings, in order to override refusals.

The American Psychiatric Association's *Model guidelines*[40] recommend that incompetency to make treatment-decisions be one of the requirements for involuntary hospitalization. Utah has incorporated such a requirement into its commitment statute,[41] but there are as of yet no comprehensive data to indicate whether or not patients who otherwise meet the commitment criteria are in fact not committed because they are judged competent to refuse treatment. While such an approach eliminates the ethical dilemma posed by hospitalization for preventive detention, it creates others; patients who are competent to refuse treatment but sufficiently disordered that they cannot care for themselves outside a hospital or other structured setting would be denied such a setting, and might continue to pose a danger to themselves or to others under a strict interpretation of such a standard. Such patients would thus be denied the benefits of the asylum function, which is again becoming somewhat respectable in the wake of the problems of deinstitutionalization.[42]

## Involuntary commitment to general hospitals

In addition to community-based treatment, the movement which has been called 'decarceration' by Scull[43] has led to increased reliance on treatment in psychiatric units in general hospitals as compared with public mental hospitals, as part of a normalization process both for the patients themselves and for psychiatrists within the medical community. While it is clear that such hospitals are now treating an increased number of mental patients, it is equally clear that many provide only open wards, and avoid treating involuntary patients wherever possible. Psychiatrists at such facilities hail the superiority of their resources, but complain that uncooperative patients disrupt the environment for other patients and tie up valuable staff time in paperwork and testimony.[44] Such clinicians are faced with the ethical dilemma of denying their demonstrably greater treatment-capacities to the most disturbed patients in the community, or of sacrificing some of the benefits of their settings for voluntary patients in order to accept the challenge of treating involuntary patients. To the extent that they eschew committed patients, they only increase the demands on dwindling resources at public hospitals.[45]

## Involuntary commitment to out-patient treatment

The community mental health movement has been characterized from its inception by a greater emphasis on a psychosocial than on a medical model of mental disorder.[46] Part of this philosophy has been a greater attention to individual patient autonomy than had characterized the treatment approach in public hospitals, and, as with psychiatrists in general hospitals, a concomitant preference for voluntary treatment on the part of staff. While most community mental health centre psychiatrists have shown little hesitation in initiating involuntary hospitalization, they have been less receptive to accepting responsibility for patients committed to treatment at their facilities,[47] particularly with the increased likelihood of liability for the behaviours of their patients in the post-*Tarasoff* era.[48] As states experiment with out-patient commitment criteria based on prevention of deterioration rather than sequestration of dangerousness, out-patient psychiatrists are faced with a conflict between provision of treatment in a less restrictive (if still coercive) setting which might maintain remissions of psychotic disorders and thus avoid unnecessary hospitalization, and violation of their own principled dislike of coerced treatment. To the extent that out-patient facilities accept the responsibility of treating committed patients, they will also be increasingly subject to community pressure to control deviant but non-dangerous behaviour on the part of their clientele—pressure previously diffused through hospitalization.

## The 'deprofessionalization' of mental health service-delivery

Although community mental health centres and public mental hospitals were initially directed by psychiatrists, responsibility for administration and an increasing proportion of direct service has shifted to non-medical mental health professionals.[49] A growing number of states now permit licensed psychologists to perform commitment evaluations,[50] and many of the day-to-day decisions about patient-care (including the administration of such controversial procedures as seclusion, restraint, and involuntary medication) are made by nurses and other allied health professionals, albeit usually under the aegis of orders written by physicians.

There are several reasons for this diffusion of responsibility; first, the maldistribution of psychiatrists is nowhere more evident than in the public mental hospitals,[36,51] which continue to be the treatment sites for the majority of involuntarily hospitalized patients. Second, the growing challenge from non-medical mental health professionals to the psychiatric hegemony over the provision of mental health services, while primarily aimed at private in-patient and out-patient practice, has affected public hospitals as well.[52] The substitution of professional for hospital medical staff organizations by accrediting agencies has led to the assumption of many duties formerly restricted to physicians by non-physicians.[24] Third, the ever-increasing amount of paperwork required by third-party payers, accrediting agencies, and attorneys and courts has consumed significant amounts of time previously available for direct clinical services, and has not been matched by a concomitant increase in funding. Fourth, the higher salaries necessary to attract psychiatrists have led to a shift in staffing patterns, particularly in community centres which have been in financial difficulty since the withdrawal of federal funding, and which do not experience the same degree of pressure from accrediting agencies to maintain a high physician–patient ratio.

Since the only duties externally mandated to be done by psychiatrists are the prescription of medications and the signing of treatment-plans, the psychiatrists who remain in public facilities are under growing pressure to serve as signatories for such documents, without expectations that they will actually see, much less treat, patients. Some accede to these demands; others choose to practise elsewhere, resulting in further pressure on those who remain and attempt to practise responsibly.

Psychiatry as a profession has an ethical responsibility to reverse this trend and to work toward the provision of comprehensive services to the most severely mentally ill population. The dilemmas are too systemic to be resolved through the actions of individual practitioners, and need to be addressed through increased emphasis on the treatment of the chronically mentally ill in training programmes,[53] and through greater collaboration between psychiatric residency programmes and public mental health systems.[54]

## The duty to protect society

Both the American Medical Association[55] (Section 9) and the American Psychiatric Association[11] (Section 4[7]) have included since 1973 a provision for breaching the confidentiality of the physician–patient relationship, if necessary, in order to protect the welfare either of the patient or of the community. Similar provisions exist in the ethical codes of psychologists and social workers. Thus the *Tarasoff* decision in California[56] did not create a duty previously unrecognized by the mental health professionals themselves. It did, however, significantly lower the threshold for taking direct action when patients appear to pose a risk of dangerous behaviour. As a result of social trends toward protection of society at the expense of individuals' rights, current legal pressure is almost all on the side of petitioning for involuntary hospitalization rather than treatment in the community, and towards reluctance to release once hospitalized.[57]

As a result, clinicians are now faced with an increased ethical dilemma between the exercise of clinical judgement and treatment in the least restrictive setting, and the short-term protection of society (and themselves) by increased use of involuntary hospitalization and delaying releases until the responsibility can be passed to judges at commitment review hearings.

## Criminalization of involuntary hospitalization

A number of authors have provided data in support of the hypothesis that when legal or financial barriers to involuntary civil hospitalization are erected, the prevalence of mentally disordered persons in gaols and prisons increases.[58,59] After the passage of restrictive civil commitment laws in the 1970s, there was also a significant increase in the numbers of persons hospitalized for evaluation of, or treatment to, competency to stand trial.[60,61] There is little that mental health practitioners can do directly to prevent the arrests of such persons and their placement in gaols, prisons, and forensic hospitals. Such placements pose significant ethical problems, however, particularly in the case of mentally disordered persons who have been arrested specifically because they do not meet their jurisdiction's dangerousness criteria for civil commitment, or in order to avoid expending county funds on their treatment.

Competency to stand trial evaluations comprise the majority of forensic admissions in many states. Since the criteria for competency to stand trial are not synonymous with those for clinical recovery sufficient to permit discharge from hospitals, a significant number of patients are capable of returning to court as competent to proceed before their clinical conditions improve sufficiently to warrant discharge. Clinicians are therefore faced with a choice between adhering to the legal parameters of the commitment, or keeping patients longer in order to provide maximally effective treatment, knowing that if they choose the latter, they are helping to perpetuate the inappropriate use of the criminal justice system in order to bypass legal or economic barriers to civil commitment.

Space does not permit discussion here of the other significant ethical problems in the treatment of mental patients which have arisen recently within the criminal justice system, and which are largely due to the different goals of the correctional and mental health systems. The most troubling, if the least frequent, is that of providing clinically appropriate treatment to condemned inmates in order to restore their competency to be executed.[62]

Another significant problem, particularly in the Soviet Union,[63] is the use of commitment to psychiatric hospitals in order to prevent political dissidents from having a public forum for their views, and at the same time to discredit those views by branding them as the product of mental illness. Robitscher[64] has described such uses of commitment, admittedly on a smaller scale, in the United States; and I have discussed more recent examples in the context of competency to stand trial.[65] It continues to be important for psychiatrists to avoid being used as instruments of political policy in such ways.

## The international perspective

Many of the problematic changes in the way in which involuntary hospitalization is practised which have been brought about by constitutional challenges in the courts in the United States have begun to appear in other countries as well, although more frequently based on legislative rather than judicial mandates. Statutory change in Italy in 1968 permitted voluntary psychiatric hospitalization for the first time. Further changes in 1978 encouraged use of general rather than public psychiatric hospitals by limiting the use of the latter to cases of relapses of major mental disorders. It also moved away from a dangerousness standard by restricting the 'commitment for menace' provisions of the 1904 law to criminal patients. These changes reduced admissions to public hospitals by a much greater number than the concomitant increase in general hospital psychiatric units, and also led to a decrease in the percentage of involuntary admissions nationwide to 25 per cent by 1984, with much lower percentages in some areas. As in the United States, deinstitutionalization appears not to have been accompanied by the establishment of sufficient community resources to provide effective treatment for all those released from, or not admitted to, psychiatric in-patient facilities.[66]

In England, the trend toward 'legalism', which had been supported by legislation, was reversed in 1959 by a new statute which removed many of the legal safeguards for patients.[7] Subsequent concern for patients' rights under the revised statute led in 1983 to a partial return to a legal framework for commitment. Criteria for involuntary hospitalization still included a mental disorder requiring hospitalization for treatment; commitment of patients with personality disorders or other non-psychotic disorders under *parens patriae* grounds is permitted only if treatment is likely to produce improvement in the condition. The admission and discharge process is still controlled by clinicians, rather than by courts. Mental Health Review Tribunals were established which are required to review admissions and continued hospitalizations at regular (if lengthy) intervals; patients are provided with legal assistance for these hearings.

Under the 1983 Act, patients have the right to refuse 'hazardous, irreversible or not fully established' procedures. Psychosurgery and hormonal treatments cannot be given without the consent of the patient *and* the concurrence of two physicians. Electroconvulsive therapy and psychotropic medication, however, may still be given without patient consent if one independent physician concurs with the treating psychiatrist. Critics of the revisions argue that they did not seriously challenge medical hegemony, as without experienced and aggressive mental health attorneys, the Tribunals appear likely to continue to defer to medical opinions.[67] The criteria for admission are still largely expressed in clinical terms, and there is little effective limitation of the involuntary use of electroconvulsive therapy or medications.

In Canada, a constitutionally-based Charter of Rights and Freedoms was passed in 1982 which appeared to provide for more formal judicial oversight of the rights of mental patients, including their right to refuse treatment. Because of the Canadian tradition of parliamentary supremacy over the judiciary and the conservatism of the Supreme Court, however, the provisions of the Charter are felt to be unlikely to lead to the types of formal judicial procedures found in the United States. The right to refuse treatment is generally conceptualized under an informed consent rather than a rights analysis.[68]

In eight out of ten Canadian provinces, as well as in England, Scotland, Australia, and New Zealand, statutes authorize clinicians to treat involuntarily committed patients with psychotropic medication without consent. In Ontario, patients may be given treatment (except psychosurgery) without their consent if authorized by the Regional Review Board after a hearing at which it is determined that such treatment is in the patient's best interests. In Nova Scotia, if the admitting psychiatrist deems the patient to be 'incapable of consenting', substituted consent may be obtained, without a hearing, from a guardian, the nearest relative, or the Public Trustee. The patient does, however, have the right to appeal against the psychiatrist's determination of incompetency to the Provincial Review Board. Similar procedures exist in South Australia. Formal guardianship procedures may also be used to override patients' refusal of treatment; but, as in most United States jurisdictions, the complexity of the procedures militates against their use for the limited objective of providing involuntary treatment with psychotropic medication.[68]

Spain still operates under a 1931 Act which was more concerned with the economics of institutions than with patient rights, although 1978 revisions to the Spanish constitution do address issues such as the right to refuse treatment and informed consent. The government controls the system, whose primary function appears to be protection of the public. Involuntary hospitalization is generally reserved for dangerous patients, but the decisions to commit and to discharge are made by psychiatrists. The government may refer cases to the courts for disposition, but such referrals are rare.[69]

Segal has investigated the results of the statutory changes discussed above on the characteristics of patients committed in the United States, England and Wales, and Italy.[70] As a result of the dangerousness criteria predominant in the United States since the mid-1960s, in-patient censuses decreased, but shifted dramatically toward young males. The reverse has been true in Italy, while in England and Wales, where the criteria did not change significantly between 1963 and 1988, patient demographics did not change appreciably.

It can be anticipated that as other countries adopt policies and procedures similar to those established in the United States, they will increasingly be faced with the same ethical dilemmas.

## Potential solutions to current ethical dilemmas in involuntary commitment

The dilemmas discussed above do not admit of easy resolution. Both the American Psychiatric Association and the American Academy of Psychiatry and the Law are in the process of revising their ethical codes in response to changing conditions of practice; the duration of the review process such changes must undergo is testimony to the difficulty of the process.

Legal scrutiny of psychiatric practice, always more intense when governmental power is used to restrict personal freedom, has increased significantly in the past three decades in the United States, and may be expected to increase in other countries as well in the near future. While psychiatrists have traditionally (and with some justification) resisted such oversight, it also has the potential to provide support as well. Many hospital-based psychiatrists have found that proactive consultation with in-house advocates or ombudsmen can be of assistance in resolving ethical conflicts, and also may be a useful source of support for reform measures designed to obtain the additional resources necessary to provide effective treatment. External reviewers, such as the Joint Commission on Accreditation of Hospitals and the Health Care Financing Administration, which is responsible for Medicare reviews, may have significant impact on funding

funding decisions at the state level, and should be considered potential allies rather than adversaries.[71]

Although external review of patient's treatment-refusal may be time-consuming (particularly if judicial review is required), it also provides a forum in which to share the ethical burden of decision-making in problematic situations, such as those of patients suffering from the early signs of tardive dyskinesia who decompensate clinically without anti-psychotic medication. The major problem caused by external review is delay in the provision of treatment; here, psychiatrists can have an impact at the legislative level by working to mandate more timely hearings.

Since no profession has demonstrated the ability to police itself adequately, the judicial system may also provide external reinforcement for efforts within the psychiatric profession to improve the ethical standards of its members. Paradoxically, the increased litigiousness of United States society has hindered efforts at self-policing, since practitioners who are sanctioned by their own professions frequently seek redress in the courts, discouraging psychiatrists and other professionals from engaging in serious review of their colleagues' conduct for fear of spending valuable clinical time in court, even if they are provided with immunity from personal liability. Clinicians also fear that individual actions taken outside the normal physician–patient relationship, such as warning potential victims of their patients, or reporting unethical conduct on the part of colleagues, might involve them in allegations of breach of confidentiality, libel, or slander. Statutory provisions such as those in effect in a number of states to provide immunity for therapists against liability in warning potential victims or initiating commitment[72] or in reporting colleagues alleged to have sexually abused their patients[29] are examples of such legislative support for ethically appropriate clinical behaviours.

As the conditions under which psychiatrists practise, particularly in the involuntary treatment of patients, are increasingly regulated by courts and legislatures, the profession is forced to adopt (or at least to practise under) a code of ethics not of its own making. It is therefore essential that organized psychiatry, both at the state and national level, become increasingly proactive in helping to shape the regulations with which it must live. And in order to achieve the profession's goal in this manner, psychiatrists must learn to operate in the foreign environment of the law, to understand the legal viewpoint, and to be prepared to compromise, rather than to hold to an absolutist clinical position which is increasingly unacceptable to judges and legislatures.[73] It is also necessary for psychiatrists to devise research to collect relevant data to support their positions, rather than to continue to base their arguments on authority and ideology.

Diamond[74] has distinguished between professional ethics (those promulgated by an organized profession) and personal ethics, based on an individual's own ethical code. Given the lack of specificity of the American Psychiatric Association's ethical code with respect to involuntary commitment, and the increasing complexity of regulations surrounding it, it is incumbent on each psychiatrist to become aware of the pitfalls and conflicts involved in the provision of such treatment, and to strive to resolve them both individually and collectively.

## References

1 Ennis, B. J.: *Prisoners of psychiatry: mental patients, psychiatrists, and the law.* New York, Harcourt, Brace, Jovanovich, 1972.
2 Miller, R. D., Ionescu-Pioggia, R. M. and Fiddleman, P. B.; The effect of witnesses, judges, and attorneys upon civil commitment in North Carolina: a prospective study. *Journal of Forensic Sciences* 28:829–38, 1983.
3 Gutheil, T. G., Rachlin, S., and Mills, M. J.: Differing conceptual models in psychiatry and law, in *Legal encroachments on psychiatric practice*, ed. S. Rachlin. (New Directions in Mental Health Services). San Francisco, Jossey-Bass, 1985.
4 Chodoff, P.: Paternalism versus autonomy in medicine and psychiatry. *Psychiatric Annals* 13:318–20, 1983.
5 Kaplan, L. V. and Miller, R. D.: Law, psychiatry and rights. Presented at the 15th International Congress of Law and Mental Health, Jerusalem, Israel, June 26, 1989. In preparation.
6 Strauss, L.: *Natural right and history.* Chicago, University of Chicago Press, 1953.
7 Rachlin, S.: One right too many. *Bulletin of the American Academy of Psychiatry and the Law* 3:99–103, 1975.
8 Miller, R. D. and Fiddleman, P. B.: Emergency involuntary commitment: a look at the decision-making process. *Hospital and Community Psychiatry* 34:249–54, 1983.
9 Monahan, J.: The prediction of violent behaviour: toward a second generation of theory and policy. *American Journal of Psychiatry* 141:10–15, 1984.
10 American Psychiatric Association: *Amicus curiae* brief in *Estelle* v. *Smith.* 451 US 454, 101 S.Ct 1866 (1981).
11 American Psychiatric Association: *Principles of medical ethics with annotations especially applicable to psychiatry.* Washington DC, American Psychiatric Press, 1978.
12 Givelber, D. J., Bowers, W. J., Blitch, C. L.: *Tarasoff,* myth and reality: an empirical study of private law in action. *Wisconsin Law Review* 1984:443–97, 1984.
13 Stone, A. A.: *Law, psychiatry and morality: essays and analysis.* Washington DC, American Psychiatric Press, 1984.
14 Hiday, V. A.: Reform commitment procedures: an empirical study in the courtroom. *Law and Society Review* 11:652–66, 1977.
15 Treffert, D. A.: The right to refuse treatment. Presented at the Spring Scientific Meeting of the Midwestern Chapter of the American Academy of Psychiatry and the Law, Madison, WI, 15 April 1989.

16 Sosowsky, L.: Explaining the increased arrest rate among mental patients: a cautionary note. *American Journal of Psychiatry* **137**:1602–5, 1980.

17 Huber, G. A., Roth, L. H., Appelbaum, P. S. and Ore, T. M.: Hospitalization, arrest or discharge: important legal and clinical issues in the emergency evaluation of persons believed to be dangerous to others. *Law and Contemporary Problems* **45**:99–123, 1982.

18 Morse, S. J.: A preference for liberty: the case against involuntary commitment of the mentally disordered. *California Law Review* **70**:54–106, 1982.

19 Chu, F. D. and Trotter, S.: *The madness establishment.* New York, Grossman, 1974.

20 Miller, R. D., Bernstein, M. R., Van Rybroek, G. J., and Maier, G. J.: The right to refuse treatment in a forensic patient population: six-month review. *Bulletin of the American Academy of Psychiatry and the Law.* **17**:107–19, 1989.

21 Weinstein, R. M.: Mental patients' attitudes toward mental hospitalization: a review of quantitative research. *Journal of Health and Social Behaviour* **20**:237–58, 1979.

22 Szasz, T. S.: Voluntary mental hospitalization: an unacknowledged practice of medical fraud. *New England Journal of Medicine* **287**:277–8, 1972.

23 Dabrowski, S., Gerard, K., Walczak, S., *et. al.*: Inability of patients to give valid consent to psychiatric hospitalization. *International Journal of Law and psychiatry* **1**:437–41, 1978.

24 Joint Commission on the Accreditation of Hospitals: *Accreditation manual for hospitals.* Chicago, JCAH, 1984.

25 *Rennie* v. *Klein.* 462 F. Supp. 1131 (D.N.J., 1978); 476 F.Supp. 1294 (D.N.J. 1979).

26 Miller, R. D., Maier, G. J., and Kaye, M.: The right to remain silent during psychiatric examination in civil and criminal cases: a national survey and an analysis. *International Journal of Law and Psychiatry* **9**:77–94, 1986.

27 Appelbaum, P. S. and Gutheil, T. G.: *Clinical handbook of psychiatry and law.* New York, McGraw-Hill, 1982.

28 Miller, R. D. and Weinstock, R.: Conflict of interest between therapist–patient confidentiality and the duty to report sexual abuse of children. *Behavioural Sciences and the Law* **5**:161–74, 1987.

29 Gartrell, N., Herman, J., Olarte, S., Feldstein, M., Localio, R., and Schoener, G.: Sexual abuse of patients by therapists: strategies for offender management and rehabilitation, in *Legal implications of hospital policies and practices*, ed. R. D. Miller (New Directions in Mental Health Services). San Francisco, Jossey–Bass, 1989.

30 Schmid, D., Appelbaum, P. S., Roth, L. H., and Lidz, C.: Confidentiality in psychiatry: a study of the patient's view. *Hospital and Community Psychiatry* **34**:353–5, 1983.

31 *Estelle* v. *Smith.* 451 US 454, 101 S.Ct 1866 (1981).

32 Birnbaum, M.: The right to treatment. *American Bar Association Journal* **46**:499–505, 1960.

33 *Wyatt* v. *Stickney.* 344 F.Supp. 373 (M.D. Ala, 1972).

34 Rachlin, S.: Toward a definition of staff rights. *Hospital and Community Psychiatry* **33**:60–1, 1982.

35 Solomon, H.: Presidential address to the American Psychiatric Association. *American Journal of Psychiatry* **115**:1–9, 1958.

36 Talbott, J. A.: Why psychiatrists leave the public sector. *Hospital and Community Psychiatry* **30**:82, 1979.

37 Brakel, S. J., Parry, J. and Weiner, B. A.: *The mentally disabled and the law*, 3rd edn. Chicago, American Bar Foundation, 1985.

38 Appelbaum, P. S.: The right to refuse treatment with antipsychotic medications: retrospect and prospect. *American Journal of Psychiatry* **145**:413–19, 1988.

39 Zander, T. K.: Plaintiff's brief in *Wisconsin ex rel. Jones* v. *Gerhardstein*. 141 Wis.2d 710, 416 N.W.2d 888 (1987).

40 American Psychiatric Association: Guidelines for legislation on the psychiatric hospitalization of adults. *American Journal of Psychiatry* **104**:672–9, 1983.

41 Utah Code, Annotated Chapter 64–7–36.

42 Bachrach, L. L.: Asylum and chronically ill psychiatric patients. *American Journal of Psychiatry* **141**:975–8, 1984.

43 Scull, A.: *Decarceration: community treatment and the deviant—a radical view*, 2nd edn. New Brunswick NJ, Rutgers University Press, 1984.

44 Leeman, C. P.: Involuntary admissions to general hospitals: progress or threat? *Hospital and Community Psychiatry* **31**:315–18, 1980.

45 Miller, R. D.: Psychiatric units in general hospitals: élitism revisited? *Hospital and Community Psychiatry* **32**:804–5, 1981.

46 Baker, F. and Schulberg, H. C.: The development of a community mental health ideology scale. *Community Mental Health Journal* **3**:216–25, 1967.

47 Miller, R. D.: Outpatient civil commitment of the mentally ill: an overview and an update. *Behavioral Sciences and the Law* **6**: 99–118, 1988.

48 Miller, R. D., Luskin, R. L., Starrett, D., Bloom, J. D. and Weitzel, W.: American Psychiatric Association Task Force Report no. 26: *Involuntary commitment to outpatient treatment*. Washington DC, American Psychiatric Press, 1987.

49 Fink, P. J. and Weinstein, D. P.: Whatever happened to psychiatry? The deprofessionalization of community mental health centers. *American Journal of Psychiatry* **136**:406–9, 1979.

50 Drude, K. P.: Psychologists and civil commitment: review of state statutes. *Professional psychology* **9**:499–506, 1978.

51 Knesper, D. J. and Pagnucco, D. J.: Estimated distribution of effort by providers of mental health services to US adults in 1982 and 1983. *American Journal of Psychiatry* **144**:883–8, 1987.

52 Miller, R. D.: Recent developments in antitrust: challenges to medical autonomy, in *Legal implications of hospital policies and practices*, ed. R. D. Miller. (New Directions in Mental health Services). San Francisco, Jossey-Bass, 1989.

53 White, H. S. and Bennett, M. B.: Training psychiatric residents in chronic care. *Hospital and Community psychiatry* **32**:339–43, 1981.

54 Zwerling, J.: The public hospital system as a nexus between government and the university, in *State mental hospitals: problems and potentials*, ed. J. A. Talbott. New York, Human Sciences Press, 1980.

55 American Medical Association: *Principles of medical ethics*. Washington DC, American Medical Association, 1957.

56 *Tarasoff* v. *Regents of the University of California*. 118 Cal. Rptr. 129, 529 P.2d 553 (1974); 17 Cal.3d 425, 551 P.2d 334 (1976).

57 Huber, G. A., Roth, L. H., and Appelbaum, P. S.: Hospitalization, arrest or discharge; important legal and clinical issues in the emergency evaluation of persons believed to be dangerous to others. *Law and Contemporary Problems* **45**:99–123, 1982.

58 Steadman, H. J., Cocozza, J. J., and Melich, M. E.: Explaining the increased arrest rate among mental patients: the changing clientele of state hospitals. *American Journal of Psychiatry* **135**:816–20, 1978.

59 Whitmer, G.: From hospitals to jails: the fate of California's deinstitutionalized mentally ill. *American Journal of Orthopsychiatry* **50**:65–75, 1980.

60 Dickey, W.: Incompetency and the nondangerous mentally ill. *Criminal Law Bulletin* **16**:22–40, 1980.

61 Rachlin, S. and Stokman, C. L. J.: Incompetent misdemeanants—pseudocivil commitment. *Bulletin of the American Academy of Psychiatry and the Law* **14**:23–30, 1986.

62 Miller, R. D.: Evaluation of and treatment to competency to be executed: a national survey and an analysis. *Journal of Psychiatry and Law* **16**:67–90, 1988.

63 Bloch, S.: The political misuse of psychiatry in the Soviet Union, in *Psychiatric Ethics*, 2nd edn, ed. S. Bloch and P. Chodoff. Oxford, Oxford University Press, 1990.

64 Robitscher, J.: *The powers of psychiatry*. Boston, Houghton Mifflin, 1980.

65 Miller, R. D. and Germain, E. J.: Evaluation of competency to stand trial in defendants who do not want to be defended against the crimes charged. *Bulletin of the American Academy of Psychiatry and the Law* **15**:371–79, 1987.

66 Arata, A., Del Brenna, A. M., Lo Nano, D., and Sorbo, S.: The therapy of mental disorders in Italy: the role of hospitals after the 1978 reform. *International Journal of Law and Psychiatry* **7**:207–14, 1984.

67 Shapland, J. and Williams, T.: Legalism revised; new mental health legislation in England. *International Journal of Law and Psychiatry* **6**:351–69, 1983.

68 Gordon, R. and Verdun-Jones, S. N.: The right to refuse treatment: commonwealth developments and issues. *International Journal of Law and Psychiatry* **6**:57–73, 1983.

69 Calcedo-Ordonez, A. and Florez, J. A.: Law and psychiatry in Spain. *International Journal of Law and Psychiatry* **5**:413–18, 1982.

70 Segal, S. P.: Civil commitment standards and patient mix in England/Wales, Italy, and the United States. *American Journal of Psychiatry* **146**:187–93, 1989.

71 Rachlin, S.: Litigating a right to treatment: *Woe* is me. *Psychiatric Quarterly* **60**:182–92, 1988.

72 Felthous, A. R.: *The psychotherapist's duty to warn or protect*. Springfield IL, Charles Thomas, 1989.

73 Miller, R. D.: Who's afraid of forensic psychiatry? *Bulletin of the American Academy of Psychiatry and the Law*, in press.

74 Diamond, B.: *The ethics of expert witness testimony*. Critical issues in American Psychiatry and the Law, Vol. 8, ed. R. Weinstock and R. Rosner. New York, Plenum Press, 1990.

# 14

# The ethics of deinstitutionalization*

*Roger Peele*

## Introduction

The deinstitutionalization of the psychiatrically ill since 1955 raises a number of ethical issues. First I shall present a chronology of the development of deinstitutionalization in the United States, then list the value conflicts inherent in the major forces playing a role in deinstitutionalization. I shall end with a discussion of the specific issues facing psychiatry and others involved in deinstitutionalization.

## Chronology of deinstitutionalization in the US

### 1955

The number of patients in public mental hospitals in the United States peaks at 550 000.

Sociologist Erving Goffman studies patients at St Elizabeth's Hospital, a 7000-bed public institution in Washington DC, and puts forward the thesis that some signs and symptoms of psychiatric illness are not part of the illness itself but are the result of being in an institution.[1] Goffman is referring to what we would call today defective (or negative) signs of schizophrenia. The better the institution ('better' in the sense of structuring and filling the patient's days and evenings) the more likely—according to Goffman—that the institution would produce these defective signs of schizophrenia. Goffman's work remained unchallenged for over twenty years.[2]

The US Congress authorizes a Joint Commission on Mental Illness and Health to make recommendations on how to meet the needs of the psychiatrically ill.

### 1958

American Psychiatric Association President Harry Solomon writes:[3]

I do not see how any reasonably objective view of our mental hospitals today can fail to conclude that they are bankrupt beyond remedy. I believe, therefore, that

---

* *Editors' note*: Although this chapter focuses almost exclusively on the situation in the United States, the editors believe that the ethical issues arising from deinstitutionalization in that country can be applied usefully to comparable situations emerging elsewhere.

our large mental hospitals should be liquidated as rapidly as can be done in an orderly and progressive fashion.

## 1960

The Supreme Court rules in *Shelton* v. *Tucker* (a case not involving the psychiatrically ill) that

Even though the government purpose be legitimate and substantial, that purpose cannot be pursued by means that broadly stifle fundamental personal liberties when the end can be more narrowly achieved.[4]

From this decision would arise the principle of placing patients in the 'least restrictive alternative', often in preference to hospitalization.

## 1961

The Joint Commission's report, *Action for mental health*, is published.[5] The seven volumes contained many recommendations, including:

- no public hospital should have more than 1000 beds
- clinics should be established for each 50 000 population catchment area

Gerald Caplan's *An approach to community mental health* is published.[6] It captured the thinking of many in calling for a preventive psychiatric approach that would treat illness in the community, and thus prevent the need for hospitalization. Caplan championed both primary and secondary prevention based upon psychoanalytic explanations of the cause of psychiatric illness.

Thomas Szasz's *The myth of mental illness* is also published.[7] While his concept that mental illness is a harmful metaphor was not accepted by many, it did contribute to a widespread feeling that voluntary treatment should be questioned.

## 1963

President Kennedy sends a message to Congress entitled 'Mental illness and mental retardation'. This results in Congressional passage of legislation calling for the creation of community mental health centres and federal improvement grants for public mental hospitals. The passage of this legislation was based to some extent on testimony that community support would evolve as an alternative to institutional care and treatment. However, no scientific evidence for such a supposition was presented.

The psychiatrically ill become eligible for aid under the federal programme *Aid to the Disabled*. This later becomes Supplemental Security Income (SSI) and Social Security Disability Insurance (SSDI), under which federal payment is eventually made to hundreds of thousands of mentally ill patients for the purpose of assisting them to live outside institutions.

### *1964*

Federal regulations associated with the 1963 legislation call for community mental health centres to provide:

1. In-patient services
2. Partial hospitalization services
3. Out-patient services
4. Twenty-four-hour emergency services
5. Consultation and education services

Note that these requirements do not provide for a community support system to replace services that had been provided by the institution.

### *1965*

Medicare and Medicaid programmes are passed by the US Congress. These two programmes contain major discriminations against funding for the psychiatrically ill that will influence deinstitutionalization. Medicare will provide only 190 days of in-patient care during a person's life, and only $500 of clinical treatment at 50 per cent co-payment. Medicaid will cover treatment in psychiatric departments of general hospitals but not in psychiatric hospitals, although under certain circumstances it will cover nursing-home costs. These federal programmes offer opportunities for the states to receive federal dollars for the care and treatment of the psychiatrically ill previously provided for in state psychiatric institutions. Moving elderly patients from such institutions to nursing homes, and relying on psychiatric units of general hospitals for acute care, reduces the costs to the state. This presents major ethical issues for clinicians as discussed below under the heading 'Value issues in transinstitutionalization'.

### *1966*

The US Court of Appeals for the District of Columbia rules in *Lake* v. *Cameron* that a patient is not to be involuntarily hospitalized if an alternative that does not infringe upon his or her rights to liberty (community placement) can be found.[8] This decision follows from the logic of *Shelton*, viz., that before Ms. Lake could be admitted to a hospital involuntarily, it had to be established that a less restrictive alternative was not available.[4]

### *Late 1960s*

Federal government champions governance in the hands of citizen boards, since 'local control' is regarded as less suspect than control by state, county, or city. This concept and the partial intrusion of the federal government in the early 1960s has the effect of dividing responsibility for the chronically psychiatrically ill among a multitude of parties, thus leaving no agency—federal, state, county, city, or 'local'—in full charge.

The number of the psychiatrically ill in public psychiatric hospitals drops below 400 000.

### 1970

In the 1960s chronically ill psychiatric patients are transinstitutionalized into single-room occupancies ('SROs'); but gradually the number of such units available in the United States declines from 2 000 000 in 1970 to 1 000 000 by 1987.

### 1971

*Wyatt* v. *Stickney*, a 'right to adequate treatment' suit in Alabama, calls for improved staffing and many other changes in Alabama's public mental and retardation institutions.[9] Alabama responds by decreasing the number of patients, i.e. deinstitutionalizaling patients to the community or transinstitutionalizing patients to nursing homes in order to improve staff-to-patient ratios.

### 1972

In *Lessard* v. *Schmidt*, a Wisconsin court rules that the only grounds justifying involuntary treatment are dangerousness to others or self.[10] Although not binding elsewhere, this decision helps set a tone that makes it more difficult to hospitalize the psychiatrically ill involuntarily.

The Joint Commission on Accreditation of Hospitals (JCAH), renamed the Joint Commission on Accreditation of Health Organizations (JCAHO) in 1987, establishes separate standards for psychiatric hospitals. JCAHO standards encourage deinstitutionalization in two ways: (1) standards generally are easier to achieve with a relatively small number of patients; and (2) these standards expect planning for community placement outside the institution from the moment each patient is admitted.

The number of the psychiatrically ill in public mental hospitals drops below 300 000.

### 1974

The *Tarasoff* decision by the California Supreme Court requires clinicians to warn potential victims that patients may be planning to harm them.[11] This decision becomes the rule in many states, discouraging clinicians from assuming responsibility for dangerous patients.

### 1975

The Supreme Court's decision in *O'Connor* v. *Donaldson* ultimately results in a psychiatrist being successfully sued for $20 000 because he sent papers to courts asking that a patient remain committed to a Florida institution.[12] The psychiatrist was found at fault even though the courts had agreed to the psychiatrist's recommendation thirty times previously that Mr Donaldson should be hospitalized. This decision increased the sense among hospital psychiatrists that they could be held legally liable for prolonged patient hospitalization. For the psychiatrist working in thinly staffed public settings, the simplest way to avoid both professional liability for inadequate treatment on the one hand and civil liability for deprivation of liberty on the other, was to discourage admissions or, if the patient was admitted, to facilitate rapid discharge.

In *Dixon* v. *Weinberger*, the District of Columbia Circuit Court finds that hundreds of St Elizabeth's Hospital patients have a right to community placement in a 'least restrictive setting'.[13]

Federal CMHC legislation adds seven more requirements to the five services already expected of CHMCs (see under 1964, above):

6. Screening of patients prior to admission to public mental hospitals.
7. Follow-up care for those released from mental hospitals.
8. Development of transitional living facilities for the mentally ill.
9. Children's programmes must be developed.
10. Programmes for the elderly must be developed.
11. Drug abusers' programmes must be developed.
12. Alcohol abusers' programmes must be developed.

These changes recognized that the original five requirements were inadequate. Numbers 6, 7, and 8 were intended to help improve the care and treatment of patients leaving institutions.

## 1977

The number of psychiatrically ill in public psychiatric institutions falls below 200 000.

## 1979

In *Rogers* v. *Okin*, the Massachusetts Supreme Court, relying on the Massachusetts constitution, begins a series of rulings that will have the effect of involving courts in decisions about the involuntary administration of medications.[14]

## 1981

The Omnibus Budget Reconciliation Act changes federal support to meet less specific federal requirements. Towards the end of the Carter Administration (1977–81) proposals were developed that had called for massive federal help to reach the deinstitutionalized psychiatrically ill. However, under this Omnibus Act the Carter Administration proposals were not implemented; also, the gradual increasing of federal responsibility for the psychiatrically ill that had been evolving since 1963 was reversed. After almost three decades of federal leadership and initiatives in planning for the needs of the psychiatrically ill, the federal government suddenly withdraws, leaving leadership and planning to the states.

The decrease in federal support of low-income housing contributes to the decline in low-cost housing at a rate of about 300 000 units per year in the 1980s.[15]

### 1986

In testimony before Congress, the National Institute of Mental Health presents estimates of the location of adult schizophrenics as follows:[16]

| State mental hospitals | 104 800 (6%) |
| Nursing homes | 73 500 (5%) |
| Acute-care in-patient units | 225 400 (14%) |
| Out-patient | 269 000 (17%) |
| Unknown | 937 300 (58%) |

This testimony highlights the results of deinstitutionalization in the United States. The total in state institutions is less than 120 000, down from 550 000 in 1955.

By the 1980s, studies of the homeless suggest that two-thirds of the homeless are psychiatrically ill, one-half of those being people with substance-abuse disorders (including alcoholism). Fuller Torrey has pointed out that even if one accepts the lowest estimates for the number of people who are homeless, twice as many of the psychiatrically ill are on the streets as in state mental hospitals.[16]

### Experience in Great Britain

In Great Britain, deinstitutionalization has also produced an increase of the homeless mentally ill.[17] In December 1986 a survey of the homeless found 56 per cent of them had been treated for psychotic disorders, and 34 per cent had psychotic symptoms the night that they were seen. The number of hospital beds is decreasing at the same time that the number of hostel beds, a resource for the discharged psychiatrically ill in the community, is also shrinking.

One study reported that the psychiatrically ill who were in-patients received more meals and baths, and had a fuller social and entertainment life, than did those who had been returned to the community.[18]

## Deinstitutionalization and values

The values influencing the events of the chronology have a number of sources:

1. The mental health professions
2. The legislative branches
3. The executive branches
4. The judiciary
5. Lay organizations
6. Accreditation bodies

While these six sources of values contributing to deinstitutionalization share some attitudes, each also has contributed some values unique to the process.

## The mental health professions

In the early nineteenth century, psychiatry had a belief, embodied in what was called 'moral therapy', that people suffered from illnesses caused by exposure to immoral conditions in the community. It followed that treatment should remove the patients from these immoral settings and place them in moral settings where they would be cured. In the first half of the nineteenth century this approach did result in claims that the majority of patients were 'cured'. In the second half of the century, for various reasons, moral therapy was discarded, and institutions caring for these patients became warehouses for patients, not treatment-centres. The profession, in an effort to become more 'scientific', adopted the hypothesis that the psychiatrically ill suffered from brain diseases, not from the corrupting influence of the community.

The conditions existing in these institutions were often seen as inhumane, and periodic calls for reform were heard from the 1870s through to the 1940s. In the 1950s, the call for reform of the institutions was changed to a call for abolition of the institutions (see Solomon's remarks, cited under the heading *1958* above). Some key professionals took a position opposite to that of the early nineteenth century. Instead of conceiving of the mentally ill as suffering from the corrupting influence of the community, with the cure being placement in institutions with a moral setting, they held that the mentally ill suffered from the institutional environment itself, and that they could be cured by being placed in the warm bosom of the community. The medications discovered in the early part of the 1950s made it possible to carry out such a transfer of patients; but the new policy itself was never subjected to the empirical scrutiny to which the medications were subjected. The profession seems to require a scientific process when thinking of medications, but not when thinking of policy.[19] In Great Britain there also have been complaints that deinstitutionalization is taking place without research or monitoring of the process.[18]

While Wyatt and others state that 'scienceless had led to homeless', other professionals continue to champion the proposition that institution-alization is harmful. As late as 1989 Mosher and Burti maintained:[20]

Reducing our reliance on in-patient hospital care is justified on a number of grounds:

1. *Humanitarian*. Because these institutions treat persons as objects, basic human qualities like individuality, autonomy, independence, and the sense of personal responsibility are undermined. Reducing their use will prevent this process of dehumanization.

2. *Moral*. Hospitals are known to cause the iatrogenic disease 'institutional-ism' . . . . Not using hospitals will keep the prevalence of these syndromes to a minimum.

3. *Economic*. Because in-patient care consumes 70 per cent of mental health dollars, reducing its use will allow the support of badly needed, more effective, and more normalizing community programmes.

4. *Scientific*. Nineteen of 20 studies comparing in-patient psychiatric hospitaliza-tion with a variety of alternative forms of care found the alternatives as effective, or more so, and less costly . . . . These studies also found hospitals to be habit-forming; hospital-treated patients tended to recycle through the hospital, whereas alternatively treated clients did not.

Thus, clinicians and the professional policy-makers continue to face the charge that hospitalization is harmful for their patients. The belief of Mosher and Burti is not fully shared by the majority of psychiatrists. For example, many of them regard as suspect any statement that talks of the 'mentally ill' as a single entity. The advances in medicine usually involve distinctions that define which patients will benefit, which will be harmed, and which will neither be benefited nor harmed. When Mosher and Burti clarify which patients will be helped by hospitalization, and which will be harmed, their position will be more accepted.

## The legislative branches

Saul Feldman has pointed out that there is a Darwinian process in the legislative process. Thousands of bills are submitted in the legislative hopper, and only a few emerge.[21] For a legislative proposal to survive, legislators must be convinced that it offers great hope of establishing a social good or abolishing a social evil. Those championing the community mental health centres before Congress in the 1950s and 1960s gave assur-ances that the development of centres would achieve a positive revolution in psychiatric care.[16]

## The executive branches

Public institutions operate within the bureaucratic ethos of loyalty to the hierarchy, as well as with expectations of efficiency, competence, expertise, accountability, and neutrality. The executive branch characteristically attempts to achieve these goals through the development of departments that have very specific accountabilities stated through regulations.

This departmentalization within the executive creates ethical problems that contribute to deinstitutionalization and erect barriers to the care and treatment of deinstitutionalized patients. Usually a government department has limited resources. Therefore, if accountability can be narrowed, quality care can be achieved for the smaller number for whom the department is still accountable. While state public institutions previously had provided all the board, housing, social, vocational, recreational, and health care, including psychiatric treatment, that the psychiatric patient in the hospital needed, accountability for the psychiatrically ill in the community became unclear and fragmented because of the departmentalization of government. The psychiatrist in government programmes may have to face the following kinds of questions with ethical implications:

- Should the psychiatry department's hospital agree to assume responsibility for a person who needs housing and who is also dependent on alcohol when the housing authority refuses to give the person housing until the alcoholism is cured?

- Should the psychiatry department's hospital agree to assume responsibility for a person who needs treatment for leukaemia and is also disabled from schizophrenia when the general hospital claim that the patient's schizophrenia makes him unmanageable on their oncology unit?

In these two cases, who should be primarily accountable for the patient—housing, health, or psychiatry? As a rule, none of them will assume responsibility for the person's total welfare—only for their department's area of accountability. To deal with this problem, case-managers are used to achieve comprehensiveness of care to make up for divisions of authority; but case-managers, especially in large impersonal urban areas, cannot save psychiatrists from having to make painful decisions about care and treatment. Many people with psychiatric disorders have a long list of problems that involve many authorities. Because of his limited scope, the psychiatrist must decide whether to bend the regulations that pertain to his department and serve the patient, or adhere to the regulations and refuse services. In the two cases above, is it ethical to tell such persons that we will not hospitalize them and can only see them in the psychiatric clinic when that refusal might contribute to the psychiatrically ill being homeless or dying? Yet, to bend the department's regulations to hospitalize all of these people spreads resources thinner for those who do qualify for hospitalization.

Compounding the departmentalization of services is the state–city–county split that has occurred in many areas. In the 1960s federal efforts denigrated the state responsibility, and made it difficult for states to assume responsibility for the psychiatrically ill, leading to additional fragmentation of services for the psychiatrically ill. Examples that have occurred in some states include:

- limiting the state authority to patients with non-organic disorders, and turning over the care of those with organic diagnoses to local general hospitals;

- limiting admissions to committed patients only, and not allowing patients to enter public institutions voluntarily, conceptualizing voluntary patients as the responsibility of the private hospitals;

- excluding patients who have substance-abuse disorders even if their primary diagnosis is another psychiatric disorder, conceptualizing these patients as the responsibility of state or local drug and alcohol agencies.

These three forms of departmentalization of authority can pose difficult ethical questions for the psychiatrist. In the first case, should one select a diagnosis of schizophrenia for an organic patient to make him eligible for care at the state institution? In the second case, should one commit a patient who is quite willing to volunteer, in order to make him eligible for hospitalization? In the third case, should one 'forget' to list phencyclidine-abuse disorder in a man who also has schizophrenia?

In these three examples, if the psychiatrist does decide to 'fudge' the facts to get help for the patient, he may be setting a climate for additional regulations, which will aim to increase the bureaucratic barriers so as to keep the psychiatrist neutral, bringing about increased regulations that often will be applied to all psychiatrists. Using our 'forgetting' a patient's substance-abuse disorder to avoid making the patient ineligible for admission to a state hospital as an example, the bureaucracy may try to correct this 'forgetting' by requiring drug-free urines for all admissions to its state psychiatric hospitals. Thus, 'humanistic' efforts, efforts that compromise the neutrality expected in a bureaucracy, can lead to increased costs for all as a result of compensatory efforts to ensure that neutrality.

Departmentalization takes place in Great Britain, where local authorities have no responsibility for involuntary psychiatric patients, although they will provide services for the co-operative patient.[18] Furthermore, in Great Britain, if a chronically psychiatrically ill person lacks a home address or has an address outside a hospital's catchment area, this can be used as a reason to deny responsibility.[17] As in other countries, the British police are often delegated the task of trying to resolve the problems of the deinstitutionalized psychiatrically ill, but the police too are limited by departmentalization when trying to resolve the situation of a specific person who is not 'considered to be "mad enough" for admission to hospital or "bad enough" for prison'.[18] In both Great Britain and the United States homeless families with children have become a major focus of concern in the late 1980s. For example, a survey of London's homeless 'households' found that 60 per cent had children.[22]

In summary, the departmentalization within executive branches makes it difficult for the psychiatrically ill to gain access to government services in the first place, and to receive comprehensive services should they gain access.

## The judiciary

The values of the judiciary have had a substantial effect on deinstitutional-ization and public psychiatric administration. To understand this influence, it is useful to compare three aspects of the ethos of the judiciary and of medicine:

1. Whereas the judiciary pursues its factual determinations formally, adversarially, and with rules of evidence, medicine pursues its factual determinations informally, co-operatively, and scientifically. A major change in public psychiatry over the past three decades is the increase of the adversarial climate, making it more difficult to retain the psychiatrically ill in institutions and to reach those in the streets[23] (see Chapter 13). Whereas the major goal of the judiciary is to achieve justice, the major goal of medicine is to restore health. There is an inherent conflict here, but the public administrator finds that this conflict has increased enormously since the 1960s.

2. Whereas the judiciary's concern about *error* is expressed in the statement that it is better that ten people go free than that one innocent person be punished, medicine's concern about *error* is expressed in the statement that it is better that ten people be hospitalized unnecessarily than that one person should not be hospitalized and should die. Here we have a classical ethical dilemma, illustrating the difficulty in making unequivocal moral judgements in these complex matters. As the judiciary seems to perceive hospitalization, or even the involuntary giving of medications, as a form of punishment, hospitalization and effective treatment become more difficult. This judicial colouring of public psychiatry has contributed to deinstitu-tionalization through making it more difficult for physicians to be responsi-ble for the psychiatrically ill.

3. Whereas the judiciary has to assume there is free will to preserve a sense of culpability, medicine has to assume deterministic models to achieve therapeutic predictability. (Every therapeutic act involves a pre-diction as to what the act will produce. That prediction may be based upon empirical evidence, or may be based upon a concept of the illness. Such a concept cannot allow free will at any of its syllogistic junctions, because

that would remove predictability, and thus deprive it of therapeutic useful-ness.) The psychiatrist wanting to assume responsibility for the psychiatric-ally ill will need to face this assumption that people have free will whenever they are dealing with the courts.

*Example*: A 56-year-old man hospitalized for 21 years with schizophrenia is on a ward that is crowded, smelly, and physically dangerous for him because some younger men pick on him. He is told that they have a place in a group home for him, but he says that he does not want to go. He is placed in the group home over his objections, and, after he has been there three months, his social worker finds that he is being underfed and has lice, and decides that he should be rehospitalized. He objects, but is removed and brought back to the hospital. Five weeks later a very attractive group home is found for him and he objects to being placed there.

This patient's wish to avoid change is typical of many people with schizophrenia, an illness whose symptoms include fear of newness (neophobia) that leads to their rejection of change even when all objective criteria would suggest that they would be more comfortable in the newer setting. In the process of deinstitutionalization, clinicians typically placed patients in the community against their wishes. Neophobia contributes to the pattern by which people with schizophrenia prefer shelters or their place in the streets to public housing or psychiatric hospitals.

Many have argued that mental hospitals can provide more freedom for some patients than available community alternatives,[24,25] and some mental health professionals have argued that the goal should not be the least restrictive alternative, but the most optimal setting for the patient.[24,26] But generally the judiciary has adopted the principle of least restrictive setting for all mental patients, meaning 'not in the hospital'. In the face of limited resources, clinicians will implement this principle in order to reduce patient-loads, even though they do not believe it to be sound—but it serves other interests, as we have pointed out above, to reduce the total patient-load.

### Lay organizations

Lay organizations as a rule supported the move towards deinstitutionaliza-tion throughout the 1950s and 1960s, as they continued their historic call for reform. This changed somewhat in the 1980s, with the formation of the National Alliance for the Mentally Ill (NAMI), an organization composed primarily of families of patients with schizophrenia or bipolar disorders. With NAMI's growing influence, the values of the families became part of the conflicting values within which the public psychiatrist has to work. Their influence has contributed to a fading of belief in psychosocial causes of schizophrenia, and a questioning of deinstitutionalization when it places the responsibility of the care of the patients on their families.

## Accrediting bodies

Accrediting bodies mandate standards of care and treatment for psychiatric institutions that are costly, and often difficult for them to achieve. Many public hospitals go for years without attaining JCAHO accreditation. The American Psychiatric Association has taken the position that no one should be *forced* into such institutions for treatment, that is, that unaccredited institutions should only admit voluntary patients. Yet most unaccredited public hospitals have many involuntary admissions carried out by psychiatrists who 'have no other choice'.

## Ethical issues

The history of deinstitutionalization and the conflicting values of the parties that influenced the policies and decisions that contributed to deinstitutionalization raise a number of ethical issues. Firstly, we will address some generic aspects of these conflicting values, and then the ethical dilemmas inherent in some specific forms of deinstitutionalization and transinstitutionalization. Lastly, we will discuss the ethical issues faced by those serving patients already deinstitutionalized.

While many patients are discharged from psychiatric hospitals into supportive settings, and the illnesses of other patients are resolved to the point that little support is needed, thousands of patients have been discharged into inadequate settings or into the streets. Have these discharges been unethical? Before addressing this question, we need to describe the phenomenon known as 'treating the census'.

'Treating the census' refers to the need frequently felt on public psychiatric wards to reduce the census so that the remaining patients on the units have some hope of receiving adequate attention and treatment. Otherwise, when the number of patients exceeds the ward's approved number of patients, the situation becomes unmanageable, and patient-care suffers. In addition to the psychiatrist's wish to have a reasonable number of patients, the pressures from superiors and from the ward staff also contribute to a felt need to say, for example, 'let's discharge four patients today'. There are units that have no discretion as to the number of patients, usually admission units; and these are the ones that feel most of the pressure to treat the census. Patients are discharged before they are 'ready' or before arrangements are made for the community supports that are needed. In addition to direct discharges, other means are used to reduce the census. For example, if a psychiatrist is sluggish in discharging patients rapidly enough to avoid a crushing number of on-the-unit patients, staff may allow patients to elope, or set up situations that lead patients to be released 'against medical advice'. While some public systems are not overburdened and do not have this problem, it is probably fair to say that all public psychiatric services in large urban areas in the United States are overburdened at some times, and must deal with the temptation to discharge patients prematurely.

These discharges swell the population of the psychiatrically ill homeless who are on the streets. They contribute to the feeling on the part of patients that they were not welcome in the public psychiatric service, and not wanting to experience that rejection again contributes to their determination to remain on the streets.

Treating the census rather than fully treating the patient raises ethical issues. Which value should apply—medicine's tradition of treating the individual, based on each patient's need, or the need of an organization to husband its limited resources? While patients or others may be harmed if they are discharged too soon, wards that are overcrowded are dangerous. Here the psychiatrist faces the question of whether to be loyal to the patient or to the organization. The psychiatrist can be 'heroic', holding the patients until their illness has diminished to the level where it can be supported by the community—an approach that may even result in the unit being allocated more resources to meet patients' needs more fully. (However, our applause should wait until we know the source of those additional resources. They may come from another hard-pressed in-patient programme that is squeaking less.)

The considerations that lead the psychiatrist to 'deinstitutionalize' the patient are summarized below:

- the need to treat the census;
- the ethos that decries the 'institutionalism' to which the mentally ill are subject, and maintains that they should be removed from institutions to avoid their adverse effects;
- legal barriers to involuntary hospitalization;
- the judiciary's implementation of the 'least restrictive setting' principle;
- the need to keep the number of patients at a minimum in order to provide optimal treatment for a few, so that accreditation standards can be maintained;
- the principle that the community should assume responsibility for the patient—and that discharging patients will 'force them' to become responsive. Not to discharge patients postpones adequate public understanding and adds an element of dishonesty to public policy. Note the use of patients to achieve change that is considered desirable by some.
- the principle that fiscally it is in the state's interest to have the patient in the community at little cost to the state, or in other institutions that will receive federal funds, thus reducing the impact on the taxpayers of the state.

● a reduction in legal liability which generally results. While some discharges can increase liability, fear of liability tends to increase the felt need to treat a few well rather than many inadequately.

There appear to be no ethical guidelines for the public psychiatric policy-maker on the extent to which one can exclude patients from a programme in order to force responsiveness on the part of another agency. Does one exclude patients only when one knows that such a tactic will produce a response for these patients, or when one knows that such a move will produce a positive response after a single patient has suffered? Or is it all right to allow many patients to be harmed or to suffer if one has some hope of an eventual change in public policy? Or would it be ethically correct to adopt such a tactic even when the prospects for change are not hopeful, or, in fact, virtually hopeless?

There appear to be no ethical guidelines for the degree to which one should preserve or increase the effectiveness of a programme by exclusion. While some are condemned with 'you are trying to establish a good programme through only admitting good patients', there are many situations that beg for limitations in order to save a worthy programme. How many patients with schizophrenia and substance-abuse, for example, should a substance-abuse programme admit? Should they be allowed to exclude all? How many such patients should a programme treating schizophrenia be expected to take? While some of these questions can be answered programmatically, the questions nearly always raise an ethical question as to the degree to which exclusiveness is appropriate.

One solution exists in theory: to define the responsibilities of a unit geographically. A programme's responsibility can be defined in terms of the problem (for example, an alcoholic programme), in terms of non-pathological factors (for example, a Hispanic programme), in terms of the therapeutic approach (for example, a therapeutic community programme), or in terms of geography (for example, all patients from Montgomery County). The definition of responsibility employed by community mental health centres is geographic. In the 1960s many public hospitals adopted a form of organization called 'unitization', which meant that for each unit of the hospital responsibility was defined geographically. This approach did clarify responsibility, and undoubtedly helped avoid some irresponsible deinstitutionalization; but it also tended to make it hard for staff to develop clinical skills in depth and to evolve specialized programmes, because of the psychopathological heterogeneity of the population being served.

## The issue of futility

If psychiatry had a value system that allowed it to decide when further treatment was futile, it would then be easier for public policy-makers and clinicians to address this issue. This, in turn, would help answer questions about how much institutionalization is needed. If the assumption is accepted that all patients are treatable and their treatment plans should include how they are to be transferred to the community, the consequence is that psychiatry never faces up to the question about what to do with the patient for whom psychiatric treatment is futile. Part of the difficulty is the lack of any practical definition of 'when is it futile to continue treatment' except for some organic brain-disorders. Does one decide that medication treatment is futile after a schizophrenic patient has been treated with 18 medications or combinations of medications without any benefit, or does one wait until one has tried 25? How many different types of psycho-therapy and/or medications should be tried in a patient with depressive neurosis (dysthymia) before one concludes that further treatment would be useless?

Some have called for asylums to address this question of futility.[23,27,28] Yet there are practically no programmes in public psychiatric hospitals that are identified as asylums. Since 'asylum' is a concept rather than a location, it can exist as a group home in the community rather than on the grounds of a public psychiatric hospital, and placement in a group home is what happens to some patients for whom treatment is 'futile'. But this happens without the acknowledgement of futility, and the ethics of addressing futility is not mentioned in public policies.

## Value issues in transinstitutionalization

While we do not know the exact number of public psychiatric institution patients who have been deinstitutionalized through transinstitutionaliza-tion, it probably numbers in the tens of thousands. It is estimated that 700000 nursing-home patients have psychiatric problems, while from 5 to 20 per cent of prison inmates are estimated to be psychiatrically ill. Board-ing homes constitute another site for transinstitutionalization, although some argue that boarding homes represent a real return to the com-munity. Transinstitutionalization is attractive to mental health agencies, first, because it reduces their number of patients, and second, because patients removed from the institution are often ones labelled 'non-responders', who do not make good use of their resources. When the patient is transferred from the state hospital to a nursing home, costs are reduced for the state, because the nursing home is usually less expensive than the hospital, and the state can be reimbursed by about 50 per cent for the cost of the patient's nursing-home stay by the federal government through Medicaid.

Transinstitutionalization of patients raises a number of ethical questions. For the patient, the move may be an improvement in living conditions; but often it is not. Can transferring a patient to another institution that offers less comfortable conditions, less freedom, less psychiatric support ever be justified? Can it be justified when the move frees up resources that will help other patients? Can it be justified on the basis of improving the morale of staff who no longer have to work with a patient for whom treatment will be futile and who will negatively affect the climate of therapeutic effectiveness? Can it be justified on the grounds that a court decision has held that the public psychiatric institution in question is the most restrictive setting for the psychiatrically ill, and any move is seen as meeting the goal to 'deinstitutionalize' the patients? Can it be justified because 'the court says so', even though the psychiatrist knows the patient will be less happy, less free, less well-served psychiatrically, and sometimes have his life threatened ('moving old trees can be lethal', as some find that there is an increased mortality when the elderly are moved)? Can it be justified on the political basis that the state wants to reduce the cost of care of the psychiatrically ill to the state taxpayer, and proposes to do so through reaching Medicaid federal dollars?

## Values in transferring the patients to their families

Deinstitutionalization often involves the transfer of patients from the institution to the family.

*Example*: Mr S.S., aged twenty-seven, has been in and out of hospitals since the age of eighteen, usually being discharged to his home. On three occasions he has been tried in group homes, from where his threatening behaviour and unpredictable and unexplained two- to three-day disappearances resulted in his being returned to the hospital. The ward decides again to try to place him with his 48-year-old severely diabetic mother and 53-year-old father, a blue-collar family with limited financial resources. The parents want to do what is right for their son, but question their ability to work effectively with him, since they have failed frequently in the past, and group homes have also failed. Furthermore, they do not believe that the parents represent the long-term solution, since they are likely to die before their son.

How much is the psychiatrist justified in using his influence to push for transfer of this patient to the family, since he is likely to be quite trying periodically, even with close monitoring by the clinic? The psychiatrist in this situation faces a number of ethical dilemmas. Should he accede to the patient's wish to return home? Or to the agency's generic wish that patients should be transferred back to the community, and the ward staff's wish to keep the number of patients on the ward reasonable? During the 1960s and 1970s psychiatrists frequently pressed to discharge the patients to families less resourceful than Mr S.'s, totally destroying the quality of life of those families. (Here we are talking about families that basically cared and wanted to do the 'right thing', and believed that the psychiatrist knew what was right.) Sometimes families were pressed to accept family therapy, implying family blame.[29] Ethical? During the 1980s, NAMI's influence has helped to change the values involved in such deinstitutionalization; but there are no ethical guidelines for the psychiatrist as to the appropriate course of action.

## Deinstitutionalization and AIDS

In Chapter 15 the issue of confidentiality arising with patients who are HIV-positive or have AIDS is discussed. Some HIV-positive multiple-problem patients, especially psychiatrically ill adolescents, present major questions in trying to maintain confidentiality when dozens of people may be involved in the care of the patient in an institution—for example, other health agencies, special education agencies, and social service agencies, in addition to the psychiatric clinic. The act of deinstitutionalization itself may raise substantial issues.

*Example*: Alice, aged twenty-six, is admitted for phencyclidine psychosis manifested by her screaming that she has to jump out of the window of her fourth-floor apartment. She is confused, agitated, and incoherent. She was a heroin addict in her early twenties, who switched to phencyclidine and crack in her mid-twenties. This combination of drugs produces a prolonged period of confusion and erratic behaviour. After five weeks she becomes lucid and pleasant and wants to be discharged to return to her occupation—prostitution. Her HIV test comes back positive. It is pointed out to her that returning to prostitution could be lethal to her clients, but she is used to the life-style that prostitution provides, and refuses to consider relinquishing it. She does promise to have each of her clients use a condom.

Should she be discharged? What is the difference between returning typhoid Mary to the kitchen and returning HIV Alice to the street corner? In today's climate of deinstitutionalization, no one seriously proposes that she be retained in the hospital on mental health grounds. This can be rationalized on the grounds that her spreading the HIV virus is a public health, not a mental health, problem, even though it is well known that the public health agency has no power to control her.

## Ethical issues faced by the psychiatrist on assuming responsibility for deinstitutionalized patients

Our focus in this chapter has been on the conflict in values inherent in the deinstitutionalizing of the psychiatrically ill, but we want to at least note that there are ethical issues also for the psychiatrist responsible for patients who want to avoid returning to the institution. Successful community

placement requires an assertive approach in which one uses many resources to retain the patients in the community. Ethical issues commonly
arise, such as the following:[30]

- Any effort by even voluntary patients to terminate treatment or miss
  appointments is regarded as psychopathological, not a patient's right to
  free choice (see our point above about there being no place for the
  concept of free will in dealing with patients), and is dealt with as psychopathological.

- Retaining the patient in the community may involve staff showing
  up unannounced and intruding into the patients' lives to make the point
  that the latter should keep their clinic appointments, an intrusion that
  may be quite uncomfortable for patients, just as it would be for non-
  patients—and may be persisted in after the patient has requested that
  they cease.

- Bribing/blackmailing/encouraging the patient to come to the clinic by
  having an agreement with the patient's fiscal resource that the patient's
  funds will be retained at the clinic and doled out with each clinic appointment that is kept.

- Contacting landlords, police, employers, or relatives about a patient
  when the patient has not given permission that information be divulged
  to anyone. Simply contacting these people to ascertain the patient's
  status amounts to informing them that the patient is on the clinic's rolls.

## Summary

Deinstitutionalization has been the major public psychiatric event of the
last half of the twentieth century. While hundreds of thousands of patients'
lives have become fuller, freer, and more productive, other hundreds of
thousands have been abandoned or transinstitutionalized. Although improved psychopharmacological agents have made deinstitutionalization
possible, the driving force has been a change in values. These changes in
values have placed many public psychiatrists in ethical situations that have
no satisfactory answers.

## References

1 Goffman, E.: *Asylums: essays on the social situation on mental patients and
  other inmates.* New York, Doubleday, 1961.
2 Peele, R., Luisada, P. V., Lucas, M. J. *et al.: Asylums* revisited. *American
  Journal of Psychiatry* **134**:1077–81, 1977.
3 Solomon, H. C.: The American Psychiatric Association in relation to American
  psychiatry. *American Journal of Psychiatry* **115**:1–9, 1958.

4 *Shelton* v. *Tucker*. 364 US 479, 81 S Ct 257, 5L Ed 2d 231 (1960).
5 Joint Commission on Mental Illness and Health: *Action for mental health: final report of the Joint Commission on Mental Illness and Health 1961*. New York, Basic Books, 1961.
6 Caplan, G.: *An approach to community mental health*. New York, Grune and Stratton, 1961.
7 Szasz, T. S.: *The myth of mental illness*. New York, Harper, 1961.
8 *Lake* v. *Cameron*. 364 F 2d 657 (1966).
9 *Wyatt* v. *Stickney*. 325 F Supp. 781 (MD Ala 1971); enforced by 344 F Supp. 373, 376, 379–385 (MD Ala 1972).
10 *Lessard* v. *Schmidt*. 349 F Supp. 1078; 379 F Supp. 1376; 413 F Supp. 95 S Ct 1318 (Wisc. 1972).
11 *Tarasoff* v. *Regents of University of California*. 529 P 2d 553 (Cal 1974); 551 P 2d 533 (Cal 1976).
12 *O'Connor* v. *Donaldson*. 95 S Ct 2486 (Fla 1975).
13 *Dixon* v. *Weinberger*. 405 F 2d 974 (DC Cir. 1975).
14 *Rogers* v. *Okin*. 478 F Supp. 1342; 634 F 2d 650, cert. gr. 101 S Ct 1972; 451 US 906, 68 L Ed 2d 293 (Mass 1979).
15 Institute of Medicine's Committee on Health Care of Homeless People: *Homelessness, health, and human needs*. Washington DC, National Academy Press, 1988.
16 Torrey, E. F.: *Nowhere to go: the tragic odyssey of the homeless mentally ill*. New York, Harper & Row, 1988.
17 Lowry, S.: Caring for the homeless. *British Medical Journal* **298**:210–11, 1989.
18 Lowry, S.: Concern for discharged mentally ill patients. *British Medical Journal* **298**:209–10, 1989.
19 Wyatt, R. J. and DeRenzo, E. G.: Scienceless to homeless (editorial). *Science* **234**:1309, 1986.
20 Mosher, L. R. and Burti, L.: *Community mental health: principles and practice*. New York, Norton, 1989.
21 Feldman, S.: Out of the hospital, onto the streets: the overselling of benevolence. *Hasting Center Report* **13**:5–7, 1983.
22 Delamoth, T.: 250 years of solicitude. *British Medical Journal* **298**:211, 1989.
23 Chodoff, P.: Involuntary hospitalization of the mentally ill as a moral issue. *American Journal of Psychiatry* **141**:384–89, 1984.
24 Bachrach, L. L.: Is the least restrictive environment always the best? Sociological and semantic implications. *Hospital Community Psychiatry* **31**:97–103, 1980.
25 Brooks, A. D.: Mental health law, in *The administration of mental health services*, 2nd edn, ed. S. Feldman. Springfield, IL, Thomas, 1980.
26 Perr, I. N.: The most beneficial alternative: a counterpoint to the least restrictive alternative. *Bulletin of the American Academy of Psychiatry and the Law* **6**:4–7, 1978.
27 Lamb, H. R. and Peele, R.: The need for continuing asylum and sanctuary. *Hospital Community Psychiatry* **35**:798–802, 1984.
28 Bachrach, L. L.: Asylum and chronically ill psychiatric patients. *American Journal of Psychiatry* **141**:975–8, 1984.

29 Hatfield, A. B.: What families want of family therapists, in *Family therapy in schizophrenia*, ed. W. MacFarlane. New York, Guilford, 1983.
30 Diamond, R. J. and Wikler, D. I.: Ethical problems in community treatment of the chronically mentally ill, in *The training in community living model. A decade of experience*, ed. L. I. Stein and M. A. Test. New Directions for Mental Health Services, no. 26. San Francisco, Jossey-Bass, 1985, pp. 85–93.

# 15

# Confidentiality in psychiatry

*David Joseph and Joseph Onek*

'Whatsoever I shall see or hear in the course of my profession . . . if it be what should not be published abroad, I will never divulge, holding such things to be holy secrets.'

—Hippocratic Oath.

'Three people can keep a secret if two of them are dead.'

—Benjamin Franklin, Poor Richard's Almanac.

## Introduction

Medicine has always stressed the importance of confidentiality, but the practice of psychiatry, even more than of other branches of medicine, depends to a significant degree upon an assumption of confidentiality between patient and doctor. Confidentiality, which can be defined as entrusting information to another with the expectation that it will be kept private, is closely related to 'confidence, confession, trust, reliance, respect, security, intimacy, and privacy'.[1] Although doctors and their patients place a high value on the establishment and maintenance of the confidential relationship, confidentiality has been such a central aspect of the practice of medicine and psychiatry that its importance is often taken for granted, and its maintenance is frequently less than rigorous.

The extent to which information confided by a patient is actually non-disclosable is regulated to a considerable extent by law. State privilege statutes establish when a psychiatrist must or must not testify concerning patient information in judicial or administrative proceedings. Reporting laws, such as those for child-abuse, often require psychiatrists to disclose patient information to state officials. In many states there are statutes or judicial decisions regulating such areas as disclosure of patient information to insurance companies or collection agencies. The imposition of a duty to warn the potential victim of a dangerous patient represents a well-publicized example in which state tort (damage) law may regulate disclosure.

The regulation of confidentiality required by the legal system interacts closely with the regulation imposed by professional ethics. Whenever legal requirements such as those to report child-abuse or undue familiarity override the principle of confidentiality, ethical norms are modified. At the same time, the ethical norms of psychiatry can constitute the basis for decisions regarding legal obligations. When considering whether the disclosure of patient information by a psychiatrist constitutes a breach of the psychiatrist's fiduciary duty or a breach of his implied contract with the patient, a court is very likely to accord great weight to the ethical norms of the profession.

The ethical aspects of confidentiality can be more clearly delineated by considering its relationship to privacy and privilege. Privacy can be narrowly defined as 'the freedom of the individual to pick and choose for himself the time, circumstances and particularly the extent to which he wishes to withhold from others his attitudes, beliefs, behavior, and opinion',[2] or more broadly defined to encompass an individual's 'right to personal autonomy and freedom'.[1] If one uses the latter definition of privacy, then confidentiality can be considered to be one of many aspects of privacy. If one employs the former definition of privacy, then confidentiality becomes 'co-extensive'[1] with privacy.

Privilege is a legal concept which refers to the right of an individual to control which information, communicated in confidence, can be revealed in a judicial or administrative proceeding. Although the privilege protecting communications between priest and penitent, lawyer and client, and physician and patient has long been an integral aspect of our social structure, the concept of privileged communications runs counter to the tradition of common law, which holds that the courts have access to all relevant information.[3] Privilege exists only when established by specific legal statute, and statutes, especially those pertaining to the practice of psychotherapy, differ considerably from one state to another. Although there have been legal challenges by psychiatrists[4] and recommendations to make it mutual,[5] the right to waive privilege belongs to the individual and not to the physician.

Originally, the law's only concern with confidentiality was in the context of privilege in judicial proceedings. But because of breaches of confidentiality by physicians, and because of 'the right of defendants to secure justice, the needs of insurers to guarantee equity and prevent fraud, and the desire of society to protect itself from future violent acts'[6] the law has devoted increasing attention to the limits of confidentiality. Psychiatrists in turn have progressively looked to the law to provide guidelines for standards of conduct. Although thoroughly understandable, the wish for the law to answer most ethical questions is doomed to disappointment. Quen has noted that only non-lawyers believe that 'there is an abstraction called the law which is reliable, predictable, and standard, Actually, the law, even in statute, means only what the last judge who interpreted it said it means.'[7] Although overstated, this point of view correctly emphasizes that there are limits to how much guidance can be expected from the law. Moreover, the legal system is unlikely to consider even a small fraction of the many situations in which the disclosure of confidential information may occur. The *Guidelines on confidentiality* of the American Psychiatric Association[8] delineate many situations in which psychiatrists will need to use ethical principles in reaching decisions about patient care. The management of confidentiality on a day-to-day basis is much more a matter of professional ethics than of legal requirements. It is precisely for this reason that psychiatrists and mental health professionals need to examine and reassert ethical norms.

The necessity of confidentiality in a psychotherapeutic relationship was initially based on theoretical assumptions, but recent research[9-15] has confirmed the importance of confidentiality to patients and their therapists. The shared value of confidentiality notwithstanding, given the realities of modern medical practice, and especially of hospital medicine, confidentiality has been called, a 'decrepit concept'.[16] The importance of health-care teams, increasing subspecialization with multiple consultations, and the role of third-party payers have contributed to an increased tension between the patient's wish to maintain maximum confidentiality and his desire to receive the best possible care.[14,16] While some[17,18] have argued for absolute confidentiality, these factors, in concert with the legal obligations imposed on psychiatrists in such areas as commitment and child-abuse[19] have resulted in what Stoller[20] has aptly called 'relative confidentiality'.

Although psychiatrists and mental health professionals are well aware that absolute confidentiality is a fiction, patients are strikingly uninformed about the circumstances under which confidentiality can and cannot be compromised.[12,15] Psychiatrists must therefore assume the ethical responsibility to be candid with each patient at the outset of treatment about the realities of maintaining confidentiality. Psychiatrists need to be expert about their professional discipline, but they also need to be knowledgeable about the laws regulating confidentiality. Where relevant, it is important to inform patients about the possibility of compelled disclosure in situations of contested wills, custody proceedings, and personal-injury suits, and to make them aware of the legal and ethical requirements under which the psychiatrist is required to disclose information in instances of imminent harm to self or others, including child-abuse. An early emphasis on this aspect of confidentiality underscores the seriousness which is accorded confidentiality and strengthens the therapeutic alliance.

When considering confidentiality psychiatrists must be aware that, by virtue of involvement in a personal injury suit or other litigation, any patient's records may be made public in a court-room proceeding. Furthermore, patient records may have to be disclosed to insurance companies and other third parties, as well as to the patient himself. These ever-present possibilities routinely create difficult ethical considerations regarding which information to enter in the official patient record.

## Confidentiality and office management

In the daily conduct of psychiatric practice, whether in a private office, group practice, psychiatric clinic, or hospital, psychiatrists affect patients' privacy and confidentiality by a number of subtle actions. Offices may be constructed with a separate entrance and exit to reduce the possibility that patients will see each other. If this is not the case or if the waiting-room is shared among several psychiatrists, a patient may habitually be late to protect his confidentiality (privacy) by time when architecture does not do it for him. Although a particularly significant concern for individuals well-known to the public, this is more important to many patients than may be apparent. Psychiatrists have become so inured to the elimination of anonymity in shared waiting-rooms that the practice of announcing a patient's given name is rarely seen to be an unnecessary compromise of confidentiality. When seeing a patient for the first time, one can avoid this particular compromise of confidentiality by announcing, 'I'm Dr Hamilton'; and for subsequent appointments one can enter the waiting-room without mentioning the name of the patient to be seen next.

Telephoning a patient at work poses a similar dilemma. Some, wishing to preserve as much of the patient's confidentiality as possible, will identify themselves as 'Michael Hamilton', concerned that 'Dr Hamilton' will arouse curiosity in the individual answering the phone. Patients may be hesitant to request that the psychiatrist calling at work should not identify himself by name, and it is useful to ask how the patient would prefer the situation to be handled. The telephone-answering machine has created a new set of problems regarding confidentiality. One woman, whose family knew she was seeing a psychiatrist, was outraged when he left a message on her home answering machine regarding the proper dosage of medication, despite the fact that she had been urgently calling him for this information. She considered this to be confidential information, to which no one else should have been privy without her permission. When two psychiatrists share the same telephone number and answering machine, all messages are automatically shared. Although patients could leave a message such as 'Please have Dr Hamilton call 244-5000', this seems unlikely to occur, in part because these subtle breaches in confidentiality have become so commonplace as to be overlooked and/or accepted by both patients and psychiatrists.

Careless storage of records commonly jeopardizes patients' confidentiality. Regardless of legal statutes, psychiatrists have an ethical obligation to ensure that patients' clinical and billing records as well as appointment books are securely stored. In hospitals and clinics where offices are cleaned at night, psychiatrists may forget that material left on desks or in unlocked drawers is readily available to unauthorized persons. The very need to keep so many routine behaviours in mind makes it surprisingly difficult to maintain the maximum degree of confidentiality.

Additional issues arise from the use of ancillary personnel such as secretaries, accountants, and bill-collection agencies. Patients who have little apparent concern over being seen by the secretary may be displeased should the secretary write the bill, even if it does not contain a diagnosis. Issues of confidentiality are much greater when secretaries transcribe histories and process notes. This is especially troublesome in clinics and hospitals, where the individual psychiatrist may have little role in the selection of the secretary, and where the importance of confidentiality may not receive the formal emphasis and repeated reinforcement required for consistent maintenance. In such situations psychiatrists can easily ignore the ethical responsibility to ensure that ancillary personnel are thoroughly educated and trained in the importance of maintaining confidentiality.

Depending upon the state, psychiatrists may be legally required to inform a patient in advance that an unpaid bill will be submitted to a collection agency or become the basis of a lawsuit. Regardless of legal requirements this course is consistent with ethical principles. In addition, the patient's confidentiality can be most effectively safeguarded by supplying the agency or court with the minimum amount of information necessary to secure payment, and by sanitizing billing records before they are given to an accountant.

## Confidentiality and conversations about patients

Like other physicians, psychiatrists talk about their patients. In many instances such talk is in the service of patient-care (a kerbside consultation); in others it is more in the interest of relieving anger, guilt, or some other internal state, or achieving some personal end such as self-aggrandizement. However, questions may arise even in instances in which talking about a patient might appear to have no ethical dimension. As an example, a general practitioner who has referred a patient for a psychiatric evaluation meets the psychiatrist at a party, and inquires about the patient. Some psychiatrists believe that unless express informed consent has been given, even to indicate whether or not the patient is under treatment violates the patient's confidentiality. Others take the position that such a response would reflect 'a misuse of confidentiality' that was 'absolutely discourteous'.[21] Given the actual way in which contemporary medicine is practised, and in view of research regarding patients' attitudes toward confidentiality, it seems reasonable to assume that patients expect some discussion about them, and trust that their physicians will exercise proper judgement regarding which information to convey and which to keep private. None the less, when a patient is referred by another professional, a routine request for permission to talk with the referring individual implicitly underscores the psychiatrist's commitment to confidentiality without interfering with the sharing of appropriate information.

Written reports to a referring physician which will be included in a patient's permanent file and are likely to be read by others raise ethical issues about which information to include. However, oral reports may also pose questions about confidentiality. For example, a patient with headaches, splenic flexure syndrome, and depressed mood was referred by his general practitioner for a psychiatric consultation, which revealed a dysthymic disorder and a family history of depression, denied anger with a controlling wife, alcohol-abuse, and homosexual concerns. None of this material had been conveyed by the referring physician. If the patient gives general permission for the release of information, what should be conveyed in writing, what should only be conveyed orally, and what should not be shared at all? In addition to determining what is essential in assisting the referring physician to provide the best medical treatment, it is important to keep it in mind that the personal historical material belongs to the patient. If the patient does not wish the psychiatrist to reveal his alcoholism, a finding clearly of importance to his medical treatment, the psychiatrist can conduct a brief psychotherapeutic intervention with the goal of exploring the patient's refusal—a decision which may have been motivated by the avoidance of shame. From an ethical perspective, in the face of continued refusal, the final decision about what is conveyed belongs to the patient. By ensuring that the patient reads and approves any letter, both confidentiality and the therapeutic relationship can be protected.

When patients in psychotherapy are referred to a psychiatrist for a psychopharmacological or other consultation a different kind of ethical problem regarding confidentiality can arise. In one instance, a man in weekly psychotherapy with a psychologist for treatment of a depression which followed a mild left-sided cerebral infarction was referred for an evaluation of the advisability of antidepressants. The referring psychologist spoke with the psychiatrist about the patient, and the patient, after getting a good response from an antidepressant, took 'a vacation' from psychotherapy. A month later he 'confessed' to the psychiatrist that one of the issues he had been dealing with in psychotherapy was a past incestuous relationship with his daughter. The psychologist and the patient had chosen to keep this information confidential, with the result that the psychiatrist's understanding of the case was significantly limited. If a patient refuses permission for certain important information to be shared with the consultant, the referring professional may decide not to proceed with the consultation.

Gossip is a more insidious, but no less serious, threat to confidentiality. Gossip can be viewed as a 'triangular sociopsychological relationship involving the exchange of tales about others, fostering intimacy, discharging hostility, and attended by a feeling of pleasure',[22] and the gossiping psychiatrist has been the focus of considerable attention.[23-26] The functions of gossip include a mastery of anxiety, a search for intimacy, the re-enactment of childhood sexual curiosity, self-aggrandizement of one's talents, or, by extension, the talents of one's children (patients), a search for admiration, and an attempt to manage envy. For psychiatrists, gossip also counteracts the profound psychological deprivation that is an inherent aspect of the professional requirement to keep so great a part of one's life private. From the perspective of confidentiality, when the psychiatrist gossips, internal conflicts have resulted in the unilateral breaking of the fiduciary trust with the patient. The compromise of confidentiality which occurs, regardless of whether the patient's identity is revealed, is likely to have subtle therapeutic as well as ethical ramifications.

The maintenance of confidentiality can be especially difficult with regard to the psychiatrist's own family. When a psychiatrist is preoccupied with an anxiety-provoking case such as a suicidal patient, conflict exists between the wish to explain his preoccupation and the wish to protect the confidentiality of the patient, who may actually call and identify himself by name. Ethically, psychiatrists are obliged not to talk in any detail with their own families about patients, especially those patients who may be identified by their family members in social or professional situations.

## Confidentiality and patient records

Patients tell psychiatrists their most intimate thoughts, and physicians possess a natural inclination to record all relevant information in the patient's record. Psychiatrists need to exercise considerable discretion about entering private information in the official patient record. In clinics and hospitals it is obvious that many individuals have access to the records, but it is easy to overlook the fact that some staff may know the patient and that the seriousness with which confidentiality is maintained will vary greatly among them. Furthermore, any patient records may have to be turned over in the course of personal injury, child-custody, or other litigation, or at the request of insurance companies. On the other hand, in hospitals it is often essential that clinical staff have access to some very private information, and thorough records contribute to better patient-care. Given the inherent tension between making information available to treating staff and maintaining patient confidentiality, psychiatrists need to consider carefully just which personal data must be included in the record. Caution should be given to detailing marginally useful information about third parties, and descriptions of a patient's impulses and fantasies which have not resulted in overt behaviour. If there is a necessity to record such information, it can be kept separate from the official patient-chart, reviewed periodically, and, if appropriate, destroyed.

Particular care is necessary with respect to records that are likely to be the subject of litigation. For example, if a patient has been involved in an automobile or occupational accident, the record should not include the patient's thoughts about his blameworthiness—thoughts which may not be accurate. If, for some reason, these are included, the psychiatrist should clearly indicate any doubts about the accuracy of the speculations.

## Confidentiality and requests for information from third parties

Since the importance of maintaining the confidentiality of patients' records is such a central tenet of psychiatry, it may come as a surprise that the peer-review process established between the American Psychiatric Association and the Aetna Insurance Company initially did not require that the patient provide consent before the treating psychiatrist filed the Mental Health Treatment Report.[27] It is also noteworthy that a recent Medicaid audit required that copies of patients' records be sent to a central agency.[28] These two occurrences underscore the serious difficulties regarding patient confidentiality which frequently result when a third party is involved.

Requests from third parties (insurers, employers, schools, licensing agencies, etc.) regularly pose conflicts regarding confidentiality. In Chapter 21, Chodoff has elaborated upon the conflicts inherent in psychiatrist–patient–third party relationships. With regard to the issue of confidentiality, additional difficulties stem from the fact that patients usually sign a general statement of consent for the release of information. Since patients are likely to believe that they have only agreed to the release of relevant information, it becomes the responsibility of the psychiatrist to clarify with the patient what information will be supplied. As Robitscher[29] has emphasized, the problem becomes especially thorny if the patient is no longer in treatment. The psychiatrist:

does not feel he has the right not to release information after the patient has authorized the release, but he feels he is being forced into an unprofessional stance in retailing (detailing) confidences. It places the therapist at times in a position where he has to divulge information harmful to the patient—a violation of the Hippocratic injunction to do no harm—or alternatively, has to give a false picture of the patient to the inquirer. It raises a complicated informed consent question: if the patient had not been coerced, or if he knew what was going to be divulged, would he have signed the release of information form. It blackmails the therapist into giving information, because if he refuses as a matter of policy, discretion, or conscience to give information, he may be blocking the professional progress of his patient or at least it may lead to the inference that there is something to hide. [pp. 234–5]

By assisting patients to structure the consent, psychiatrists can protect them from acting in ways which might well not be in their self-interest. Even when provided with a signed release which specifies the information to be revealed, psychiatrists should attempt to consult with former as well as current patients about what is going to be released. After such consultation, patients may choose to revoke their release. Some psychiatrists refuse on principle to provide information regarding current or former patients in situations such as government security clearances. If the government agency has resources to conduct an independent psychiatric examination, such a refusal may not be harmful to the patient, and may contribute to a relationship more supportive of psychotherapy.

If the psychiatrist is planning to send a report to the institution or agency, this should be made absolutely clear at the outset. In general, patients should be informed about the specifics of the actual information that is being conveyed, and should be provided with an opportunity to discuss this information. In cases in which the psychiatrist believes that it will be harmful for the patient to know full details, discretion is both ethically and clinically indicated. Furthermore, psychiatrists need to be aware that receiving institutions will manage issues of confidentiality very differently. A survey of state mental hospital directors and directors of mental health centres determined that identifying data were routinely reported to state offices in the following way: 30 per cent submitted names, 31 per cent addresses, and 25 per cent social security numbers; 51 per cent submitted one or more of these.[30] In contrast, a study of psychotherapists working in mental health facilities specifically for medical students found a strong reluctance to break confidentiality.[31] Given the disparity between the expectations of patients, the values of psychiatrists, and the procedures of institutions, the psychiatrist is ethically obliged to clarify what information will be conveyed, and become informed about the institution's handling of confidential material.

## Confidentiality and disclosures in the public interest

Psychiatrists frequently become aware of information which, if disclosed in the proper manner, would benefit the public. A dramatic and not uncommon situation is created when a psychiatrist learns that his patient has had sexual relations with a previous therapist, but does not wish to bring charges or to bring the matter to the attention of the local ethics committee. When a patient reports sexual relations with a former therapist, psychiatrists should be aware that several state laws require the reporting of such information regardless of the patient's wishes. In the absence of such laws, psychiatrists are under no legal obligation to report the behaviour. While exploration of the patient's reservations about reporting is therapeutically indicated, many considerations (not wishing the spouse or family to know, avoidance of a public investigation) might result in a decision to take no action. In such instances it would also be unethical for the psychiatrist to pressure the patient, directly or implicitly, to pursue a more aggressive course of action. If the patient gives consent for the psychiatrist to contact the former therapist or licensing board, the decision whether the psychiatrist should act on the information gained within the confidence of the therapeutic relationship poses an ethical problem. Of course, the patient, herself, if she wishes, can notify the appropriate authorities.

A different conflict regarding confidentiality and undue familiarity may be encountered in institutional settings. A hospitalized patient tells her psychiatrist that another psychiatrist on the ward has had sex with her. She refuses to take the matter up with the administrator of the ward and will not permit her psychiatrist to discuss the matter with anyone. In this instance the psychiatrist has an exceedingly difficult ethical dilemma—to protect his patient's confidentiality or to protect other patients for whom he has clinical responsibility with whom the psychiatrist might also be having sexual relations or might in the future. As an initial step, focused discussion and psychotherapy with the patient should be undertaken in the hopes that she will take action herself or will grant permission for the psychiatrist to pursue a specific course of action. If neither of these result, given the psychiatrist's responsibility for an identifiable group of patients, some unilateral action by the psychiatrist is ethically permissible. Speaking directly with the psychiatrist in question, informing the impaired physician's committee, consulting with the hospital's ethics committee, or speaking with the hospital administrator are reasonable options. Regardless of which course of action is followed, ethics require that the patient should be fully informed of the psychiatrist's decision.

Not all conflicts regarding disclosure in the public interest concern undue familiarity. A less dramatic situation is created when the psychiatrist learns from his patient, a social worker in a psychiatric hospital, that the ward psychiatrist is billing insurance companies for time not actually spent with patients, information which the patient does not wish to report for fear of retaliation. In this instance, for the psychiatrist to institute any action based on his patient's report would violate the patient's right to keep this information confidential, and would constitute unethical behaviour, even though it would protect the ethical standards of the profession. A unique situation was described by Chodoff,[32] who learned of an instance in which a psychiatrist became aware that his patient was considering politically defecting with sensitive material. In this instance a concern for national security was in conflict with the commitment to maintain the patient's confidentiality. Even in a case such as this, the question whether the danger posed to the public warrants disclosure is a difficult one.

## Confidentiality with patients dangerous to themselves or others

Since the *Tarasoff* decision in 1974,[33] psychiatrists have been faced with the possibility of liability for the violent conduct of their patients towards third parties. One major problem inherent in the *Tarasoff* decision is the ascription to psychiatrists of a predictive ability with regard to dangerousness which is greater than is justified by current knowledge. As a result of this decision psychiatrists have been forced into a role strongly at odds with their therapeutic commitment to patients' confidentiality and their wish to avoid becoming involved in acts of social control. There are, none the less, circumstances in which the psychiatrist's conviction that a patient will carry out a dangerous act is strong enough to warrant breaking confidentiality. Four such situations involve suicide, homicide, AIDS, and child-abuse.

### Suicide and homicide

The ethical issues involved in cases of suicidal and homicidal patients have been discussed elsewhere in this volume (Chapters 8 and 12). With specific regard to questions of confidentiality, psychiatric ethics do not preclude informing family members of a suicidal patient's intent, or notifying the potential victim of a homicidal patient. The degree of conviction necessary to justify disclosure will vary among psychiatrists, but if the data support it, the clinical decision to break confidentiality is justified. When such a decision has been reached, it is important to keep in mind that, in addition to safeguarding patients' confidentiality, psychiatrists also have the responsibility of informing patients when their own actions are jeopardizing their confidentiality. They have the additional ethical responsibility of attempting to develop with the patient a course of action so that the breaking of confidentiality, like its establishment, can be a mutual process. The thoughtful and creative interventions described by Roth and Meisel[34] in *Tarasoff*-type clinical situations can serve as a model for the management of potential homicidal and suicidal cases, as well as instances of child-abuse and AIDS. Although the psychiatrist may ultimately have to act without the patient's participation or consent, efforts to involve the patient ensure the maintenance of ethical standards despite the breaking of confidentiality.

### The paedophile: an example of child-abuse

Although state law requires the reporting of child-abuse, ethical issues regarding confidentiality can arise when the patient is not currently abusive or when, in the course of therapy, the psychiatrist learns that in the past the patient abused a child who is no longer a minor. To open an investigation of past abuse can be extremely stressful for the victim, regardless of the fact that the abuse occurred many years previously.[35] A similar dilemma is faced by the psychiatrist who learns that his adult patient was abused as a child. If, as is likely, the state reporting laws do not cover such instances, the decision regarding the reporting and investigation of the abuse belongs to the patient, provided, of course, there is no evidence to suggest current paedophilic activity on the part of the alleged abuser. When the patient is a potential paedophile and a camp counsellor, schoolteacher, or youth-group leader, implementing the duty to warn can be difficult. In the absence of concern about a particular child, one must ascertain whether the duty to warn pertains to all the children, to the organization, or both. From an ethical perspective, unnecessarily alarming both parents and children is most certainly not a benign intervention. Informing the institution, rather than the class of individuals who might be affected, is a restrained but effective course of action.

## AIDS

The current AIDS epidemic has given rise to many ethical issues.[36–38] In some states, psychiatrists are required to report all cases of HIV positivity to public health authorities. But ethical issues involving confidentiality arise whenever people who are at high risk for AIDS or are HIV-positive are sexually involved with unknowing partners.[39] Guidelines pertaining to such situations have not been provided by statute or case-law in most states. Although the American Psychiatric Association has developed a policy regarding confidentiality and disclosure for patients with AIDS,[40] at present a specific course of action will need to be evolved by each psychiatrist in his own clinical setting. Absent state laws to the contrary, the American Psychiatric Association takes the position that it is ethically permissible for psychiatrists to warn partners or identifiable potential partners that a patient is HIV-positive, provided that the patient has been encouraged to provide the warning himself, has failed to do so, and is informed what information will be shared and with whom. The issue, however, continues to be actively debated.[41,42] Since the 'duty to warn' put forth in the initial *Tarasoff* decision was superseded by the 'duty to protect',[43,44] ethics require that informing the partner of the patient's positive HIV status must be accompanied by thorough education about AIDS and its prevention.

Hospital psychiatrists are frequently confronted by a number of complex problems regarding the confidentiality of a patient's HIV status.[45,46] Should a psychiatrist repect the wish for confidentiality of a non-psychotic, well-controlled man who does not wish other staff to be informed of his positive HIV status? How should a patient who is HIV-positive and sexually active on the ward be managed if he refuses to share this information with all patients? A depressed, HIV-positive man is to be transferred to another hospital for rehabilitation following a mild cerebral infarction, but will not consent to release of information regarding his HIV status. Can the psychiatrist ethically convey this knowledge without the patient's permission? A butcher is hospitalized for an acute adjustment reaction with depressed mood. He has used intravenous drugs in the past, and is HIV-positive. If he refuses to inform his employer, what is the psychiatrist's ethical responsibility?

Although the ethical issues resulting from AIDS are serious and complicated, they are confronted more often by general practitioners than by psychiatrists. However, as many as 25 per cent of individuals in the early stages of HIV infection manifest subtle dementia on neuropsychological testing, and 33 per cent will show a mild to severe dementia during the course of their illness.[47] Because of this and because many other individuals at risk for AIDS are initially treated in mental health facilities, psychiatrists may be the first to test the patient for HIV infection. Both clinically and ethically it is desirable to obtain the patient's consent and to elaborate the course of action resulting from a positive test prior to the testing. In addition, a careful assessment of organic impairment is an essential aspect of the evaluation of the AIDS patient, not only from the perspective of thoroughness, but also to assess the patient's ability fully to comprehend the implication of his illness and to give informed consent.

## Confidentiality and psychiatric genetics

Some hereditary medical illnesses such as Huntington's disease and Wilson's disease may present with psychiatric symptoms and confront the psychiatrist with a difficult ethical dilemma. A man seeks psychiatric treatment for depression and is found to have Huntington's disease. Recently married, he refuses to inform his wife, fearing that she will elect not to have children. In such cases, despite the pain that would be inflicted on the mother and child should offspring develop the disease, in the absence of an imminent and definite threat, any disclosure by the psychiatrist would, in our opinion, be difficult to justify. This position of non-disclosure reflects the high degree of restraint which is frequently required to prevent concern and compassion from overriding the patient's fundamental right to regulate the disclosure of personal information.

## Ethics, confidentiality, and the treatment of children

In this book Chapter 16 provides a thorough overview of the ethical issues which arise in psychiatric treatment of children. When working with children, the ethical principles which guide the psychiatrist's management of confidentiality in the treatment of adults need to be significantly modified.

Until they achieve a sense of themselves as separate, autonomous individuals, children do not develop a mature sense of confidentiality. Young
children believe that their parents know their private thoughts and feelings, and may be concerned that their secrets are revealed through their
secretions (for example, nocturnal emissions, urine, faeces).[25] Before the
age of seven, children operate by pre-logical cognition, and cannot achieve
the sense of personal responsibility essential to an understanding of confidentiality.[48] Even by the age of twelve, when children begin to think
according to the principles of formal operations, that level of cognition
may only be achieved in areas where they have regular practice. Erikson
has stressed that 'morality, ideology and ethics must evolve in each person
by a step by step development from less to more differentiated and insight-
ful stages . . . Developmentally speaking, we must . . . differentiate between an earlier *moral* conscience and a later ethical one.'[49] Kolansky[50]
has noted that if promised total confidentiality, a young child may actually
become more rather than less anxious. This is especially true of pre-school
and latency children, but may at times even be true of adolescents. Thus
the point of view that confidentiality is an inherent good in therapeutic
relationships cannot automatically be applied to work with children. Ethical
behaviour requires that the psychiatrist evaluate what, if anything, about
confidentiality should be explained to the child, rather than pursue the
abstract goal of promising total confidentiality. The decision of when to keep
or when to break confidentiality must be reached anew not only with each
child, but also in each instance in which the issue occurs with the same child.

Although the clinical situation will differ, a thorough discussion with
parents about the management of confidentiality is essential. In theory, the
person who provides consent for the treatment has access to anything
discussed between child and psychiatrist. In practice, however, the therapeutic communications with the child are confidential, and the psychiatrist
determines what, if any, information will be shared with parents. Clarification with the parents at the outset that the child's therapy is confidential
and that the disclosure of information conveyed by the child will depend
upon clinical judgement is not only ethical, but may eliminate a future
conflict that might result in the parents' discontinuing the child's therapy
abruptly and against the psychiatrist's advice. Sometimes the content of a
child's therapy may be indirectly communicated. As Lipton[51] has noted,
the nature of the questions which a child psychiatrist asks of parents during
the course of therapy indirectly reveals some of the subjects discussed by
the child.

Child psychiatrists take a range of positions with regard to the confidentiality of sessions with parents. Although a psychiatrist might promise to
keep the material of parental sessions 'confidential', such information
cannot be isolated from the psychiatrist's thinking. Family secrets are

secrets only in the sense that they have not been explicitly divulged, and, in actuality, are 'known', and strongly influence family functioning and the experience of the child. Similarly, the information which parents convey must influence the way the psychiatrist listens and responds to the child. Ethically, child psychiatrists who wish to keep private some information conveyed by parents, need to explain that, regardless of whether it is directly communicated to the child, such information will have some impact upon treatment. It would seem prudent to emphasize that clinical judgement will determine what material from sessions with parents is directly discussed with the child.

Although legal issues are central in child-custody cases, ethical issues concerning confidentiality frequently arise. Control of all information about the child's treatment generally belongs to the parent who has the legal responsibility to give consent for the treatment. For example, the custodial parent may refuse permission for the psychiatrist to provide the non-custodial parent with any information regarding the child, even though the child might be spending the summer with that parent. The psychiatrist, believing that a consultation with the parent would benefit the child, is in the ethical dilemma of depriving the patient of the maximum therapeutic benefit in order to conform with the law. The problem is further compounded in work with young children, to whom it may be almost impossible to explain the situation adequately. Ethics dictate that the psychiatrist be prepared to work intensively with the custodial parent, and, if necessary, to request that the court intervene on the child's behalf and permit appropriate disclosures to the non-custodial parent.

## Ethics, confidentiality, and adolescents

Issues of confidentiality are nowhere more fluid and complex than in the psychiatric treatment of the adolescent, who may have the legal right (depending on the state) to be responsible for the decisions regarding the disclosure of confidential material, but whose psychological immaturity compromises his ability to make the best choices regarding its management.[52] Although the child's ability to conceptualize confidentiality evolves gradually, by twelve to fifteen most children understand and value the concept.[53] By this age they have passed from Piaget's stage of moral realism to the stage of moral relativism, and have acquired the sense of personal responsibility essential to the development of ethical standards and full understanding of confidentiality. At this point they can also recognize its importance in psychotherapy.[48]

In addition to the striking variability in the degree to which adolescents understand confidentiality, the kinds of issues which they bring to the psychiatrist are often much more serious than those brought by younger

children. Assuming that an adolescent has the right to consent to treatment
without parental permission, and therefore has the right to control the
maintenance of confidentiality, what ethical course of action shall the
psychiatrist pursue if the child informs him of plans to run away; what is
ethically indicated if he admits that he has moved from the occasional use
of marijuana to the frequent use of cocaine, but refuses permission for the
psychiatrist to discuss these issues with the parents? Should a psychiatrist
maintain the confidentiality of a thirteen-year-old girl who plans to have
sex with her seventeen-year-old boyfriend while the parents are away for
the weekend? How shall one respond to reports of parental nudity if the
patient refuses permission to raise the issue with them? How does one
discuss confidentiality with a teenager who knows full well his legal rights
at the outset of treatment? Given that the psychological development of
adolescents may lag significantly behind the legal rights achieved by
chronology alone, it seems prudent to be realistic regarding confidentiality.
Frank explanation of the psychiatrist's wish to respect the patient's rights
and at the same time protect the treatment and the patient's welfare will
provide a framework for resolving issues of confidentiality should they
arise. Crucial in such a dialogue is the complete assurance that confidentiality will not be broken without prior discussion with the patient.

## Ethics, confidentiality, and group, family, and couples therapy

Groups by their very nature are public, and group therapy can be conceptualized as 'a form of communal living where there is little privacy
among its members, and privacy is not a value. Outside the group, however, isolation and privacy prevail.'[54] Additional problems with establishing and maintaining confidentiality result from the permeability of
group boundaries, and the fact that the responsibility to maintain confidentiality is shared by all members, and therefore necessarily diluted.[26] To
these problems are added the human proclivity to gossip and the fact that
in most states the law has not definitively forbidden the breaking of confidentiality by group members. Given these obstacles to the maintenance
of confidentiality, psychiatrists have employed a number of mechanisms.
Among these are (1) using first names only; (2) urging group members to
see themselves as co-therapists, thereby increasing their sense of responsibility; (3) discouraging or forbidding meetings of group members outside
the psychotherapeutic setting; (4) rigorous analysis of any breaks in confidentiality; and (5) terminating treatment of anyone who breaks confidentiality,[55] and (6) the establishment of a contract regarding confidentiality.

In group settings no psychiatrist can responsibly assure the degree of
confidentiality which can be maintained in work with a single person. The

group psychotherapist, not his patients, has a professional code of ethics which is based on confidentiality.[54] Group members will need relatively frequent reminders of the importance of confidentiality,[56] especially given the multiplicity of forces which work to weaken it. This is true even for 'closed' groups in which no new members are added for the duration of the group. As discussed in the above consideration of the confidentiality of meetings with the parents of a child in psychotherapy, it is impossible for the psychiatrist to be unaffected by the information which a group (or family or couples) psychotherapy patient might discuss in an individual session.[57] We believe that ethical responsibility requires the psychiatrist to explain this clearly to the patient.

To a significant degree, these issues pertain to family therapy as well as to group therapy. Further difficulties arise because the developmental maturities of the members of the family are so disparate. Young children, for example, cannot be expected to maintain confidentiality over private matters (for example, alcoholism, violence, and infidelity); and it is therefore important to clarify this with the parents before the beginning of therapy. The therapist also has the responsibility of ensuring the confidentiality of the parents with respect to the children.[58]

## Confidentiality when patients are seeing more than one therapist

In contemporary psychiatric practice it is not unusual for patients to be treated by more than one therapist. When a patient sees one person for psychotherapy and another for pharmacotherapy, the two treatments are somewhat discrete. By contrast, when a patient is seeing one person in individual psychotherapy and another in couples or group psychotherapy, the treatments clearly overlap. In both situations initial discussions between the two therapists are often indicated, and, depending upon the patient and the manner of practice of the therapist, ongoing communication may be desirable. Permission given for an initial sharing of information does not automatically pertain to future discussions. In one instance, a woman in individual psychotherapy entered a group specifically devoted to the treatment of adults who had been sexually abused as children. She freely gave permission for her therapists to consult prior to her entering the group. After several months, the group therapist called the individual therapist to convey some concern about the nature of the patient's participation in the group. The individual therapist asked whether the patient had given permission for the call, and, upon learning that she had not, ended the conversation. The patient, on learning of the group therapist's call, was angered, both because her permission had not been asked and because she had been unaware of the therapist's concern.

In general, this type of communication is best conceptualized as one would any other release of information. As such, it needs to be clearly structured with the patient beforehand. For example, a man in couples treatment had discussed his extramarital affair only with his individual therapist. The couple's therapist requested and was granted permission to speak with the individual therapist, who postponed the conversation until he had discussed what information the patient wished to be kept confidential. To avoid just such a dilemma many individual psychotherapists would refuse any discussion at all. Whether or not one takes this position, whenever possible, permission for discussion should be asked in each instance and the specific information to be disclosed should be clarified prior to each discussion. In addition, ethics dictate that the specifics of each discussion should be shared with the patient. This course of action is prudent, because the information belongs to the patient and because the information conveyed will affect the thinking and behaviour of the therapist. Therefore, when discussing a patient with another therapist, one should share only those thoughts which one would not have any hesitation in discussing directly with the patient.

## Confidentiality and writing and speaking

The inclusion of detailed clinical material in oral presentations and in the psychiatric literature presents the psychiatrist with the unavoidable ethical dilemma of protecting the patient's confidentiality while at the same time avoiding a reduction of the material's scientific merit by excessive disguise. Even if written with the utmost attention to the disguise of identifying data and with all due discretion, a detailed case-study raises:

serious questions about its effect on the patient in relation to his social milieu. Even if these can be discounted, we must still consider the implications with respect to persisting transferential attitudes towards his [former] analyst. We know that they do exist and they must be taken into account. To have one's analyst become one's biographer must acquire a significance difficult to define over the long run.[59]

Stoller in a provocative and thoughtful discussion of this problem quotes a patient whose case-vignette had been published without her knowledge:

'You said,' she stated, 'it hadn't hurt me, that you were justified because I couldn't be identified' (I recall that slightly differently: I believe I said it need not have hurt her because she could not be identified, thereby ignoring, in the comfort of proper ethics, her more complex experience . . .) 'How could you know that by not informing or warning me or whatever that you were transgressing that sacred boundary, the infinite trust I placed in you.' [p. 382][20]

Stoller, who allows patients to read and edit any detailed report, emphasizes the problem of obtaining truly 'informed consent' from a patient whose transference strongly influences the freedom to refuse. If the patient is currently in treatment, the ability to give informed consent may be especially affected by the transference. In such a situation patients should be encouraged to consult with another psychiatrist regarding publication, and this consultation might be paid for by the author. When writing about patients in the mental health field whose friends and colleagues can be expected to read the psychiatric literature, the need for disguise is especially great. When the identity of the author will make identification of the patient more likely, the article might be published under a pen name. Lipton[51] reported a situation indicative of the extreme caution that one must take in writing about patients. In the instance he described, an analyst in a study-group presented a case. A member of the study-group, without asking or informing the presenter, used the case in an article. The patient's father read the case, recognized his son as the patient, and informed him of the article. The patient was predictably furious with his analyst. It seems clear that a psychiatrist intending to publish a detailed case history must obtain the patient's consent. We believe that meaningful consent requires that the patient should read the actual material and then give permission for publication. If the psychiatrist thinks that it would be detrimental to the patient to read this material, ethics would indicate that it should be excluded from the publication.

Finally, we draw attention to the ethical issues involved in the large case-conference in which patients agree to be interviewed and the issue of giving informed consent for taped sessions which are to be used in the future for 'educational purposes'. With regard to taping, the consent should be as specific as possible with respect to the circumstances in which the tape will be used. If the patient is currently in treatment, a consultation with an independent psychiatrist will maximize the likelihood that the consent is free and fully informed. Furthermore, the consent should be renewed on a periodic basis. As emphasized by Graham in Chapter 16, this is especially important with regard to children and adolescents who may wish to prevent disclosure when they come of age. Since confidentiality is significantly compromised and devalued whenever patients are interviewed or tapes are played before large audiences, one needs to be certain that the information could not be effectively conveyed in a less revealing fashion. In addition, psychiatrists should remind members of the audience of their obligation to leave if they know the patient or anyone in his family.

## Ethics, confidentiality, and psychiatric education

Psychiatric education invariably involves discussion of residents' private thoughts and feelings, and the relationship between psychiatric supervisors and their students is likely to elicit stronger transference responses than between students and teachers in other medical or non-medical settings. Furthermore, members of the psychiatric faculty may be in possession of important information about residents, which they have acquired under confidential circumstances. These factors contribute to ethical issues regarding the maintenance of confidentiality which are encountered in procedures of admission, patient-care, supervision, and evaluation.

Admissions committees regularly face ethical choices regarding the confidentiality of material pertaining to applicants. In one instance, a committee member had treated an applicant for a serious depression on several occasions. He had significant reservations about the applicant, who had not informed any interviewers of the treatment. Concerned that the applicant, the applicant's patients, and the residency would be adversely affected should the applicant matriculate and later decompensate, he was faced with the ethical conflict between his responsibility to the patient (applicant), the residency programme, and the community. He considered this information to be confidential, and ultimately chose to keep it private. Admissions committees must routinely decide whether to inquire about an applicant from a former therapist. Should such a request be made, it would be the responsibility of the therapist, in consultation with the applicant, to determine what, if any, information should be shared with the committee. From an ethical perspective, however, such a request places the committee in the position of asking the applicant to violate a basic tenet of the psychiatrist–patient relationship. Furthermore, since the committee has significant control over the applicant's future, it is questionable whether truly informed consent can be given.

There is considerable disagreement regarding the ethical obligation of psychiatric residents (or psychiatrists) to inform patients when their cases are being supervised. Medical and surgical patients receiving care in a teaching hospital expect their cases to be used for educational purposes; but psychiatric patients treated by residents or other students may not be aware that the details of psychotherapy sessions will be discussed with another person on a regular basis. Psychiatrists have taken broadly divergent positions on this topic,[60-62] ranging from the opinion that telling the patient about supervision represents an unanalysable parameter which unnecessarily burdens him with the therapist's problems (for example, feelings about being in training) to the point of view that the supervisor should be present at the initial interview, and that the role of the supervisor should be clearly explained. Since a high value is placed on confidentiality in therapeutic relationships, and since decisions to break confidentiality are generally made by the patient or with his knowledge, a unilateral and ongoing compromise of confidentiality, such as is inherent in supervision, would seem to require prior discussion with the patient. Confidentiality, however, is more than an end in itself; confidentiality is protected to further the success of the treatment. With many patients, especially those who are suspicious or overtly psychotic, complete candour may sacrifice the therapeutic alliance on the altar of confidentiality. In arriving at what is ultimately a clinical decision, the psychiatrist must weigh the impact of disclosure. Should the psychiatrist elect to discuss the issue of supervision, patients may subsequently displace their mistrust from therapist to supervisor—a development requiring therapeutic exploration. Even in such circumstances, the candour of the therapist in informing the patient of the supervisor's role will underscore the seriousness with which the therapist views the subject of confidentiality, and will help to repair any rift in the therapeutic alliance. Should patients inquire whether their cases are supervised, ethics would dictate a frank and open discussion of the subject. Psychiatrists who are in psychotherapy themselves may often discuss patients with their therapists. However, to inform patients of this compromise of confidentiality would be honest, but almost always countertherapeutic.

Additional issues of confidentiality are also inherent in the process of supervision. Psychiatric educators are so accustomed to the importance of supervision that 'it is difficult for them to see it as impinging on trainees' privacy and therefore on their security within the training program'.[63] Especially when exploring residents' personal reactions to their patients, supervisors will acquire considerable information which may be only marginally relevant to their evaluation, and which should therefore be kept confidential. Supervision, which can be considered to be the 'psychotherapy of work',[64] is rooted in education and in psychotherapy, thus creating the ethical issue of confidentiality for the supervisor and concerns about the degree of disclosure of personal information for the supervisee. Moreover, residents frequently experience significant conflict about how much of the patient's identifying data should be revealed to the supervisor—the patient's full name or the names of others mentioned by the patient, a particularly thorny problem when the patient is well-known or is involved with a well-known individual. While each resident-supervisor pair must make its own decision regarding this matter, we consider the nature of supervision to be such that the resident is not required to maintain the confidentiality of material revealed in therapy. In fact, if the resident does not feel required to edit the patient's material, the supervision may be freer and more productive. As do psychotherapists, supervisors may have to discontinue supervision if they know the patient or someone important in the patient's life.

The evaluation of residents, and especially candidates in psychoanalytic institutes, poses difficult problems of confidentiality.[65-67] One analytic institute which adopted a principle of strict confidentiality, completely separating a candidate's analysis and evaluation, was unable to adhere to this principle, and broke confidentiality in a number of ways, some overt, others more subtle.[65,66] Although the maintenance of confidentiality may be more difficult in psychoanalytic institutes (it is institutionalized when the analyst reports on the progress of the patient to the committee evaluating candidates' progress), it is not easy in psychiatric residencies, especially those in smaller communities where a member of the faculty may be treating one of the residents. Compromises of confidentiality are exemplified by the following:

1.  Dr Smith, member of the psychiatric faculty, hears from a patient that a resident exhibited immature and unprofessional behaviour by mocking Dr Smith at a party. Without informing the resident in question, Dr Smith enters a note in the record which is not available for review by the resident.

2.  An analyst hears from a psychoanalytic candidate in treatment some highly negative comments about another candidate; he participates in the second candidate's evaluation, introducing the material but protecting the source by invoking confidentiality.

3.  A resident confides to a faculty member that he is seriously depressed, and clinically he appears quite paranoid. He is referred to a psychiatrist not associated with the residency, whom he can see for treatment. Although the resident's work is satisfactory, the degree of his paranoia gives the faculty member significant concern. Can he ethically discuss his concerns with the faculty without the resident's knowledge or permission?

4.  A resident informs the director of residency training that a respected, long-time supervisor from the community has made repeated explicit sexual overtures. She wishes to be transferred to a different supervisor, and does not want the director to speak to the supervisor or to inform the faculty of the reasons for the change. The director, convinced of the accuracy of the report, accedes to her wishes and assigns her to a different supervisor. Ethically, what courses of action are open to him regarding the supervisor whose future absence from the list of supervising psychiatrists would be certain to attract attention?

While each of these situations is complicated by the involvement of a third party, the faculty, ethical principles dictate that confidentiality should be broken only if absolutely necessary, and only after discussion with the party conveying the confidential information. This approach seems applicable in institutional and educational situations, as well as in clinical work.

## Responding to material heard in confidence from the patient

When psychiatrists hear certain material within the confidential boundaries of the therapeutic relationship, several ethical problems may be created. One category of situations concerns the degree to which psychiatrists can ethically use information which the patient conveys within the therapeutic setting; a second concerns possible actions which the psychiatrist might take in response to information about a patient from a third party.

Laws regulating insider trading apply to information acquired in treatment. A psychiatrist who invests or makes other business deals on the basis of insider information obtained through the psychotherapeutic relationship can be found guilty of insider trading. Thus, when the president of a small firm whose stock is traded publicly informs his psychiatrist that his company is going to be bought out, the psychiatrist cannot act on this information himself, nor can he convey it to others. But laws regulating insider trading do not pertain to decisions which the psychiatrist might wish to make on the basis of a non-insider stock tip offered him by a patient who has had great success with investments. However, a psychiatric code of ethics might require that this information should not be used for any investment decisions by the psychiatrist. If conveyed to the patient, any investment decision will significantly alter the nature of the therapeutic relationship. If the recommendation proved successful, the patient might wish or feel obliged to offer other suggestions. It is not inconceivable that he could reasonably expect to be reimbursed for his professional advice by a fee reduction or 'free hour'. If unsuccessful, he might feel guilty and seek to make amends or avoid expressing hostility. Even if the psychiatrist never informs the patient that he acted on the investment suggestion, the relationship with his patient will be affected. Good advice might lead him unconsciously or even consciously to encourage the patient to provide other investment information. If the tip proved to be a poor one, the psychiatrist's disappointment and resentment would be likely to find a means of expression within the therapeutic relationship. As strictly as the psychiatric boundary is regulated by concern for privacy and confidentiality, so strictly is it governed by the implicit understanding that the psychiatrist's sole interest in the patient is to provide treatment and to further the achievement of therapeutic goals. Using information acquired in the therapeutic relationship to make specific investment decisions cannot help but alter the nature of the psychiatrist–patient relationship, and therefore has ethical ramifications.

Based on what their patients tell them, psychiatrists inevitably do engage in a wide range of extratherapeutic actions which are within the boundaries of ethical behaviour. In the field of finance, for example, a psychiatrist cannot be expected to ignore general information regarding interest rates which his banker patient tells him in the hopes of earning the psychiatrist's admiration or affection. Similarly, attending a movie, reading a book, or eating at a restaurant on the suggestion of a patient do not cross the line separating ethical from unethical action. But psychiatrists need to keep in mind that every such action may have an impact, even if minor, on the relationship between them and their patients.

## Responding to confidential material heard in another setting of relevance to the patient

Numerous situations occur in which the psychiatrist learns in a confidential relationship of information of significant importance to a patient. We believe that these instances of 'reverse confidentiality' merit serious consideration. In smaller communities, for example, or in psychoanalytic institutes in which a limited number of psychiatrists are available to treat the same population, the psychiatrist is routinely faced with the ethical problem of how to handle material about one patient which is conveyed to him by another. How should a psychiatrist respond to the report from Mr A that Mr B (another patient) is abusing drugs if Mr A is unwilling to inform Mr B that he has told the psychiatrist, and is also unwilling to be identified as a source of information. Unless the danger to the patient is considered to be extremely severe, unilateral breaking of Mr A's confidentiality seems unwarranted, and the psychiatrist and Mr A must attempt to resolve the issue therapeutically. A different type of problem is presented by participation in the activities of professional ethics committees. A psychiatrist, who is a member of the local psychiatric ethics committee, learns that his patient's daughter is about to enter treatment with a psychiatrist who he knows will definitely be expelled from the local psychiatric society for having had sexual relationships with a patient. In this instance the psychiatrist has conflicting fiduciary responsibilities—one to maintain the confidentiality of the proceedings of the ethics committee, the other to protect his patient's daughter. An ethical (and legal) solution to this situation might be to express serious reservations about the daughter's psychiatrist, without identifying the specifics or the source of one's doubts.

Another situation, also more common in small or circumscribed communities, but not infrequent in any psychiatric practice, is created when a patient describes intimate details of the life of someone whom the psychiatrist knows well. While it is an everyday occurrence for a psychiatrist to hear confidential material about named third parties, there is an inherent ethical conflict if the third party is the psychiatrist's close friend. In such instances, professional ethics dictate that the psychiatrist consider referring the patient to someone else—a step which, from a therapeutic perspective, will allow the treatment to proceed without the difficulties inevitably faced by the psychiatrist who is forced to listen to material which the friend might wish to keep private.

# Conclusion

In psychoanalysis and in most psychiatric treatments, 'one of the understandings about confidentiality is that the analyst wields no power in the life of the patient other than the power of psychoanalysis itself. Confidentiality embodies the recognition of a power never to be used.'[64] Although confidentiality has been shown to be highly valued by psychiatrists and patients, its boundaries are assaulted from without by many forces, and threatened from within by the human urge to gossip, the therapeutic need for periodic consultation, the educational and scientific requirement that clinical case material be made available for discussion, and the need to protect against such potential harms as suicide, homicide, and child-abuse. Current and future legal statutes and judicial decisions may provide some guidelines for psychiatrists. In most contexts, however, ethical norms rather than laws will be the primary source of guidance towards solutions which respond to the specific situation while maintaining the basic principle of compromising as little confidential material as possible. Since absolute confidentiality, however desirable in principle, is a fiction, psychiatrists need to act with candour in discussing the limitations of confidentiality. This is especially true in light of the demonstrated misconceptions which patients have about the degree to which their therapeutic communications can be kept private. Absolute candour, however, may not always be in the patient's interest. Where disclosure is not required by law, clinical judgement will determine whether the patient's treatment will be positively or adversely affected by informing him of breaches in confidentiality. Regardless of whether consent is required, the very nature of confidentiality obliges the psychiatrist to reveal only the degree of information which is necessary. When disclosure will have a direct impact on the patient, as in instances of suicidal and homicidal intents, ethics require that the patient be informed that confidentiality is going to be breached.

We are only too aware of the effort required, and, in the case of writing and speaking, of the sacrifice which may be entailed in the ethical maintenance of confidentiality. However, the psychiatrist's primary responsibility to the welfare of his patient merits this degree of vigilance and care in the safeguarding of the patient's confidentiality.

# References

1 Winslade, W. J. Confidentiality in *Encyclopedia of bioethics*, ed. W. T. Reich. New York, Free Press, 1978, pp. 184–200.
2 Shah, S. T. Privileged communications, confidentiality and privacy. *Professional Psychology* 1:56–69, 1969.
3 Knapp, S. and Vandecreek, L. *Privileged communications in the mental health professions.* New York, Van Nostrand Reinhold, 1987.

4  *In re Lifschutz*. 85 Cal. Rptr 829, 476 P.2d 557 Cal. Sup. Ct 91970).
5  Everstine, L., Everstine, D. S., Heymann, G. M., *et al.*: Privacy and confidentiality in psychotherapy. *American Psychologist* **35**:828–40, 1980.
6  Applebaum, P. S. Confidentiality in psychiatric treatment, in *The American Annual Psychiatric Review*, ed. L. Grinspoon. Washington DC American Psychiatric Press, pp. 327–34, 1982.
7  Gilmore, M. and Shear, K.: Ethical and legal considerations of confidentiality in the treatment of hospitalized health professionals. *Psychiatric Quarterly* **50**:237–45, 1978.
8  American Psychiatric Association: Guidelines on confidentiality. *American Journal of psychiatry* **144**:1522–6, 1987.
9  Jagim, R. D., Wittman, W. D., and Noll, J. O.: Mental health professionals' attitudes toward confidentiality, privilege and third-party disclosures. *Professional Psychology* **9**:458–66, 1978.
10 Lindenthal, J. J. and Thomas, C. S.: Consumers, clinicians and confidentiality. *Social Service and Medicine* **16**:333–5, 1982.
11 Lindenthal, J. J. and Thomas, C. S.: Psychiatrists, the public and confidentiality. *Journal of Nervous and Mental Disease* **170**:319–23, 1982.
12 Schmid, D., Appelbaum, P. S., Roth, L. H., and Lidz, L.: Confidentiality in psychiatry: a study of the patient's view. *Hospital and Community Psychiatry* **34**:353–5, 1983.
13 Appelbaum, P. S., Kappen, G., Walters, B. Lidz, C., and Roth, L. H.: Confidentiality: an empirical test of the utilitarian perspective. *Bulletin of the American Academy of Psychiatry and The Law* **12**:109–16, 1984.
14 Lindenthal, J. J., Thomas, C. S., and Ghali, A. Y.: A cross cultural study of confidentiality. *Social Psychiatry* **20**:140–44, 1985.
15 McGuire, J. M., Toal, P., and Blau, B.: The adult client's conception of confidentiality in the therapeutic relationship. *Professional Psychology* **16**:375–84, 1985.
16 Siegler, M.: Confidentiality in Medicine—a decrepit concept. *New England Journal of Medicine* **307**:1518–21, 1982.
17 Slovenko, R. and Usdin, G. L.: The psychiatrist and privileged communication. *Archives of General Psychiatry* **4**:431–44, 1961.
18 Dubey, J.: Confidentiality as a requirement of the therapist: technical necessities for absolute privilege in psychotherapy. *American Journal of Psychiatry* **131**:1093–6, 1974.
19 Plaut, E. A.: A perspective on confidentiality. *American Journal of Psychiatry* **131**:1021–4, 1974.
20 Stoller, R. J.: Patients' responses to their case reports. *Journal of the American Psychoanalytic Association* **36**:371–92, 1988.
21 Fink, R.: Viewpoint. *Psychiatric News*, 3 Feb. 1989, p. 18.
22 Rosenbaum, J. E. and Subrin, M.: The psychology of gossip. *Journal of the American Psychoanalytic Association* **11**:817–31, 1963.
23 Medini, G. and Rosenberg, E. H.: Gossip and psychotherapy. *American Journal of Psychotherapy* **30**:452–6, 1976.
24 Olinick, S. L.: The gossiping psychoanalyst. *International Review of Psychoanalysis* **7**:439–45, 1986.
25 Caruth, E. G.: Secret bearer or secret barer? *Contemporary Psychoanalysis* **4**:548–62, 1985.

26 Lakin, M.: *Ethical issues in the psychotherapies*. New York, Oxford University Press, 1988.
27 Rosner, B. L.: Psychiatrists, confidentiality and insurance claims. *Hastings Center Report* **10**:5–7, 1980.
28 Schwed, H. J., Kuvin, S. F., and Baliga, R. K.: Medicaid audit: crisis in confidentiality and the patient–psychiatrist relationship. *American Journal of Psychiatry* **136**:447–50, 1979.
29 Robitscher, J.: *The powers of psychiatry*. Boston, Houghton Mifflin, 1980.
30 Noll, J. O. and Hanlon, M. J.: Patient privacy and confidentiality at Mental Health Centers. *American Journal of Psychiatry* **133**:1286-8, 1976.
31 Lindenthal, J. J., Amaranto, E. A., Jordan, T. J., and Wepman, B. J.: Decisions about confidentiality in medical student mental health settings. *Journal of Counseling Psychology* **31**:572–5, 1984.
32 Chodoff, P.: Personal communication, 1988.
33 *Tarasoff v Regents of the University of California* 529 P.2d 553 (1974).
34 Roth, L. H. and Meisel, A.: Dangerousness, confidentiality and the duty to warn. *American Journal of Psychiatry* **134**:508–11, 1977.
35 Kelly, R. J.: Limited confidentiality and the pedophile. *Hospital and Community Psychiatry* **38**:1046–8, 1987.
36 Ginzburg, H. M. and Gostin, L.: Legal and ethical issues associated with HTLV-III diseases. *Psychiatric Annals* **16**:180–5, 1986.
37 Kelly, K.: AIDS and ethics: an overview. *General Hospital Psychiatry* **9**:331–40, 1987.
38 Dyer, A. R.: AIDS, ethics and psychiatry. *Psychiatric Annals* **18**:557–81, 1988.
39 Eth, S.: The sexually active, HIV infected patient: confidentiality versus the duty to protect. *Psychiatric Annals* **18**:571–6, 1988.
40 American Psychiatric Association: AIDS policy: confidentiality and disclosure. *American Journal of Psychiatry* **145**:541–2, 1988.
41 Perry, S.: Warning third parties at risk of AIDS: APA's policy is a barrier to treatment. *Hospital and Community Psychiatry* **40**:158–61, 1984.
42 Zonana, H.: Warning third parties at risk of AIDS: APA's policy is a reasonable approach. *Hospital and Community Psychiatry* **40**:162–4, 1984.
43 *Tarasoff v. Regents of the University of California*. 131 Cal. Rptr 14, 17 Cal. 3d 425, 551 P.2d 334 (1976).
44 Weinstock, R.: Confidentiality and the new duty to protect: the therapist's dilemma. *Hospital and Community Psychiatry* **39**:607–9, 1988.
45 Carlson, G. A., Greeman, M. and McClellan, T. A.: Management of HIV-positive psychiatric patients who fail to reduce high risk behaviors. *Hospital and Community Psychiatry* **40**:511–4, 1989.
46 Zonana, H., Norko, M., and Stier, D.: The AIDS patient on the psychiatric unit: ethical and legal issues. *Psychiatric Annals* **18**:587–93, 1988.
47 Price, R. W., Sidtis, J. J., and Navia, B. A.: The AIDS-generation complex, in *AIDS and the nervous system*, ed. M. G. Rosenblum. New York, Raven, 1988.
48 Green, J. and Stewart, A.: Ethical issues in child and adolescent psychiatry. *Journal of Medical Ethics* **13**:5–11, 1987.
49 Erikson, E.: Psychoanalysis and ethics—avowed and unavowed. *International Review of Psychoanalysis* **13**:409–15.
50 Kolansky, S. K.: Personal communication, 1989.

51 Lipton, E. L.: Considerations concerning discussions and publication of case histories—delivered at the meeting of the American Psychoanalytic Association. New York, 17 December 1988.

52 Perr, I. N.: Confidentiality and consent in psychiatric treatment of minors. *Journal of Legal Medicine* **4**:9–13, 1976.

53 Kobocow, B., McGuire, J. M., and Blau, B. I.: The influence of confidentiality conditions on self disclosure of early adolescents. *Professional Psychology* **14**:435–43, 1983.

54 Slovenko, R.: Group psychotherapy: privileged communication and confidentiality. *Journal of Psychiatry and Law* **5**:405–66, 1977.

55 Gutheil, T. G. and Appelbaum, P. S.: *Clinical handbook of psychiatry and law.* New York, McGraw-Hill, 1982, Chapter 1.

56 Davis, K. L.: Is confidentiality in group counseling realistic? *Personnel and Guidance Journal* **58**:197–201, 1980.

57 Hines, P. M. and Hare-Mustin: Ethical concerns in family therapy. *Professional Psychology* **9**:165–71, 1978.

58 Margolin, G.: Ethical and legal considerations in marital and family therapy. *American Psychologist* **37**:788–801, 1982.

59 Stein, M. H.: Writing about psychoanalysis. *Journal of the American Psychoanalytic Association* **36**:105–24, 1988.

60 DeBell, D. E.: A critical digest of the literature on psychoanalytic supervision. *Journal of the American Psychoanalytic Association* **11**:546–75, 1963.

61 Cavenar, J. O., Rhoades, E. J., and Sullivan, J. L.: Ethical and legal aspects of supervision. *Bulletin of the Menninger Clinic* **44**:15–22, 1980.

62 Hassenfeld, I N.: Ethics and the role of the supervision of psychotherapy. *Journal of Psychiatric Education* **11**:73–7, 1987.

63 Betcher, R. W. and Zinberg, N. E.: Supervision and privacy in psychotherapy training. *American Journal of Psychiatry* **145**:796–803, 1988.

64 Scharff, D. E.: Personal communication, 1973.

65 Dulchin, J. and Segal, A. J.: The ambiguity of confidentiality in a psychoanalytic institute. *Psychiatry* **45**:13–25, 1982.

66 Dulchin, J. and Segal, A. J.: Third party confidences: the uses of information in a psychoanalytic institute. *Psychiatry* **45**:27–37, 1982.

67 Kernberg, O. F.: Institutional problems of psychoanalytic education. *Journal of the American Psychoanalytic Association* **34**:799–834, 1986.

# 16

# Ethics and child psychiatry

*Philip Graham*

## Introduction

Many ethical issues of importance in mental health and illness in adults are also of relevance in the child. However, there is a considerable number of issues special to children, and it is these that will be emphasized in this chapter. Certain broad differences of principle will first be outlined, and consideration will then be given to diagnosis, treatment, child protection, the child and the law, research, and teaching.

The child's welfare is the responsibility of his parent or parents. He is assumed to be under the control of his parents, and this applies to health care as well as to other aspects of the child's life. Ethical issues frequently arise for the child psychiatrist when parents are not exercising their responsibility for the child's welfare appropriately, or when the child, though still the parent's responsibility, is not in fact in their control. Parents may not look after their children properly for a variety of reasons, and often many factors are pertinent in an individual case. It is important to remember also that there may be genuine conflict between the child's interests and those of his parents. For example, the interests of a mother with schizophrenia might well best be served by her continuing to look after her child, but the child's interests might require that a substitute placement be found as soon as possible. In contrast, a severely aggressive child might be best looked after at home from his point of view; but the mental health of his parents might be best served by his removal. Psychiatrists, psychologists, and paediatricians not infrequently find themselves in an ethical dilemma posed by these considerations.

Further complexities in ethical issues concerning children stem from the fact that, in childhood, intelligence and moral judgement are in a state of constant development.[1] The child's increasing understanding as he matures means that those concerned need continually to reappraise this capacity when decisions affecting his welfare are required. In the mentally handicapped child (and adult) a prolonged, sometimes permanent state of immaturity of understanding and moral judgement exists. Here it seems appropriate to take account of mental rather than chronological age when deciding how much weight should be given to the child's own contributions.

Children are subject to different constraints from those experienced by adults. Compulsory schooling and the prohibition of full-time paid employment are examples. Such rules and regulations are seen by adults as necessary for the process of socialization; but it is important to acknowledge not only that older children themselves may, not unreasonably at times, take up negative attitudes towards these constraints, but also that many adults are ambivalent about the values to which children are directed. These broader issues relating to the status of the child, socialization, and values will not be discussed further in this chapter, but they are of general importance.

# Diagnosis

Various aspects of the diagnostic process in child psychiatry (and indeed in psychiatry in general) have been called into question from both a practical and an ethical point of view. Concerns have been expressed in particular over the negative effect of specific diagnostic labels, and over the value and justification of screening programmes to identify disturbed and slow-learning children.

## The diagnostic process

Although diagnosis has long been accepted by many psychiatrists as a central feature of medical and psychiatric procedure in childhood, opinion has differed regarding the proper nature of the diagnostic process and the value attributed to it. The need to classify disorders is clearly necessary as a form of shorthand communication between professionals and as a pointer to particular treatment; but there has been increasing dissatisfaction with the notion that a diagnostic label is anything like an adequate guide to management. Thus Rutter[2] comments: 'The decision regarding care or placement must take into account social impairment, persistence of problems and availability of suitable treatments as well as the diagnosis of type of disorder. Not all people with a particular disorder require the same action and individual differences must be taken into account so that services are tailored to individual needs (rather than slotting individuals into pigeon holes which offer a diagnosis cum treatment package).' A diagnostic process which does not entail obtaining information along these lines is incomplete and unsatisfactory as a basis for action.

Therefore psychiatrists who give an opinion having only obtained an incomplete picture are in a doubtful ethical position. Two problems arise here. The first is that lack of time and pressure of work often mean that the psychiatrist is faced with difficult choices—seeing a few patients properly (and leaving others unseen), or a larger number incompletely. Secondly, some forms of therapy require the patient or family rather than the psychiatrist to set the pace of the sharing of information. Protagonists of these approaches suggest that 'rushing' family members, and asking leading questions, merely raises resistances inhibiting the transmission of accurate information. There is some work available, however, to suggest that such fears are misplaced.[3]

*Diagnostic labelling*

Ethical concerns about the effects of diagnostic labelling revolve around two main issues—the use of inaccurate, inappropriate, or misleading labels, and the potential negative effect of a label on the quality of the child's life.

The debate about inappropriate labelling has centred mainly around the use of the terms 'hyperkinetic syndrome', 'attention-deficit hyperactivity', and 'conduct-disorder', to describe states in children whose 'disability' can arguably be seen as unwillingness to conform to the norms of behaviour regarded as desirable by their parents and teachers;[4] but the issues are relevant to other diagnoses. Inability to concentrate, overactivity, impersistence, and disruptive behaviour are indeed statistically somewhat loosely associated with minor electroencephalographic abnormalities and other signs of neurophysiological dysfunction; but in many cases the causal nature of this association has not been adequately established. Strong criticisms have been mounted[5,6] over the alleged use of medical labels to describe social problems, and of the consequent tendency, to be discussed below, to prescribe medication as a form of social control. Box,[6] for example, referred to the 'increasing employment of medical solutions to school problems which are essentially moral, legal and social', and accuses the school medical system of attempting to screen, prevent, and treat non-organic behaviour disagreements.

Ethical problems related to labelling are not limited to diagnoses such as attention-deficit hyperactivity and conduct-disorder in which social norms are contravened. The application of a diagnosis implies the presence of pathology, and the assumption of pathology may be misleading and indeed unhelpful in a wide range of situations in which it is currently assumed to be present. A teenage girl who is sad, miserable and anxious, off her food, and insomniac following the break-up of a precious relationship with a boyfriend may not be helped if a psychiatrist makes a diagnosis of major depressive disorder and prescribes antidepressant medication, rather than providing support, understanding, and counselling. Of course a diagnosis of depression should not inevitably lead to the use of medication; but the reality is that shortage of time, the expectations of patients, and the persuasive effect of drug-company literature mean that this is often the outcome. The medicalization of misery is of course not just an ethical issue in child psychiatry; but there are special dangers in childhood, for if a pattern of medicalizing feelings is established in childhood, there is every reason that it will continue into adulthood.

The ethical position of the child psychiatrist involved in the diagnosis of behaviour problems which largely revolve around deviant and troublesome behaviour is certainly fraught with difficulty. It is probably easier if the psychiatrist limits his attention to those severe disorders which, one might assume, would result in maladaptation even to a better than average, if not to an optimal, domestic or school environment. Many would also argue that the psychiatrist's task when faced with nonconformity and deviance involves not only adequate assessment of the child, but also a full appraisal of the environment in which the child is apparently, and perhaps only apparently, creating difficulties. Assessment of a child who shows disruptive school behaviour should therefore include a consideration of the teaching methods used and of the means applied to achieve class-room control. These issues are further discussed later in relation to treatment.

The negative effects of the application of labels are fully discussed by Hobbs,[7,8] who forcefully makes the point that a diagnostic tag like 'mental retardation' can stick to a child for life, and adversely affect his opportunities. However, labels can obviously exert positive as well as negative effects. A child upon whom inappropriate and unhelpful pressure has been placed may be given a learning programme much *more* suited to his needs and abilities once a label of 'brain-damage' has been attached to his disorder. Excellent facilities for autistic children may only open their doors to a child once this label has been assigned to him. Further, the use of labels can be viewed as a pragmatic as well as an ethical issue. Is there good evidence that labels act to the detriment of children? Findings are not clear-cut. In a frequently quoted study conducted by Rosenthal and Jacobson,[9] children were given randomly assigned intelligence scores which were then passed on to their teachers. At the end of an academic year children who had been allocated low scores were achieving significantly less well than those allocated high scores. However, various attempts to replicate the study[10] have not obtained such clear-cut findings, and even in the original study the results held for younger but not for older children. Research has also been done on the effects of labelling children as offenders, by comparing the outcome of boys charged and found guilty of certain offences with that of boys who had shown equally serious antisocial behaviour, but who had not been involved in criminal proceedings. Here the evidence[11,12] tends to support the hypothesis of negative effects from labelling.

Most psychiatrists would be appropriately wary of the use of diagnostic labels when communicating with people whose attitude to such labels was uncertain or unknown. In an interview with a parent or teacher, a psychiatrist should regard it as an essential part of his job to explain the terms he uses and to ensure that these are understood, at least at the time of the interview. I must admit, however, that this is a counsel of perfection; in practice once a report has been dispatched the psychiatrist often has little control over the way his words are interpreted. The issue of confidentiality is, of course, of considerable relevance in this context.

## Screening

With improved resources and better screening instruments there has been an increased tendency to screen groups of children for the presence of developmental delay and behaviour disturbance. Again there is a danger both that children will be inappropriately labelled and that expectations of services may be raised in parents' minds when in fact none are available. I would regard it as necessary to ensure that those involved in screening programmes, including parents, are made aware of the limitations of screening methods. Moreover it is unethical to institute such programmes unless services are adequate to treat children who are identified as having some problem. These types of issues have been taken so seriously that recent authoritative advice[13] suggests that it is inappropriate to screen routinely for behaviour problems in the general population. In my view it would be most unfortunate if such advice led to the abandonment of the continuation of behaviour screening, so long as there is careful monitoring of its effects.

## Treatment

Ethical questions in the provision of treatment in child psychiatry are of major importance because many forms of treatment currently offered have uncertain benefits.[14] Where existing therapy is clearly beneficial, as, for example, in the use of the bell and pad in nocturnal enuresis, consideration of ethical issues is limited to the adequate explanation of side-effects and the need for the psychiatrist's awareness of the dangers of symptom-suppression or symptom-substitution. When, as in the case of the example given, these aspects have been investigated, and it has been concluded that the issues are straightforward, ethical factors will have been adequately dealt with. Unfortunately most treatment in child psychiatry does not fall into this desirable category, and a careful assessment of the risks and benefits involved is necessary.

Many psychiatrists believe—though their belief is regrettably little acted upon—that the application of treatment of unproved efficacy brings with it an ethical obligation to conduct evaluative research. Certainly it can be convincingly argued that the lack of this research is morally less defensible than the conduct of research using untreated control subjects, and this issue is further discussed in Chapter 19. As the situation exists at present, the various forms of treatment in children produce problems of their own, and these different forms will therefore be considered separately.

*Medication*

The use of stimulant medication in children presenting with overactivity, distractibility, impersistence, learning disabilities, and other behavioural or cognitive deficits is partly a result and partly a cause of the delineation of the hyperkinetic syndrome and attention-deficit hyperactivity, the nature of which has already been mentioned in this chapter. It is well-established that methylphenidate and dexamphetamine-sulphate can produce improved performance in learning tasks in laboratory research, and that they can also reduce distractibility, impersistence, and disruptive behaviour in the class-room.[15,16] This effectiveness is not limited to children diagnosed as hyperactive, but has been shown, at least in the laboratory situation, to enhance performance in normal children.

The widespread use of stimulant drugs has nevertheless been criticized, especially by Schrag and Divoky[5] in the United States, and by Box[6] in Britain. Their arguments are similar to those that have been employed against the use of the hyperkinetic syndrome label, and as these have been discussed earlier they will not be rehearsed now. However, the objections to the label are clearly reinforced if, as has been contended, one result is that children are inappropriately drugged into mindless conformity by the use of medication. Thus, according to Box, 'school children by the million in America, and by tens of thousands in this country (the United Kingdom) are being put on long-term programmes of drug therapy simply because their behaviour does not fit in with the requirements of schools'. Although the figures quoted are in all likelihood grossly exaggerated, there is no doubt that a very large number of American children, and perhaps a small but not insignificant number in Britain, are treated with stimulant drugs in order to reduce behaviour which, *inter alia*, is creating difficulties for teachers and other pupils.

Sedgwick[17] pointed out, in a thoughtful reply to Box, that the question of the number of children on medication is largely irrelevant. If the treatment *is* effective, the smaller number of children being treated in Britain may be due not to any praiseworthy concern for children, but to the neglect of the needs of the poorly achieving child. The first issue to determine is whether, for the individual child, the disadvantages of medication are clearly outweighed by the benefits. Further, the possible change in attitude of other children, parents, and teachers if the behaviour of the treated child is improved cannot be regarded as unimportant. Especially if behavioural change can be achieved in no other way, the diminution of rejection by teachers and peers as a result of reduced disruptiveness on the part of the child could be seen as a clear benefit to him. If this benefit, however, was not accompanied by improved learning ability, or was achieved only at the cost of the child's becoming depressed and apathetic on the drug (a not infrequent occurrence), the use of medication might well be regarded as unjustified.

The criticism levelled most ferociously against the use of stimulants is less pertinent than other points that should be made. The first of these relates to the efficacy of alternative forms of treatment. Wolraich and his colleagues[18] have demonstrated that for certain types of behaviour associated with the 'hyperactive child' syndrome, behaviour-modification can be as effective as, and in some cases superior to, drug therapy, and it is now authoritatively suggested[19] that cognitive-behavioural therapy is the first choice for motivated children of normal or superior intelligence. Obviously dangers of stimulant medication, such as medicalization of social problems, side-effects, and dependence, should lead to cautious and judicious use of drugs, and only after other less harmful measures have failed. The second issue concerns the possibility that the use of medication may discourage the therapist from trying to understand the child's feelings and behaviour. Finally, there is the question of what degree of severity of the problem justifies the prescribing of stimulants. Differences of opinion on this last point probably account for the hitherto much more widespread use of stimulants in the United States than in Britain.[20] Most British child psychiatrists reserve medication for severely over-active disruptive children, even in the knowledge that stimulants improve concentration and performance in less severe cases and in normal children. In so far as this policy has been rationally considered by British psychiatrists it is probably the result of a calculation that the known and unknown risks of medication outweigh potential benefits in all but the seriously handicapped child. The view is also taken that it is no part of the psychiatrist's job to smooth out normal variations in learning ability, especially when a lower level of concentration is often accompanied by greater vivacity, curiosity, and explorativeness, all of which have their own appeal, and may be lost with exposure to medication. Failure to demonstrate[21] long-term improvement in learning ability or behaviour as a result of the use of drugs is a further discouragement to their application in less severely affected children.

Before leaving the subject of physical methods of treatment, it is worth mentioning the use of more drastic procedures such as electroconvulsive therapy and temporal lobectomy. Again the questions of efficacy and risk require much thought, particularly in the light of the possibility of long-term and perhaps permanent damage resulting from these physical manipulations of the brain. If a child's psychiatric condition, however, is very severe, it is unreasonable to place these measures out of his reach merely because of age. On a visit to the Soviet Union I was assured that the use of electroconvulsive therapy was illegal in children under the age of sixteen; if this is the case, the admittedly extremely rare but not unknown case of a pubescent child with a prolonged catatonic illness would be deprived of the most effective available treatment. Although the presence of seriously aggressive behaviour in a child with intractable temporal lobe epilepsy may appropriately be regarded as an additional reason for considering temporal lobectomy, the use of psychosurgery must surely be regarded as a highly questionable procedure. Aggression as an indication for psychosurgery is discussed further in Chapter 10.

Surgical sterilization of promiscuous mentally handicapped teenagers has also been the subject of controversy. In Britain the Department of Health and Social Security has recommended a consultation procedure before sterilization is undertaken in a child under the age of sixteen.[22] A report of a working group on medical/ethical problems[23] suggests that this recommendation should also apply to mentally handicapped people over the age of sixteen. The working group concluded that, in a female, only 'proven parental incapacity' (a woman has had a child and signally failed to provide adequate parental care) coupled with an inability to manage contraceptives constitutes sufficient justification for sterilization. It suggests that male promiscuity should be controlled by appropriate drugs rather than by surgery.

Many American states have now enacted legislation to deal with this matter. There is also a need for legislation in the UK (and elsewhere) on this issue, as case-law is in some confusion, and the matter should probably no longer be left to be decided by individual judges.[24]

## Psychotherapy

Individual and family psychotherapy are probably the most common forms of treatment used in child psychiatry, and there is evidence for their efficacy in a range of emotional disorders and certain psychosomatic conditions.[14] Ethical problems facing the psychotherapist include the uncertain benefits and the danger of the subtle indoctrinating nature of the techniques used, and the potential neglect of, and lack of respect for, parental concerns (in individual child therapy) or individual development (in family therapy). Green and Stewart[25] have considered ethical issues in relation to treatment in child and adolescent psychiatry in some detail.

The uncertainty of psychotherapy's benefit provokes the question of the degree to which parents and their children should be informed about the chance of being helped by this treatment. Honest disclosure is advantageous in that it enables parents to decide whether they are prepared to accept treatment in the light of the costs involved (for example, therapists' fees, time off work, the child's time out of school). The issue may prove more complicated, since parents sometimes opt out of therapy ostensibly for these material reasons, but in fact because they suspect, perhaps justifiably, that therapy will be painful to them and to the child. There are advantages in the therapist's pointing to the likelihood of such pain occurring at the onset of treatment. The usefulness of relatively brief, focused treatment embarked upon on a 'contract' basis for a specified number of sessions is attractive; but the view of many therapists is that not all psychiatric conditions in childhood are likely to respond to such brief measures. The issue is clearer where it has been reasonably established, as in the case of interpretative psychoanalytic therapy for childhood autism, that a treatment is probably of no benefit.[26]

In this case it is obligatory for the therapist to point out the evidence explicitly, and, if he undertakes such intervention, to indicate its experimental and non-therapeutic nature.

The indoctrinating quality of different forms of psychotherapy—the overt or covert process in which the therapist imposes his values on his patient—has been frequently discussed (for example, in relation to child-guidance work, by Blumenfeld[27]). The issues here in the therapy of children and families are scarcely different from those in the treatment of adults (see Chapter 8). In so far as family therapy—especially in work with disturbed children—is becoming increasingly popular, it is worth examining some of the specific ethical problems associated with this form of treatment; this issue has recently been the subject of a substantial systematic review.[28] Family therapists, by virtue of their emphasis on the need to treat individuals as family members, risk undermining existing family structures that do not fit into their preconceived notions as to how a family should function. It is, for example, common practice for family therapists to insist that the father attends treatment sessions. His participation may lead to an alteration in family functioning, whereby his paternal role and authority are undermined; this is especially the case in working-class families, in which division of responsibilities between parents tends to be clearly defined. Most family therapists are well aware of this danger; but a danger it remains. Many parents are reluctant to divulge criticism of their children to the therapist in front of them, and hesitate to do so. The practice of family therapists, however, is to encourage expression of such negative feelings, in the reasonable belief that the child knows what the parent feels anyway, and that unless there is an honest acknowledgement of these aspects of communication, little progress in improving family relationships is likely. The risk exists that parents will develop a habit of negative thinking about their children which they would otherwise not have adopted. Another issue concerns the therapist's use of certain potent procedures. Techniques such as family sculpting and paradoxical injunction in family therapy may sometimes be practised without the therapist's awareness of the degree to which he is engaged in paternalistic manipulation.[29]

I do not need to emphasize the importance of clinical research in contributing to a greater understanding of the risks and benefits of family therapy, which in turn will no doubt clarify the ethical problems mentioned.

Finally, the limiting nature of each form of psychotherapy when practised in an exclusive manner warrants comment. In individual therapy with children it is common practice for material disclosed by the child to be kept secret from the parents on the grounds that the child will not produce this material once he knows his parents will be informed. This exclusion raises anxieties in them, and it is arguable whether therapy of this type should be undertaken unless concomitant discussion occurs with parents and they are fully agreeable. There is a danger that parents are persuaded to consent when they may be exercising accurate judgement in their concern that their child's individual therapy will be associated with an undermining of their own authority. A converse problem arises in family therapy when, because the child is not given an opportunity to express his feelings privately to the therapist, he may not disclose his concerns about, for example, physical violence to himself or between his parents, or sexual abuse, which may be at the root of his problems. Many practitioners who have a preference for either individual or family therapy acknowledge the advantages in providing an opportunity for both individual and family sessions to occur, at least during the initial phase of assessment.

## Behaviour-modification

Ethical aspects of behaviour-modification have been usefully discussed in the context of its application in single-case research design,[30] and in treating problems in gender-identity. In gender-identity treatment, Rosen and his colleagues[31] make the point that parents and mental health professionals often have to decide whether a particular outcome can really be regarded as beneficial. In general the element of manipulation involved in behaviour-modification is more overt than in psychotherapy, and may therefore, paradoxically, be less open to unconscious abuse. On the other hand, the very effectiveness of the procedures involved, as, for example, in the achievement of class-room control with disruptive and aggressive pupils, raises additional questions similar to those I have discussed when considering medication. Achieving an atmosphere of tranquillity in the class-room through behavioural methods (or with drugs), can hardly be regarded as justified unless, as a result, improved opportunities are created for learning, which enable children who are the target of these therapeutic measures to benefit as well as their class-room colleagues. Intervention which leads to behaviour control without positive effects on the children towards whom it is directed, is clearly open to objection.

## Special educational and hospital in-patient provision

While until recently the availability of separate educational provision for disturbed and slow-learning children was seen as advantageous to such children, and indeed as a form of positive discrimination, attitudes have swung noticeably. It is now thought preferable to educate children with exceptional needs as far as possible alongside ordinary children, in order to ensure minimal stigmatization and as much of a normal school experience as is feasible. In the United States, this changed attitude is reflected in various State and Federal laws (for example, Public Law 94/142); and in Britain in similar legislation (for example, the 1981 Education Act) and in official government documents such as the *Warnock Report*.[32] Nevertheless there is almost universal agreement that *some* special separate provision continues to be necessary and desirable, at least for severely handicapped children. In so far as psychiatrists have responsibility for advising on educational needs, they are involved in decisions which have a distinctly ethical component, regarding, for example, the desirability of a separate school placement for a disruptive child who is benefiting from his current education, but is disturbing others; or the wisdom of placing a child in a special residential school, because, while special schooling is necessary, the limited resources of the education authority have led to no suitable day placement being available.

There is often considerable, and, I would say, highly understandable, pressure from teachers on psychiatrists for them to use their influence to facilitate the removal of extremely difficult children and adolescents to special educational or even hospital institutions. Conflicts between health, education, and social service departments as to where responsibility for the placement of a difficult child lies often place the child psychiatrist in a problematic ethical dilemma.[33] In this situation the psychiatrist needs to ask a number of questions, and to ensure that they are being honestly answered by all concerned—including, of course, himself! Have all possible measures been tried in order to keep the child in an ordinary school? For example, has the employment of additional staff been envisaged? If this possibility has been rejected as too costly an alternative, has the local authority concerned made realistic comparisons between the actual costs and those of a special-school placement? Will placement outside the ordinary school really help the child? If not, has this been stated openly to the parents and teachers concerned, so that there is no doubt in anyone's mind for whose benefit removal from the ordinary environment is planned? How aware is the child himself of the real reasons for the proposed placement? Bruggen and his co-workers[34] have shown that posing these sort of questions, in relation to proposed admission to an adolescent psychiatric unit, can actually form a focus for therapeutic work. Although many psychiatrists will feel that this approach is inappropriate in some clinical situations, there is no doubt that it can in others shed light on the real reasons for parents' requesting admission for their child or adolescent.

The question of involuntary commitment of children to hospital on grounds of mental illness has been discussed by Hoggett[35] in relation to British procedure, by Roth[36] in the United States, and more generally by Tooley.[37] In Britain, unless the child's parents have legally forfeited their rights, their consent to commitment cannot be overridden by the contrary wishes of their child if he is under the age of sixteen.

Although the UK 1983 Mental Health Act applies to children and adolescents, in practice its provisions are rarely used for children under the age of sixteen years. Nevertheless, ethical issues do arise in relation to articulate young adolescents who take a different view from their parents and psychiatrists about the need for in-patient treatment. In these circumstances, it seems ethically appropriate to listen carefully to what the young people have to say, to acknowledge the strength of their views, and then, in the light of what they say, to apply, in partnership with parents, the principles enunciated in the Mental Health Act concerning compulsory admission. Where parents refuse to allow treatment which is clearly necessary for the safety of their child (as, for example, in the case of a dehydrated and emaciated fourteen-year-old suffering from anorexia nervosa), then it seems both legally and ethically desirable to invoke legal powers available for the protection of children (in the UK by the use of Place of Safety or Care Orders) rather than mental health legislation.[35]

## Research

The lack of established knowledge about the cause, prevention, and effective treatment of child psychiatric disorders highlights the need for research to be vigorously pursued. Indeed it is not difficult to argue that, with current knowledge so slender, the conduct of research is ethically more justified than unevaluated clinical practice. Some practitioners who participate in both research and clinical work are more comfortable in their research activities than in applying treatment of dubious validity in possibly spurious attempts to alleviate suffering. The majority find validation in their clinical activities in the subjective sense of meaning and helpfulness they derive from their interaction with families and children. The ethical dilemma here is not special to child psychiatry.

Most ethical issues affecting research in children are similar to those which occur in adults, and are dealt with elsewhere in this book (see Chapter 19). However, there are special problems in children concerning the ethical principles that researchers should consider, as well as different issues in relation to informed consent. Helpful ethical guidelines in the conduct of research involving children have been recommended by working parties of the British Paediatric Association[38] and the Institute of Medical Ethics.[39] Although these working parties mainly concern themselves with research on physical disorders and physical methods of investigation, the principles they set forth are readily applicable to the study of psychiatric conditions and to the use of psychological techniques.

The chief principle which should underlie ethical judgements in research entails consideration of the risk–benefit ratio. Risks of causing 'physical disturbance, discomfort or pain or psychological disturbance for the child or his parents' are classified as negligible (less than those occurring in everyday life), minimal, more than minimal but not definitely harmful, and harmful. The main problem in psychological research is that it is extra-ordinarily difficult to assess risks in advance. A psychiatric interview (for example, in an epidemiological survey in which a child is asked among other items about his concerns, anxieties, and fantasies) could be seen, and indeed has been seen, either as a non-intrusive benign procedure involving negligible risk (compared for example to the everyday experiences of exposure to insensitive criticism from parents, teachers, and peers), or as a potentially highly disturbing event leading to prolonged distress because previously suppressed material is now exposed with little or no attempt to make it meaningful for the child. In general, follow-up studies suggest that research interviews with children are either experienced as trivial events or as pleasurable or helpful; but it would be surprising if the occasional child were not seriously upset. There do not appear to be any systematic studies along these lines, but there is no reason why this should be so. Smith,[40] for example, carried out a one year follow-up of a group of seven-year-old children who had been venepunctured for research purposes, and found very few after-effects. The results of systematic follow-up of psychiatric-research interviewing of children would be of great interest.

Another risk of research especially pertinent to children is the possibility that a treatment offered, which in normal clinical practice would not have been made available, might become associated with maladaptive behaviour which would not otherwise have occurred. Thus, an investigation involving the use of medication may lead to a habitual pattern of tablet-taking to solve problems of living. This particular problem has arisen in studies of the use of stimulants for over-activity and of hypnotics for sleep-disorders in infancy. The investigator has an obligation, when offering treatment that is not requested, to ensure that it is undertaken only where there is a strong likelihood of its being efficacious (unfortunately a rare event in child psychiatry), or where the parents (and the child if he is of sufficient age) are highly motivated to accept treatment. Thus, in one study of the value of hypnotics for severe sleep-disorder, only children whose parents were unambiguously motivated were entered in the trial.

The benefits of research can be considered in terms of whether they involve the child or family studied, or only other children. Research offering no benefit to the child—non-therapeutic research—is legal in English law,[41,42] and indeed without this type of work it would be impossible to establish norms on physiological and psychological parameters in children without problems. The value of knowledge which accrues from the investigation of normal children should not be underestimated; many a child with a temporary disturbance such as nocturnal enuresis has been saved intrusive and even harmful treatment by a knowledge of the wide prevalence of the condition in the general population, and of its good prognosis without intervention.

We face a major problem in applying the principle of the risk–benefit ratio because the magnitude of the benefit is always uncertain. Thus, a hypothesis regarding the aetiology of childhood autism might involve the examination of cerebro-spinal fluid. The likelihood of a positive finding might be exceedingly small; but, if such a result were obtained, understanding of the nature of the condition could be significantly advanced. The people most qualified to evaluate the chance of benefit are the investigators and their colleagues working in allied fields; but, for understandable reasons, they may be influenced by their enthusiasm for the work to over-estimate likely benefit and underestimate potential risk. It is for this reason, among others, that the establishment of ethical committees or similar bodies, whose task is to adjudicate as impartially as possible on the basis of the risk–benefit principle, is so essential. It is clearly important that, when ethical committees consider research involving children, at least some of their members should be aware of the special problems inherent in research in this age-group. The *Institute of Medical Ethics Report*[39] recommends that an ethics committee dealing with projects concerning children should require investigators to explain the research project to parents or guardians, and, where a project involves greater than minimal risk, to provide a brief, simply-written explanation to parents. In these circumstances consent should be obtained in writing. The committee's considered judgements are of particular relevance in the case of institutionalized mentally handicapped or mentally ill children, who may lack an independent advocate. An investigation, for example, of the administration of hepatitis virus to mentally handicapped children at Willowbrook State School was heavily criticized[43] on the grounds that the procedure was of no possible benefit to these children. The procedures adopted in the Willowbrook study would probably not have gained the acceptance of an independent scrutiny; the lesson learned is that investigators, even those with the best possible motivation of increasing knowledge and improving preventive measures, can be helped by independent guidance when their procedures appear even slightly questionable.

There is general agreement that parental consent should be obtained before any research procedure is carried out in children and adolescents under the age of sixteen. Consent should only be sought after a full explanation of what the research will entail, and this should involve an honest disclosure of both likely risk and potential benefit. No specific age has been established in Britain at which the child himself must provide consent in addition to his parents; but the Institute of Medical Ethics Working Party[39] pointed out that a large majority of children aged fourteen or over have the necessary competence to give consent, and that most children aged seven or over understand enough to be able to give or refuse assent. They recommended that non-therapeutic research procedures should not be carried out if a potential child subject aged seven to fourteen years refuses assent to it.

While the risk exists that children's altruistic motivations might be inappropriately 'played upon', there is perhaps an even greater danger that children may be debarred from altruistic activity because of the overprotective attitudes of adults. Moreover, where altruistic behaviour has occurred it may also be considered ethically desirable for public acknowledgement of this fact. For example, in an investigation involving the donation of deciduous teeth for estimation of their lead content the six- or seven-year-old children donors were given a badge depicting a child with a large dental gap, and the message 'I gave a tooth'. I would regard as ethically undesirable the situation in parts of the United States where clinical research involving children is virtually impossible because of an overriding concern for their rights. Advances in knowledge for the ultimate benefit of the afflicted necessitate inconvenience to be experienced by individuals who do not themselves suffer; and the privilege of participating in such activity should, I believe, not be denied to children who will benefit from the experience.

## Teaching

To be effective, clinical instruction sometimes requires live demonstration of diagnostic and treatment techniques. However, most psychiatrists would argue that situations in which children are interviewed about the nature of their feelings and problems in front of an audience of medical or other students are not ethically appropriate. The introduction of one-way screens and video-recording has made the demonstration of clinical skills and clinical phenomena less intrusive, but has brought its own ethical difficulties.

Clinical teaching should involve the minimum of interference, and parents (as well as children, to the limits of their understanding) should be informed of the status of observers, and of the degree of confidentiality that will be exercised. The opportunity to meet the observers behind one-way screens is important when there is a possibility that a student is personally acquainted with the child and family, especially if it is not clearly understood that acquaintances should not observe. Similarly, presentation of video material requires special concern in the case of children, since they may outgrow their problem, while a record of their abnormality is retained. Parents' consent to preservation of video-recordings should not be allowed to override the right of the child to decide the fate of the material when he reaches an age at which he is capable of appreciating its nature. Automatic destruction of video-recordings after a defined period, say five years, is another, perhaps more feasible, and preferable alternative.

One controversial aspect of teaching is the degree to which parents should be informed of the trainee status of doctors, social workers, psychologists, and psychotherapists who participate in the diagnosis or treatment of their children. It could, paradoxically, be argued that because some research findings indicate that trainees have greater success in certain conditions than their trained counterparts, parents should be warned if their children are to be seen by experienced professionals! Most child psychiatrists would agree that, as in other fields, where an establishment is used for training purposes parents should be informed of this fact, and assured that, if their children are to be seen by trainees, adequate supervision will be provided by experienced staff. The quality of this supervision is of course in itself an issue which has ethical implications.

## Child protection

The paramount requirement for normal emotional and intellectual development in children is parental care of high quality. Many ethical questions face the psychiatrist, when, for a variety of reasons, care has become or threatens to become of a kind which ranges from suboptimal to deplorable.

Concern regarding parents who are unable to provide adequate care and protection for their children raises numerous ethical issues, many of which may involve child and indeed general psychiatrists. Inadequacy of care is now usually classified according to the form of 'child-abuse' that is involved. The psychiatrist may well be involved in the assessment of any of these—physical abuse, sexual abuse, emotional neglect or abuse, or Munchausen's syndrome by proxy.

### Assessment and diagnosis

The diagnosis of physical abuse is usually within the province of the paediatrician, who will have to judge whether childhood injuries could have been accidentally caused or are more likely to have been deliberately inflicted. Paediatricians, social workers, and the police are likely to be involved in the initial stages of diagnosis of child sexual abuse, failure to thrive (a common accompaniment of emotional neglect), and Munchausen's syndrome by proxy. However psychiatrists, because of their special skills in interviewing and understanding family dynamics, may be involved in all of these situations.

A psychiatrist may become aware of the possibility of abuse as a result of information he obtains during treatment. A girl may, for example, give hints of a sexual relationship with her father. In these circumstances, the psychiatrist is under a duty to impart such information to a colleague, usually a member of the social services department, so that further assessment can be considered. Professional confidentiality is, of course, breached by such action; but it is encouraged by professional organizations concerned with confidentiality issues.[44] It is important to remember that, in the UK at any rate, responsibility for the safety of the child lies not with the doctor or psychologist, but with the social services department. Where unresolved conflict occurs, the final responsibility lies with the judicial system. It is not ethical for a doctor or psychologist to take responsibility for the safety of a child without involving those who have statutory duties in this respect. Another difficult ethical issue arises when paediatricians suspect abuse, but have no clear proof, and believe that the interviewing skills of a psychiatrist may be helpful in clarification. In these circumstances, should parents be told of the true reasons for a psychiatric referral, or is it ethically acceptable to indicate only that the psychiatrist is being asked to give an opinion on the mental health of the child or the parents? Most would believe that referrals should not occur for covert reasons; but if the well-being of the child is the paramount consideration, the issue is not a simple one.

A psychiatrist may be requested for an opinion on the likelihood of abuse where previous interviewing has failed to elicit information on which a clear judgement, one way or the other, can be based. This is particularly likely to arise with young children in whom sexual abuse is suspected, when skilled psychiatric interview, and other techniques such as specialized doll play, may be helpful. The psychiatrist does however need to be aware of the limitations of information obtained in fantasy play, to avoid leading questions as far as possible, and to consider carefully the various alternative reasons why children might provide circumstantial information. Professionals using these techniques need special training, and this should include some consideration of the importance of their own attitudes in coming to conclusions. Both denial and over-eagerness to identify abuse have clearly led to a significant number of diagnostic mistakes in the past. Children do make false accusations, although this is probably unusual; and, more commonly, professionals who prefer not to listen have failed to respond to calls for help from children who have clearly indicated the fact that they are being, or have been, seriously abused. Ethical issues in relation to sexual abuse have been considered by Jones.[45]

If abuse is diagnosed, and in other situations such as marital breakdown where a child's future care is concerned, a psychiatrist may be involved in providing advice on the best placement for the child. Abusing parents only suffer from formal mental illness in a relatively small minority of cases; but personality problems and difficulties in making and maintaining close relationships are very common in parents whose quality of child care is called in question. In assessing 'fitness to parent'[46,47] general psychiatrists therefore have to do a great deal more than decide whether or not the parent has a mental illness. In cases of marital dispute over the custody of children, and in circumstances where children have been removed from their biological parents and there is disagreement as to whether they should be returned, child psychiatrists also need to take into account a wide variety of factors; among these the child's attachments, the potential capacity of the adult concerned to provide long-term affectionate care, and his willingness to acknowledge responsibility for his actions in the past and to accept professional help in the future, are of special relevance.

Psychiatrists may be asked to provide an opinion by a wide variety of different agencies—social service departments, parents, foster-parents, solicitors acting for one parent in a marital dispute; but it is important that they remember that their first duty is to the child. In most countries, as in the UK, this task is made easier by the fact that the law insists that where there is a conflict of interests between parents and children, the child's interest is paramount. One way in which psychiatrists can ensure their reports are used appropriately is to insist before they give an opinion that, whatever their findings, their report must be made available in full to all those involved in a dispute.

The psychiatrist may be consulted by a couple, one of whom has had a psychiatric problem, who are seeking advice about embarking on parenthood. More commonly, he may not be consulted by them, but find himself uncertain as whether to discourage, for example, a husband and wife whose severe personality disorders, in all likelihood, disqualify them from competent parenthood. Most psychiatrists are reluctant to accept as part of their job the provision of such unsolicited advice. I regard it as reasonable to promote discussion about parenthood, since inevitably those couples most in need of discouragement are least likely to seek or heed advice.

A related ethical dilemma occurs when a psychiatric opinion is sought in a decision about termination of pregnancy. Psychiatrists opposed to termination on religious grounds may regard it as necessary to disclose their views before examining the patients; but unfortunately this does not always occur. Since psychiatric grounds for termination are open to wide interpretation, it is worthwhile from a child psychiatrist's point of view to indicate the dismal social and psychological outcome of children whose mothers requested termination and were refused it.[48]

Serious psychiatric disorders in the post-partum period pose ethical problems when the interests of mother and new-born conflict. Close contact between the two may benefit the mother but place the child at risk, resulting in a most difficult situation. A knowledge of the bonding process may assist the psychiatrist who faces this problem. A realistic appraisal of the mother's capacity to provide adequate parenting in the future is also important. A large body of psychiatric opinion holds that the child's interests are paramount. Thus, if a mother suffering from chronic schizophrenia or a severe personality disorder is judged as probably unfit to provide adequate parental care, the child's interests will be served best by a prompt move towards permanent substitute care, involving long-term fostering or, preferably, adoption. An ethical problem is associated with the possibility, however slight, that the mother will cope and wishes to keep the child. Should she be encouraged? There is in these circumstances an undesirable tendency for a doctor who has known the mother for some time, and become identified with her interests, to overlook the likely fate of the child.

## The child and the law

Since ethical aspects of forensic psychiatry are covered elsewhere in this book (see Chapter 18), mention will be made here only of issues which relate specifically to children. I should first note that the responsibility accorded to children for criminal offences they have committed varies with age. Thus in England and Wales a child under the age of ten cannot be charged with any criminal offence, although over the age of eight suspicion of an offence can be grounds for instituting proceedings which may result in the child's removal from parental care. Between ten and thirteen years children can be charged with a criminal offence, but it must be proved that they knew their actions were wrong. From the age of fourteen a child is assumed to be responsible for his acts, and from seventeen years he or she is subject to the full process of the law.

Psychiatrists who advise the court on how to deal with a child offender are of course likely to be less concerned with the retributive and deterrent element of the judicial decision than in the question of whether the court is acting in the interests of the child and his or her family. It is a matter of argument whether the psychiatric report should be limited to information relevant to the making of this decision, or whether psychiatrists should impart any knowledge (assuming they have it) of the nature of the offence which might lead the court to alter its view of the offence's gravity. Most psychiatrists would feel that, in order to provide a report which will prove helpful to the court and to the child, they need to interview the parents as well as the child, and also to have access to any reports from his school. In circumstances where information from parents is obtained by social workers or probation officers, the psychiatrist's view will be limited by lack of direct contact. The status of reports based on such partial material might be regarded as dubious, and it is therefore essential for psychiatrists to indicate the basis on which they are providing their opinions.

It is often unclear to the child and family, and sometimes regrettably to the psychiatrist, for whose benefit a psychiatric report is being prepared. If the court's question is whether the child is or was suffering at the time the offence was committed from some form of mental disorder, the report may well be seen as serving the court. If on the other hand the need is for information to enable the court to understand the background, the report is more likely to be of benefit to the child. Most psychiatrists who prepare reports appreciate that their submissions may serve both purposes, and make this explicit to the child and his family. In the case of a conflict of interests the interests of the child should take priority over those of the court, as long as this does not involve untruthfulness or any danger to society.

An interesting issue which may involve the court and is specific to childhood is school truancy. Truancy in general is the business of the school welfare officer and the court; but school-refusal stemming from anxiety lies within the province of the child psychiatrist, the school psychologist, and the social worker. A situation does arise in school-refusal in which collusion between parents and child is so great, and the prospects of successful treatment by conventional psychiatric means are so small, that the psychiatrist may wish to institute legal action in order to achieve an enforced separation. The ethical basis for bringing legal action is fragile; psychiatrists should therefore limit their actions to a clear statement that they can see no objection on psychiatric grounds why legal measures should not be adopted.

## Conclusion

Ethical issues concerning the mental health of children need to be seen in a broad context. The fact that children are developing organisms gradually becoming capable of taking greater responsibility is relevant not just to mental health issues, but also to physical health, education, and social welfare. The same can be said of dilemmas posed by the fact that the state invests parents with responsibility for the care of children, but that many parents provide most unsatisfactory care for their children—who, nevertheless, may well love them, need them, and be unwilling easily to accept substitutes for them. There is an increasing and welcome tendency, when decisions need to be taken, for children's views to be canvassed, heard, and taken into account. This tendency can only work for the benefit of children, who, by the time they become adults, should feel competent to make decisions for themselves, as well as to entrust gradually increasing responsibility for decision-making to their own children as they, in turn, become mature enough to do so. It is a principal task of mental health professionals to facilitate this process.

## References

1 Graham, P.: Moral development, in *Developmental psychiatry*, ed. M. Rutter. London, Heinemann, 1980, pp. 339–53.

2 Rutter, M.: Classification, in *Child psychiatry, modern approaches*, ed. M. Rutter and L. Hersov. Oxford, Blackwell, 1976, pp. 359–84.

3 Cox, A., Hopkinson, K. F., and Rutter, M.: Psychiatric interview techniques. II Naturalistic study: eliciting factual information. *British Journal of Psychiatry* **138**:283–91, 1981.

4 Bosco, J. J. and Robin, S. S. (ed.): *The hyperactive child and stimulant drugs*. Chicago, University of Chicago Press, 1976.

5 Schrag, P. and Divoky, D.: *The myth of the hyperactive child*. New York, Pantheon, 1975.

6 Box, S.: Hyperactivity: the scandalous silence. *New Society*, 1 December 1977, pp. 548–60.

7 Hobbs, N.: *The future of children*. San Francisco, Jossey-Bass, 1975.

8 Hobbs, N.: *Issues in the classification of children*. San Francisco, Jossey-Bass, 1975.

9 Rosenthal, R. and Jacobson, J.: *Pygmalion in the classroom: teacher expectation and pupils' intellectual development*. New York, Holt, Rinehart, and Winston, 1968.

10 Brophy, J. E. and Good, T. L.: *Teacher–student relationships: causes and consequences*. New York, Holt, Rinehart, and Winston, 1974.

11 Gold, M. and Williams, J. R.: National study of the aftermath of apprehension. *Prospectus* **3**:3–12, 1969.

12 West, D. J.: *Delinquency: its roots, careers and prospects*. London, Heinemann Educational, 1982.

13 Hall, D. M. B. (ed.): *Health for all children*. Oxford, Oxford University Press, 1989.

14 Graham, P.: *Child psychiatry: a developmental approach*. Oxford, Oxford University Press, 1986.

15 Cantwell, D. and Carlson, G.: Stimulants, in *Paediatric psychopharmacology: the use of behaviour modifying drugs in children*, ed. J. S. Werry. New York, Brunner–Mazel, 1978.

16 Conners, C. and Werry, J. S.: Pharmacotherapy, in *Psychopathological disorders of childhood*, ed. H. Quay and J. S. Werry. New York, Wiley, 1979, pp. 336–86.

17 Sedgwick, P.: *New Society*, 5 January 1978, p. 31.

18 Wolraich, M., Drummond, T., Salomon, M., O'Brien, M. and Sivage, C.: Effects of methylphenidate alone and in combination with behaviour modification procedures on the behaviour and academic performance of hyperactive children. *Journal of Abnormal Child Psychology* **6**:149–61, 1978.

19 Schachar, R. J. and Taylor, E. A.: Clinical assessment and management strategies, in *The overactive child*, ed. E. Taylor. Oxford, Blackwell Scientific Publications, 1986, pp. 236–56.

20 Bosco, J. J. and Robin, S. S.: Hyperkinesis: prevalance and treatment, in *Hyperactive children: the social ecology of identification and treatment*, ed. C. K. Whalen, and B. Henker, New York, Academic Press, 1980, pp. 173–90.
21 Quinn, P. and Rapoport, J.: One-year follow up of hyperactive boys treated with imipramine and methylphenidate. *American Journal of Psychiatry* **132**:241–5, 1977.
22 Department of Health and Social Security. Sterilisation of children. DS 333/75. London, HMSO, 1975. Unpublished.
23 Working Group on Current Medical/Ethical Problems. Sterilisation of the mentally handicapped. *Lancet* **ii**:685–6, 1979.
24 Bainham, A.: *Children, parents and the state*. London, Sweet and Maxwell, 1988, pp. 138–42.
25 Green, J. and Stewart, A.: Ethical issues in child and adolescent psychiatry. *Journal of Medical Ethics* **13**:5–11, 1987.
26 Rutter, M.: Infantile autism and other pervasive disorders, in *Child and adolescent psychiatry: modern approaches*, ed. M. Rutter and L. Hersov. Oxford, Blackwell Scientific Publications, 1985, p. 558.
27 Blumenfeld, A.: Ethical problems in child guidance. *British Journal of Medical psychology* **47**:17–26, 1974.
28 Walrond-Skinner, S. and Watson, D. (eds): *Ethical issues in family therapy*. London, Routledge and Kegan Paul, 1987.
29 Lindley, R.: Family therapy and respect for people, in *Ethical issues in family therapy*, ed. S. Walrond-Skinner and D. Watson. London, Routledge and Kegan Paul, 1987.
30 Kazdin, A.: Single case research design in clinical child psychiatry. *Journal of the American Academy of Child Psychiatry* **22**:423–432, 1983.
31 Rosen, A. C., Rekers, G. A., and Bentler, P. M.: Ethical issues in the treatment of children. *Journal of Social Issues* **34**:122–36, 1978.
32 Department of Education and Science. Special educational needs. Report of the Committee of Enquiry into the Education of Handicapped Children and Young People. London, HMSO, 1978.
33 Sutton, A.: Legal and ethical problems in child psychiatry. *Bulletin of the Royal College of Psychiatrists* **13**:193–4, 1989.
34 Bruggen, P., Byng-Hall, J., and Pitt-Aikens, T.: The reason for admission as a focus of work on an adolescent unit. *British Journal of Psychiatry* **122**:319–29, 1973.
35 Hoggett, B.: *Mental health law*, 2nd edn. London, Swet and Maxwell, 1984.
36 Roth, L. H.: Mental health commitment: the state of the debate 1980. *Hospital and Community Psychiatry* **31**:385–96, 1980.
37 Tooley, K.: Ethical considerations in the involuntary commitment of children and in psychological testing as a part of legal procedures. *Mental Hygiene* **54**:484–9, 1970.
38 Working Party on Ethics of Research in Children: Guidelines to aid ethical committees considering research involving children. *British Medical Journal* **280**:229–31, 1980.
39 Nicholson, R. (ed.): *Ethics and medical research in children*. Oxford, Oxford University Press, 1987.
40 Smith, M.: Taking blood from children causes no more than minimal harm. *Journal of Medical Ethics* **11**:127–31, 1985.

41 Skegg, P. D. G.: English law relating to experimentation on children. *Lancet* **ii**:754–5, 1977.
42 Dworkin, G.: Legality of consent to non-therapeutic medical research on infants and young children. *Archives of Diseases in Childhood* **53**:433–6, 1978.
43 Ethics in research (editorial). *British Journal of Hospital Medicine* **2**:759, 1968.
44 General Medical Council: *Annual Report*. London, General Medical Council, 1987, p. 15.
45 Jones, D. P. H.: Some reflections on the Cleveland affair. *Association of Child Psychology and Psychiatry News* **10**:13–18, 1988.
46 Oates, M.: Assessing fitness to parent, in *Taking a stand*. London, British Agencies for Fostering and Adoption, 1984, pp. 29–41.
47 Schoettle, W. C.: Termination of parental rights—ethical issues and role conflicts. *Journal of the American Academy of Child Psychiatry* **23**:629–32, 1984.
48 Forssman, H. and Thuwe, I.: One hundred and twenty children born after application for therapeutic abortion refused. *Acta Psychiatrica Scandinavica* **42**:71–88, 1966.

# 17

# Ethics and psychogeriatrics

*Catherine Oppenheimer*

This chapter considers some general issues concerning elderly people, and goes on to discuss areas of specific ethical interest. The specific topics are, for the most part, structured around an imaginary case history (Miss A).

## Who are the elderly?

Why is there a separate chapter in this book on elderly people? Old age *in itself* does not mark off a person as ethically different in any way from someone in middle age or youth. But many circumstances which do give rise to specific ethical problems—circumstances such as physical illness, mental incapacity, dependence on help from others, and vulnerability to cruelty or exploitation—become statistically commoner in people as they grow old. Discussion of our responsibilities towards 'the elderly' frequently focuses on people in such circumstances. Hence the proper image of an old person as healthy, independent, and fully able to protect himself, is constantly subject to erosion. This is an example of the halo effect—the halo of disability conferred on all the elderly.

The halo effect operates also in another direction. 'Old age' refers to an ill-defined age-group that can span the years from sixty-five to ninety-five or more. The difference between people aged ninety-five and sixty-five may be at least as great as that between a fifty-five-year-old and a twenty-five-year-old. The use of a single category to encompass the whole range will obscure the vast differences between people at different parts of this age-band, let alone the difference between individuals irrespective of age. The real problems faced by many ninety-year-olds may falsely be attributed also to sixty-five-year-olds, simply because of the 'elderly' label that they bear. As an example, take the gloomy predictions about the 'burden of the elderly', expected to grow ever more onerous into the next century.[1] Talk of the widening imbalance between the economically dependent elderly and the economically productive young is grounded in assumptions about social organization, as well as in biological fact. The ratio between the elderly and the young could be altered, at the stroke of a pen, without violating any biological truth, by shifting the boundary between them at retirement age from sixty or sixty-five to seventy or seventy-five.

The tendency to view the elderly as a homogeneous mass is related to another tendency, also hard to avoid—viewing old age too much from the perspective of youth. Illnesses are generally written about by people other than those who experience them; and the same is true of old age. Perhaps this is less true now than formerly, and in both fields there are groups and individuals whose voice can be heard. What they say is of the greatest importance, but they do not absolve the rest of us from the task of remembering those who cannot speak out, and recognizing that their views are not necessarily represented by the articulate ones. Few surveys are yet available that directly examine the wishes and attitudes of elderly people. Mostly it is younger people who write about the problems experienced by elderly people. Perhaps this does not matter where the material is strictly factual; but where feelings, beliefs, or rights are at issue, there is much room for subjectivity and unexamined assumptions to infiltrate the arguments. The likely sources of untested assumptions are the professionals' second-hand experience of old age, through their observation of the old people they have cared for, and possibly also of relatives and friends. In addition, their opinions are liable to be coloured by their beliefs and wishes about their own future old age. (This last statement is in itself an untested assumption—it is one of the clichés of gerontology, but I know of no empirical support for it. In practice, one may often hear passionate arguments about the right way to care for an elderly person that come down in the end to statements of the form 'if I am like that when I am old, then I hope . . .').

We should question how accurately one can look into one's own future in this way: would we accept a view of middle age that emerged from a discussion among teenagers? The imaginative leap of empathetic understanding is a technique widely used in psychiatry and psychotherapy; but it is safe only when tempered by corrective information from the person being empathized with. The problem with old age—our own or others'—is that such corrective information may be difficult or impossible to get.

The potential injustice to elderly people contained in the assumptions that are made about them because they are seen as old rather than individual is an injustice built into social institutions. The remedy prescribed for damaging stereotypes is to 'accord respect to the individual'; but this phrase takes us only part of the way. Do you respect me as a human being with universal human attributes, or as a person of advanced age and therefore worthy of respect, or as myself—unique me? You cannot respect me (uniquely) without knowing who I am.

Where a person holds all the information that needs to be known about her, and can communicate it to others, there is no problem in respecting her individually. (Or at least there is no ethical problem: the practical difficulty of giving enough time and attention to allow proper communication is often neglected, and so people's individuality is lost.) Different issues arise when the person cannot speak for herself, and the information on which respect for her should be grounded has to be sought elsewhere. The two common sources of such information are the person's relatives, and the people currently looking after her, such as nurses or care staff in a home. Very probably the relatives will speak from their knowledge of how she was in earlier times, and they may make inferences about her likely attitudes to her present state from what they know of her feelings and her statements earlier in life. On the other hand the care staff currently looking after her will make inferences based on their knowledge of her as she is now, and on their experience of other old people who have passed through their care. These two frameworks of perception may or may not agree, because the sources of their assumptions are different, and the attempt to 'respect the individual' may founder on the problem of determining who the individual is. Is she the person we meet now, expressing herself (obscurely perhaps) in her current behaviour, or is she the person who was quite different before, and who, for sixty years or more, would not have wished to be what she is now?

There are two further points that should be mentioned concerning assumptions made about old age. Each involves a problem of labelling, and the clutch of attitudes that goes with each label. These labels are 'ill' and 'helpless'.

Psychiatric illness is common in old age, and diagnosis can be harder to make than in young people. The psychiatrist experienced in old age may therefore set his threshold for detecting illness rather lower for the elderly than he does for younger people. Non-medical people involved in a particular problem may give impetus to this process, if their anxieties can be relieved by attaching a medical label to the problem. The responsibility for solving it is then transferred to medical institutions, which may appear to have powers (such as the power to admit compulsorily to hospital) that others do not. This is the pressure that tends towards a medical labelling of problems.

There is an equal but opposite risk that, out of the laudable wish to preserve old people's freedom and to avoid such labelling, signs of illness may be misinterpreted, and the ill old person may be denied necessary and effective treatment. Depressive illness is an example of a condition whose ambiguous boundaries make it particularly subject to these conflicting pressures. The harm done by not diagnosing depression when it is present is almost equalled by the harm that may result from diagnosing it when it is not. Alzheimer's disease in its early stages can also be difficult to diagnose. In this case, however, there exists as yet no recognized effective treatment for the condition, so that the consequences of missing the diagnosis may be less severe, and time can be allowed to clarify the situation.

The other label concerns helplessness. Old people are frequently limited in one aspect or other of their lives, and thereby obliged to accept help from someone. The more they accept outside help, the more their lives become public to others. At the extreme comes institutional life—residential care or a hospital ward. This affects only a small minority of elderly people at any one time; but it is an experience that many will go through, and it will enter into their calculations for their future. Furthermore, many elderly people experience lesser breaches of their privacy, with the entry of helpers (such as care assistant, district nurse, or bath-attendant) into their lives at home.

The painful process of subjecting oneself to public scrutiny may happen at any age; but for younger people it is more likely to be a transient experience. In old age, once begun it is likely to continue. The surrender of privacy in accepting outside help brings with it other surrenders. The old person must share with other clients in the help being offered, and fit in with a system that is shaped by the requirements of care-givers as well as the needs of the cared-for. Other people's perceptions of her life will guide her future, and she risks being seen as helpless in areas where help is not needed.

In this, the elderly have common cause with young disabled people. The person in the wheelchair is assumed not to be capable of speaking for herself, just as anyone over a certain age is expected to need the protection of society. The very existence of special categories of people (geriatricians, social workers in elderly-care teams, members of Age Concern) sets apart the group whose rights they wish to affirm. It is a process that tends to reduce all people under the label to the lowest common denominator. Mrs Amanda Smith, aged seventy-five, who delivers meals on wheels and campaigns for a local day-centre for the elderly, has a clear sense of her own identity. It is very different from the view of those who recognize her only as one of the many old ladies who burden society today.

## Specific ethical issues

The classical issues of medical ethics—the limits to autonomy, paternalism, the continuity of the individual, the postponement of death—are everyday matters to those who work with elderly people with psychiatric illness. They arise in many different forms, and often their resolution is determined by the individual circumstances of the case. Rather than engaging in lengthy general discussion, it seems more instructive to tie them to the story of a single imaginary elderly person.

## Competence and autonomy

Miss A is seventy-three, a retired schoolteacher, who has always been regarded as a bit of an eccentric in her village. She rarely speaks to others, and does most of her shopping by telephone; and her only companion is her beloved dog. Recently her neighbours have contacted the local social services office: 'She has been coming into our garden at night and picking our flowers; we know that the grocer who delivers her food has not been paid for months, and she looks so dirty and neglected nowadays. What's more, she is still driving her car. It cannot be safe—you must do something.'

Arguably, dementia in old age is the greatest single source of ethical problems in the elderly—not only for those who suffer from dementia, but also for those who are suspected of suffering from it. While sufferers gradually lose the capacity to safeguard their own interests, the onset of this illness is often insidious. Hence all old people are liable to come under suspicion, and to be treated as needing protection even when they do not. The situation becomes more complicated when the old person is believed to pose a risk to others as well as to herself. Neighbours may fear that when she sets fire to her flat, they too will go up in flames. The wandering old man who gets knocked down in the road has inflicted harm on the driver as well as himself. Old people who are drivers themselves raise particularly acute problems.[2] The risk of involvement in accidents increases in drivers over seventy years old; but the risks of social isolation are also higher for elderly people without transport. People who have driven all their lives and who value the independence it has given them, and who do not recognize their failing skills, will fight passionately to preserve their 'right to drive'. Family influence may sometimes be enough to persuade elderly risky drivers to give up driving; but where this is not so, and the driver will not accept advice from others, active intervention may be needed. Possible interventions range from the least formal (and arguably most coercive), such as removing car-keys or a vital part of the car engine, to the formal reporting of the driver to the licensing authority.

How can we ensure that elderly people in general are not subjected to needlessly imposed intervention, and how can we decide at what point the offer of help is appropriate? That point may be as difficult to decide when the old person welcomes help, as when she rejects it. In other words, what are the proper limits to paternalism and to the exercise of autonomy?[3]

Resolution of this question often hinges on the issue of competence—a concept easy to invoke but difficult to define. Competence is not a unitary state.[4–6] It makes sense only in relation to particular tasks that have to be carried out by the person whose competence is being judged. Someone who can no longer organize her own financial affairs may nevertheless be regarded as competent to give instructions that someone else shall organize them for her. (In Britain, the legal instrument known as the 'enduring power of attorney' may be implemented by a person who is not competent at that point to manage the details of her affairs, so long as she is known to understand the implications of the power that she is conferring.) Someone who cannot safely look after herself at home may well be perfectly competent, in a residential setting, to choose what dish she would like for supper and whether she wishes to sit in the garden when it is fine. Brody,[6] in a helpful discussion of competence, identifies the following 'capacities that constitute the patient's competency to participate in health care decision making':

(1) the ability to receive information from her surroundings;

(2) the capacity to remember the information received;

(3) the ability to make a decision and give a reason for it;

(4) the ability to use the relevant information in making the decision; and

(5) the ability to assess the relevant information appropriately.

Descriptively, this list is helpful in understanding the elements that enter into a decision, and how the process may be hampered by a variety of psychiatric conditions, such as altered consciousness, memory impairment, or depression. But does it then follow that people impaired in any of these capacities should not take part in any decisions about their health care? That would be far too stringent an exclusion. It would be tantamount to saying that autonomy belongs only to those who are perfectly well. The alternative approach, where any of these capacities are in doubt, is, as Ratzan suggests,[7] to operate within a modified paternalism—to set up the conditions for a 'protected milieu of autonomy', where the patient's scope for participating in decisions is kept as wide as possible, consonant with the limitations imposed by cognitive or other handicaps.

Such an analysis lays upon the doctor or other professional a heavy, threefold responsibility:

1. To judge where the patient's choice is necessarily constrained, and where it should be free.

2. To offer honest choices, rather than pseudo-choices. For example, pseudo-choice is offered where the professional operates a covert rule that makes only one of the options permissible, or where information presented to the patient about the options is selectively limited to favour one of them. Moreover, when choice is offered, then the outcome of the patient's choice should not be made grounds for questioning the competence of the patient. (There may be a case for arguing, as Brody does,[6] that if the patient's choice is seen as seriously aberrant, her competence on other grounds should be re-examined.)

3. To find ways of presenting choice to the patient that circumvent as much as possible the obstacles posed by her illnesses or handicap.

This last point, the importance of presenting information to patients in a way that takes into account their ability to grasp it, is one that has not yet been fully discussed in the literature. To some extent discussions on obtaining informed consent for participation in experiments does touch on the issue. For example, Weintraub[8] discusses the use of methods such as video-presentations and group discussions to augment the conventional ways of giving information about experiments, so as to allow maximum informed choice by the participants. Such methods address the problem of competent elderly people who may have to grapple with a body of detailed information in unfamiliar territory.

With patients suffering from dementia the problem is different. For them one must maintain maximum choice in the face of language disorder, memory loss, the inability to hold two alternative possibilities in the mind at the same time, and the difficulty of forming a conceptual view of the future. In the field of mental handicap, professionals are accustomed to the idea of dissecting tasks into manageable steps; but comparable developments have not yet taken place in the professional literature in dementia. In everyday practice, however, it is common for manoeuvres to be used to try and make choice as available as possible for demented patients. Let us return to Miss A, and suppose that we have decided that it would be helpful if she could be introduced to day care. When this is discussed with her she declines it. But what actually did the offer of 'day care' mean to her? Many community psychiatric nurses at such a point would take pains to become acquainted with her, and, when they had gained her trust through repeated visits, might invite her to come for an outing with them. During the outing or a subsequent one, they might then call in at the day centre for a cup of tea.

If Miss A seemed to enjoy that visit, then the same manoeuvre might be repeated until she had become accustomed enough to the new setting to be willing to go by ordinary means of transport.

Was this an underhand manoeuvring of a vulnerable person, or a fitting stratagem which, respecting her autonomy, enabled her to make an informed concrete choice when she was no longer able to make an abstract one?

## Compulsory help

Now suppose that Miss A has not been offered day care, and is still at home. One day she drives her car into the wall of her garage. She is uninjured, but the car will no longer go, and she abandons it. Eventually the general practitioner is able to persuade her to let him examine her at home. The house is cold and filthy, and he finds rotting food in the kitchen. The dog looks ill and neglected, and Miss A has lost weight. Though she is not unfriendly to him, she refuses to accept any help from him or from anyone else, arguing vigorously that it is her right to live as she pleases. Visits by a social worker and a psychogeriatrician do not add much to this picture, beyond establishing that Miss A has slight memory impairment, with some disorientation in time, and poor insight. She is suspicious, but there is no evidence of a paranoid state or other functional illness such as depression. The diagnosis made by the psychiatrist is of an early dementia, with features suggesting impairment of frontal-lobe function.

Reluctantly Miss A agrees that a home help may visit her, but when she comes Miss A will not allow her to touch anything in the home, and only rarely eats the food that is prepared for her. After a few weeks Miss A refuses to let the home help in altogether. Over the next few months, in the face of increasing anxiety about Miss A's health and safety, the professionals involved (general practitioner, social worker, and psychogeriatrician) decide that, whatever Miss A's wishes, they have to intervene.

The ethical problems raised by involuntary admission to hospital are discussed elsewhere in this book (Chapter 13). In the psychiatry of old age, an important practical distinction is made between functional illness (such as depression, mania, and paranoid state, which reflect a temporary disturbance of brain function, often amenable to treatment) and organic conditions such as the various dementing illnesses, which mostly arise from damaged or degenerating brain tissue, and are usually irreversible.

Where elderly people suffer from functional psychiatric illness there are no new ethical problems attributable merely to the patient's age. If treatment can be given to her at home then that is preferable to admitting her to hospital; and voluntary admission is preferable to compulsory. Ultimately the same good reasons as at a younger age (such as risk to the patient or others, failure of insight and compliance, or the need for close nursing care) may in the end make involuntary admission the proper choice of action. The likelihood that the patient herself will, on recovery, agree with the need for admission (will give 'retroactive informed consent') also makes the choice a reasonably comfortable one, ethically speaking, for the professionals to take.

The case is different when the patient suffers from a dementing illness. There are two aspects to this. First, compulsory admission to hospital is less appropriate for dementia than for functional illness. Admission will not cure the disorder, and hospitals are not necessarily the best sources of the care that is needed. Where a patient with dementia is willing to accept help, it is usually much better to support her at home than to admit her to hospital; and the presumption must be that the same balance of benefits would apply to the unwilling patient, if only help could be delivered to her at home. The legal powers that could compel people to receive care, and the appropriate place for providing such care, will be discussed further when we return to Miss A.

The second aspect in which irreversible organic illness differs from functional illness is this. In dementia, it is difficult to make the same clear distinction between a person and her illness that we make when we compulsorily treat functional illness. There is no real prospect of receiving retroactive informed consent from the patient for decisions that have been imposed on her. Although it is often a comfort to see such a patient manifestly happier and less anxious when she is safely in hospital, that is not the same as receiving her consent.

The case is further complicated when the person is engaged in some slowly self-destructive behaviour such as heavy drinking, where it is unclear whether her cognitive impairment is playing a part in her failure to understand the grave consequences of her actions. One would not normally treat a patient compulsorily for alcoholism, however risky her behaviour, because the assumption is made that that is the way she chooses to behave. But if a person with an alcoholic dementia continues to drink heavily, to what extent can one assume that she has made a free choice to jeopardize her future in that way?

Let us return to Miss A's case, where the professionals have decided that some intervention must be made. Frequently in such a situation the psychiatrist will be seen as the person with the legal powers (in Britain, under the Mental Health Act of 1983) to intervene, and pressure will be put on him to act accordingly. For his part the psychiatrist may feel that hospital has little to offer Miss A, and may wish that the general practitioner and the social worker had their own legal power to overrule Miss A's views for her own good, compelling her to accept food, warmth, and personal care at home. In some states of the USA there exists the power of 'out-patient commitment'; but in Britain there is no comparable form of power to enforce any care outside hospital. Under the Mental Health Act 1983 guardianship (possibly vested in the local social services department) may allow the guardian some limited power to determine where a person lives, and oblige her to allow access to the guardian. The extension of such powers, so as to allow imposed treatment of people outside hospital, has been proposed and debated, but at present is viewed with great caution in Britain.[9]

Would a legal mechanism to impose help on a person at home make this ethical issue any easier? It is generally accepted that wherever care has to be imposed on an involuntary patient, the least coercive measure possible should be used. It is interesting, then, to ask which would be perceived as more coercive: removal to hospital or the introduction of strangers into the person's home? Possibly there is good reason why admission to hospital has remained the most widespread method for taking legal control of people's lives for medical reasons. Arguably, the violation of privacy and the potential for abuse are less, and the opportunities for formal checks on the control exerted over the patient are greater, in an institution staffed by many people than in a scatter of private homes into which only one staff member goes at a time.

These ethical issues are brought out most sharply in the context of legal measures for imposing care.[10] But they also cannot be ignored in the much commoner situations where demented people at home, in day centres or hospitals, or getting in and out of cars and ambulances, are coaxed and urged without benefit of legal status as detained patients, in ways that make them unhappy, anxious, or angry. The justification for these actions is that they serve the long-term interest of the patients. If the home help can wash and dress Miss B every morning then she can stay at home; if Mr C goes to day care then his wife can manage to go on looking after him for months and years to come. It is the inability of the patient with dementia to grasp long-term issues that hampers her participation in such decisions, and places such responsibility on others to judge the choices correctly for her. Responsibility is not less when the imposition of decisions is formally unsupervised: the docile person needs to be defended from over-management as much as the prickly person needs to be defended from negligence.

## Investigations and research

We return to Miss A. All attempts to support her at home have failed. She has a brother living in another part of the country, who for years has visited her regularly every few months. He too has noticed her memory and competence failing over the last few years, and is anxious that everything possible should be done for her. Miss A is eventually compulsorily admitted to hospital: a painful occasion, with Miss A carried bodily to the ambulance, and the neighbours peering out of the windows. The dog is found a home by the social worker. Fortunately Miss A now accepts care from the nurses, and seems to be reasonably content on the ward.

The consultant is happy to make a presumptive diagnosis of Alzheimer's disease on the basis of her history and the earlier assessment he made of her at home. The senior registrar, however, wishes to carry out full investigations, to exclude any treatable cause of dementia. Staff at the nearby teaching hospital are engaged in research into dementia, and wish to carry out a detailed psychological interview and computerized tomography on every demented patient entering hospital. They approach Miss A's doctors to ask if they may perform these investigations on her.

Treatable causes of dementia are rare in old age, relative to the frequency of the major dementing illnesses (Alzheimer's disease and multi-infarct dementia). It is therefore common in British psychogeriatric practice, whenever a typical clinical history is obtained, to omit some investigations (such as computerized scanning or a lumbar puncture) that would be regarded as essential by neurologists investigating a younger patient with a probable dementing illness. It is important to ask whether this practice is dictated by a restraint on resources, or by a consideration of the balance of benefits to the patient. Routine investigations such as blood tests are not in question; but the discomfort and anxiety of procedures such as radiological investigation must be justified by the likely benefit to be obtained. The benefits may include the unusual gain of discovering a treatable condition, or a more intangible gain felt by the staff looking after a patient when they have a much clearer idea of the condition they are dealing with.

Whenever the clinical picture is untypical then the balance of benefits is shifted towards more thorough investigation; and this shift will be accelerated by the trend toward earlier referral of patients with possible dementia, since there will not have been time for the typical progression of the history of illness to have occurred before the referral is made. In addition to those considerations, it will probably not be long before potential treatments for Alzheimer's disease will alter the balance decisively, and will make an early and certain diagnosis of the disease essential.

Research projects set up a different balance of benefits.[11] In pursuit of a sensible research question, as part of a well-constructed study, investigations (such as an exhaustive psychological interview) which would make no material difference to the individual patient's prognosis could nevertheless yield great benefit to similar patients in future. Is it right to ask elderly patients to participate in such studies?

There is now a substantial literature in this area,[7,8,11,12] with two clear themes. The first theme is that elderly people who are able to decide for themselves would be subjected to an unjust diminution of their autonomy were they to be denied the opportunity of participating in such studies.

Old people are just as likely as young people to have the altruism, curiosity, or scientific enthusiasm to encourage them to participate in research, and they should be enabled to do so provided that they are judged to be fully informed and fully able to decide, free of any coercive influences.

The second theme concerns research with non-competent patients. On a strict view, only those who freely consent may participate in research. But then no patient with dementia may be a research subject, no clinical research on dementia may be done, and all hope of a better future for people with dementia must rest on other lines of enquiry. It is generally agreed that this view is too strict, and that research into diseases which, like dementia, impair patients' competence to participate freely in research ought not to be unnecessarily hampered. Many people would wish when well to give advance consent for participation in such research in the event of their developing a dementing illness; and patients' relatives are often willing that they should take part in research.

The exact mechanisms by which such patients might participate, and through which their rights could be safeguarded, are still unclear. In Britain, any investigator engaging in clinical research must submit his project to the scrutiny of local research-ethics committees; but there is not yet any mechanism for ensuring uniformity of procedure or principles among these different ethics committees.[13]

Certain safeguards appear to be generally agreed: only research which could not be carried out in any other way should be undertaken in demented patients; the disadvantages and risks to the patient should be minimal, and balanced against the benefits to be gained by future patients; and the researcher should not be linked in any way to the team responsible for the care of the patient, so that they are able to make an objective decision on behalf of the patient. Whether or not relatives should decide on behalf of a non-competent patient is still unclear, though it is customary for them to be consulted. The validity of proxy consent is discussed by Reich[11] and by Ratzan.[7] In Britain, the publication of a draft code of practice[14] for the Mental Health Act 1983 provoked energetic debate over the ethics of research in non-competent patients.[15–17]

### Treatment, restraint, and risk

Miss A has by now become very difficult to care for properly on the ward. She is withdrawn and suspicious, and liable to hit and scratch the nurses when they help her to wash and dress. With the progression of her dementia, her command of language is severely impaired; but sometimes it seems that she is saying that she is in prison, and being tortured by the nurses.

The ward staff disagree about whether she should be given sedation. Dr L considers that she has a paranoid illness related to her dementia, that she has delusions that distress her, and that she needs treatment for the relief of that illness. Nurse M believes that it is wrong to put a patient under chemical restraint just because she is difficult to nurse. Dr N says that unless Miss A's aggressiveness can be controlled then she will never be able to live outside hospital. In this context it is important to point out that major tranquillizers can be seen as having both a specific therapeutic effect on psychotic symptoms, and a general effect of tranquillizing and calming disturbed behaviour.[18]

When a person is no longer able to participate in decisions about the medication that she receives, and cannot even report on her own symptoms, the prescriber is reduced to basing major decisions about treatment purely on the behaviour of the person. It then becomes important to think clearly about the reasons for treatment, and for whose benefit the treatment is being undertaken. There are several dimensions to this. Firstly, the dimension of normal or pathological. One may regard a person as voluntarily acting in accordance with their personality and their wishes, or one may regard them as involuntarily ill, their behaviour driven by the illness, and needing to be relieved by treatment. Secondly, the dimension of nuisance or risk. Using tranquillizing medication to reduce risk to a patient may be felt to be justifiable; but the point at which risk to the nurses caring for the patient can reasonably be dealt with by medication is much harder to determine. Thirdly, the issue of wider versus narrower freedoms. One may see the use of sedation as a trespass on a person's liberty, and therefore refuse to use it to control disturbing aspects of behaviour. Is it possible that other important freedoms have thereby been lost? For example, maybe the disturbed behaviour can be managed satisfactorily on a psychogeriatric ward, but will be beyond the competence of staff in a nursing home. So the patient is denied the opportunity of moving to a nursing home, where in other respects the quality of her life may be very much better than on a psychogeriatric ward.

Many of the same arguments apply to the use of physical restraints (such as straps, cot sides, special chairs). But there are also differences. Medication carries a special ambiguity in that it possesses the aspect both of specific therapy and of non-specific control. Restraint is very much more likely to be perceived by the patient as painful, frightening, or humiliating, and to create distressing conflicts for the nurses who administer it.[18,19] Nevertheless, it is precisely the obtrusiveness of physical restraint that also makes it possible to maintain strict safeguards on its use. By contrast it is much easier to engage in covert or self-deceiving use of chemical restraint under the guise of treatment. In Britain acceptance of overt physical restraint is less ready than in the United States.[20,21] But subtler forms of physical restriction, such as the use of doors secured in ways too complicated for demented people to open, are almost universal in psychogeriatric units. Justification for such devices ought always to be regarded as provisional, not forgetting that all patients on a ward, not only those especially at risk, are restrained by such measures. In addition, the risks attached to restraint must be remembered. When people climb over cot sides they have further to fall.[21]

### The elderly patient and her family—the question of dual loyalty

In framing the story of Miss A to link specific ethical issues, we have bypassed the question of the patient's family, and particularly those families that are closely involved with the care of the elderly person with psychiatric illness. Troublesome ethical issues related to patients in their family setting are common in psychogeriatrics, and such situations bring out in acute form the principle, important at all ages but particularly in old age, that no patient should be considered in isolation, but should always be seen in his social context.

On Miss A's ward there is a patient, Mrs B, aged 80, who was admitted for assessment of her agitation. She is not demented, but has always been an anxious person; and since suffering a myocardial infarct two years ago she has been continually preoccupied by fears about her health, and can talk of nothing else. She lives at home with her husband, who is eighty-four, and very frail with severe emphysema. Since her infarct he has looked after her and carried out most of the housework; but now he is refusing to have her home again. 'I cannot look after her any more. It worries me to death. If she has another attack, what can I do? You have no idea what it has been like these last two years.' Mrs B is looking forward to going home. 'I must be with my husband. I will be all right dear, he will look after me.' The couple have been offered extra help at home, but both have refused: Mrs B sees no need for it, Mr B cannot see how it would help. 'What is the use? Unless someone is there night and day, I shall not stop worrying for a moment.'

This situation and its variants are familiar to everyone who works with the elderly. Sometimes the relationship between two people has always been bad, and the onset of illness, and the consequent professional assumption of responsibilities towards one partner, create a longed-for opportunity for the other partner to escape. In effect, there is divorce by hospital admission. Sometimes the relationship was previously very good, but illness in one or both partners has created intolerable strains that cannot be resolved by the introduction of help from outside. The anxiety and guilt engendered by the dependence of the other partner may be impossible to relieve. It is usually such anxiety, or the loss of emotional contact with the ill relative, rather than the physical aspects of an illness, that cause the relationship to give way.

The professionals in such a situation find themselves forced into the position of arbiter. Mrs B has a right to live in her own home; but if the hospital discharge her home they cannot ignore the consequences to Mr B. Should they say that their responsibility is solely to Mrs B (their patient), and that somebody else must worry about her husband? If they agree that Mrs B cannot reasonably expect her husband to look after her now, and that her judgement is faulty if she believes that he can, are they then justified in making different arrangements for her discharge from hospital —such as finding her a place in a residential home?

Mrs C, aged eighty-three, is moderately demented and lives with her son. They are visited regularly by the community psychiatric nurse, who observes that the son has difficulty in managing his mother. He admits to getting exasperated with her, but turns down all offers of practical help. One day Mrs C has a black eye. Her son says that she fell, and Mrs C agrees with him. When she is offered day care or a short spell in hospital she refuses, saying that she wants to stay at home with her son. A case-conference is held. The different professionals involved with Mrs C pool their information, and agree that they can only continue to remain on the alert for the moment. Two weeks later Mrs C is badly bruised on her arm. She half-admits to the community nurse that her son held her tightly by the arm; but the following day she denies this.

Is this the moment when the professionals should intervene, and should they remove Mrs C from her son's care? Physical abuse of elderly people by those caring for them is something that has become widely recognized only in recent years.[22] The major problems arise where there is suspicion but no proof of injury, and where the old person insists on remaining with the carer who is suspected of abusing her. At the time of writing Britain has no formal provision for the investigation or management of such cases, by contrast with suspected child-abuse. Recent interest in the topic[23] makes it probable that such procedures will gradually be agreed upon.

Mrs D lives with her son and daughter-in-law and their two teenage boys. Her son brought her to live with them three years ago, after his father died. Over the years she has become unable to look after herself, and now the daughter-in-law has to help her with all her personal care. She trails around the house all day, and will not let her daughter-in-law out of her sight. The boys have come to hate their grandmother, and spend as much time as they can away from home. The son regards it as a matter of course that his mother will remain with them. His wife is terrified that she is losing her sons, and that her marriage is breaking up under the strain.

The main theme in these different family patterns is the same: what boundary should the psychiatrist (or psychiatric nurse, or social worker) set to their responsibility, when the life of an old person who is their primary concern is unavoidably bound up with the lives of other people?

It is impossible to see the identified patient in isolation, ignoring the family setting. On the other hand, neither would it be right for the professional to adjudicate among different members of the family. What then is the professional role? He or she may feel under pressure to make judgements about the reasonableness or otherwise of family members (is Mr B really too frail to cope now? Is Mr D expecting too much from his wife?); about the risks that people pose to each other (should Mrs C's wish to stay with her son be overridden?); and about the duties that family members owe each other (should young Mrs D put her sons' needs above her mother-in-law's?). Theoretically, the professional should be assisting the family to make these decisions for themselves; but one key reason why it may not be possible to avoid active involvement in decisions is the professional's control over resources. For example, the decision to admit one of these patients to hospital may have profound consequences for her future.

Such consequences may have little to do with events that take place in hospital, and a great deal to do with the impact of the admission on the family system outside. Admission removes the patient from the family situation, allowing it to settle to a new equilibrium, which subsequently resists the reintroduction of the patient. Admission identifies the patient as ill, and therefore to be treated in a different way from other family members, with different and maybe lesser rights. It marks out the patient as someone needing an institutional setting, and therefore to be placed in a different institution when hospital care is no longer offered. This is an area where the symbolic power of the psychiatrist extends way beyond its legitimate base—the training that enables him to diagnose and treat disease.

## Resources

Miss A has been found a place in a private nursing home. It is expensive. Her brother is unhappy to see her savings disappear in this way, and is apprehensive about what will happen when they run out. But he accepts the decision because Miss A seemed to like the nursing home when she first saw it, and she has settled well there. The care is good, the staff believe in using little medication and much affection, and Miss A is happy. A year later the owner of the home sells up to a consortium, and soon changes in the home begin to appear. A much stricter regime is introduced.

The staff are angry with Miss A when she is difficult. She becomes progressively more tense and irritable, and begins to hit the other residents. The medical officer for the home prescribes sedation, and Miss A spends most of the day slumped half-asleep in a chair. The brother contacts her former psychiatrist, and begs him to intervene.

Does the psychiatrist have a duty to intervene here? Should he take Miss A out of this hostile environment; and, if so, does he not also have a duty to the other residents there, all equally unhappy and at risk? Major difficulties arise for professional staff who work within a fragmented and uncoordinated system of provision for vulnerable elderly people. The variety of sources of funding (partly from the state and partly from the private sector) is associated with marked variability in the standards of care, with only weak control being exerted over these standards by either statutory or market mechanisms. The power of the professionals to influence the standards of care obtaining in the different establishments to which their patients go is very limited. The power of the market to maintain these standards is limited also. Even for competent and fit elderly people it is difficult to exert a full power of consumer choice in conditions of residential care. Having once made the decision to move into a home, the psychological barrier to revising that decision and moving again is for most people immense. People with dementia are doubly vulnerable. First, their illness makes it difficult for them to exercise choice, and it is likely that somebody else will do so on their behalf. Second, the dementia makes it impossible (or difficult) for them to adapt to their environment—they need an environment capable of adapting to them.

The mechanisms whereby a society should provide for its dependent elderly citizens raise ethical issues on a political rather than an individual plane.[24] Whether provision should largely be made by individuals for their own futures, or by families for their own elderly relatives, or whether resources should be pooled through systems of taxation and benefits, is a basic question under this head. At an individual level painful situations are created when elderly people who had expected to provide some inheritance for their children (in most cases, by leaving their houses to them) are obliged instead to use those resources to finance their own care in residential or nursing homes. The professional who advises, contrary to the patient's wishes, that such care is necessary cannot then feel comfortable that he is safeguarding his patient's autonomy. A further twist is thus added to the family dilemmas mentioned in the previous section, especially where a family's perception of what society should provide for their elderly is different from the situation which obtains in reality.

For the psychiatrist, the role of agent or interpreter for social arrangements to which he owes no personal conviction is uncomfortable, and at some point must become ethically untenable. Then what? Should the professionals attempt, in the role of citizen, to alter the arrangements that society has put in place? Should they resign from working in a system to which they cannot assent?

The manner in which society allocates its resources to the elderly in preference to other groups has been debated within the frameworks of health economics and of social justice (critically reviewed by Avorn[25] and Silver[26]). There is a tendency in such debates to consider, at least by implication, the elderly as an expensive burden, a group set aside from the rest of society. A valuable counterbalance is provided by Daniels,[27] who takes as his starting-point the recognition that old age is a part of everybody's life. In thinking about old age, we are thinking about ourselves. It is only by freezing a slice in time that the elderly can be seen as something different from 'us'. This simplification does not do justice to Daniels's argument. Anyone interested in this area should read his book.

The argument that the elderly have had 'a fair innings', and that it is right that resources should now be devoted to younger people, rests on the kind of narrow view attacked by Daniels, if not on pure thoughtless prejudice. It is, for example, usually untrue (unless one is thinking purely of number of years accumulated) that people now aged eighty have had a 'fair innings' when compared with people now twenty years old. The opposite is much more likely to be true: that they endured hardship in their youth which present-day young people have been spared, and that they now are entitled to a little compensating benefit.

Likewise, the argument for narrow limits on health-care expenditure for those with existing disability or a shortened life expectation has no sound ethical foundation.[28] (This is the argument for distributing resources according to a formula (QALY) based on the Rosser index, a crude and inappropriate[29,30] estimate of overall disability.) One could more persuasively argue that those whose misfortune it is to be afflicted with ill health ought not on that account to be additionally burdened by economic discrimination. There *are* legitimate reasons for limiting some treatments for some illnesses where there is pre-existing disability; but they are different arguments, and will be considered in the next section.

## Quality of life

Miss A has been brought back to the hospital from the nursing home while a better home is sought for her. During the winter there is a flu epidemic on the ward, and Miss A develops broncho-pneumonia. Her brother asks that this should not be actively treated: 'she has no quality of life now, and her life ought not to be prolonged'. But the nurses feel differently. 'Not treating the chest infection will only prolong the period of illness and discomfort. She will not necessarily die from it, and if she recovers without treatment she will have suffered unnecessarily during that time.'

The quality of a person's life is the phrase most often invoked when trying to decide how actively to treat an illness occurring in someone already seriously disabled by another condition. It is a dangerous phrase, in that it easily slides from describing the effect of the patient's disability into appraising the person's value—their value to themselves or to other people. Then, by a further step, it slides into assessing (or appearing to assess) whether life or death is better for them. Pearlman and Spear[31] report a vivid discussion of this area. The phrase 'quality of life', used in the sense of 'value of life', makes it almost impossible to arrive at rational decisions about treatment. There is no morally valid basis for making such an appraisal of the relative values of lives.

There is, however, a more manageable (and ethically more appealing) way of tackling the decision about treatment of incidental illness in a person with major disability. This is to consider the implications of the person's pre-existing disability in terms of the *ceiling* that the disability sets to the benefit likely to be gained from treatment. A person with retinal degeneration is not likely to derive major benefit from a cataract operation, because the limit to her vision is set by the retinal condition. A severely demented person who is an energetic walker within the hospital ward may benefit much more from a hip replacement after fracture than would a person chairbound by severe respiratory disease—even though in other respects people might be inclined to say that the quality of the demented person's life was less than that of the person with respiratory disease, who can still read, listen to music, enjoy visits from his friends, and plan his future.

Thus the likely benefits and risks from any given treatment have to be considered in the context of the *specific* disabilities that each person has, rather than in the context of a vague overall guess at the value that might be set on their continuing existence.[32,33] One problem with following this preferred criterion is the purely practical one that there is often insufficient information to allow an accurate judgement to be made (a problem, incidentally, which is inherent in the QALY approach also).

In the absence of clear data, decisions are made on hunch or prejudice, and are framed in terms of ethical principles (*should* elderly people be subjected to cardiopulmonary resuscitation?) Where data are available, a different question can be asked. The answer turns out to be that age itself is not a determinant of survival after cardiopulmonary resuscitation, though pre-existing illness and disability are.[34,35] The issue then is: to what extent is my patient comparable to the patients in this group, and how good are his personal chances of surviving after cardiopulmonary resuscitation?

There is a growing number of studies of surgical and other procedures in old age, which carry the same message. It is the specific risks of the procedure, and the specific disabilities of the patient, that are important. Age itself is irrelevant. Evans[36] puts this message most forcefully.

Even where better empirical data are available, there is still the question about the odds which any patient would wish to choose for himself. In practice choices are often made on behalf of patients, and they are not given the opportunity of deciding for themselves. For example, in Bedell and Delbanco's study[37] even physicians who believed in discussing matters with their patients had rarely done so; and they proved to be poor predictors of their patients' real wishes.

In another investigation[38] elderly people in hospital were asked to judge whether hypothetical contemporaries of theirs ought to be resuscitated or not. A diversity of opinions was expressed. The crucial point, however, was that the vast majority of the patients felt that elderly people should have these issues discussed with them, and that they should have the opportunity of saying how they felt about resuscitation for themselves. It is very probable that a person's wish to maximize her chances of survival or not will depend on individual personal factors that have little to do with measurable disability.[39] This question has not been systematically studied among the elderly, but is touched on in an interesting analysis of people withdrawn from dialysis.[40] Among the group of competent diabetics, those who opted to discontinue dialysis, and therefore die, did not apparently differ in complications or social situation from those who wished to continue with dialysis.

## Advance directives, and 'death with dignity'

Miss A was not given antibiotics. She recovered none the less from her chest infection; but she is weak, and spends much of her time asleep. She is uninterested in food, though with coaxing she will accept nutritious drinks. Her swallowing is poor, and sometimes she chokes.

The conscientious ward doctor is concerned that she is becoming dehydrated, and wishes to give her intravenous fluids. The nursing staff think that she is dying, and ought to be given opiates, though she is not apparently in pain. Her brother is informed of her condition, and decides to stay for a few days in a nearby hotel so as to visit her more frequently. He feels strongly that his sister would not have wished either for intravenous fluids or for unnecessary medication; and his view of her wishes is respected. The staff make it possible for him to spend most of his time on the ward with her. She dies peacefully in his company on his third day there.

In the previous section we considered some examples of conditions occurring in the elderly where the costs and benefits of treatment can be weighed up with a degree of objectivity, and where better empirical information can improve the quality of the decisions made.

Quite a different kind of equation arises in situations where death is regarded implicitly as a benefit, rather than as a cost, of any intervention or non-intervention. A searching discussion of the issues is given in Hilfiker's classic paper.[41] Many people (though not usually those who choose to work with the psychiatrically ill elderly) regard severe dementia with some horror, and death as a vastly preferable state.[42,43] The indignities of dementia, and the wish for 'death with dignity' on behalf of the old person, are often presented as the opposite arms of a decision in such discussions.

This horrified view of dementia is associated with two misconceptions. One is the belief that demented people are kept alive by active medical intervention; whereas in fact many demented people are physically very robust, and rarely need medical intervention of any kind.[44] The other belief is that the indignity associated with dementia can be relieved only by death; whereas in fact much indignity is created by inadequate and ignorant care, and 'is as much a function of the environment as [of] the patient'.[45] The belief that death is preferable to the demented state also strays into discussions of euthanasia, though in fact most serious proposals for euthanasia confine the territory strictly to those who are competent to make a choice for death. Non-competent people are usually specifically excluded from proposals for legalized euthanasia.[46]

A different approach to the issue comes from the practice of advance directives, or living wills.[47] Though the detail of this procedure varies from place to place, both in the US and more recently in the UK there is an acceptance that many people wish to put on formal record certain decisions taken in advance concerning their medical treatment at a time when they become unable (for example, because of mental incapacity) to express any current decision.

These decisions are generally not seen as legally binding at the time that they become relevant. It is accepted that a person may not be able fully to foresee any future state of mind;[41] that people should not cut themselves off from the possibility of altering their views even if they cannot fully express the altered view; and that no one can bind another to act contrary to the latter's own ethical principles. Consequently the writer of an advance directive can never do more than entrust a future attendant with the duty of trying to fulfil the writer's wishes in the light of circumstances at the time. For the attendant (medical or otherwise) attempting to make decisions on behalf of a non-competent patient it is likely to be very helpful to have concrete evidence about the attitudes and feelings of that person before the non-competent state came about—most especially if other sources of information (such as relatives) are in doubt or in conflict.

Related to the advance directive is the proxy decision. Relatives may be asked to assist in a decision that the patient can no longer make for himself. But Wray's study[48] suggests that the family are much more likely to be consulted over decisions *not* to treat than over decisions to treat actively in demented patients.

Brody[49] comprehensively analyses the role of the family in such decisions. The relatives' role is not to take over the decision for the patient, but rather to give guidance about what the patient himself is likely to have wished.[5] For many relatives this attitude comes naturally; and, while different members of the family may disagree on what they themselves want, they may still be able to agree on what their father, for example, would have wished. Such substituted judgements raise difficult issues,[49] and relatives have been found to be poor at guessing an elderly person's wishes.[50]

As in other periods of life (for example with handicapped new-born children) decisions about administering or withdrawing treatment fall into a different category from those concerning the basic requirements of life, especially food and drink. At the point when the elderly patient no longer willingly takes food very difficult decisions have to be made, especially by the nursing staff.[51,52] There are problems both of appraisal (is the patient refusing food because she cannot manage to swallow, because she is depressed, because she is angry with me, or because she has consciously chosen to die?) and with the perception of duty (if she adamantly refuses, should I leave her in peace but unfed, or torment her with unwanted food?).

The availability of mechanical methods of nutrition (such as nasogastric tube or intravenous feeding) probably only compounds these dilemmas. Not only do they create discomfort and burden for the patient, but they also divert nursing attention from other important aspects of care—the risk is that the tubes will be nursed, not the patient.[52] Norberg and colleagues vividly discuss[51] these issues, and focus on the anxiety and conflict that the nurse experiences if she sees it as her duty exclusively to keep the patient alive. The hospice movement has taught us that concentration on achieving a good death for the patient in its due and proper time allows, paradoxically, for a much more optimistic focus to management. This applies as much to the later stages of dementia as to other conditions.

The perspective that prefers a good death to simply death may also be helpful in decisions about treatment of incidental illness (see above). Sometimes the chances of survival offered by a treatment are less important than the effect it may have on the likely manner of death. For example, where an elderly person with an acute abdomen is thought likely to die under anaesthetic it may still be worth considering whether that death is better than dying with unrelieved obstruction of the bowel.[44] In other words, management of a foreseeable, though not certain, death has an honourable place in any treatment plan.

The manner of death is likely to matter greatly to the relatives. For their sakes alone it is important that careful thought be given to the management of death. Most people, as they look ahead towards their own deaths, fear burdening their relatives, and want to be remembered well. The final days of a dying old person are likely to be vividly remembered by the relatives. A death which caused them to feel angry, helpless, guilty, or bitter may overshadow the memories of the person's earlier life.[53,54] The last gift of a dying person to her family is the memory of a good death, in which they were able to play their proper part. It is the duty of those who care for elderly people to make it possible for that gift to be made.

## References

1 Thomasma, D. C.: Freedom, dependency and care of the very old. *Journal of the American Geriatrics Society* **32**:906–14, 1984.

2 Graca, J. L.: Driving and aging, in *Ethical issues in the care of the elderly*, ed. D. W. Jahnigen and R. W. Schrier, pp. 577–89. Clinics in Geriatric Medicine **2** (3). Philadelphia, Saunders, 1986.

3 Harris, J.: Professional responsibility and consent to treatment, in *Consent and the incompetent patient: ethics, law and medicine*, ed. S. R. Hirsch and J. Harris, pp. 37–47. London, The Royal College of Psychiatrists, Gaskell, 1988, p. 43.

4 Gostin, L. O.: Observations on consent to treatment and review of clinical judgment in psychiatry: a discussion paper. *Journal of the Royal Society of Medicine* **74**:742–52, 1981.

5 McCullough, L. B.: Medical care for elderly patients with diminished competence: an ethical analysis. *Journal of the American Geriatrics Society* **32**:150–3, 1984.

6 Brody, B.: *Life and death decision making.* New York, Oxford University Press, 1988, pp. 100–3.

7 Ratzan, R. M.: Being old makes you different: The ethics of research with elderly subjects. *Hastings Center Report* **10**: 32–42, 1980.

8 Weintraub, M.: Ethical concerns and guidelines in research in geriatric pharmacology and therapeutics: individualisation, not codification. *Journal of the American Geriatrics Society* **32**: 44–8, 1988.

9 Wattis, J. P.: Should refusal of therapy lead to institutionalisation? *Geriatric Medicine* **18**:35–6, 1988.

10 Gray, J. A. M.: 'Section 47': an ethical dilemma for doctors. *Heath Trends* **12**:72–4, 1980.

11 Reich, W. T.: Ethical issues related to research involving elderly subjects. *The Gerontologist* **18**:326–37, 1978.

12 Warren, J. W., Sobal, J., Tenney, J. H., *et al.*: Informed consent by proxy. An issue in research with elderly patients. *New England Journal of Medicine* **315**:1124–8, 1986.

13 Institute of medical ethics: Research ethics committees. *Institute of Medical Ethics Bulletin* **18** (suppl. 2): 1–19, 1986.

14 Department of Health and Social Security: Mental Health Act 1983: Section 118. Draft Code of Practice. London, HMSO, 1985.

15 Langley, G. E.: A threat to psychiatric research? *British Medical Journal* **293**:133–4, 1986.

16 Murphy, E.: Psychiatric implications, in *Consent and the incompetent patient: ethics, law and medicine*, ed. S. R. Hirsch and J. Harris. London, Royal College of Psychiatrists Gaskell, 1988, pp. 65–73.

17 Kendell, R. E. and Langley, G. E.: Comments on ethics of research with dementia sufferers. *International Journal of Geriatric Psychiatry* **4**:239–46, 1989.

18 Robbins, L. J.: Restraining the elderly patient, in *Ethical issues in the care of the elderly*, ed. D. W. Jahnigen and R. W. Schrier, pp. 591–9. Clinics in Geriatric Medicine **2** (3). Philadelphia, Saunders, 1986.

19 Strumpf, N. E. and Evans, L. K.: Physical restraint of the hospitalised elderly: perceptions of patients and nurses. *Nursing Research* **37**:132–7, 1988.

20 Royal College of Nursing (Working Group of the Forum for Nurses Caring for the Elderly Mentally Ill): Focus on restraint: guidelines on the use of restraint, in the care of elderly people. London, RCN, 1987.

21 Lancet (editorial): Cotsides—protecting whom against what? *Lancet* **ii**:383–4, 1984.

22 Eastman, M.: *Old age abuse*. Age Concern, England, 1984.
23 Tomlin, S.: *Abuse of elderly people—an unnecessary and preventable problem*. British Geriatrics Society, 1989.
24 Roberts, A.: Serious gaps in care of the elderly. *British Medical Journal* **229**:682, 1989.
25 Avorn, J.: Benefit and cost analysis in geriatric care. Turning age discrimination into health policy. *New England Journal of Medicine* **310**:1294–1301, 1984.
26 Silver, G. A.: The old, the very old, and the too old. *Lancet* **ii**:1453, 1987.
27 Daniels, N.: *Am I my parents' keeper? An essay on justice between the young and the old*. Oxford, Oxford University Press, 1988.
28 Harris, J.: QALYfying the value of life. *Journal of Medical Ethics* **13**:117–23, 1987.
29 Stein, R. E. K., Gortmaker, S. L., Perrin, E. C., *et al.*: Severity of illness: concepts and measurements. *Lancet* **ii**:1506–9, 1987.
30 Donaldson, C., Atkinson, A., Bond, J. and Wright, K.: QALYs and long-term care for elderly people in the UK: scales for assessment of quality of life. *Age and Ageing* **17**:379–87, 1988.
31 Pearlman, R. A. and Speer, J. B.: Clinical conferences: quality-of-life considerations in geriatric care. *Journal of the American Geriatrics Society* **31**:113–20, 1983.
32 Loewy, E. H.: Treatment decisions in the mentally impaired: limiting but not abandoning treatment. *New England Journal of Medicine* **317**:1465–9, 1987.
33 Edmunds, L. H., Stephenson, L. W., Edie, R. N. and Ratcliffe, M. B.: Open-heart surgery in octogenarians. *New England Journal of Medicine* **319**:131–6, 1988.
34 Bedell, S. E., Delbanco, T. L., Cook, E. F. and Epstein, F. M.: Survival after cardiopulmonary resuscitation in the hospital. *New England Journal of Medicine* **309**:569–76, 1983.
35 Gulati, R. S., Bhan, G. L. and Horan, M. A.: Cardiopulmonary resuscitation of old people. *Lancet* **ii**:267–9, with correspondence 685, 794, 1983.
36 Evans, J. G.: Curing is caring. *Age and Ageing* **18**:217, 1989.
37 Bedell, S. E. and Delbanco, T. L.: Choices about cardiopulmonary resuscitation in the hospital. When do physicians talk with patients? *New England Journal of Medicine* **310**:1089–93, 1984.
38 Gunasekera, N. P. R., Tiller, D. J., Clements, L. T. S-J. and Bhattacharya, B. K.: Elderly patients' views on cardiopulmonary resuscitation. *Age and Ageing* **15**:364–8, 1986.
39 Levinson, A-J. R.: Termination of life support systems in the elderly: ethical issues. *Journal of Geriatric Psychiatry* **14**:71–85, 1981.
40 Neu, S. and Kjellstrand, C. M.: Stopping long-term dialysis. An empirical study of withdrawal of life-supporting treatment. *New England Journal of Medicine* **314**:14–20, 1986.
41 Hilfiker, D.: Allowing the debilitated to die. Facing our ethical choices. *New England Journal of Medicine* **308**:716–19, and also correspondence following: *New England Journal of Medicine* **309**:862–3, 1983.
42 Robertson, G. S.: Dealing with the brain-damaged old—dignity before sanctity. *Journal of Medical Ethics* **8**:173–9, 1982.
43 Robertson, G. S.: Ethical dilemmas of brain failure in the elderly. *British Medical Journal* **287**:1775–7, 1983.

44 Murphy, E.: Ethical dilemmas of brain failure in the elderly. *British Medical Journal* **288**:61–2, 1984 (letter).

45 Wattis, J. P. and Tyre, N.: Ethical dilemmas of brain failure in the elderly. *British Medical Journal* **288**:62, 1984 (letter).

46 Angell, M.: Euthanasia. *New England Journal of Medicine* **319**:1384–50, 1988.

47 Lazaroff, A. E. and Orr, W. F.: Living wills and other advance directives, in *Ethical issues in the care of the elderly*, ed. D. W. Jahnigan and R. W. Schrier, pp. 521–34. Clinics in Geriatric Medicine, 2 (3). Philadelphia, Saunders, 1986.

48 Wray, N., Brody, B., Bayer, T., *et al.*: Withholding medical treatment from the severely demented patient. Decisional processes and cost implications. *Archives of Internal Medicine* **148**:1980–84, 1988.

49 Brody, B.: Life and death decision-making. New York, Oxford University Press, 1988, pp. 30–2 and elsewhere.

50 Emanuel, E. J.: What criteria should guide decision-makers for incompetent patients? *Lancet* **i**:170–1, 1988.

51 Norberg, A., Norberg, B. and Bexell, G.: Ethical problems in feeding patients with advanced dementia. *British Medical Journal* **281**:847–8, 1980.

52 Lo, B. and Dornbrand, L.: Guiding the hand that feeds. Caring for the demented elderly. *New England Journal of Medicine* **311**:402–4, 1984.

53 Anonymous: When experience does not help. *British Medical Journal* **297**:1686–7, 1988.

54 Witherington, E.: De profundis. *British Medical Journal* **298**:1654, 1989.

# 18

# Ethics and forensic psychiatry

*Jonas Rappeport*

## What is forensic psychiatry?

Pollack, who has discussed this issue at length, distinguishes two distinct areas in which the professions of psychiatry and law interact.[1] The broader one involves legal issues touching upon the practice of psychiatry. These include commitment, guardianship, the right to treatment, and the right to refuse treatment. The term 'forensic psychiatry' should be limited to the actions of psychiatrists in assisting the law to carry out some of its responsibilities. Included are what Pollack calls 'psychiatry for legal purposes', covering issues such as criminal responsibility, competency at the time of a crime, testamentary capacity, child custody, and others where psychiatric opinions are sought by the law to help the law arrive at decisions. Many psychiatrists do not make this distinction, and are likely to designate as forensic psychiatry all facets of psychiatric involvement with the law. This chapter will focus on ethical problems that arise mainly in Pollack's narrower definition of forensic psychiatry.

The word 'forensic' comes from the Latin *forum*, and in the context of forensic psychiatry refers to the fact that the psychiatrist's report is made public, that the relationship between psychiatrist and client is not private and therapeutic, but open to the scrutiny of others. The ancient forums have today become the legislature and the court-room. They furnish psychiatry an opportunity to assist the law in maintaining a safe and orderly society.

Because the psychiatrist's forensic role is quite different from his usual medical one of serving an individual patient, questions have been raised as to whether it is ethical for a psychiatrist to serve a third party, the law. Who is being helped—the patient, the lawyer, or the court? This question became pertinent after the law accepted the idea that physicians specializing in mental disorders had something to offer in cases in which insanity or criminal responsibility were at issue. Before this time such cases were decided without such aid. One of the earliest cases to utilize the testimony of mental health experts was the *McNaghten* case of 1843. Gradually psychiatric specialists were introduced into court proceedings as experts, a trend which became established early in the twentieth century.

The early forensic psychiatrists were aware of the ethical issues that faced them in their effort to assist the law. They expressed concern about using the physician's role to obtain information for non-therapeutic purposes, as well as about other ethical problems inherent in forensic work. These concerns have been voiced more recently by, among others, Szasz,[2] Bazelon,[3] Robitscher,[4] and the APA Task Force on Sentencing.[5] Robitscher, for instance, has stated 'The psychiatrist is the most important non-government decision-maker in modern life, and he has much more power than most government officials.'[4] The psychiatrist has power to recommend to the court that a defendant be given a life sentence or even the death penalty; that a defendant be considered not guilty by reason of insanity or incompetent to stand trial; or that a deceased's will be invalidated. He can recommend the annulment of a marriage, or who should have custody of the children of a disrupted family. True, the psychiatrist only renders an opinion, and the final decision is that of judge or jury. Nevertheless, we should not underestimate the importance sometimes given to his opinions. To accept these grave responsibilities without careful adherence to ethical guidelines would represent a serious departure from the physician's usual ethical posture. The role of psychiatrist in working with the court and the law has been challenged by Thomas Szasz, who asserts that we abuse our power regularly, and, in fact, that we have no place in assisting the law.[2] Judge David Bazelon believes that such a role is legitimate, but that it requires real expertise; he accuses psychiatrists at times of pretending to have expert knowledge when in fact they do not.[3] Because our society is increasingly concerned about human rights, the law has increased its monitoring of the mental health system, since abuses have occurred and do occur there. Psychiatrists need therefore to become more knowledgeable about legal theories and concepts. Most psychiatric testimony is presented to courts not by individuals who consider themselves specialists in forensic psychiatry, but by general psychiatrists who are called upon from time to time for this purpose. Therefore it is urgent that guidelines about ethical issues should be established. This chapter should contribute to further discussion on the ethics of forensic psychiatry. Because of my lack of experience in the British and other legal systems, my discussion will focus mainly on the American scene; but I hope that the points made and the issues discussed will be of sufficient significance to merit the attention of psychiatrists everywhere. I am aware, however, that the relationship between physicians and patients in the United States is more on a contractual basis than in all other parts of the world. The generally accepted paternalistic role of the physician towards the patient has been replaced in the United States by patient's rights and patient autonomy and independence. To a lesser extent, other democratic countries are adopting some of these reforms. Currently there are active

patient-rights movements in both Canada and Britain. The recent establishment of a Bill of Rights in Canada has added a legal basis for new
patient rights.[6]

This contractual relationship raises various ethical issues for the
psychiatrist. Commitment hearings requiring testimony based on the
patient's communications to the psychiatrist raise confidentiality issues.
The increase in such adversarial hearings exposes psychiatry to greater
scrutiny, and raises additional issues concerning our credibility.

The right-to-treatment and the right-to-refuse-treatment movements
have raised issues which have been good and bad for both psychiatrists and
their patients. Patients have more autonomy, they participate in treatment
decisions, and therapeutic abuses can be avoided. This is particularly true
where decisions are made jointly by patients and their care-givers. However, placing treatment decisions into a judicial model has generally not
proved very productive. It is very costly and delays treatment, and it may,
therefore, not to be in the patient's best interests. Many ideas expressed in
this chapter are my own, and they may not suit others. They have been
influenced by my teachers and colleagues, particularly Doctors Robert
Sadoff and Irwin Perr, who originally worked with me in studying the
need for the development of ethical guidelines for forensic psychiatry
at the request of the American Academy of Psychiatry and the Law.
Following our original development of proposed guidelines in 1979, the
Academy's Ethics Committee, under the guidance of Henry Weinstein
MD, worked diligently to produce the *Ethical guidelines for the practice of
forensic psychiatry*.[7] These were approved by the Academy's membership in May 1987. Since the Academy does not itself hear ethical complaints, these guidelines have been given to the American Psychiatric
Association Ethics Committee for their guidance. In the future, attempts
will be made to integrate the guidelines into the APA's ethical principles.[8]
I plan to quote the AAPL *Ethical guidelines* where appropriate in this
discussion.

One question requiring attention is: Who should establish ethical guidelines for any professional group? Should it be done in an evolutionary
manner, by fiat, or by majority vote? Perhaps only general guidelines are
required, which would allow each person to evolve his own ethics, to be
judged by his peers when challenged (see Chapter 3). Or, after such
guidelines are formulated, those more knowledgeable about ethical issues
might develop operational ethical principles. The latter could then be used
by peer-review and ethics committees in their deliberations concerning
specific forensic problems. Many psychiatrists give little consideration to
ethical principles when testifying, despite the fact that they are sensitive to
problems of confidentiality in their relationship with patients. Nevertheless,
it is clear that, with increasing involvement in forensic matters, psychiatrists'

behaviour in specific situations may be challenged on ethical grounds, and they may be brought to account.

In the *Preamble*, the AAPL *Ethical guidelines* say:

The American Academy of Psychiatry and the Law is dedicated to the highest standards of practice in forensic psychiatry. Recognizing the unique aspects of this practice which is at the interface of the professions of psychiatry and the law, the Academy presents these guidelines for the ethical practice of forensic psychiatry.

A part of the *Commentary* to the *Preamble* says:

Forensic psychiatry is a sub-specialty of psychiatry in which scientific and clinical expertise is applied to legal issues in legal contexts embracing civil, criminal, correctional or legislative matters; forensic psychiatry should be practiced in accordance with guidelines and ethical principles enunciated by the profession of psychiatry.[7]

## Do we qualify as experts?

Before examining specific areas, we should discuss the issue of how expert are our opinions. Are we capable of informing the court about the true level of our knowledge, or is the legal system such that the court is not always cognizant of what we do, and do not know? Judge Bazelon has stated, with reference to the criminal justice system:

it is essential that the decision-maker not have the issues of state power and individual liberty obscured by testimony which over-reaches the bounds of the witness's legitimate expertise ... it is essential not only that the decision-maker confront what relevant information is known but that it also be aware of what is unknown ... Lastly, in evaluating the psychiatric and other information provided, the decision-maker must be able to see clearly the extent to which such information may be colored by individual and institutional bias.[9]

Similarly, in a recent article on ethics in mental health care, Roth states: 'Expert testimony by mental health professionals may fail to distinguish fact from opinion, e.g. abuse of psychiatric testimony concerning the prediction of violence and application of the death penalty; problems of conclusory testimony and double agentry in the handling of sex offenders.'[10]

Rules of evidence are so constructed that witnesses must be qualified as experts before they can render opinions. Some who may not be adequately qualified are nevertheless accepted as experts. Standards for determining the qualifications of an expert differ in medicine and in law. Of course, if a doctor consciously misrepresents his training or experience, it is a serious matter, not only unethical but fraudulent.

Psychiatric expertise has also been criticized by Ziskin, whose book on psychiatric and psychological testimony is well-used by attorneys.[11] In a recent article, Faust and Ziskin say 'The involvement of psychologists and psychiatrists within the legal arena continues to grow rapidly but remains highly controversial. Studies show that professionals often fail to reach reliable or valid conclusions and that the accuracy of their judgements does not necessarily surpass that of law persons, thus raising substantial doubt that psychologists or psychiatrists meet legal standards for expertise.'[12] Other critics—Ennis and Litwach among them—have also raised questions about whether psychiatric testimony meets the standard of expert testimony[13] which they believe should determine if it is ethical for psychiatrists to testify in the court-room. These positions opposing psychiatric testimony have not been generally accepted, and psychiatrists continue to be called upon to assist the court. In *Ake* v. *Oklahoma*, the Supreme Court stressed the importance of the defence having a psychiatrist available.[14–16]

I believe that we can testify honestly and effectively. While our ability to make accurate diagnoses is limited, the advent of DSM III and DSM III R has increased our reliability.[17,18] It is our job to make clear to the judge or jury that our expertise encompasses a more complete understanding of an individual than that of the average lay person, and that this goes beyond mere diagnosis. We must make this clear on direct examination and, certainly, on cross-examination. Since we cannot control the questions we are asked on cross-examination, some of our opinions will not be challenged to the extent that they should be in an adversarial system. The judge or jury will therefore not have a true picture of the limitations of our knowledge. What should we do if the cross-examining lawyer does not do a good job? Is it our responsibility to clarify? Most would say that we are acting ethically as long as our replies do not imply knowledge that we lack, and as long as we do not purposely try to confuse the issue. If we answer honestly, our doubts or the limits of our knowledge should be evident.

Halleck,[19] Halpern,[20] and Bazelon[21] all believe that psychiatrists do not have the specific expertise to evaluate competency to stand trial or criminal responsibility. They argue that participation in this part of the criminal-justice protocol represents an unethical role for psychiatrists. Furthermore, they believe it is embarrassing and degrading to participate in it. Why should we be embarrassed by differing opinions? Orthopaedic surgeons and other specialists disagree in their testimony in personal injury and malpractice cases. Perhaps the greater publicity given to 'insanity' cases means greater exposure to scrutiny? Are we embarrassed to let the public know that the state of our art is such that we do not know everything, and that there are different schools and theories in psychiatry?

Even if our opinions amount to no more than an educated guess, the law needs whatever expertise we can furnish. Although some may object to the educated-guess concept, we have no insanity tests of our own, only those of the law. Like any other experts called on by the law for assistance, we can refer to a related body of knowledge. However, as Bazelon again emphasizes, it is imperative that psychiatrists go only as far as that knowledge will allow: 'The danger ... is that psychiatric participation in these decisional processes may slide by imperceptible degrees into psychiatric assumption of responsibility for the ultimate decisions themselves. Rather than confining themselves to those aspects of the problem for which they have expertise, psychiatrists may be seduced into taking responsibility for making judgements or assessing facts about which they have no special competence.'[21]

If our opinions are educated guesses, we face an ethical problem similar to that discussed previously with regard to our responsibility to make clear the limits of our diagnostic ability. Who is responsible for making this clear, the psychiatrist, or the lawyer who cross-examines us? If we function solely as a consultant to those who employ us, what is our ethical duty? If the opposing lawyer does a poor job of ferreting out the weaknesses of our opinions via cross-examination, should we do his job for him?

Unfortunately, psychiatrists sometimes transgress the limits of psychiatric knowledge. I have heard such statements in staff conferences as 'That blankety-blank committed such a horrible offence, he's got to be responsible. I don't care how crazy he is.' A psychiatrist is understandably not insulated against having strong personal feelings. Is it not unethical to participate in a case when such feelings are generated?

With reference to expert qualifications, the AAPL *Guidelines* say:

Expertise in the practice of forensic psychiatry is claimed only in areas of actual knowledge and skills, training and experience.

### Commentary

As regards expert opinions, reports and testimony, the expert's qualifications should be presented accurately and precisely. As a correlate of the principle that expertise may be appropriately claimed only in areas of actual knowledge, skill, training and experience, there are areas of special expertise, such as the evaluation of children or persons of foreign cultures, or prisoners, that may require special training and expertise.[7]

## Opinions without examination

What should a psychiatrist do when he is asked to render an opinion about an individual he has not examined, as when a will or a death payment on a life-insurance policy is challenged? The patient is dead; only those who knew him remain. The information they offer may enable the psychiatrist to form an opinion as to the deceased's mental state when he wrote his will.

In some situations, such as after suicide, psychological autopsy may help clarify the deceased's mental state. Sometimes the psychiatrist may not be permitted by law (or legal manoeuvre) to examine a living person, but must instead render an opinion from data based on other sources. Generally, a physician does not give his opinion unless he has examined the patient.

Impartially and the adequacy of the clinical evaluation may be called into question when an expert opinion is offered without a personal examination. While there are authorities who would bar an expert opinion in regard to an individual who has not been personally examined, it is the position of the Academy that if, after earnest effort, it is not possible to conduct a personal examination, an opinion may be rendered on the basis of other information. However, under such circumstances, it is the responsibility of the forensic psychiatrist to assure that the statement of his opinion and any reports or testimony based on this opinion clearly indicate that there was no personal examination and that the opinion expressed is thereby limited.[7]

The APA Ethics Committee was asked:

*Question:* A psychiatrist testifies for the State in a criminal case about the competency of the defendant. He based his testimony upon medical records and did not examine the defendant nor have his approval to render an opinion. Was this ethical?

*Answer:* Yes. See Section 7, Annotation 3 (APA) (116).

Confusion has arisen by taking the second sentence above and not connecting it to the first sentence as was intended. It is common for forensic experts to offer opinions, as was done according to the question. Further, it would be too great an extension of the 'Goldwater rule' to say that a person, by being a defendant in court, has entered into '... the light of public attention.' This annotation was developed to protect public figures from psychiatric speculation that harms the reputation of the profession of psychiatry and the unsuspecting public figure (September 23, 1983).[22]

It is clear therefore that this does not interdict the rendering of clinical impressions (not a diagnosis) without examination when requested by the courts. However when speaking to the press caution is certainly advisable. When involved in a notorious forensic case, it is tempting to seek self-aggrandizement and publicity by openly discussing the case. In some circumstances the public has a genuine need for information and understanding, which may reduce anxiety in the face of stories about the horrible and frightening crimes. The ethical line here is a narrow one.

A related ethical issue involves a psychiatrist's statements about a dead patient. Robert Moore has stated:

When we speak of the dead ... our ethical principles are less clear. Privilege disappears with death so that the psychiatrist is not compelled legally to maintain confidences after the death of his patient or examinee. However, what is ethical may be beyond what is legal . . . lacking absolute guidelines, the psychiatrist should ask himself some questions before he makes public statements about deceased patients or examinees: Who will be harmed? Who will benefit? Are the benefits to society and my profession of great enough value to justify the balance of the two questions above? Why do I really want to do this?[23]

While Moore is referring to the deceased and to the problem of the psycho-historian, similar considerations apply to a notorious criminal defendant.

It is ethical to render an opinion (clinical impression and prognosis) based on a review of records, reports, and letters, under certain conditions, but *such opinions should never be rendered if it is at all possible to examine a person directly*. As thorough as records might be, personal examination is far better. Secondly, in those situations where a personal examination is not possible, it must be made completely clear that the opinions expressed are based only on a review of records and other information. Is it the responsibility of the psychiatrist to see that the judge or jury understands these limitations when he testifies, or can he let the responsibility rest with the cross-examiner? It would be unusual for the witness to state spontaneously that the patient was not examined unless asked by the lawyer. Goldzband's[35] policy is to inform the lawyer who requested his evaluation that he must reveal this fact on direct examination. I agree with this position, because this particular circumstance is so fraught with the possibility of misunderstanding.

## Confidentiality

Perhaps the most important problem in forensic psychiatry, as in psychiatry generally, is the issue of confidentiality. It appears evident that in court cases information obtained from a patient by a physician could be used against the patient's 'best interests'. A number of troubling questions immediately arise. What are the best interests of a murderer? Has the psychiatrist obtained information without the former's full understanding that it might be used to his detriment? Has the interviewee given truly informed consent? Is informed consent possible under the circumstances, and is it our responsibility or that of the patient's lawyer? Will the psychiatrist be able to obtain information he needs and still have a fully informed and consenting patient? Is the examinee a 'patient' or an 'individual being examined' when we interview him for his lawyer or the court?

A serious potential for abuse of the relationship between doctor and patient exists whenever a forensic interview is conducted. It is imperative that the patient should be clearly informed whose servant the interviewer is. The latter should advise the examinee: 'I represent the prosecutor, or the court, or your lawyer (whichever is appropriate); I am here to examine you in order to determine your competency to stand trial; if I report that you are so mentally ill that you cannot stand trial, you will go to a hospital; I may need to report to the court anything that you tell me; if there is something you don't want me to report, call this to my attention, and I will then have to use my judgement.' This makes the forensic interview totally different from the usual therapeutic relationship, where confidentiality is the rule. Although we may try to help the patient deal with the law, our help is quite different from that which we give in our more usual treatment role. Therefore, it is imperative that the interviewer knows just what are the limits of confidentiality, and these must be conveyed to the individual examined. In some situations it is possible to guarantee the patient full confidentiality (under the lawyer's 'work-product rule'). This varies in different jurisdictions, and should be promised only under the assurance of the patient's lawyer. Such exceptions, however, do not invalidate the usual rule—that to pretend that the usual doctor–patient role is in effect during a forensic examination is patently dishonest and unethical.

The AAPL *Guidelines* refer to this issue, in part, as follows:

Respect for the individual's right of privacy and the maintenance of confidentiality are major concerns of the psychiatrist performing forensic evaluations. The psychiatrist maintains confidentiality to the extent possible given the legal context . . . .

## Commentary

The forensic situation often presents significant problems in regard to confidentiality. The psychiatrist must be aware of and alert to those issues of privacy and confidentiality presented by the particular forensic situation. Notice should be given as to any limitations.

For example, before beginning a forensic evaluation, the psychiatrist should inform the evaluee that although he is a psychiatrist, he is not the evaluee's 'doctor'. The psychiatrist should indicate for whom he is conducting the examination and what he will do with the information obtained as a result of the examination. There is a continuing obligation to be sensitive to the fact that although a warning has been given, there may be a slippage and a treatment relationship may develop in the mind of the examinee.

The psychiatrist should take precautions to assure that none of the confidential information he receives falls into the hands of unauthorized persons.

The psychiatrist should clarify with a potentially retaining attorney whether an initial screening conversation prior to a formal agreement will interdict consultation with the opposing side if the psychiatrist decides not to accept the consultation.

In a treatment situation, whether in regard to an inpatient or to an outpatient in a parole, probation, or conditional release situation, the psychiatrist should be clear about any limitations on the usual principles of confidentiality in the treatment relationship and assure that these limitations are communicated to the patient. The psychiatrist should be familiar with the institutional policies in regard to confidentiality. Where no policy exists, the psychiatrist should clarify these matters with the institutional authorities and develop working guidelines to define his role.[7]

Special problems may arise when the psychiatrist is engaged by the prosecutor. Has the psychiatrist's 'medical presence' seduced a defendant to confess or reveal evidence previously unknown to the prosecutor? Should the psychiatrist warn the subject not to tell him certain information? What is the proper use of such information? Is it unethical to tell the prosecutor? What if the patient was not adequately warned? Should the doctor testify about information he obtained in this fashion? In a recent instance, a forensic psychiatrist examined an offender for the defence. He believed that under the law his notes were totally confidential and privileged. Upon reading the report, the prosecutor subpoenaed his voluminous notes. The psychiatrist resisted the subpoena, but was advised that his interpretation of privileged communications law might be incorrect, and that the notes might have to be submitted. He went to court to fight. The judge insisted on his statutory right to review the notes, and, after doing so, decided that the material was too inflammatory and that the prosecutor did not have the right to it. In many American states the psychiatrist's notes would be subject to a subpoena and discoverable by the prosecution. Was the doctor unethical, implying a guarantee when not absolutely sure? It is imperative that we act most cautiously, even if the result is a less thorough evaluation.

The AAPL *Guidelines* recommend:

The informed consent of the subject of a forensic evaluation is obtained when possible. Where consent is not required, notice is given to the evaluee of the nature of the evaluation. If the evaluee is not competent to give consent, substituted consent is obtained in accordance with the laws of the jurisdiction.

Some of the Commentary related to this is:

It is important to appreciate that in particular situations, such as court ordered evaluations for competency to stand trial or involuntary commitment, consent is not required. In such a case, the psychiatrist should so inform the subject and explain that the evaluation is legally required and that if the subject refuses to participate in the evaluation, this fact will be included in any report or testimony.

With regard to any person charged with criminal acts, ethical considerations preclude forensic evaluation prior to access to, or availability of legal counsel. The only exception is an examination for the purpose of rendering emergency medical care and treatment.

Consent to treatment in a jail or prison or other criminal justice setting must be differentiated from consent to evaluation. The psychiatrists providing treatment in these settings should be familiar with the jurisdiction's rules in regard to the patient's right to refuse treatment.[7]

## The pre-arraignment evaluation

The ethics of the pre-arraignment psychiatric examination are a matter for concern. Several years ago a problem arose in Southern California when it was discovered that a district attorney routinely arranged for a psychiatrist to interview suspected offenders as part of the interrogation procedure, prior to arraignment. Many believed that this violated the rights of the alleged offenders and constituted unethical psychiatric practice.

Was the prosecutor using the psychiatrist's humanitarian role in order to obtain information for prosecutory purposes, or to use at trial to counter an insanity plea? Was the psychiatrist relying on the police (or prosecutor) to inform the defendant that he had a right not to speak to the doctor? Was the defendant competently and knowingly waiving that right?

The issue was considered by various committees of the American Psychiatric Association, each group rendering a different opinion. Goldzband has discussed the issues involved in detail.[24]

In the case of *Estelle* v. *Smith*, Dr Grigson examined Mr Smith for competency to stand trial without the knowledge of Mr Smith's attorney. Of more serious concern in that case was that the doctor later testified in the penalty (death) phase of the trial, giving evidence based on what he had learned in the pre-trial competency evaluation. The Supreme Court said:

The admission of the doctor's testimony at the penalty phase violated the respondent's Fifth Amendment privilege against compelled self-incrimination, because he was not advised before the pre-trial psychiatric examination that he had a right to remain silent and that any statement he made could be used against him at a capital sentencing proceeding.[25]

Section 9 of the American Medical Association *Principles of medical ethics with annotations especially applicable to psychiatry* reads:

Ethical considerations in medical practice preclude the psychiatric evaluation of any adult charged with criminal acts prior to access to, or availability of, legal counsel. The only exception is the rendering of care to the person for the sole purpose of medical treatment.[7]

Why is this such a problem? A person is arrested, read his rights, and is interrogated. In walks the friendly psychiatrist (sent by the prosecutor). He introduces himself as a doctor and sits down to talk to the person in order to discover his mental state now and at the time of the crime. The individual having been interrogated (an experience which probably would make most people anxious) may wish to share his innermost feelings with the psychiatrist; it may be to his benefit to reveal what is going on in his mind now and what was going on in his mind at the time of the crime. Such information may be most useful in a defence of not guilty by reason of insanity. On the other hand, the information could be damaging. Another opinion is that it is right for the psychiatrist to examine the suspect only after his arraignment and on the request of his lawyer. While arraignment occurs promptly, defence counsel's request for an examination may be delayed weeks, possibly months, allowing the development of secondary defences and elaboration of thoughts and feelings which may obscure the original condition.

Might it not be better for a psychiatric interview to be done at the outset? The answer to this question may depend on the conditions under which the prosecutor's psychiatrist operates. Does he always relay to the defence lawyer everything the individual has told him? Is his orientation prosecutory, defence, or non-adversarial? Does the defence lawyer always know that such an evaluation was conducted? Does the evaluation protect society in any way? By delay, the defendant could be coached to fabricate a psychosis. On the other hand, he might recover completely from an acute psychosis and have genuine amnesia for the episode, thus seriously impairing his ability to convince the court of his insanity at the time of the crime. Had he been examined earlier, the psychiatrist could have reported on his condition at the time of arrest. This is a complicated issue. While pre-arraignment examination before the defendant has obtained a lawyer may benefit the defendant, and also the public by assisting the prosecution, its potential for abuse is so great that it cannot be condoned. Instead, we should encourage the defence lawyer to request an evaluation as soon after arrest as possible. Under no circumstances should the examination be done without his knowledge. Of course, this position does not preclude any necessary *treatment* prior to appointment of counsel.

## The insanity plea

Involvement in the insanity plea is considered the hallmark of forensic psychiatry. Psychiatry receives most exposure through media coverage of sensational trials. Whenever a heinous crime is committed, the insanity plea is considered by the defence. Of those examined to determine criminal responsibility, almost 90 per cent are considered responsible. Of the remaining 10 per cent, less than 0.5 per cent are found 'not guilty by reason of insanity'.[26,27] Nevertheless, our participation at this stage of the criminal justice process serves an important role.

The ethical issue of concern with regard to psychiatric participation in the insanity plea is how to formulate the opinions which determine our evaluation.

Is the sole determinant of responsibility the presence or absence of psychosis? In my view, diagnosis alone is inadequate to determine the question of responsibility; the defendant's thought process and their relationship to the crime must also be considered. There are situations, although they are rare, where a person suffering from a personality disorder may appear to be not responsible. The APA statement below differs with this.

After the trial in the case of *US* v. *John Hinckley*, the APA Insanity Defense Work Group recommended: '... the terms mental disease or mental retardation include only those severely abnormal mental conditions that grossly and demonstrably impair a person's perception or understanding of reality and that are not attributable primarily to the voluntary ingestion of alcohol or other psychoactive substances.'[28]

## Testifying

A prominent American forensic psychiatrist, Bernard Diamond,[29] refuses to testify if his testimony will harm an individual he has examined; therefore he is never called upon by the prosecution, a situation which he gladly accepts. When he testifies for the defence, his attitude is brought to the jury's attention, as it should be. Is it proper for a psychiatrist to participate in a trial where his testimony might cause the defendant to be punished? An important dictum in medicine is *Primum non nocere*, 'First do no harm'. A psychiatrist who testifies that a defendant is dangerous, cannot be helped by treatment, and will always be a danger to society, is by such testimony encouraging the jury to request the most severe sentence—even the death penalty if this is applicable. Is he doing harm? If the psychiatrist is consultant to a lawyer or to the court, and not a physician treating a patient, then the dictum does not apply. (It is a matter of opinion whether incarceration is harmful.) Is this a role for a psychiatrist? What about his responsibility to the community? Should society not also receive his help? After all, we do not make a decision, but only render a scientific opinion. The decision is that of the court. We only present our understanding of an individual and his behaviour for the court's consideration. It could be argued that good citizens—judges and jurors—should have expert assistance in reaching their decision. Judge Bazelon believes the psychiatrist should stay in the court-room: 'Total retreat, to my mind, is neither a desirable nor a viable option ... Unquestionably, inclusion of the psychiatric perspective often enhances the sophistication with which such public and private decisions may be reached.'[3] If we have a role, then we must render the best opinions that we can, recognizing that the opinion may be used in a way that the defendant does not regard as beneficial.

How strongly should we press our opinion when testifying? Should we conceal our limitations or take the opportunity to inform the court about them? A wishy-washy witness is not useful; but one who is so self-assured that he admits to no possibility of bias, error, or limitation is not credible. A witness who attempts honestly to present his opinion without either exaggeration or self-depreciation is likely to be the most effective. Halleck says:

There is considerable agreement among psychiatrists who do a lot of courtroom work that a psychiatrist can comfortably sustain a truly adversarial role only until he is actually sworn in as a witness. In preparing his report, in reviewing the attorney's case, in anticipating cross-examination, and in anticipating and contradicting testimony of other expert witnesses, the psychiatrist can fully commit himself to the cause of his employer . . . Once the psychiatrist is sworn in, however, and takes the witness stand, he should cease to view himself as an adversary. At this point he becomes a servant of the court. This point cannot be over-stressed. The psychiatrist when testifying must have the psychological flexibility to initiate a modest change in his identity . . . When he takes the witness stand the psychiatrist becomes a person committed to the process of truth-seeking no matter how the truth may conflict with his own ideologies. At this point the psychiatrist should not be reluctant to reveal information that may be adverse to his client's interest. He should never make any effort to embellish his testimony in a manner which leads to even minor distortions of information.[30]

In dealing with impartiality and objectivity, the AAPL *Guidelines* suggest:

The forensic psychiatrist functions as an expert within the legal process. Although he may be retained by one party to a dispute in a civil matter or the prosecution or defense in a criminal matter, he adheres to the principles of impartiality and objectivity. His clinical evaluation and the application of the data obtained to the legal criteria are performed in the spirit of such impartiality and objectivity. His opinion reflects this impartiality and objectivity.

*Commentary*

The adversarial nature of our Anglo-American legal process presents special hazards for the practicing forensic psychiatrist. Being retained by one side in a civil or criminal matter exposes the forensic psychiatrist to the potential for unintended bias and the danger of distortion of his opinion. It is the responsibility of the forensic psychiatrist to minimize such hazards by carrying out his responsibilities in an impartial and objective manner.

The practicing forensic psychiatrist enhances the impartiality and objectivity of his work by basing his forensic opinions, his forensic reports and his forensic testimony on all the data available to him. He communicates the impartiality and objectivity of his work and the soundness of his clinical opinion by distinguishing, to the extent possible, between verified and unverified information as well as between clinical 'facts', 'inferences' and 'impressions'.[7]

## Pre-trial

Once we have made the decision to testify, other problems arise. In order to present convincing scientific evidence, it is necessary to discuss in detail the past history and current reactions of the defendant, and to present some psychodynamic understanding of what was going on in him at the time of the crime. Is it proper for the defendant to hear the testimony about the examination? If he were a person evaluated for treatment, one might not discuss these matters with him; but the law states appropriately that the defendant has a right to hear the testimony of all witnesses; he must be able to instruct his lawyer about the accuracy of the information presented. Is it unethical for us to participate under such conditions? We present a formulation which we believe correct but which the defendant may totally reject or find frightening, confusing, or disorganizing to himself or to his family. I do not believe that such testimony is unethical. In a situation where the law must prevail, the defendant has to choose. Does he want psychiatric testimony or not? If he does, then he risks hearing unpleasant things. Experience indicates that most defendants can deal with such testimony. However, some cannot. Strasburger describes such a situation, and suggests strategies for minimizing any harm.[31] Miller has recently suggested that these problems can be avoided by sharing the information prior to trial.[32]

## Pre-sentence

When undergoing a pre-sentence psychiatric examination, the defendant may admit guilt for crimes for which he has never been charged. Can this information be used by the prosecution as the basis for new charges? Probably not; however, the prosecutor could start a new investigation. Is it ethical to include such information in a report, considering the influence it might have on the judge? What about the psychiatrist's responsibility to the judge and the community? What about the expert's professional integrity if he 'covers up'? Did the patient fully understand the relationship, and know what use would be made of the information he divulged? I cannot offer specific answers to these thorny questions; solutions depend on the many variables peculiar to each case. Perhaps, with apologies to Shakespeare, 'To thine own self [and thy profession] be true' is the best we can do until clearer guidelines are established.

Are we acting unethically when our pre-sentence recommendations are not based on firm data? Our ability to predict future behaviour and the effectiveness of treatment may be based on very limited knowledge. It is important to convey the reasons for our opinions and to eliminate personal bias. We also have responsibility to be well acquainted with the professional literature.

## The death penalty

After conviction for a capital crime, some jurisdictions require an immediate hearing before the same jury to determine whether the sentence should be life imprisonment or death. In Texas, for example, the psychiatrist is asked about the defendant's propensity to commit violent crimes and also about his treatability. In the Smith case in Texas, Dr James Grigson testified: 'It's my opinion that really Mr Smith does not have any regard for another human being's property or for his life, regardless of who it may be.' He stated further, 'We don't have anything in medicine or psychiatry that in any way at all modifies or changes their behaviour.'[33] The defendant had only one previous conviction, for possession of a small quantity of marijuana. The psychiatrist's testimony was based on an examination of Smith for competency at the judge's request prior to his murder trial. Smith had co-operated, but was not told that the assessment was for any reason other than to determine competency; his lawyers were not aware of the examination. After conviction the case was appealed and the appellate court ruled, 'A defendant may not be compelled to speak to a psychiatrist who can use his statement against him at the sentencing phase of a capital trial.'[34] If prosecution desired such an examination, the court added, the defendant should be warned about the use of the findings and have the 'guiding hand of counsel'.

Could Dr Grigson's opinion be considered a breach of ethical principles? He rendered an opinion on data obtained under the guise of another purpose, without informing the patient, and his opinion had little or no scientific validity. In any event, the case should serve as a warning how easily one can become involved in questionable activities. In forensic work, it is imperative always to bear in mind the circumstances under which information is obtained. Death-penalty testimony also raises, in bold relief, the previously discussed issue of 'doing harm'.

## Ethical issues in civil law

Many situations in civil litigation need careful scrutiny for the presence of ethical problems. The one which has caused me most concern involves custody evaluations, where often the psychiatrist is only able to examine one party to the custody suit. For example, the mother may be his patient, and he is asked to report on whether she is psychologically sound enough to have or retain custody of her children. Her lawyer, of course, would like the psychiatrist to include a negative opinion about the competing spouse, whom the doctor has not examined or perhaps has seen only briefly in connection with the wife's therapy. Any definite reference by the psychiatrist to the husband's capacity as a father is unethical. It is proper to indicate that, on the basis of experience with the mother, there is nothing which would cause question about her competence as a mother. However, it is unethical to offer an opinion on the father based on statements made by his wife. Her statements are very likely to be self-serving.

Suppose the father displayed sick or inappropriate behaviour during the limited therapeutic contacts described above. Should the psychiatrist mention these and indicate that such behaviour indicates that this man may not be an adequate father? If this is done, it is the psychiatrist's responsibility to make clear that this impression is not the result of a complete and thorough examination. Statements contained in psychiatric reports may be given exaggerated significance by advocates in an adversarial procedure; opinions should therefore be based only on solid data. Goldzband discusses this issue in greater detail in his recent book *Custody cases and expert witnesses*.[36]

The AAPL *Guidelines* say:

In custody cases, impartiality and objectivity require that all parties be interviewed, if possible, before an opinion is rendered. When this is not possible, or, if for any reason not done, this fact should be clearly indicated in the forensic psychiatrist's report and testimony. Where one parent has not been seen, even after deliberate effort, it may be inappropriate to comment on that parent's fitness as a parent. Any comments on that parent's fitness should be qualified and the data for the opinion be clearly indicated.[7]

## Malpractice

Psychiatrists frequently produce definitive and declaratory statements that a physician being sued practised below the appropriate standard of care which are based on the patient's statement alone, or, conversely, statements that the physician practised within the standard of care which are based solely on the physician's statement. This seems to me to be as wrong as rendering an opinion in a custody case about the parenting skill of the parent who was not examined based on the words of the examined parent. How can one be definite about what happened when the facts are in dispute? Is it not unethical to make definitive statements under these circumstances?[37]

## Personal injury

Personal injury or tort cases can lead to ethical problems, particularly because money is involved. What should be included in a psychiatric report after examining an allegedly injured individual? What should the psychiatrist do when the patient, claiming that his back was hurt during a fall in a restaurant, relates that he also injured his back two years prior to the restaurant fall while painting at home? If such a statement is included, the patient's lawyer may ask to have it deleted. Is it unethical to do so? If the patient has understood the purpose of the examination, then all his disclosures must be reported. Keeping such information secret, in my opinion, represents collusion, and is unethical, and probably illegal.

Irrelevant personal data can be eliminated; however, even here careful judgement is required. See the previous discussion on confidentiality and the AAPL *Guidelines*.

A similar problem arises when the patient lies in the examination, and does not furnish pertinent information. On the witness stand the psychiatrist may then be presented with the missing facts, for example, 'Doctor, did you know that Mr. Jones also injured his back two years prior to the current accident when he fell off a ladder while painting his house?' Indicating unawareness of such an occurrence, the expert witness would be shown proof that it occurred, and then would be asked, 'Doctor, would knowledge of this change your opinion as to the causal relationship of the recent accident to his back problems?' The answer would then have to be 'Yes, it certainly might.'

Another problem is the possibility that pejorative or 'undesirable' information in a report might be used to coerce a patient into settling a case. One example is a statement that the patient was previously treated for syphilis contracted while on an excursion to the red-light district, a matter totally unrelated to the issue in hand. The patient may have willingly spoken of this, despite his knowledge of what it could be used for, because he wanted the psychiatrist to have a full understanding of his medical history. Or it might have been obtained from other medical records. The patient may have asked the examiner not to mention the information. Perhaps he holds an important public position, and would not want such information to become public, especially in the court-room. If it were included in the report he might be forced to settle the case to keep it from being revealed. The psychiatrist has a responsibility, even in the forensic setting, to protect the patient when ethically permissible. I suspect that at times we do this by unconscious selection of what we recall. Again, this is an issue that must be decided on a case-by-case basis, as is illustrated by the examples I have given here; not to include the patient's statement that he had previously fallen off a ladder would represent omission of a significant fact; omission of the information about previous syphilis would not.

In the United States, unlike Britain, lawyers operate on a contingency basis in personal-injury cases. Since the lawyer is usually responsible for the charges of the psychiatric examination and report, he might prefer that the examining psychiatrist also accept such an arrangement. However, participation in any contingency-fee arrangement is prohibited by ethical tenets of both the American Medical and Psychiatric Associations. It should be made clear at the outset, therefore, that the lawyer is responsible for the psychiatrist's fee upon receipt of the report. Some psychiatrists are willing to agree to hold the litigant responsible for charges; but this could be a veiled type of contingency.

The AAPL *Guidelines* say:

Contingency fees, because of the problem that these create in regard to impartiality and objectivity, should not be accepted. On the other hand, retainer fees do not create problems in regard to impartiality and objectivity and, therefore, may be accepted.

Is it proper for the psychiatrists employed by opposing sides in litigation to confer with each other? Most lawyers oppose 'collaboration' or discussion unless prior arrangements have been made. Although informal discussion between colleagues is a standard procedure in medicine, it is not in law. Here the psychiatrist's duty is to the lawyer, and he should abide by his wishes. Legal practice is totally different from medical practice. Law is both adversarial and proprietary, and opinions are guarded; whereas the essence of medicine is its openness and its free communication among colleagues.

A psychiatrist may occasionally find himself briefly involved in consultation with a lawyer, and discover that he cannot be of help. If later he is called upon by the other side to participate in the case, it would be improper for him to do so unless the first lawyer releases him—a highly unlikely prospect.

## Forensic hospital practice

Many ethical questions arise in forensic hospital practice. While non-criminal patients may be confined involuntarily in an ordinary mental hospital, patients treated in forensic psychiatric institutions are there on an even more clearly involuntary basis. They are there by court order, either having been found not guilty by reason of insanity, or being evaluated for this plea, or because they have been transferred from a less secure hospital.

The inadequate treatment offered in many forensic psychiatric hospitals is a pressing issue for all psychiatrists (see Chapter 21). If a patient is to be exposed to adverse conditions beyond a certain limit, should we refuse to co-operate in procedures which might result in his confinement in such sub-standard institutions? If we note these poor standards, should we not speak out?

Strong community or political pressure may be exerted on a forensic psychiatrist not to release a patient because of the community's unreasonable fear. In a study of the staff's decisions to release or not to release forensic patients, Thornberry and Jacoby[38] found evidence of 'political predictions'. They believed that the medical opinions were affected by socio-political considerations. Is it not unethical and a dereliction of responsibility to capitulate to such pressure when the psychiatrist has concluded that the patient is no longer dangerous? A hospital superintendent once confided to me that he had obtained a job and accommodation for one such patient, and engineered an 'escape' for him. Several superintendents have obtained releases by arranging a hearing with a judge—one more receptive to professional opinion than another judge, who said, 'I don't care how well he is, he is going to stay in the hospital as long as I hear the case.' Whether or not such efforts are justifiable or ethical, I cannot say. Medicine has an honourable tradition of not responding to social or political pressure in making judgements. The same tradition should apply in these forensic situations, unless we wish to follow the example of certain Soviet practices (see Chapter 24).

The treatment of those who have been found not guilty by reason of insanity and who have been committed may cause problems if the hospital personnel disagree with the verdict. For example, the hospital psychiatrist may believe the patient was responsible for his behaviour, and may have testified to that effect. How does this doctor now treat a patient for an illness that he does not believe exists? Does he merely 'warehouse' the patient, because he views him as a malingerer, or does he attempt to treat him responsibly, and with as open a mind as he can? It is obvious that any course but the latter would be unethical. A policeman shot and killed a boy whom he thought was about to shoot him. No gun was found on the boy. The policeman was found not guilty by reason of insanity, relying on testimony by defence psychiatrists that he suffered from an epileptic disorder. The hospital staff, having found no such disorder, and in fact no evidence of mental illness, wanted to release him almost immediately. The court, however, insisted that the patient receive treatment, or at least extensive observation.

## The forensic psychiatrist in the prison

Difficult problems arise when psychiatrists work in prisons, particularly if they lack a clear contractual relationship with the institution, and do not make their position clear to the patient (inmate). It might be tempting for such psychiatrists to align themselves with the administration, and to ferret out possible riots, smuggling of contraband, or other illegal acts. Perverting the role of therapist in this manner is certainly improper. On the other hand, some psychiatrists tend to identify with the prisoner, align themselves not with, but against, the administration, and offer inmates a level of confidentiality which they cannot guarantee. In one such situation the warden, following a murder within his institution, attempted to obtain the psychiatrist's records so that he could get more information about the suspect. The psychiatrist believed, incorrectly, that he had a confidential relationship with the inmate, and that the records were in his control. However, no psychiatrist employed in that institution had ever established such a contract with the warden, and the psychiatrist's records were turned over. Was the doctor irresponsible in not gaining a prior clarification of this issue, and in believing that he could walk into a public institution and set his own ground rules? For instance, what should one do when an inmate in individual therapy reveals that he is currently involved in an escape plan? Is it ethical to report this to the prison authorities? The answer might depend on the psychiatrist's contract with the patient and with the administration. At the very least, it would be a difficult problem, particularly if the incipient escape or riot plan could cause injury to others.

## Summary

Forensic psychiatry is not a field into which a psychiatrist should step without a good deal of forethought. It contains many ethical pitfalls. The contract of the forensic psychiatrist is essentially not with the patient, but with the latter's lawyer or the court. In fact, the 'patient' is not really a patient in the usual doctor–patient sense. This needs to be made clear to the examinee at the outset. Another house is being entered, not the house of medicine but that of law—with its different motives, goals, and rules of conduct. In medicine we communicate openly, in the law we may not. In medicine we listen to everything, and may discuss it with colleagues. In law, the attorney by whom we are employed may not want us to do this. He may even wish us to omit information which he believes will harm his client; we may want to omit material which we feel is irrelevant. We may be tempted to say too much or too little, or in our zeal advance ideas and theories which have no foundation, or allow our personal bias to appear as professional opinion. These are only some of the ethical problems which arise in the forensic arena. Weinstock recently surveyed a group of forensic psychiatrists on their perception of ethical issues.[39]

I have raised more questions than I have provided answers. Forensic psychiatry as a sub-specialty is in its infancy. The American Academy of Psychiatry and the Law has provided ethical guidelines which are helpful; but they are not always able to supply clear-cut ethical positions. Hopefully experience and discussion will assist in the reduction of these difficult problems. I have undertaken to give my opinion when I have felt justified in doing so. Certainly the most important maxim for the psychiatrist is not to take advantage of the doctor–client relationship by encouraging the subject to talk without making it absolutely clear whom he represents and what use will be made of the information. Forensic work gives the psychiatrist an opportunity to assist people in a way which is different from that of the therapist, and to assist society through the law; but it can also put one in a position to do much harm. As George Moore once said: 'The difficulty in life is the choice.'

# References

1 Pollack, S.: Forensic psychiatry, a specialty. *American Academy of Psychiatry and the Law Bulletin* **II**:1–6, 1974.

2 Szasz, T.: *Psychiatry justice.* New York, Macmillan, 1975.

3 Bazelon, D.: The role of the psychiatrist in the criminal justice system. *American Academy of Psychiatry and the Law Bulletin* **6**:139–46, 1978.

4 Robitscher, J.: *The powers of psychiatry.* Boston, Houghton Mifflin, 1980.

5 Report of the Task Force on the Role of Psychiatry in the Sentencing Process, in *Issues in forensic psychiatry*, pp. 191–200. Washington DC, American Psychiatric Association, 1984.

6 Rappeport, J.: Belegaled: mental health and the law in the United States, 1986. *Canadian Journal of Psychiatry* **32**:719–27, 1987.

7 *Ethical guidelines for the practice of forensic psychiatry*, ratified 5/87, American Academy of Psychiatry and the Law, Baltimore, MD.

8 American Psychiatric Association: *The principles of medical ethics with annotations especially applicable to psychiatry.* Washington DC, APA, 1988.

9 Bazelon, D.: The role of the psychiatrist in the criminal justice system. *Bulletin of the American Academy of Psychiatry and the Law* **6**:145, 1978.

10 Roth, L. N.: To respect personal families and communities: some problems in ethics of mental health care. *Psychiatry Digest* **40**:17–26, 1979.

11 Ziskin, J.: *Coping with psychiatric and psychological testimony*, 4th edn. Marina del Rey, CA, Law and Psychology Press, 1988.

12 Faust, D. and Ziskin, J.: The expert witness in psychology and psychiatry. *Science* **241**:31–5, 1988.

13 Ennis, B. J. and Litwach, T. R.: Psychiatry and the presumption of expertise: flipping coins in the courtroom. *California Law Review* **62**:693–752, 1974.

14 *Ake* v. *Oklahoma*, 470 US 68 (1985).

15 Appelbaum, P. S.: In the wake of Ake: the ethics of expert testimony in an advocate's world. *Bulletin of the American Academy of Psychiatry and the Law* **15**:15–25, 1987.

16 Rachlin, S.: From impartial expert to adversary in the wake of Ake. *Bulletin of the American Academy of Psychiatry and the Law* **16**:1–9, 1988.

17 *Diagnostic and statistical manual of mental disorders*, 3rd edn (DSM III). Washington DC, American Psychiatric Association, 1980.

18 *Diagnostic and statistical manual of mental disorders*, 3rd edn revised (DSM III). Washington DC, American Psychiatric Association, 1987.

19 Halleck, S. L.: *Psychiatry and the dilemmas of crime.* Los Angeles, University of California, 1971.

20 Halpern, A. L.: Use and abuse of psychiatry in competency examinations of criminal defendants. *Psychiatric Annals* **5**:4, 1975.

21 Bazelon, D.: The role of the psychiatrist in the criminal justice system. *Bulletin of the American Academy of Psychiatry and the Law* **6**:139–46, 1978.

22 *Opinions of the Ethics Committee on the principles of medical ethics with annotations especially applicable to psychiatry.* Washington DC, American Psychiatric Association, 1985.

23 Moore, R. A.: Right for the dead (guest editorial). *Psychiatric News* 21 March 1980.

24 Goldzband, M. G.: Pre-arraignment psychiatric examinations and criminal

responsibility—a personal Odyssey through the law and psychiatry west of the Pecos. *Journal of Psychiatry and Law* **4**:447–666, 1976.

25 *Estelle* v. *Smith* 451 US 454, at 454 (1981).
26 Rappeport, J. R.: The insanity plea: getting away with murder? *Maryland State Medical Journal*, March 1981.
27 Monahan, J. and Steadman, H.: *Mentally disordered offenders: perspectives from law and social sciences*. New York, Plenum, 1983.
28 Insanity Defense Work Group, American Psychiatric Association: Statement on the insanity defense. *American Journal of Psychiatry* **140**:6, 1983.
29 Diamond, Bernard: Personal communication, 10 July 1980.
30 Halleck, S. L.: Law in the practice of psychiatry, a handbook for clinicians. New York, Plenum, 1980.
31 Strasburger, L. H.: 'Crudely, without finesse': the defendant hears his psychiatric evaluation. *Bulletin of the American Academy of Psychiatry and the Law* **15**:229–33, 1987.
32 Miller, R. D. and Germain, E. J.: Should forensic patients be informed of evaluators' opinions prior to trial? *Bulletin of the American Academy of Psychiatry and the Law* **17**:53–59, 1989.
33 *Smith* v. *Estelle* 602 F 2d 694, at 697.
34 *Smith* v. *Estelle* 602 F 2d 694, at 708.
35 Goldzband, M. G.: *Custody cases and expert witnesses*, 2nd edn. New York, Harcourt Brace Jovanovich, 1985.
36 Goldzband, M. G.: *Custody cases and expert witnesses: a manual for attorneys*, 2nd edn. Clifton, N.J., Prentice-Hall Law & Business, 1988.
37 Sadoff, R.: Personal communication, 20 September 1989.
38 Thornberry, T. P. and Jacoby, J. E.: *The criminally insane*. Chicago, University of Chicago Press, 1979.
39 Weinstock, R.: Perceptions of ethical problems by forensic psychiatrists. *Bulletin of the American Academy of Psychiatry and the Law* **17**:189–202, 1989.

# 19

# Ethics and psychiatric research

*John Wing*

In the last chapter of his intellectual autobiography,[1] Karl Popper explains, paraphrasing Wolfgang Köhler, why few scientists care to write about values: 'The reason is simply that so much of the talk about values is hot air.' A value is involved every time a practical and immediate problem has to be solved or a decision made and there is no satisfactory substitute for rational consideration of the pros and cons of each issue. We evolve general ethical guidelines or principles (which differ, however, in different societies) in order to avoid having to think out the rights and wrongs of every possible alternative before taking everyday decisions; but they must always be open to challenge and to rational argument.

Many ethical theorists reject this common-sense approach to ethics. Comte, who created positivism, and Marx, who created dialectical materialism, are prime examples. They thought, though for quite different reasons, that they could forecast, far ahead of events, the way that human society would evolve. Once the predictions had been made, the task of the politician was to ensure a smooth transition towards the inevitable future. The criterion of morality, therefore, was whether an action was or was not likely to bring forward the golden age; the end justified the means.[2]

Plato, who was a historicist of rather a different kind, created a system of ethics that has been much admired; but he was able to propose the establishment of a correctional institution where those with atheistic views would be incarcerated for a period of five years in order to be given appropriate instruction. 'And when the time of their imprisonment has expired, if any of them be of sound mind let him be restored to sane company, but if not, and if he be condemned a second time, let him be punished with death.' The idea that the state should designate what is healthy and what is sick is part of what the author who has brought this Platonic equation of insanity and dissent to our notice calls 'social psychiatry'.[3] Although this concept of social psychiatry is unrecognized in Europe it is important for psychiatrists everywhere to understand the nature of the claims that can be made in their name; for example, that radical social reconstruction based on freeing the people from 'surplus repression' will solve the ills of Western societies.[4] If such theories were seriously applied the outcome could not be guaranteed to be more democratic than in Plato's *Republic*. Another example of historicist morality applied to psychiatry is discussed in Chapter 24.

The authors in this volume are unlikely to espouse any of these extreme ideologies. They will no doubt adopt a broadly liberal stance; regarding the rights of individuals (in this case, patients) as more important than the rights of agents who might claim to be acting for the good of society and therefore, in the long run, for the good of the individuals who constitute society. Robert Neville has made an attempt to look at the recommendations of one modern commision of enquiry into ethical issues[5] through the eyes of a modern equivalent of a seventeenth-century Puritan divine.[6] The exercise is not wholly convincing, but the notion that each individual is flawed, and in order to achieve grace has to seek the common good rather than his own necessarily incomplete fulfilment, is indeed still latent in modern Western societies. Such a sense of responsibility is shown by those who carry kidney-donor cards and by those who regard it as their duty to take part in research projects if their reasonable scruples can be overcome. Perhaps this individual responsibility is insufficiently recognized in debates on the ethics of clinical and research practice.

This introduction may serve to remind the reader that the ethical aspects of research are no more controversial than the ethical apsects of any other subject. In particular, the ethics of clinical research depend almost completely on the ethics of clinical practice. Every clinical decision ought to involve an experiment. The practice of medicine focuses on one individual patient at a time, but the physician is always trying to learn something that may benefit others as well. Current methods of treatment depend on experience of past methods. Research in this sense is a normal part of practice, and is a value to be preserved. Ethical problems are most likely to arise when treatment is based on theories which have been insufficiently tested to discover whether they have harmful consequences, or when the theories are virtually untestable because they are stated with insufficient clarity and detail. The scientific testing of diagnostic and therapeutic claims is therefore itself a moral imperative.

There is nowadays a fairly general acceptance of the view that new drugs should not be introduced without being tested. There is no similar consensus in respect of social treatments, most of which become firmly adopted before they have been thoroughly examined. The harm that may come from the application of misguided social theories, or the misapplication of sensible theories, is at least as great as any harm that can follow the prescription of a harmful drug or an unnecessary course of psychotherapy. In fact, it can be much greater, since harmful social practices can become institutionalized into the structure of a complete psychiatric service. The 'custodial era' in psychiatry, although it was not as black as it has sometimes been painted, nevertheless illustrates how the practices inherent in the concept of the 'total institution' can become generally and uncritically adopted, even though many of them were quite unnecessary and demonstrably harmful.

Medicine (or any other activity) would come to a full stop if every decision had to be monitored by an ethical committee. What then constitutes an experiment of sufficient substance to warrant such an opinion being obtained? Who is to judge when some item of practice ought to be referred to a committee? When does clinical practice become 'research'?

Before attempting to answer these questions, I will consider three main practical problems that ethical committees are always concerned about; the balance of good and harm to which a patient may be exposed, what constitutes informed consent, and confidentiality.

## The balance of good and harm

### The principle of least harm

The central ethical principle in clinical practice is that doctors must not knowingly act against the interests of their patients and must take all reasonable steps to ensure that they do not do so unwittingly. Doctors have to decide, first of all, whether their expertise can be applied to any of the problems brought to them by the patient. If one of these problems does seem to be explicable in terms of some medical theory or theories ('diagnosis'), they then have to weigh the consequences of advising the patient to accept further investigation or treatment based on the predictions of that theory. This means balancing the advantages and the disadvantages of giving the advice against those of not giving it, in the light of knowledge that is rarely complete and may be conflicting. This uncertainty is particularly great in psychiatry; first, because disease theories are not as well developed as in other branches of medicine, and secondly, because many of the problems brought by patients arise out of difficulties in everyday life to which disease theories have almost no relevance at all. It is the doctor's duty to be as well informed as possible. Some of the most reasonable criticisms of psychiatric practice have arisen because psychiatric expertise has been applied to people who were not mentally ill or because treatments (physical, psychological, and social) have been applied without the psychiatrist's being aware that they could have harmful effects. This has often been due to the fact that the necessary research has not been undertaken. The more the relevant theories have been subjected to rigorous tests, the better-informed doctors can be, and the less likely are they to cause unwitting harm.

Apart from the ethical obligation on any doctor to be as well equipped as possible for clinical practice, no special ethical issue is raised by accidental or unforeseeable damage and, in any case, there is provision through the courts for deciding issues of negligence. There are, however, circumstances in which the possibility of doing damage may be accepted because of the likelihood of a greater good. The amputation of a gangrenous foot is a case in point; by losing a foot the patient may save the rest of a limb. The fact that phenothiazine medication helps to prevent acute relapses in schizophrenia, at least in the short term, is so important to the welfare of patient and relatives that some uncertainty as to whether there will be harmful side-effects in the longer term is accepted (see Chapter 9).

It is at the growing-points of clinical practice, where the balance of good and harm is not yet clear, that the most difficult decisions have to be made, and the advice of disinterested colleagues may be most helpful. Even here, as in the case of the first heart-transplants, and the introduction of new forms of medication for schizophrenia and the manic and depressive disorders, the decision had to be made by physician and patient together, each trusting the other's judgement after a consideration of the risks and possible benefits.

## Risk and benefit from research projects

The vast majority of research projects do not involve any probability of serious harm coming to those involved. The 1978 United States National Commission investigating what measures were needed to protect mentally disabled subjects of biomedical and behavioural research was persuaded that there was no risk at all in one-third of projects, and a 'very low' risk of only minimal stress or embarrassment, or minor medical complications (a bruise after taking blood, for example), in nearly all the rest. Fewer than 5 per cent of projects involving the mentally disabled presented more risk than this.[5] My own experience of an ethical committee confirms this.

The Royal College of Physicians of London[7] gives as examples of minimal risk the measurement of height and weight, the collection of a sample of urine, and taking a single venous blood sample from an adult. Two kinds of minimal risk are specified. The first is where the level of psychological or physical distress is negligible, although there might be a chance of a transitory mild headache or feeling of lethargy. 'The second is where there is a very remote chance of serious injury or death, analogous to the very remote risk of travelling as a passenger on public transport.'

Benefit may be expressed as an advantage to the individual patient, either in the short term or in the longer term, because of the improved knowledge of that patient's condition that is likely to result from a study in which a group of patients with the same condition are taking part. Benefit may also accrue to society as a whole. In practice, benefit 'stands for the combined probabilities and magnitudes of several possible favourable effects'.

A distinction is often drawn between 'therapeutic' and 'non-therapeutic' research, depending on whether or not a patient stands to benefit directly from a proposed intervention. The same principles of analysis of risks and benefits apply in each case, as does the requirement to obtain informed consent and to preserve confidentiality. But Ethical Committees might reasonably conclude that the benefit would have to be very substantial to justify more than minimal risk in the case of non-therapeutic research.

## The ethics of clinical trials

This still leaves a number of awkward situations in which the possible harm from a given procedure comes closer to outweighing the benefit expected from it. In such circumstances there would appear to be an ethical duty to carry out a clinical trial. But a clinical trial itself, if it is to yield the maximum information, demands that the effects of receiving the treatment should be compared with the consequences of receiving the procedure previously accepted as the best, and the latter may also entail risks as well as possible benefits. Helmchen and Müller-Oerlinghausen call this dilemma the paradox of the clinical trial: 'First, it is unethical to use treatment the efficacy of which has not been examined scientifically; second, it is also unethical to examine the efficacy of treatment scientifically.'[8] In fact, no paradox is involved, only a complication in drawing up the balance between good and harm. But it is a complication that must always be considered, not only in research projects but whenever clinical practice is innovative rather than routine. The question of what good (or prevention of harm) may come to *other* patients than the specific individual under consideration for treatment is not only of legitimate but of obligatory, though secondary, concern to the doctor. The value of considering the ethical aspects of projects with an avowedly research aim is that such issues become explicit.

The British Medical Research Council, in an influential paper, specified the principles that should guide medical research workers setting up trials of treatments or methods of prevention which require control groups.[9] The value of such designs is that they speed up the acquisition of knowledge concerning the advantages and disadvantages of new methods. The more representative the group of patients selected for the trial, and the more random the allocation of patients to experimental or control groups, the more useful will be the information gained.

The research worker is concerned to ensure that the trial is conducted in accordance with strict scientific principles and it must therefore be considered whether this motivation (excellent in itself) is compatible with the overriding necessity to assess the balance of good and harm and inform the patient accordingly. It is not suggested that research workers will knowingly give inaccurate information in order to persuade patients to enter a trial; but the possibility of unconscious bias cannot be discounted. Undoubtedly the safest procedure is that the patient's own clinician should not be involved in the research and that he should not undertake the discussion necessary to decide consent. If this is not possible, as may be the case in small University departments, there should always be an independent clinician available who can undertake this important responsibility and who can be given authority to advise the patient where the balance of good and harm lies.

The issues involved in deciding whether and how to obtain 'true consent' will be discussed below; but they are nowhere clearer than when procedures are involved that are not of direct benefit to the individual asked to take part in the project. The possibility or probability that an investigation will be of benefit to humanity or posterity is no defence in the event of legal proceedings. Nor can an individual consent to be harmed: 'The individual has rights that the law protects and nobody can infringe those rights for the public good.'[10]

## Informed consent

### What is informed consent?

There will be no disagreement with the general rule that people chosen to participate in research projects should be told frankly what the risks and benefits are likely to be and what the purpose of the research is. There are, however, many difficulties in the way of achieving completely informed consent.

First it is impossible for the clinician to tell the patient (or client) everything that is in his mind. He must select. Secondly, the patient can only rarely be as well informed as the clinician. Even when, in exceptional cases, the patients are themselves doctors, have taken a second opinion, looked up the textbooks, consulted the original papers, obtained the best statistics as to cure-rates and side-effects and so on, they will usually still need advice as to the best course of action. Most patients, of course, do not wish to go to such lengths. They simply want advice. Thirdly, even if it were feasible to spend a very long time with each patient, attempting to inform him of all the ins and outs influencing some particular recommendation, it would often be undesirable to do so on ethical grounds, since the patient might well receive the impression that the clinician was unwilling to take responsibility, and therefore come to doubt the value of the advice. Finally there is the difficult question of gauging how far the patient can understand an explanation of why a particular treatment or course of action is recommended rather than all the various alternatives available to the clinician. In the last resort, the matter is one of whether the patient can trust the clinician or not.

## Must consent always be obtained?

Occasionally, telling patients that they are to take part in a trial may actually be contra-indicated. 'For example, to awaken patients with a possibly fatal illness to the existence of such doubts about effective treatment may not always be in their best interest; or suspicion may have arisen as to whether a particular treatment has any effect apart from suggestion and it may be necessary to introduce a placebo into part of the trial to determine this.'[9] An important example of the latter situation arises when a treatment has become generally adopted because it is believed, on the basis of its proved efficacy in ameliorating an acute disorder, that it has longer-term preventive value, even though this has *not* been demonstrated. It is precisely in such situations that the dangers of adverse reactions developing after long periods of administration are most apparent.

This was the problem, for example, with long-term maintenance medication with the phenothiazines. Was it justifiable to inform a patient, after he had been taking the medication for a long time, that it was uncertain whether it was effective and uncertain whether it was dangerous? The result might very well be to destroy his trust in a form of preventive medication that might be both effective and safe. The ethical problem can only be resolved by the clinician, in the light of his scientific knowledge and his acquaintance with the individual patient. In a recent trial of fluphenazine decanoate, the psychiatrists concerned decided that it was ethically correct to include certain of their patients without obtaining their informed consent.[10] A colleague objected to this trial (and indeed to all trials) on 'ethical' grounds; but he was assuming that his personal faith in the drug's efficacy and safety ought to have been shared by the clinicians who allowed their patients to take part in the trial. The fact that his faith was not so shared is not a matter for ethics at all, but for rational argument about evidence.[11]

This and other trials have shown a superior preventive effect of drug over placebo in the short term, and, taken together with other scientific data about the interaction between social and pharmacological treatments, they allow a much better informed decision to be made by psychiatrists in future. They do not, however, answer the question as to whether dangerous side-effects might develop in the longer term; and thus some ethical doubt remains, in clinical practice, about the duration of therapy.

## Consent by children

In many countries, children below the age of eighteen are regarded as incompetent to give consent to treatment. Recent judgements in England have modified the situation somewhat, particularly above the age of six-teen, and even below that age if the child is capable of understanding what is proposed. In such circumstances the consent of parent or guardian is not essential.[12] For example the child might be away from home, or there might be a conflict of interest between parent and child. Nevertheless, it would be most unusual for a doctor to treat a child under sixteen without the consent of parent or guardian.

In the case of children who are not competent to give consent, the parent's duty to act in the best interests of the child can reasonably be interpreted to mean that the investigator can properly rely on the consent of parent or guardian. Nevertheless, behavioural refusal by the child should lead to reconsideration by all parties as to whether to proceed.

Other important precautions are that no research should be undertaken on children that can as readily be carried out with adults, and that it should only be concerned with risks or problems that are of relevance to those taking part.

### Consent in the mentally incapacitated

In the case of people who are incapacitated by reason of mental retarda-tion, mental illness, coma, or dementia, there is no provision in English law that allows a proxy to give consent on their behalf. By the same token, there is no provision against such a practice. In countries whose legal systems were derived in part from English common law (notably the United States of America, Canada, and Australia) the *parens patriae* jurisdiction still operates. This originated in the power and duty of the Crown to protect the persons and property of those unable to do so for themselves, including children and 'persons of unsound mind'. It has been superseded by other provisions in English law. However, we are concerned here with the ethical problems that are illustrated by legal cases rather than the specifics of the law.

The problem has been highlighted by the case of a severely mentally handicapped woman who had formed a seemingly satisfactory sexual re-lationship, but for whom, in the opinion of her doctors and relatives, pregnancy would be disastrous. Application was made to the High Court for permission to proceed with sterilization. This was granted; but the Official Solicitor, acting on her behalf and in order to test the law, took the case to the Appeal Court. Permission was again granted,[13] and the Official Solicitor then took the case to the House of Lords. The Law Lords also agreed.

The principle involved is whether the proposed operation is in the patient's best interests, in which case it is lawful, or not in the patient's best interests and therefore unlawful. It was put particularly clearly by Lord Jauncey. 'I should like only to reiterate the importance of not erecting such legal barriers against the provision of medical treatment for incompetents that they are deprived of treatment which competent persons could reasonably expect to receive in similar circumstances. The law must not convert incompetents into second class citizens for the purposes of health care.'

This is helpful in the case of therapeutic research. It is also helpful, in my view, in the case of controlled therapeutic trials that are conducted in order to discover whether a seemingly promising but untested intervention actually does have value for the persons involved. In such trials, inclusion either in the experimental or in the control group should, in the judgement of those conducting the trial and of any others responsible for its ethical conduct, provide information of value for the treatment of each person individually.

The position of non-therapeutic trials, however, remains in English law much as it was. There is an absolutist moral stance which states that no adult can give consent for another, even if that other is incapable of consent, the risk is negligible and the benefits substantial. On this basis, the law is interpreted in the narrowest and most restrictive sense possible. It may well be that the weight of public opinion (the moral consensus) would now justify departing from such an extreme ethical position. Lord Donaldson, in the Appeal Court judgement mentioned above, said in relation to therapeutic interventions:

This difficulty of decision cannot ever be removed, but it would undoubtedly be much lessened if the medical profession were to produce ethical and professional guidelines for the treatment of incompetent adults.[13]

A principled ethical case can also be made for allowing a mentally incapacitated individual to participate in non-therapeutic research within carefully defined limits.

Several professional bodies have put forward guidelines that would protect the interests of those involved, including the following:

- the risk is no more than minimal;
- the research is concerned with the problem of the patients involved and cannot be carried out with competent patients;
- the individuals themselves do not indicate objection either verbally or behaviourally;
- their relatives agree after being fully informed; and
- an Ethical Committee gives its sanction.

If there is no relative, if the risk is more than minimal, or if the research is prolonged, the Ethical Committee should approve the appointment of an independent 'patient's friend', who would make the decision to participate after informed consideration of all the circumstances.

The UK Medical Research Council's report on the ethics of research[9] ruled out any possibility of research with incapacitated people or with children. In the light of the developing moral consensus on these matters, and taking into account the considerations summarized above, the Council has set up two linked working parties to review the current situation and to make recommendations as to whether their rules should now be changed.

### Research when consent might not be freely given

When research is proposed with individuals who are under some form of constraint, such as prisoners, or employees, or people under a legal order by reason of mental disorder, the necessity for truly informed and free consent is particularly crucial. There should be no hidden pressures, as in the promise of some form of reward from which those who refuse are excluded; no victimization of those who do not participate; and no relaxation of any of the usual ethical procedures. The responsibility of an Ethical Committee is particularly onerous in such cases.

In the United States, the 1978 Report of the National Commission for the Protection of Human Subjects of Biomedical and Behavioural Research[5] is very much to the point. Proposed regulations based on this report and issued by the United States Department of Health, Education, and Welfare in 1978 were extremely detailed and specific. They provoked a storm of critical responses mostly, but not exclusively, from academic psychiatrists who objected to the seeming implication that research was intrinsically bad and to be tolerated only under stringent controls; they argued that the proposed regulations would hamper clinical research in psychiatry and thereby represented discrimination against the mentally ill as a class by denying them the fruit of new knowledge.[14]

However, as in the UK, the climate of ethical opinion has gradually changed during the past ten years. A consensus has been reached between patient-advocacy groups and researchers concerning a common set of ethical principles not dissimilar to those discussed above.


## Confidentiality

### Confidentiality in modern clinical practice (see Chapter 15)

A basic ethical principle in psychiatry is that the doctor should take all reasonable precautions to preserve the confidentiality of the information given to him by patients. Sometimes circumstances arise when this information cannot and should not be used only within the context of the personal psychiatrist–patient relationship. This creates a problem, since the information is divulged in the first place only because the patient wants advice, and there is an assumption on both sides that confidentiality will be maintained. The evidence given on behalf of the British Medical Association to a government Committee on Privacy[15] included the following statement: 'It is no longer practicable to look upon the single physician as the patient's sole confidant in any serious illness and it is assumed by public and profession alike that any contact with the complex medical machinery of today implies acquiescence in some degree of extended confidence'.

This concept of extended confidence is essential to a discussion of privacy. It is taken for granted that the immediate members of a clinical team in group practice, medical and non-medical, professional and clerical, must have access to confidential information, and that they will not abuse this trust. In Britain, the doctor in charge of the team is responsible to the General Medical Council should any ethical lapse occur. But doctors and nurses talk to each other about their patients, and often have easy access to each other's medical records, without there necessarily being any clear-cut benefit to the patient apart from general medical education. It is common for the doctor, through his professional skill, to learn something about the patient which he is reluctant to share with him, for example the presence of a fatal illness. This dilemma has been much discussed both in the medical and lay press without any resolution other than that the doctor has to use his own judgement whether or not to tell the patient. The doctor sometimes intentionally and one-sidedly breaches his confidential relationship with his patients without there being a public and professional outcry. This is presumably because in these circumstances the interests of patients are best served by allowing the physician to exercise his clinical judgement.

Behind clinical medical practice there stands an implied bond of trust between the public and the medical profession, as well as the individual patient's confidence in his own doctor. It is assumed that the actions taken by the responsible doctor are intended to be beneficial, and that no harm will result from them. These actions include the passing of confidential data to other people who, in turn, will act responsibly, since they would not otherwise be given the information. It is well accepted in practice, by both parties, that specific permission cannot be sought every time confidential information is transferred.[16]

Even if it were possible for a patient to give a blanket permission for all the acts of transfer of information from one doctor to another that are necessary in modern clinical practice, it would not protect the doctor from legal action if any harm should come from such a transfer. A patient cannot, in law, consent to be damaged. The question therefore, even in purely clinical practice, is not whether information can be transferred by the responsible doctor, or by a doctor standing in for him, without the explicit consent of the patient; the question is, under what circumstances should such transfers take place? The most likely source of a leak of information to unauthorized persons is a lack of security in the clinical

records system. An attention to security at this level is probably as important as any other. However, public concern has mainly been aroused by the
possibility of unauthorized access to medical information systems where
there is a facility for computer linking. We are not concerned here with the
administrative uses of such registers; but the security issues are much the
same as for research registers.

A statement by the British Medical Research Council pointed out:

The systematic collection and analysis of medical information has always been an
important requisite for those doctors, particularly medical officers of health, concerned with the study and control of the health of the whole population rather than
the individual patient ... The control of epidemics of infectious disease was
achieved in part through the notification of its onset in individual patients by family
doctors to the medical officers of health. Similarly, the control of non-infectious
diseases may be assisted by the transfer of medical information between doctors.
The origins of many of these non-infectious diseases may lie in early life, their
evolution is slow and insidious, and the relation between cause and effect is often
obscure and complex. The changing social habits and conditions of life in a con-
gested urban community, together with changes in industrial processes, continually
create new health hazards, such as the toxic hazards of food additives, combustion
of fuel on a new scale or of a new type of environmental pollution. Advances in the
production of new powerful therapeutic and prophylactic agents have created a
need not only to assess their effectiveness, in comparison with existing drugs or
forms of treatment, but also to maintain a continued watch for the development of
adverse reactions. [17]

There are three main categories of use of medical data for research
purposes: small research projects in which information is collected from
medical records and associated documents such as death certificates;
moderately-sized data-collection systems utilizing record linkage, such as
ongoing or *ad hoc* case registers, which are still under local medical control; and regional or national data-collection systems which allow record
linkage. The problems posed are somewhat different at each level; but
what all three have in common is that it is often impossible to gain the
patient's informed consent for each act of transfer of data. Underlying the
three categories lies a single dimension of increasing scale, complexity, and
longevity of the system of data-collection and storage. What the psychiatrist will be concerned with, therefore, is the likelihood of public benefits
accruing from each transfer of information, balanced against the possibility
of harm to the patient.

*Small-scale research projects*

In small-scale research projects the main problem is likely to be careless-
ness. Documents tend to be left lying around, and information about
identifiable patients might in this way become known to unauthorized

people. However, few research workers or assistants are likely to be involved, and there is usually one psychiatrist personally responsible for the project. The risks are much the same as those in ordinary clinical practice. The most famous case of breach of confidentiality was actually the result of a burglary at a physician's private office, so that it can hardly be argued that 'state' systems are uniquely vulnerable. Attention to security should be a part of all research projects. In particular, it is rarely necessary for identifying data to be included on documents which contain confidential material. A name–number list is much more easily kept under secure conditions than a large set of bulky files. Larger-scale collaborative projects, in which information about identified individuals is collected in a number of medical centres, pose more complicated problems, but the precautions taken locally are the same: the security of the name–number list, restriction of access to specified persons, supervision by a named doctor responsible for confidentiality, and licence by an ethical committee. It is best for data forwarded to a central office for collation to be identified by number only; it should not be necessary to hold names or other identifiers on a computer file.

*Local case-registers*

Psychiatric case-registers under local medical control have been developed for research purposes in several parts of Europe and the United States. It is necessary to collect identifying data, such as names and addresses, for two reasons. First, the name, address, date of birth, and sometimes other identifying items are needed to link records from different agencies or different occasions, so that cohort studies can be undertaken. Thus, for example, it is possible to make the vital distinction between person and event statistics (e.g. between one person being in hospital ten times and ten people being in hospital once), without which a wide range of scientific and administrative studies would be impossible. Secondly, the register can be used as a sampling frame. In general, registers in the United Kingdom do not place identifying data on the computer file, and the whole operation is small enough to be under the direct control of one doctor authorized by an ethical committee. Medical information is transferred only under very restricted circumstances, and only from one doctor to another. Identifying data are kept under conditions of strict security, and all staff who have access are fully aware of their responsibility. If an approach to a patient on the register is desired, permission is sought from the responsible clinician, and the patient's informed consent is obtained before any further inquiry is made.

These characteristics form the basis of recommendations made by the Royal College of Psychiatrists for ensuring confidentiality in medical information systems. These include the licensing of registers, the appointment of a named physician to be responsible for confidentiality, surveillance of each register by an ethical committee with non-medical as well as medical members, including some who are expert in computer security, and the adoption of a strict code of practice dealing with the conditions under which identifying data may be stored, transferred, or published.[16]

### National and regional registers

It is at national and regional registers that most recent criticism has been directed. This is not because any breach of confidentiality has in fact occurred. There has been no example of misuse of information supplied to the Mental Health Enquiry covering England and Wales during the thirty years of its operation. Names are not even given to bona-fide research workers; they must produce their own list of names, which has been obtained by permission of local clinicians.

Without identifying information, it would be impossible even to produce statistics of first admissions to psychiatric hospitals, which are the raw data required both for epidemiological and administrative purposes. The fact that the names and addresses of patients are collected in a central computer file, together with sensitive information (e.g. religion, diagnosis, marital status) leads to fears that a corrupt regime, or a few corrupt officials, would be presented with the opportunity to misuse the system. A further argument, that a well-intentioned official would allow the data to be fed into other computer systems, or would make information on named individuals available to other government agencies, must be discounted. In view of the very specific regulations, no such transfer could be regarded as anything but sinister. Such a situation is certainly not with us at present.

### Privacy regulations and the restriction of useful research

Precautions of this kind should not unduly restrict research; but protective legislation is developing in some countries to such an extent that legitimate data-gathering activities are being hampered. 'For example, in Sweden, epidemiologists are complaining that their research has been rendered tedious, time-consuming and ineffective because of the regulations governing the establishment of information systems.'[18] It is extremely expensive to break the current computer security systems, and, political corruption apart, there can be little incentive to do so in order to obtain the kind of information held in medical information systems.

Sir Richard Doll has given four examples of medical research that depended for their success 'on the maintenance of clinical records in hospitals, the existence of nosological indexes, and the willingness of doctors to provide access to their notes and to allow their patients to be followed up and, on occasions, interviewed. Sometimes they required access to industrial or other social records and very often to central registers of death or morbidity.' He points out that a proper concern over the possibility, for example, of linking records of treatment for venereal disease or psychiatric disorder with employment records, has led to a mistrust of all interchange of medical information, so that it is suggested that no such exchange should ever be made without the explicit consent of the patient.[19]

Doll quotes the statement by the British Medical Research Council: 'The Council considers that, subject to certain safeguards, medical information obtained about identified individual patients should continue to be made available without their explicit consent for the purposes of medical research.'[17] He sums up his own experience, which most research workers will endorse, as follows: 'the vast majority of people are glad to assist in medical research, even at the cost of some personal inconvenience'.

Lee Robins, a distinguished American medical sociologist, reviewed the value of long-term follow-up studies, which depended upon the ability to select unbiased samples and to obtain unbiased information about these samples throughout the period of follow-up. 'For many follow-up studies, the researcher needs access both to the subject himself and to records about him. Seeing the subject personally is valuable because the subject can provide information that has never been recorded, and he can alert the researcher to records about himself that would otherwise be missed. Record searches permit verifying the veracity of the subject's statements and also provide information he cannot supply.'[20] Robins's own research provides examples of how important such studies are in psychiatry; but she points out that access to records has been severely curtailed by the United States Privacy Act of 1974 and the Family Educational Rights Act of 1974. A report of the Privacy Protection Study Commission makes the same point.[21]

Helgason[22] has described the devastating effect of the data-protection laws in many European countries, in particular his native Iceland. Haefner and Pfeiffer-Kurda[23] have given an account of the impact of the law introduced in the state of Baden-Württemberg which led to the closure of the Mannheim register. Rothman[24] has written of 'the rise and fall of epidemiology, 1950–2000 AD'.

## The British Data Protection Act, 1984

In 1984, the British Parliament passed the Data Protection Act,[25] the aim of which is to establish and enforce a set of principles that govern the collection, storage, and processing of confidential information. Failure to comply with the provisions of the Act may result in deregistration, and, on convinction, a fine.

The Act provides for the creation of a public register of data-users supervised by a Data Protection Registrar and Tribunal. All data-users holding personal data are required to state the purpose of their registers, to give details of the data-sets held and their sources, and to provide a list of all those to whom named data are disclosed. Once registered, no other kind of purpose, data-set, or disclosure is allowed without further permission.

The rights of a 'data-subject' to see a copy of any personal record and to receive compensation if any damage is incurred are set out in detail. Certain exemptions are made from the rights of access to personal data concerning physical or mental health, and to data held only for the purposes of preparing statistics or carrying out research.

Sensibly applied, the Act and its Code of Practice provide adequate safeguards for personal information without unduly impeding epidemiological research. The code is consistent with the statement by the British Medical Research Council.[18] It may be permissible to hope that public opinion throughout the world will continue to appreciate the value of research and to accept that preserving a base for research is, with safeguards, fully compatible with respect for human rights.

## Committees on the ethics of research

### The operation of ethical committees

Research Ethics Committees were set up because of a general recognition that research on human beings should conform to principles such as those of the Nuremberg Code[26] and the World Medical Association,[27] and a conviction that investigators should not be the sole judge of their own ethical propriety. The Royal College of Physicians has recently issued an up-to-date version of their guidelines on the practice of such committees.[28]

The College suggests that membership, in addition to physicians, should include a nurse and two lay members. The Committee must be competent to decide 'whether the research is directed towards answering a worthwhile question and whether the design of the study is sound scientifically'. Such committees are now well established in the Health Districts of the UK, in Universities, and in other organizations. Their principal objective is 'to protect subjects of research from possible harm . . . in the understanding that medical research benefits society and often individuals, so that it should not be hindered without good cause'.

Grant-giving bodies, such as the Medical Research Council in the United Kingdom and the National Institutes of Health and National Institute of Mental Health in the United States, require all proposals for research to be vetted by an ethical committee, and many such committees advise research workers to submit *all* their proposed projects, although this advice does not have the force of law. Some committees specify that the decision whether to submit is left to the senior member of staff concerned, with the proviso that there is a moral obligation to consult the committee whenever there is the slightest doubt. A simple form is provided identifying the applicant, the responsible worker, and the sponsor, and including a brief description of the research and the ethical aspects involved.

Most ethical committees have now had many years of experience of considering the ethical problems raised by a wide variety of research proposals. In my own experience, while there have been a few instances in which research workers thought a committee's recommendations too cautious, there has been no single case in which they were not accepted. Research workers have the opportunity to defend their proposals if they so wish, and there is often a process of revision in order to devise a design and methodology acceptable to the committee. The lay member has had long experience of representing consumer interests, and legal advice is available as required.

Most applicants present few problems. A typical example would be the drawing of blood samples during the course of a depressive disorder in order to determine whether a chemical compound, hypothesized to be associated with severity, can in fact be found to vary appropriately in concentration. The applicant must explain why it is necessary to undertake the project; the procedure will be explained to patients, and they will be told that it will not be helpful to their own treatment but may be useful in accumulating knowledge about the nature of the condition, that there can occasionally be some temporary bruising, and that they are free to take part or not, as they choose. The committee will consider whether the applicant has met its ethical criteria, asking, for example, whether patients are capable of giving informed consent in this instance. If so, they will decide whether the probable balance of good and harm is such that they can give their approval. If the procedure were a lumbar puncture rather than a venepuncture, the committee would take into account the somewhat greater risk involved, but the principles they used would be the same.

After a time, an ethical committee becomes experienced in selecting problems that require more extended discussion because they have not previously arisen in its deliberations. When computerized tomography was introduced, for example, it was necessary for the particular indications and contra-indications to be considered in detail. The balance of good and harm is different when the procedure is used as an aid in the assessment of dementia, as a means of investigating abnormality in alcoholism or schizophrenia, and as a method of studying cerebral pathology in, say, autistic children. In the last case, the possible addition to knowledge might not be considered worth the risk to the child, even if the parents were willing to give a fully informed consent.

Another kind of issue which requires detailed consideration during the early stages of a committee's existence is the use of 'normal volunteers' in research. In most instances, the ethical problems are similar to those arising in clinical research with patients; but marginal questions do arise. For example, I have had experience of one application which sought permission to deliver a questionnaire concerning, among other things, attitudes to various sexual practices, through the letter-boxes of randomly selected houses in a particular geographical area, with a request that they should be completed and returned to the investigator in a stamped, addressed envelope. The committee's discussion turned on the problem of how far it was reasonable to expose people to such questions without obtaining their prior permission, as well as on the scientific value of this method of data-collection.

These examples, and others mentioned earlier in the chapter, indicate the way that ethical issues arise during the discussion of practical problems in research. An experienced committee develops an expertise which colleagues find impressive, and which should, one hopes, reassure the public.

## Conclusion

I believe that the general answer to the set of questions I posed at the beginning of this chapter is that no line can be drawn between innovatory clinical practice in psychiatry and more formal research investigation. Whenever there is any doubt at all, it is the duty of the responsible psychiatrist to seek the advice of an ethical committee. An inescapable concomitant of this conclusion is that there are no ethical issues specific to clinical research. Every problem that arises in research—whether it involves the balance of good against harm, a decision to undertake a laboratory procedure or to give or withhold a treatment, or to pass information to some other person—also arises in everyday clinical work.

Several bodies have put forward lists of principles that can form a useful guide to individual psychiatrists and to members of ethical committees.[5,29] However, it is necessary to distinguish between the individual psychiatrist's own decision in any given case, which must be his own moral responsibility, and a set of ethical guidelines which may be laid down by a professional or lay body in order to help him take the decision. In the last resort, the trust of the public, individually and collectively, in the psychiatric profession will depend upon the cumulative effect of a myriad decisions of the first kind. A psychiatrist must, in full awareness of the law, be free to follow conscience.

We must be clear, however, that we are dealing with individual and not group ethics. Decisions must be made in precisely the same way as they would have been if no research had been involved. One psychiatrist may believe that the value of the treatment under test has already been sufficiently demonstrated, and will therefore refuse to expose his patient to the risk of its withdrawal in a clinical trial. This decision must be respected, but it cannot be imposed on other psychiatrists who think differently. Clearly, as Helmchen and Müller-Oerlinghausen point out,[8] this will introduce biases; but a variety of designs is available to take care of this problem, and, in any case, an epidemiological approach always needs to be adopted in order to determine the limits within which the results can be generalized.[30]

Karl Popper's comment on personal responsibility for one's ethical decisions applies perfectly to psychiatrists in their roles as researchers: 'The responsibility for our ethical decisions is entirely ours and can be shifted on to nobody else; neither to God, nor to nature, nor to society, nor to history ... Whatever authority we may accept, it is we who accept it. We only deceive ourselves if we do not realize this simple point.[31]

# References

1 Popper, K.: *Unended quest: an intellectual autobiography*. Glasgow, Fontana/ Collins, 1976, p. 193.

2 Wing, J. K.: *Reasoning about madness*. London, Oxford University Press, 1978, p. 5.

3 Simon, B.: *Mind and madness in ancient Greece: the classical roots of modern psychiatry*. Ithaca, Cornell University Press, 1978, p. 187.

4 Marcuse, H.: *Negations: essays in critical theory*. Harmondsworth, Penguin, 1968.

5 National Commission for the Protection of Human Subjects of Biomedical and Behaviour Research: *Report and recommendations*. Bethesda, Department of Health, Education, and Welfare, Publication No. (OS) 78–006, 1978.

6 Neville, R.: On the national commission: a Puritan critique of consensus ethics. *Hastings Center Report*, April 1979, p. 22.

7 Royal College of Physicians of London: *Research on patients*. London, RCP, 1989.

8 Helmchen, H. and Müller-Oerlinghausen, B.: The inherent paradox of clinical trials in psychiatry. *Journal of Medical Ethics* 1:168–73, 1975.

9 Medical Research Council: *Responsibility in investigations on human subjects*. Report of the Medical Research Council for 1962–63. Cmnd. 2382. London, HMSO, 1962–63.

10 Hirsch, S. R., Gaind, R., Rohde, P. D., *et al.*: Outpatient maintenance of chronic schizophrenic patients with long-acting fluphenazine. *British Medical Journal* 1:633–7, 1973.

11 Wing, J. K.: The ethics of clinical trials. *Journal of Medical Ethics* 1:174–5, 1975.

12 *Gillick* v. *West Norfolk and Wisbech Area Health Authority and the Department of Health and Social Security*: House of Lords, 1985 3 All ER 402.

13 Judgement re 'F': Court of Appeal (Civil Division): 3 February 1989.

14 Goodwin, F.: Personal communication, 8 August 1980.

15 Home Office: *Computers and privacy*. Cmnd. 6353. London, HMSO, 1975.

16 Baldwin, J. A., Leff, J. P., and Wing, J. K.: Confidentiality of psychiatric data in medical information systems. *British Journal of Psychiatry* **128**:417–27, 1976.

17 Medical Research Council: Responsibility in the use of medical information for research. *British Medical Journal* **1**:213–16, 1973.

18 Vuori, H.: Privacy, confidentiality and automated health information systems. *Journal of Medical Ethics* **3**:174–8, 1977.

19 Doll, R.: Public benefit and personal privacy: the problems of medical investigation in the community. *Proceedings of the Royal Society of Medicine* **67**:1281–5, 1974.

20 Robins, L.: Privacy regulations and longitudinal studies. Paper read to American Association for the Advancement of Science, February 1978.

21 Privacy Protection Study Commission: *Personal privacy in an information society*. Washington DC, US Government Printing Office, 1977.

22 Helgason, T.: Data protection and problems of data confidentiality. The Icelandic experience, in *Psychiatric case registers in public health*, ed. G. ten Horn, R. Giel, W. Gulbinat, and J. Henderson, pp. 372–5. Amsterdam, Elsevier, 1986.

23 Haefner, H. and Pfeifer-Kurda, M.: The impact of data protection laws on the Mannheim case register, in *Psychiatric case registers in public health*, ed. G. ten Horn, R. Giel, W. Gulbinat and J. Henderson, pp. 366–71. Amsterdam, Elsevier, 1986.

24 Rothman, J. R.: The rise and fall of epidemiology, 1950–2000 AD. *New England Journal of Medicine* **304**:600–2, 1981.

25 *Data Protection Act*. London, HMSO, 1984.

26 *Nuremberg Code: Trials of war criminals before the Nuremberg Military Tribunals under Control Council Law*, No. 10, vol. 2. Washington DC, US Government Printing Office, 1949, pp. 181–2.

27 World Medical Association: *Handbook of declarations*. London, WMA, 1985.

28 Royal College of Physicians of London: *Guidelines on the practice of Ethics Committees in research involving human subjects*, 2nd edn. London, RCP, 1989.

29 American College of Neuropsychopharmacology: Statement of principles of ethical conduct for neuropsychopharmacologic research in human subjects, in *Legal and ethical issues in human research and treatment*. ed. D. M. Gallant and R. Force. New York, Spectrum Publications, 1978, Chapter 1.

30 Leff, J. P.: Influence of selection of patients on results of clinical trials. *British Medical Journal* **4**:156–8, 1973.

31 Popper, K. R.: *The open society and its enemies*, vol. 1. London: Routledge, 1945, p. 62 and note 18.

# 20

# Training in psychiatric ethics

*Robert Michels and Kevin Kelly*

The recent growth of interest in the ethical aspects of psychiatry began with concerns about specific issues: involuntary confinement, the distinction between treatment of mental illness and social control of deviance, the right to treatment, least restrictive settings, confidentiality, informed consent, and so on.[1,2] Initially, attention was frequently directed to some real or alleged evil or abuse, and the discussion was conducted in a 'moral' (that is, 'stamping out evil') rather than an 'ethical' framework. Since it seems unlikely that psychiatrists are inherently either more or less evil than other citizens, a discussion of their moral judgements leads to the question of how they come to be the way they are; what factors in their training or their socialization shape their ethical sensitivities and responses? A closely related theme is the role of ethics in psychiatric education; how should our knowledge about ethics influence the content and conduct of our training programmes? In view of the importance of these questions, it is curious that relatively little has been written about the teaching of ethics in psychiatry, and that both the profession and the public seem to prefer discussing the problems that psychiatrists face (and produce) rather than the methods that seem most likely to alter their behaviour.

## Can psychiatric ethics be taught?

There are several points of view about the teaching of ethics in psychiatry. Perhaps the oldest and the most widespread is that ethics cannot be taught. Proponents of this view argue that certainly psychiatrists should be 'ethical' (by which they mean virtuous), but that the only way that this can be assured is to select 'ethical' individuals and train them to become psychiatrists. The general structure of this argument is familiar to psychiatrists, since it is analogous to the view held by many physicians concerning the skills involved in the doctor–patient relationship. At least three counterarguments are important for our consideration. The first is that this position confuses ethics with morals. Ethics has to do with the way in which one thinks about and discusses moral problems and choices. A good man may not understand ethics, while a bad man might be quite sophisticated about it. Certainly we would like psychiatrists to be good people; but, as a separate goal, we would like them to understand the ethical aspects of psychiatric issues.

Secondly, a trait may have a basis in temperament, talent, or character and yet be enhanced, developed, or refined through education: musical skill, athletic ability, and the conduct of psychotherapy are all examples. It may be important to consider ethical capacities in selecting trainees, but also important to train them in ethics.

Finally, there are special problems that emerge in the consideration of the ethical aspects of psychiatry. Psychiatric ethics may be a branch of medical ethics or of general ethics; but it is a branch that has unique characteristics. There has been considerable effort devoted to the study and analysis of these issues, particularly in recent years, and it would be unfortunate if we expected each student of the field to explore these issues anew without access to the wisdom that has already been collected and formulated.

## Teaching by modelling

The second view of the teaching of ethics in psychiatry is that ethics can be taught, but only through modelling. This view would suggest that the critical problem is not selecting students, but selecting teachers. The importance of education through modelling and identification is a prominent theme in psychiatry in general, emphasized in psychodynamic, behaviourist, and developmental approaches to psychiatry. Some psychiatrists believe that most psychiatric education occurs through modelling, and almost all believe it to be important. However, accepting this proposition shifts or broadens our problem rather than solving it; we must consider how to teach the teachers as well as how to teach the students.

## Teaching by cases

The third approach considers psychiatric ethics to be an aspect of practical wisdom, taught by the case method in the discussion of specific clinical situations of practical decisions. Rounds, case-conferences, and the supervision of specific treatments form the core of most psychiatric training programmes, and ethical aspects of the psychiatrist's work can be studied in the same way as psychodynamic or psychopharmacological aspects. This approach has the virtue of bringing the teaching of psychiatric ethics into the pedagogic setting that has the trainee's greatest attention and emotional investment. One disadvantage is that ethical issues are often set aside because of the urgency of specific therapeutic problems, and there is a tendency to associate psychiatric ethics with unusual or 'tough' cases, rather than to recognize the universality of ethics as a framework for understanding professional functioning. Furthermore, this method of teaching focuses on issues related to specific patients, rather than those that emerge in consideration of broader questions of professional functioning. Ethical aspects of the relationship between the psychiatric profession and society, distribution of scarce resources, the role of the public in professional decisions, and similar matters will rarely be discussed in the context of specific cases, but they should be discussed in the course of psychiatric education. This is a general problem not unique to ethics; the same could be said about those aspects of psychopharmacology, psychodynamics, or personality development that are part of the knowledge-base of psychiatry. Finally, psychiatric educators who are excellent teachers of clinical psychiatry may not have the knowledge or interest required to teach ethics, while moral philosophers who could enrich the experience of psychiatric trainees might not be competent or appropriate as general psychiatric supervisors. It would be unfortunate if the structure of the curriculum in psychiatric ethics precluded participation by those who were most competent to teach it.

*Teaching by seminars*

The fourth approach to the teaching of ethics in psychiatry regards ethics as one of the themes of a core curriculum. A fundamental body of knowledge is taught in seminars and courses, while applications to specific problems appear in the discussion during ward rounds and supervision. This method provides exposure to the philosophical or theoretical aspects of ethics—theories of justice, concepts of right and duty, and so on; the application of these principles to the major problems of psychiatry; and experience with evaluating decisions in concrete situations. This more comprehensive approach has been recommended for the teaching of general medical ethics,[3] and employed in the few structured teaching programmes in psychiatric ethics which have appeared in the literature.[4,5,6]

# When to teach?

*Teaching in medical school*

Turning from how to teach psychiatric ethics to when the teaching should occur, we have the choice of pre-professional education, medical school, psychiatric training, or continuing education. The undergraduate period would seem to be the obvious time to develop a basis in the philosophical underpinnings of ethics, and there has been a growing interest in this subject in college curricula.[7] However, premedical preparation is so heterogeneous that courses on medical ethics in medical schools, whether required or elective, have become widespread.[3,8]

In the past two decades, medical educators have responded to a widely-held perception that the practice of medicine has become 'dehumanized', especially as a result of economic factors and the increasing use of elaborate technology,[5,9] by designing programmes to cultivate greater 'humanism' among medical students. The growth in number and variety of such programmes has been enormous,[10-14] and some have employed innovative teaching techniques.[10,15] In these programmes, ethics tends to be subsumed under the larger category of 'humanism', and psychiatry usually plays no special role. Thus, these efforts, while laudable in general, may not advance the teaching of psychiatric ethics in particular, because they tend to concentrate on cultivating good (that is, moral) attitudes and practices, rather than on cultivating critical thinking about ethical problems, and fail to address the important and complex relationships among psychiatry, medical humanism, and ethics.

Traditionally, psychiatrists have viewed themselves, and have been viewed by their colleagues in other branches of medicine, as having special interests and expertise in both humanism and ethics.[16,17] This perception is, to some extent, appropriate and useful, since that branch of medicine which deals primarily with the mind should be based on a broadly inclusive view of what it means to be 'human', and since disorders of the mind frequently compromise an individual's autonomy, a category central to ethical arguments. However, the association of psychiatry with ethics contains dangers for both fields. One danger is that both fields are often treated with the same subtle disparagement by medical school faculty and students. Many believe that there is no real expertise in these areas, and, therefore, no need for any specially trained faculty; they are seen as part of the 'art' of medicine rather than the 'science', part of the tradition shared by all physicians. Thus, everyone pays lip-service to their importance, but acts as if the subject matter were an adornment to the curriculum rather than an essential part of it.[18] Another danger is that linking psychiatry and ethics may contribute to the common confusion in clinical practice between ethical dilemmas and psychiatric problems; situations that are emotionally troubling because they embody difficult moral problems may be misidentified as presenting psychiatric questions,[19,20] while the medico-legal necessity of obtaining psychiatric consultation in cases of treatment-refusal contributes further to this blurring. Finally, there is a risk that psychiatry, eager to secure a place among the medical specialties and to be seen as scientific, will subscribe to the general distortion that ethics is intellectually 'soft', and will, for political reasons, renounce its special connection to ethics.

*Teaching in psychiatric training programmes*

The most natural setting for teaching the ethical aspects of psychiatry would seem to be during psychiatric training programmes. It is surprising that with few exceptions[12,21,22] there is almost nothing written about such teaching; and informal, anecdotal communication suggests that relatively little occurs during training other than an occasional seminar or a brief elective course. This is in spite of the fact that a number of prominent psychiatric educators have a strong interest in ethical issues.

The relatively recent growth of interest in psychiatric ethics, and the number of different subjects packed into psychiatric training, make it important not to overinterpret the failure to develop these programmes. However, there are some special problems that emerge in including the teaching of ethics in psychiatric training that are worthy of consideration. First, a great deal of this training occurs in monstrously immoral social institutions—outdated, uncomfortable, inhumane, and reflecting the stigma and fear of mental illness, as well as the political refusal to recognize and accept the inevitable costs if the mentally ill are regarded as full citizens and members of the community. The psychiatric trainee participating in these institutions—whether hospitals, community programmes, prisons, old people's homes, schools for the retarded, or the network of social services that usually fails to integrate them—feels the discomfort that has marked the entire profession's relation to the mental health system. There are several possible responses to this discomfort: guilt, anger at the profession, political activism, cynical nihilism, or withdrawal from involvement in mental health. However, whatever the specific form of the response, it is not usually a comfortable time to think about the basic ethical issues involved. Those who do become interested in such issues early in their training often tend to turn against the profession as a result. The pattern should be familiar to psychiatrists; the group try to avoid and deny the painful aspects of their roles, and those who deviate from this group norm are likely to be rebellious in other respects and rejected by the group. Fortunately, the problem seems to be diminishing in recent years, with the growing interest and awareness in the profession of the social, political, and ethical significance of its work, and, perhaps, the beginning of a recognition that consideration of these is an essential component of a training programme.

A second problem in teaching ethics in psychiatric training programmes relates to the subject matter itself. Trainees, or at least those in 'dynamically' oriented programmes that focus attention on the inner psychological world of patients, are struggling to acquire a new paradigm, to think of behaviour as determined by mental forces, wishes, fears, conflicts, and so on. This requires a suspension of their more customary framework for regarding the same behaviour, the everyday common-sense approach that includes a considerable amount of moral judgement. An important theme of psychodynamic psychiatric training is learning to suspend moral judgements in areas where they would naturally be employed. At times, this can lead to an unfortunate generalization outside the clinical psychodynamic setting, and a kind of amorality that seeks to understand all behaviour while judging nothing. Optimally, good psychodynamic training eventually leads students to recognize that in certain carefully specified clinical situations there are advantages to suspending moral judgements in order to create a field of inquiry that will make it possible to dissect the psychological determinants of behaviour—and, indeed, of morality itself. If not, the emotional atmosphere essential for the inquiry process cannot be established. Similarly, good training in ethical reasoning should lead students to recognize the advantage of temporarily suspending familiar moral judgements, so that the principles underlying these judgements can be elucidated and compared with alternative moral principles. The conflict of two such principles, or 'goods', defines an ethical dilemma, and the analysis of such a dilemma requires students to make explicit those everyday moral judgements that they have previously held implicitly or unconsciously.

Thus both ethical and psychodynamic reasoning require the suspension of familiar moral judgements, and one might think that the two would naturally reinforce each other. However, the problem in training is that a student who is struggling with the unsettling new paradigm of psychodynamics may use the more familiar paradigm of morality as a resistance, and impose moral judgements which interfere with the optimal neutrality of the psychotherapist. In the jargon of the field, ethical reasoning is confused with moral passion, and morality is used as a resistance against psychodynamic understanding. While ethics is by no means incompatible with psychodynamics, they are different, and there may be interactions between them that have educational significance. In a sense, learning psychodynamics can be like learning a foreign language, and it may be useful to stop using one's native tongue for a while. This interaction can work in both directions, and just as learning a new language can enhance one's understanding of a familiar one, so these two different frameworks for considering human behaviour can each clarify and explicate the characteristics of the other.

### Ethics in continuing education

Psychiatric education extends beyond the formal training programme, and psychiatric ethics has an important role to play in continuing medical education. Seminars and symposia have received wide attention, such as the discussion of 'the psychiatrist as double agent', co-sponsored by the American Psychiatric Association and the Institute of Society, Ethics, and the Life Sciences,[23] or the several conferences of the same Institute on ethical aspects of psychiatric treatment and research. There has also been a growing awareness of ethical issues in those psychiatrists who completed their formal training before these topics were included in educational programmes, and who now participate in postgraduate courses, although the appropriate way to introduce discussions of ethical problems into these curricula is not yet clear.[24] Those programmes which make use of case-conferences to discuss ethical issues, in a format commonly known as 'ethics rounds', usually direct these efforts to staff at various levels, including graduate psychiatrists.[2,22]

## What to teach?

### *Metaethics*

The content of the curriculum in psychiatric ethics can be considered on three levels. First is the basic introduction to ethics, the philosophical basis of moral discourse, or metaethics. If a psychiatrist is to have more than opinions on right and wrong, if he is to understand the place of these views in the larger sphere of moral reasoning, the types of justification that are being used or being discarded, and the history of these views in general ethics: in short, if he is to have an ethical understanding of his moral positions, then he must have some education in metaethics. This requirement is analogous to the need for training in basic biochemistry and pharmacology for the psychiatrist who is to understand the drugs that he is prescribing, and even to be prepared to understand those that have not yet been discovered.

Few psychiatrists are prepared to teach metaethics; if it is to be taken seriously, it requires the collaboration of philosophers, ethicists, or others with similar backgrounds. It can be taught as a distinct body of knowledge, with the advantage of emphasizing the inherent structure and relationships of the discipline itself, but with the disadvantage of being given low priority by trainees who are preoccupied with more immediate and practical concerns. Alternatively, the metaethical dimensions of specific ethical issues can be explored in the context of discussing those specific issues. For example, a discussion of the relationship between individual autonomy, involuntary treatment, and the right to treatment in psychiatric settings can be used to explore the relationship between utilitarian and absolutist modes of ethical reasoning. This second approach reverses the advantages and disadvantages of the first; the material is organized in categories that 'feel' more relevant to the students, but at the risk of diluting and fragmenting the critical issues in the underlying philosophical dialogue. There are practical problems that also must be considered: if qualified teachers are scarce, the first mode of presentation, a systematic review of ethical theory, requires less of their time, while the second format is more likely to encourage interaction between psychiatrists and professional philosophers.

## Codes of ethics and the profession

The second level of the curriculum in psychiatric ethics would involve discussions of normative rules, standards, and codes of the profession; what psychiatrists and psychiatry ought to do and why.[25-27]* This also could be taught either in a separate discussion or integrated with the teaching of specific issues in psychiatry. This level of ethics is closely related to issues of law, politics, and social policy; and their teaching can be co-ordinated in the curriculum. The teaching of rules of conduct can easily degenerate into moralistic sermons; such a fate is best prevented by serious efforts to explore professional codes or prescriptions in a metaethical framework, while at the same time considering their application to concrete situations and their practical consequences for society and for the profession.

The discussion of the codes and standards of the profession will also offer an opportunity to explore the nature of professionals and their relationship to the general society.[28] Many of the recent controversies about psychiatric ethics have focused on this theme; issues of peer-review, the psychiatrist as 'double agent',[23] and the role of the profession in responding to an individual member who breaches the professional code of ethics would all be examples.

## Specific topics

The third level of the curriculum in psychiatric ethics would be the consideration of a series of specific issues in the field. The list of potential subjects is long enough that any course would have to make selections. Possible subjects might include:

(1) the right to treatment;
(2) consent and involuntary treatment;
(3) invasive or irreversible treatments;
(4) institutions, total institutions, and deinstitutionalization;
(5) least restrictive settings and professional decisions;
(6) coercion and psychotherapy;
(7) prediction of dangerousness and the role of the psychiatrist in its prevention;
(8) children, the retarded, and the incompetent; guardianship and proxy;
(9) psychiatrist as agent of society and patient; the social and political abuse of psychiatry;
(10) behaviour-control, social engineering, and deviance;
(11) responsibility, guilt, and insanity
(12) autonomy and competence; self-determination;

* See Appendix for codes of ethics relevant to psychiatrists.

(13) performance enhancement, optimalization, and the psychopharmacology of hedonism;
(14) labelling, stigma, and the effects of diagnosis;
(15) privacy and confidentiality;
(16) distributive justice and access to health services;
(17) resource allocation and the determination of priorities;
(18) consent and risks in psychiatric research; and
(19) political activism by psychiatrists.

Each of these topics could be explored in terms of the values and choices
they entail, the history of the profession's response, the arguments that
have been presented on behalf of various positions that have been taken,
the basic ethical issues that are implicit in these arguments, and the patterns of views on the entire array of topics that reflect more general ethical
positions. Clearly, a detailed analysis of all of these subjects would con-
sume an inappropriate amount of time in a training curriculum, and selection would be required.

## Goals and objectives

The common confusion of ethics with morality leads to a fundamental
tension between different objectives, often unstated, for teaching programmes in ethics. Most students and many educators (particularly those
who have little formal exposure to ethical reasoning, but who appreciate
the difficulty and importance of ethical dilemmas) tend to see training in
ethics as a means of instilling or protecting idealism and 'human values' in
students, or of offering them humane and reasonable guidelines for resolving ethical dilemmas in practice.[5,9,15–17] Others, more inclined to value
ethical discourse as an intellectually rigorous discipline, tend to see the
objectives as educating students in the history and current status of the
discipline and cultivating habits of critical reasoning about these issues.
These different views are not incompatible, but neither are they identical;
the failure to recognize, if not to resolve, the tension between them can
seriously undermine the effectiveness of a teaching programme in ethics.
Thus, while any particular programme is likely to pursue several different
goals at the same time, the goals should be articulated as clearly as possible.
Goals related to knowledge include understanding major systems of ethical
reasoning and their similarities and differences, learning the terms and
concepts used in ethical discourse, and learning the history of the contemporary ethical dilemmas in psychiatry, with the positions and arguments that have developed around them. Among the attitude-related goals
are sensitizing the student to the ethical aspects of issues that might otherwise be seen as scientific or technical in nature, and acquainting him or her
with the subtlety and complexity of ethical reasoning, often seen by those

who are not familiar with it as little more than 'common sense'. The goals defined in terms of skill would include the student's ability to recognize ethical problems in psychiatry; to reason about them in a coherent, systematic, and useful way; and to understand the reasoning of others and participate with them in ethical discourse. Finally, the goals might involve modifying the professional behaviour of the students so that it is informed and guided by their understanding of psychiatric ethics.

The selection of goals for a specific curriculum will be determined by the stage in the student's professional education, the time available, the setting, and the faculty. Generally, programmes that aim exclusively at modifying the student's behaviour in a specific direction without attending to knowledge and attitudes have little lasting impact, while those that focus on knowledge without attention to skill have difficulty involving more pragmatically oriented students.

## Constructing curricula

Educational programmes are most successful if the students acquire knowledge that helps them to accomplish tasks in which they are currently engaged, and if they are given opportunities to apply the knowledge they are acquiring while they are acquiring it. When these principles are applied to the subject matter of psychiatric ethics, some general guidelines for constructing curricula emerge. First, although lectures about ethical issues may impart information about terms, concepts, and the history of arguments and positions, the student will gain familiarity with moral reasoning only by participating more actively through dialogue and discussion. Second, although the 'classic' issues of psychiatric ethics should be explored, and the student has much to learn about them and from participating in discussions of them, a valuable dimension is added if the underlying themes and problems are traced in the student's current professional experience. For example, the 'double agent' issue of the psychiatrist's responsibility to his patient and to society is clearly articulated in the discussions of recent problems in Soviet psychiatry (see Chapter 24) or in the judicial decisions concerning the psychiatrist's obligation to warn potential victims of violent patients. However, the question will have additional meaning to the trainee who discusses it in terms, for example, of the psychotic patient currently receiving treatment who wants to return to an occupation involving public safety for which he is not yet competent, or of the adolescent patient who is involved in sexual or drug-related behaviour that is not acceptable to family or society.

Psychiatric ethics involves intellectual areas in which psychiatrists have no special claim to expertise, and there are advantages to constructing programmes that will bring psychiatrists together with other mental health professionals, lawyers, sociologists, and philosophers, both in the student body and on the faculty.[22] The broader meaning of one's routine and daily decisions is experienced dramatically when seen through the eyes of an intelligent observer who has been socialized into a different perspective. For example, courses including psychiatric trainees and law students provide each of these groups with an opportunity to explore ethical questions in involuntary treatment or criminal responsibility that greatly enlarges the perspective that either group meeting alone would have.

Finally, like any other curriculum, attention to evaluation enriches the programme. Not only does it force the faculty to specify goals and objectives (all too often ignored when the subject matter is obviously relevant, but necessarily vague and amorphous), but it also forces a dialogue between students and faculty about these goals. Students often approach programmes in psychiatric ethics with the assumption that the intent is to teach them what to do in difficult or special situations. A well-constructed curriculum and evaluation procedure can convey that the goal is to help students identify alternatives and analyse the ethical aspects of the choices they face in their daily professional activities, to discuss these intelligently with their colleagues, and to clarify and, when appropriate, resolve differences and conflicts.

## Summary

The recent interest in psychiatric ethics has not yet produced much interest in the teaching of psychiatric ethics, but this is likely to follow. Such teaching is more likely to occur in psychiatric and continuing education programmes than in premedical or medical school curricula. It should include discussion of metaethics, or the basic principles of ethical reasoning; normative codes of professional conduct, or the rules for psychiatrists facing choices; and the specific situations and problems that interest and trouble psychiatrists today.

## References

1 Redlich, F. and Mollica, R. F.: Overview: ethical issues in contemporary psychiatry. *American Journal of Psychiatry* **133**:125–36, 1976.
2 Appelbaum, P. S. and Reiser, S. J.: Ethics rounds: a model for teaching ethics in the psychiatric setting. *Hospital and Community Psychiatry* **32**:555–60, 1981.
3 Culver, C. M., Clouser, K. D., Gert, B. *et al.*: Special report: basic curricular goals in medical ethics. *New England Journal of Medicine* **312**:253–6, 1985.
4 Hundert, E. M.: A model for ethical problem solving in medicine, with practical applications. *American Journal of Psychiatry* **144**:839–46, 1987.
5 McCartney, J. R.: Consultation-liaison psychiatry and the teaching of ethics. *General Hospital Psychiatry* **8**:411–14, 1986.

6 Salladay, S. A.: Teaching ethics in the psychiatry clerkship. *Journal of Medical Education* **56**:204–6, 1981.

7 Institute of Society, Ethics, and the Life Sciences: *The teaching of bioethics.* Hastings-on-Hudson, NY, The Institute, 1976.

8 Veatch, R. M. and Sollitto, S.: Medical ethics teaching: report of a national medical school survey. *Journal of the American Medical Association* **235**:1030–3, 1976.

9 Gorlin, R. and Zucker, H.: Physicians' reactions to patients: a key to teaching humanistic medicine. *New England Journal of Medicine* **308**:1059–63, 1983.

10 Bickel, J.: Human values teaching programs in the clinical education of medical students. *Journal of Medical Education* **62**:369–78, 1987.

11 Pellegrino, E. D. and McElhinney, T. K.: *Teaching ethics, the humanities, and human values in medical schools: a 10-year overview.* Washington, DC, Institute on Human Values in Medicine, Society for Health and Human Values, 1981.

12 Clouser, K. D.: *Teaching bioethics: strategies, problems, and resources.* Hastings-on-Hudson, NY, Institute of Society, Ethics, and Life Sciences, 1980.

13 Wolstenholme, G.: Teaching medical ethics in other countries. *Journal of Medical Ethics* **11**:22–4, 1985.

14 Pellegrino, E. D., Hart, R. J., Henderson, S. R., Loeb, S. E., and Edwards, E. G.: Relevance and utility of courses in medical ethics. *Journal of the American Medical Association* **253**:49–53, 1985.

15 Radwany, S. M. and Adelson, B. H.: The use of literary classics in teaching medical ethics to physicians. *Journal of the American Medical Association* **257**:1629–31, 1987.

16 Sider, R. and Clements, C.: Psychiatry's contribution to medical ethics education. *American Journal of Psychiatry* **139**:498–501, 1982.

17 Hayes, J. R.: Consultation-liaison psychiatry and clinical ethics: a model for consultation and teaching. *General Hospital Psychiatry* **8**:415–18, 1986.

18 Veatch, R. M., Gaylin, W., and Morgan, C. (ed.): *The teaching of medical ethics.* Hastings-on-Hudson, NY, Institute of Society, Ethics, and the Life Sciences, 1973.

19 Perl, M. and Shelp, E. E.: Psychiatric consultation masking moral dilemmas in medicine. *New England Journal of Medicine* **307**:618–21, 1982.

20 Perl, M.: Response to the articles: 'Consultation-liaison psychiatry and the teaching of ethics' by J. R. McCartney and 'Consultation-liaison psychiatry and clinical ethics' by J. R. Hayes. *General Hospital Psychiatry* **8**:419–21, 1986.

21 Bloch, S.: Teaching of psychiatric ethics. *British Journal of Psychiatry* **136**:300–1, 1980.

22 Appelbaum, P. S.: Solving clinical puzzles: strategies for organizing mental health ethics rounds, in S. J. Reiser, H. J. Bursztajn, P. S. Appelbaum and T. G. Gutheil: *Divided staffs, divided selves: a case approach to mental health ethics,* pp. 41–59. Cambridge, Cambridge University Press, 1987.

23 American Psychiatric Association and Institute of Society, Ethics, and the Life Sciences: *A conference on conflicting loyalties.* Special Supplement, April 1978. Hastings-on-Hudson, NY, The Institute, 1978.

24 Jellinek, M. and Parmalee, D.: Is there a role for medical ethics in postgraduate psychiatry courses? *American Journal of Psychiatry* **134**:1438–9, 1977.

25 Moore, R. A.: Ethics in the practice of psychiatry—origins, functions, models, and enforcement. *American Journal of Psychiatry* **135**:157–63, 1978.

26 American Psychiatric Association: The principles of medical ethics, with annotations especially applicable to psychiatry. *American Journal of Psychiatry* **130**:1057–64, 1973.

27 Michels, R.: The physician and medical education. *P&S Quarterly* **19**:13–15, 1974.

28 Michels, R.: Professional ethics and social value. *International Review of Psychoanalysis* **3**:377–84, 1976.

# 21

# The responsibility of the psychiatrist to his society

*Paul Chodoff*

Psychiatrists are citizens of the society wherein they practise their profession. As such, they have certain rights, but also, as individuals and through the organizations representing them, they must meet their responsibilities to society. In this chapter I shall discuss these rights and responsibilities, and the ethical issues arising from them.

## The rights of psychiatrists

What are the rights of psychiatrists? In my opinion, their basic right and privilege is that of practising in an area which, although difficult, is interesting and rewarding. Its rewards come in the form of intellectual stimulation and an outlet for creativity, the knowledge that one is performing a useful function in society, and a reasonable financial recompense for one's efforts. Psychiatrists certainly also have the right, and indeed the duty, to respond as effectively as possible to unfair or tendentious attacks on their profession, and to discriminatory judgement. Can psychiatrists also count on the respect of the public as one of their rewards? This is not so certain, partly because the field in which they work provokes defensive and ambivalent reactions from many people, and, more importantly, because the respect of the public can be relied on only when psychiatrists earn and deserve it by discharging their responsibilities to their fellow citizens.

## Their responsibilities

The responsibilities of psychiatrists can be subsumed under four headings: (1) to master their craft; (2) to police their ranks; (3) to be accountable to the public; and (4) to be advocates for the mentally ill.

### The responsibility of competence

The first requirement means that the public needs to be assured that the person presenting himself as a practitioner of psychiatry knows what he is doing, is well trained, and has or is acquiring relevant experience. At a minimal level, the fact that a psychiatrist has acquired a professional degree in medicine and has had residency training in psychiatry attests to some level of skill in the field. However, this obviously is not enough. Organizations representing psychiatrists require additional standards of competence from practitioners aspiring to professional recognition. This is generally accomplished through the process of acquiring credentials: by graduating from certain institutions and passing certain tests, and by attendance at continuing education courses. While the acquisition of such credentials is, for the most part, accepted and considered effective, a new and questioning climate of opinion has raised some questions about measures imposed by professional organizations. Critics charge that although ostensibly for the purpose of guaranteeing the quality of services offered to the public, these standards may also be seen as manoeuvres with the self-serving purpose of preserving a monopoly, thus increasing costs for the consuming public. An example is the sanctions previously imposed on psychiatrists or psychiatric institutions offering services through advertising. Today, of course, such advertising is a common practice in newspapers, magazines, and phone books. Another example is the recent suit mounted by the American Psychological Association against the American Psychoanalytical Association to force the latter to open its training ranks, and thus its credentials, to psychologists and social workers.[1]

One way by which the public can be assured that practitioners are honing their skills is if the latter follow treatment methods that have been proven to be effective. The ability to offer the public this reassurance varies to a certain extent between the two main treatment approaches in psychiatry—the biosomatic, particularly involving the use of psychoactive drugs, and psychotherapy. A presumption of competence can be applied to the psychiatrists in whose hands psychopharmacological treatment now rests, by virtue of their having gone through an approved residency programme with training in pharmacotherapy, and usually by their having passed formal examinations. But they also have the advantage that education and training can be monitored through controlled clinical trials of its results. Thus there is reasonable assurance that when a psychiatrist prescribes one drug rather than another for a particular clinical condition he is acting on the basis of data about its effectiveness and possible side-effects. Will this state of affairs be complicated if success crowns the recent efforts of psychologists in some states in the United States to gain legal approval, after undergoing a period of training, to prescribe psychoactive drugs in the same manner as psychiatrists? Is such a skill 'no big deal', as is stated by the foremost advocate of this change?[2] Or, as is vigorously claimed by organized psychiatry, are psychologists unequipped to understand and manage the vicissitudes and complexities of drug treatment, with consequent dire effects on their clients? In the absence of evidence in the form of data or experience this argument can easily become polemical, defending the vested interests of both groups, rather than responding to the needs of the public. It does seem that the burden of proof here lies with the psychologists, to defend themselves against the charge that they would be practising medicine without a medical education.

In the case of psychotherapy the reliability of standards that can assure the potential patient that the therapist he has chosen is reasonably competent is more problematical. It is true that psychiatrists for whom psychotherapy is a major treatment modality, like their predominantly pharmacotherapeutic colleagues, also have had residency training and usually their Boards. But how is the patient to make an informed choice in the face of the myriad schools and methods of psychotherapy? Is there any reason why this potential patient would not be as well served if he became a psychotherapeutic client of a qualified psychologist or social worker? Psychiatrists who claim that medical psychotherapy has more to offer than the psychotherapy offered by other mental health professionals need to prove their point.

Also differentiating the psychiatric pharmacotherapist from the psychiatric psychotherapist is the greater difficulty in validating psychotherapy through outcome studies than is the case with drug treatments. Studies now extant offer what seems to be conclusive evidence that, in a general way, psychotherapy is better than placebo.[3] But when it comes to matching a patient or client suffering from a particular disorder with a particular type of psychotherapy that has a good record with it, there are currently few convincing answers.[4] In the absence of such objective evidence, patients and clients have to rely on the professional credentials and reputations of therapists, without the benefit of feedback from results.

For the purposes of discussion, I have artificially dichotomized drug treatment and psychotherapy. Of course, in many instances both are offered in conjunction. Can patients who require both drugs and psychotherapy have confidence that the psychiatrist they consult will be competent in both areas? Many psychiatrists have both skills; but others will not feel appreciably more comfortable with drug prescription than will members of the other mental health professions. Any psychotherapist in such a position, MD or not, has the responsibility at least of being aware when collaborative drug treatment is indicated, and of referring the patient to an expert. A similar injunction applies to a psychiatrist skilled in drug treatment but without extensive psychotherapeutic experience when confronted with a patient for whom the latter modality is indicated.

## The responsibility to behave ethically

A profession has been defined by Eliot Friedson[5] as an occupation that has won from the public the right to regulate its own affairs. Thus, psychiatry, to maintain its recognition as a profession, must meet the second responsibility I have listed, and satisfy the public that psychiatrists can police their own ranks, at least to the extent that an offence is not so grave as to require legal sanctions. One can, of course, hope that the rigours of professional training and the supervision taking place during its course would weed out people of bad character. This, of course, cannot be guaranteed. Internal policing measures are called for in a wide range of derelictions. For example, a practitioner may be incompetent, or may be operating with improper or insufficient credentials, or under the handicap of incapacitating physical or mental illness. This is a problem faced by all branches of medicine; but when psychotherapy is the treatment modality being employed there is a particular need for vigilance, because of the seductiveness of the power that inevitably accrues to the therapist role, which can be employed in ways that are harmful rather than helpful. This is because the psychotherapeutic relationship is essentially asymmetrical. The patient shares intimate matters with the therapist; but not the other way around. Since transferential elements are certain to be present, the result is a relationship in which the patient is likely to be heavily reliant on the therapist, while the latter may acquire a considerable amount of power over the former. This enables the therapist to exploit the relationship for his own purposes. Improper sexual behaviour between therapist (usually male) and patient (usually female) is a glaring example of such exploitation,[6] but it is not the only one. A therapist can also gratify psychological needs for control or dominance, for voyeuristic or sadistic gratification, or, and I suspect even more common, for the satisfaction that derives from the imposition of one's own values on other people. The therapist's own financial gain certainly can be another motive for exploiting the relationship. In view of the resourcefulness of human cupidity, there are, unfortunately, many ways in which this kind of cheating can happen.[7] A somewhat unusual instance was reported in a recent newspaper article about a psychiatrist who had been indicted for investing in the stock-market on the basis of inside information gained from a patient. A particularly troublesome and ambiguous area in which there may be collusion for financial purposes between therapist and patient client arises in connection with third-party insurance transactions.[8]

If we accept that the psychiatric profession should do its best to abate the kinds of unethical and dishonest behaviour described above, what vehicles of enforcement are available? The usual answer, at least in the United States, lies in the peer-review and ethics committees of the psychiatric societies that have as their purpose the investigation of instances of exploitative, dishonest, or unethical behaviour.

Actions taken by these groups can be quite effective. They range from censure to expulsion from the organization and even reference to a State

Board of Licensure, with grave consequences for the practitioner's career and professional reputation. However, it must be acknowledged that there are serious limitations to the functioning of such monitoring groups. Quasi-legal bodies as they are, they are hedged about by many procedural obstacles. For the most part they are able to deal only with rather gross and specific instances of misbehaviour. Also, the dereliction must be brought to their attention, either by the offended person or by another practitioner who has knowledge of it; and this may not take place for various reasons, such as considerations of confidentiality, professional solidarity, uncertainty about the facts, and sympathy towards the accused. When confronted with such a situation any action taken by the psychiatrist should be the result of due consideration of all factors involved, including, very importantly, the patient, and the effects of such disclosure on her welfare. As experts in the multifarious ways in which human beings can disguise their behaviour and deceive themselves about their motives, psychiatrists need to be alert to the possibility that they are avoiding action because it is difficult and painful, rather than because it is not the right thing to do. Less obvious instances of the exploitation of psychiatric power—say, an excessive emphasis on hearing all the details of the patient's sexual life—are unlikely to come to an official committee's attention, or can be disguised by being attributed to differing clinical or psychodynamic views. A different kind of objection, voiced by certain critics outside the medical profession, is that these committees are subject to an inevitable conflict of interest, since the members of a professional group are judging their own colleagues. Thus, say these critics, these committees are nothing but company unions, and of little value without the addition of non-professional public representatives.[5]

The monitoring and control of unethical and dishonest behaviour on the part of practitioners constitute an ever-present responsibility for all psychiatrists, not only organizationally but individually. Possibly the most effective, though perhaps utopian, means of maintaining good conduct and the trust of the public are continuing self-exploration and a determination to ground one's relationships with patients on, as Freud said, "a love of truth precluding sham or deceit."[9]

*The responsibility to be accountable*

I turn now to a third major responsibility of psychiatrists to the society in which they practise; the need to be accountable to the public and its representatives. Accountability is a broad term with wide application. *Webster's New International Dictionary* defines accountability as 'liability to be called upon to render an account, answerable', and in this sense all of the responsibilities I am discussing can be said to be aspects of accountability. However, here I shall be somewhat more restrictive in my use of the term. The historical path trodden by the concept of accountability has been a long one.[10] It seems to have had its origin in the period when Europe was stirring from its long medieval torpor, and philosophers debated whether the divine right of the king made him accountable only to God, or whether he was a representative of the people receiving his power from them and, therefore, accountable to them. The latter meaning has, of course, won out, and is paid at least lip-service by the rulers and governing bodies of all societies, democratic or totalitarian. But not only must modern rulers be accountable, anyone holding a significant degree of power—business leaders, scientists, educators, and so forth—must conform to this requirement, and certainly this is true of the members of those professions which meddle in the fate of people, and sometimes mediate between them and the state.

For purposes of this discussion I shall consider the accountability of psychiatrists under two headings. First is fiscal accountability, the need to be straightforward and honest with patients about all monetary transactions, including fees and how they are to be paid, and, in general, the financial rules of engagement, including charges for missed sessions.[8] In the case of direct payment these negotiations are relatively uncomplicated—the patient should understand them, and he can then choose whether or not to accept them. This is not always the case when third-party payment is involved. Here the situation is more complex, and even ambiguous, for two reasons. First, and less important, the fact that part of the fee comes from an uninvolved agent may tempt the treating psychiatrist to cut corners, sometimes for his own benefit and sometimes with the collusion of the patient, rationalized as a service to him. Can a therapeutic relationship grounded in deceit of this kind be carried on effectively? Will it promote public trust?

The second and more important problem when dealing with third-party payers is that the psychiatrist, no matter what the form of treatment, is under the necessity of conveying diagnostic and other information to the insurance company. This places him on the horns of a classic dilemma between his commitment to hold everything he hears in the therapeutic encounter in absolute confidence and his obligation to answer the insurance company's questions. Without these answers treatment may be impossible, or may have to be curtailed because of a lack of coverage. It also must be acknowledged that paying agents are legitimately entitled to a certain amount of information. If this is not made available, their operations, financed by premium money, cannot be rationally planned or carried out. This does not mean, of course, that intrusive or unnecessary requests for information have to be condoned without protest. Psychiatrists have a right vigorously to defend their patients against unnecessary invasion of confidentiality and against unjust discrimination towards people in treatment for mental or emotional disorders.

Important as are the concerns about confidentiality, they are not the only reason for the reluctance of therapists to convey information to insurance companies. Other reasons include the nuisance and hassle factor. Also, diagnostic labels can be stigmatizing; the psychiatrist supplying neuroleptic drugs to a schizophrenic may fear that an accurate diagnosis will be harmful to his patient. Another more subtle source of such reluctance lies in what may be called the 'medical model' problem.[11] Patients receiving drugs for their disorders generally can be seen as being sick in a medical sense, and thus as being in conformity with the medical model, under which insurance companies operate and which they are used to dealing with. This is not as true with some patients being treated exclusively with psychotherapy. A certain number of these, by no means all or even a majority, although they may have significant interpersonal difficulties deserving of psychotherapeutic help, can be considered to be medically sick only by stretching that concept to an extent that makes it indistinguishable from normality. This is particularly true of some insight-oriented therapies, where there is a lack of clarity about such medical-model considerations as significant disability, and goals and end-points of treatment.[12] This medical-model problem, even more than questions of cost, may explain the reluctance of third-party insurance payers adequately to cover psychotherapy. Incidentally, some of these same considerations enter into the difficulty previously mentioned of validating psychotherapy through outcome studies oriented towards the results of the treatment of medical illnesses.

Psychiatrists need to be accountable not only for their financial transactions, but also in what may be called a fiduciary sense. They need to account for the considerable amount of power that has been entrusted to them not only by their patients, as has already been discussed, but also by society at large, and by the organs of state and government. Speaking of psychiatrists, Jonas Robitscher[13] claimed that in the United States they have become the most important non-governmental decision-makers in modern life, disposing of more power than most state officials.

With regard to psychiatric treatment, accountability is increasingly being called for through the doctrine of informed consent. Informed consent requires that psychiatrists convey to their patients some idea of their treatment plan and its expected effect, both positive and negative, and possibly an estimate of how long it should take. These are often difficult standards to satisfy both for practical and theoretical reasons; but in view of emerging legal sanctions, such as the *Osheroff* case, in which a depressed patient sued a psychiatric hospital because he had been treated with psychotherapy instead of drugs, they need to be taken seriously (see Chapter 8). In certain instances it may also be necessary to be clear about possible dilutions of the psychiatrists' adherence to absolute confidentiality, not only because of the third-party reasons, but in cases where violence to others may be an issue (*Tarasoff* rule).[14]

If its purpose is to maintain public confidence in psychiatry then accountability in the broad sense also obliges the profession to be clear about what it is, what it does, its capabilities, and its limits, and to make a reasonable amount of this information available to the interested public.

There is no consensus within psychiatry about these matters of definition. As a matter of fact, that the profession is currently involved in an identity crisis is widely accepted, and is a frequent source of comment and discussion. To some extent this crisis is inherent in the very nature of the work that psychiatrists do—a reflection of the reality that they must maintain as best they can an uneasy balance, with one foot in biological medicine and the other in social concerns. This characteristic has been compounded by real differences within the ranks of the mental health professions. Conflicts of direction and interest exist and are accentuated by the impact of rapidly changing customs, values, and methods of payment.

Questions about the scope and function of psychiatry which remain unsolved and confuse the public include the following: Is there a schism developing between the 'doctors' among psychiatrists and the 'therapists'? Is a medical education necessary to undertake a primarily psychotherapeutic career? Should psychoanalysis be a psychiatric subspecialty or a separate discipline?

Whom should the psychiatrist treat? Should his patients include only individuals suffering from a significant mental illness, or at least those whose disorder conforms to a reasonable definition of the medical model? Should psychiatrists attempt to divorce themselves from the constraints of that model, or should they try to redefine it? To what extent should the psychiatrist devote himself to the treatment of the 'worried well'—people suffering from discomfort or distress which is not strictly medical—or to attempts to enhance human potential? Does psychiatric concentration on this population interfere with attention to the chronically mentally ill?

How effective are psychiatric treatments? Although this question can be asked of all forms of psychiatric treatment, including drugs and somatic methods, it is most urgent with regard to the psychotherapies, as I have already indicated.

The power possessed by mental health professionals is derived not only from actual or potential patients among the public. For many years, in Western countries generally, the state has turned to experts in mental health to lend assistance in many decisions of great import to the people concerned. Help is being sought in such diverse areas as involuntary commitment procedures, custody trials, insanity pleas, research activities involving human behaviour, and sometimes even national and international politics. The fact that the state consults psychiatrists in such matters is a tribute to the respect in which they are held by the public and its representatives; but it also places them in a precarious and uneasy position. To quote the Duke in *Huckleberry Finn*, when he was invited to be tarred and feathered and ridden out of town on a rail. 'If it weren't for the honor, I might decline.' One consequence of wielding this amount of power can be an unwarranted inflation of professional egos, resulting in the kind of arrogant and ill-considered actions that occurred in the US Presidential campaign of 1964, when psychiatrists were polled about the mental stability of Senator Goldwater. A very serious responsibility accruing to psychiatrists acting in the service of the state is to balance their allegiances to individuals and to the government. Double-agent dilemmas,[15] with loyalties divided between the individual and the state, may be almost inevitable; and in extreme cases these may lead toward such monstrosities as the perversion of psychiatry for the purpose of suppressing dissent that dishonoured the USSR for many years (see Chapter 24). Yet I believe that lending assistance to the state in these decisions, with all prayerful cautions and safeguards, is a duty that cannot be shirked by members of the mental health professions.

## The responsibility of advocacy

The fourth and final responsibility of psychiatrists, no matter what their particular interests, is to serve as advocates for the emotionally disturbed and mentally ill. Fulfilling this responsibility may serve not only that segment of the public that may require psychiatric care, but also the public at large, which needs to be made aware of the problems of psychiatric patients. This advocacy role covers a wide range of subjects, from the third-party coverage of an intact patient receiving psychotherapy for emotional problems to the unkempt bag-lady eking out her existence on the city streets. For members of the former group, it must be made clear that although the suffering of such people is less obvious, and may be concealed behind an apparently normal façade, it still exists, has destructive effects on social and family lives, and eminently deserves treatment. Efforts of this kind generally are carried out at an organizational level, including negotiating with the various types of third-party payers and with legislatures to include mental health coverage and help in financing. In the United States, those patients financed through Medicare and Medicaid need help in improving the quantity and quality of their coverage.

Although this is especially true of psychotherapy, all psychiatrists place a very high value on their ability to offer the patient a therapeutic atmosphere in which the confidentiality of all communications is inviolate (see Chapter 15). Although a few dissenting voices exist, psychiatrists generally are vigorous defenders of the sanctity of confidentiality, and willingly act in its defence against various attacks. Thus, with regard to the (*Tarasoff*) duty to warn[14] that attenuates confidentiality, psychiatric efforts have been successful in refining and modifying that rule so that its threat to confidentiality is less severe. However, a grey area exists within which there may be ethical conflicts between the responsibility to advocate confidentiality and the psychiatrist's responsibility for the safety of other people.

In making the case for adequate governmental and insurance coverage for psychiatric patients or private psychiatric hospitals or in protecting their confidentiality, it must be acknowledged that psychiatrists can be seen as acting not only on behalf of their patients but also in their own interests or in the interests of the hospitals that employ them. Such motivation, however, is less likely to be operative when confronting the plight of patients with severe mental disorders who require at least some periods of hospitalization in state or Federal institutions. The quality of such care for the indigent mentally ill varies tremendously throughout the world wherever psychiatric hospitalization is practised. The responsibility to monitor such care and try to bring about improvements in it falls upon all psychiatrists. In my opinion, serious deficiencies exist in many areas of the United States with regard to effective and humane treatment of many patients with disabling mental disorders.[16] American psychiatrists can justly criticize the USSR for depriving its citizens of freedom by hospitalizing them unnecessarily; but they cannot escape the finger of blame for failing to provide mentally ill citizens with anything like the equal treatment that American values promise them.[17]

In this country psychiatric resources are far from being shared out equally; inequities exist at many levels.[18,19] A wealthy schizophrenic patient receives far better treatment than a poor one. He goes to better hospitals, receives more skilled mental health care, has access to more financial help from outside sources; and the goals of his treatment are likely to be more ambitious and better maintained than they are for the poor schizophrenic. Obviously, disparities in the levels of care on the basis of ability to pay are inherent in a capitalistic society. But such discrepancies can be morally tolerated only if they are not extreme, only if the standard of care does not fall below reasonable minimal standards of decency. All psychiatrists have a responsibility to be aware of the kind of care provided for the mentally ill in their own countries, and to do their best to bring about a more equitable distributive justice with regard to the resources available to the economically lower strata of their societies.

The subject of deinstitutionalization of the mentally ill is dealt with in Chapter 14 of this book by Roger Peele. However, I feel that I cannot close this chapter on the responsibility of the psychiatrist to his society without stressing the urgent need for psychiatrists to be advocates not only for their paying patients and for the mentally ill in state and federal hospitals. Their advocacy ought also to extend itself to try to solve or at least to ameliorate the plight of the seriously mentally ill who constitute a significant component of the homeless people wandering the streets and sleeping on gratings. Brought as they have been to the pathetic state in which they now exist by a combination of well-meaning, but, to my mind, now misguided application of civil-liberties principles and budgetary stinginess, it is the moral responsibility of psychiatrists to work towards changing both of these factors.[20]

# References

1 *Welch et al.* v. *American Psychoanalytic Association*, no. 85 CIV, 1651 (SDNY).
2 *Psychiatric News*: **24**:5. American Psychiatric Association, Washington DC, 2 June 1989.
3 Smith M. L., Glass, G. U., and Miller, T. J: *The benefits of psychotherapy and behaviour change: an empirical analysis*. Baltimore, Johns Hopkins University Press, 1980.
4 Parloff, M. B: Psychotherapy and research: an anaclitic depression. *Psychiatry* **43**:279–93, 1980.
5 Friedson, E.: *Profession of medicine*. New York, Dodd, Meade, 1972.
6 Gartell, N., Herman, J., Olarte, S., Feldstein, M., and Localio, J. D.: Psychiatrist–patient sexual contact: results of a national survey. I: Prevalence. *American Journal of Psychiatry* **143**:1126–31, 1986.
7 Towery, O. B. and Sharfstein, S. S.: Fraud and abuse in psychiatric practice. *American Journal of Psychiatry* **135**:92–4, 1978.
8 Chodoff, P.: Psychiatry and the fiscal third party. *American Journal of Psychiatry* **135**:497–510, 1978.
9 Freud, S.: *Analysis terminable and interminable*. Standard edn, Vol. 23. London, Hogarth Press, 1978, pp. 211–53.
10 Sibley, M. Q.: *Political ideas and ideologies*. New York, Harper and Row, 1970.
11 Chodoff, P.: Effects of the new economic climate on psychotherapeutic practice. *American Journal of Psychiatry* **144**:1293–7, 1987.
12 Sharfstein, S., Gutheil, T., and Stoddard, F.: Money and character disorders: on how to get the recalcitrant third party and the impossible patient to pay your bills, in *Character pathology: theory and treatment*, ed. M. Zales. New York, Brunner–Mazel, 1983.
13 Robitscher, J: *The powers of psychiatry*. New York, Houghton-Mifflin, 1980.
14 *Tarasoff* v. *Regents of the University of California*, 529P, 2d 553, 1974.
15 In the service of the state: the psychiatrist as double agent. A conference on conflicting loyalties cosponsored by the American Psychiatric Association and the Hastings Center. *Hastings Center Report* **8**(suppl):1–23, 1978.
16 Tancredi, L. R. and Slaby, A. E.: *Ethical policy in mental health care*. New York, Prodist/Heinemann, 1977.
17 Chodoff, P.: Ethical conflicts in psychiatry: the Soviet Union vs. the United States. *Hospital and Community Psychiatry* **36**:925–28, 1985.

18 Michels, R.: The responsibility of psychiatry to society, in *Law and ethics in the practice of psychiatry*, ed. C. Hofling, Chapter 10. New York, Brunner–Mazel, 1981.

19 Levine, C.: Ethics and health cost containment. Report from a Hasting Center conference. *Hastings Center Report* **9**:10–17, 1979.

20 Chodoff, P.: Involuntary hospitalization of the mentally ill as a moral issue. *American Journal of Psychiatry* **141**:384–9, 1984.

# 22

# Psychiatry in the Nazi era

*Benno Müller-Hill*

When a profession such as the psychiatric profession sets out to create its own ethics it is appropriate to remember its history. This has been attempted in the first edition of *Psychiatric ethics*. The lowest point of this past was called 'the tragic abuse of medicine during the Second World War'.[1] But no further word was said. What was this 'tragic abuse'?

- *1934–1939*: 350 000 real or potential psychiatric clients or patients are legally sterilized in Germany without informed consent, with the help of the psychiatric profession.[2,3]
- *1938–1942*: In anticipation of a law which never materializes 20 000 German Gypsies are singled out for sterilization and concentration camps by a team headed by a psychiatrist.[2,4] Many are sterilized, and more than 17 000 are killed in Auschwitz.
- *1940–1941*: 70 000 German psychiatric patients are diagnosed incurable by a team of psychiatrists. They are gassed by killer teams headed by psychiatrists. Psychiatrists try to frame a law legalizing these murders.[2,5]
- *1941–1945*: About 80 per cent of the surviving German psychiatric patients die from hunger, infections, or mistreatment in the psychiatric institutions.[2,5]
- *1940–1944*: Brain research flourishes through the murder of relevant patients.[2,5]
- *1940–1941*: The Jewish psychiatric patients are killed by gas by the same teams which kill the non-Jewish patients. When this killing by gas ends in Germany the experienced killers move in 1942 to Poland and the USSR to set up the first death-camps for the mass murder of Jews and Gypsies.[6]

There was almost complete professional silence during and after the war on these acts. General knowledge of these crimes was almost completely repressed in West Germany until the beginning of the eighties. The silence of the national and international psychiatric community allowed many perpetrators to continue psychiatric practice after the war. It is of some interest that the only existing—excellent—book published in the US on the psychiatric crimes committed in Germany was written by a former mental patient.[7] The otherwise most interesting book by Lifton[8] does not deal with academic psychiatry. It concentrates on the other medical mass murderers. An argument against the discussion of these crimes may have been that, had they actually occurred, they were specifically German, and therefore not of interest to the rest of the psychiatric community. Most recently this attitude has been questioned.[9] I will show here that some of the facts and ideas underlying these maimings and murders are still around and therefore interesting. They are:

- Many genetic diseases can be diagnosed, but often no therapy is in sight.[10]
- When an often dubious cost-benefit calculation appears to be advantageous for the community (nation), it is easily called ethical.
- The medical doctor has an obligation to the patient *and* to the community (nation). His obligation to the community (nation) sometimes (often) overrides his obligations to the patient.
- It is the duty of the medical doctor to give the best possible care for those who will eventually recuperate. Those who will never get better may be neglected, particularly when resources are (severely) limited.[11]

The social universe in which the Nazi crimes happened was constructed in such a way that the psychiatrist, like everybody else, had to follow general commands. If he accepted, he was free to choose between various evils at his own risk. For one patient saved there were always others to be destroyed. If he refused he was not endangered; others did the work. It is not astonishing that almost the whole profession chose to forget these traumatic experiences; and it may also be no accident that the writer of these pages is neither a medical historian nor a psychiatrist.

## Sterilizations against the will of patients[1,3]

The rediscovery of Mendel's laws in 1900 reinforced the notion that human pathological abnormalities might be inherited. In the realm of psychiatry, feeble-mindedness, schizophrenia, manic depression, and epilepsy were soon suspected to belong to the class of inherited diseases. Demographers spread the fear that afflicted persons had more children than sane, normal people. Thereupon many psychiatrists and anthropologists assumed that Western civilization was in danger if this process of spreading 'bad' genes was not stopped. Laws introduced in many countries allowing sterilization of such persons led nowhere to the desired mass sterilizations. In spite of the existence of various laws the number of persons sterilized remained rather small in the US.[12] The situation was similar in various European countries. In Germany for instance such a law was discussed in 1932 in the Weimar Republic. It allowed voluntary sterilization of a carefully specified group (schizophrenics, manic depressives, the feeble-minded, epileptics, and carriers of Huntington's chorea). A revised law was introduced after the Nazis gained power. Then the requirement for involuntary sterilization was to be pronounced by a court consisting of two medical doctors and one judge. The commentary to the law was written by a team consisting of the leading Munich psychiatrist Professor Rüdin and a medical and a legal official of the Ministry of the Interior.[13] University psychiatrists were not particularly eager to do the required reporting of their patients to the authorities. They feared, correctly, that they would lose patients who might be afraid to seek their help. But, by and large, the law was well-received by psychiatrists. Schizophrenia in particular left the psychiatrists the possibility of circumventing the law. After all they made the diagnosis whether a patient was schizophrenic, and thus to be sterilized, or just schizoid, and therefore to be left alone. These sterilizations began in 1934 and ended for practical purposes with the beginning of the Second World War. About 350 000 persons were sterilized (0.5 per cent of the population), and several hundreds died during the operations. It was perfectly clear to the psychiatrists and geneticists who had framed the law (among them Rüdin and Professor Fischer, director of the most prestigious research institute of human genetics (for details see Müller-Hill[2])), that it would affect some persons who did not suffer from a hereditary disease. They argued that the law was primarily for the benefit of the community (nation) and not of the individual patient. It was also perfectly clear to the authors of the law that a recessive disease would only be pushed back if the law were obeyed over several hundred years. Hitler himself wrote that such a law had to be obeyed for six hundred years to show a significant effect.[14] In the general enthusiasm of the first years of the Third Reich psychiatrists thought that everybody, healthy or ill, had to carry this out as a pledge to the unborn generations.

## Sterilization of others against their will[2]

The champions of sterilization, such as Rüdin, were not content with the law. According to their opinion a large group of clients was still missing: all those who did not fit properly into the modern industrialized state: petty criminals, the permanent jobless, beggars, prostitutes, etc. A law to allow the sterilization of this large group (estimated size: one million, or two per cent of the total population of Germany) was constantly redrafted by the Ministry of Interior, but never passed by the Government. It was to have provided essentially that two medical doctors and one high police official would decide about sterilization and transfer into a concentration camp. In anticipation of this law a study of Gypsies was monitored by the National

Institute of Health (*Reichsgesundheitsamt*) under the direction of a psychiatrist (Ritter). All Gypsies were divided into two main groups according to psychological, anthropological, and familial criteria: the real (Aryan) Gypsies (less than ten per cent) and the mixed Gypsies, presumably the descendants of the European criminal underworld. The latter were to be sterilized and—on the order of Himmler—eventually transferred to a concentration camp: Auschwitz. There, most of them (about 17 000) perished from hunger, cold, infection, and finally, gas.[2,4]

## Murder of incurable psychiatric patients by gas[2,5]

During the First World War about half the psychiatric patients held in all German psychiatric institutions died from hunger and infection. To bring order into this random process a university psychiatrist (Hoche) and a high judge and law professor (Binding) proposed, directly after the war, 'mercy killing' for incurable psychiatric patients.[15] It may be recalled that at that time virtually no therapy existed for the major forms of mental illness. Schizophrenia in particular was regarded as an irreversible process toward death. All mental patients were called 'inferior' (*minderwertig*) in textbooks or research articles. Patients in the last stages of this process were professionally called *Ballastexistenzen* ('human ballast') and *Leere Menschenhülsen* ('empty human shells'), in short *Lebensunwertes Leben* ('lives not worth living').[15]

With the beginning of the Second World War the pressure to kill all incurable, chronic psychiatric patients increased drastically. The army needed hospital beds—the psychiatrists did not resist. Legitimized by a one-sentence letter from Hitler, a murder organization was founded. The organization sent one-page questionnaires for all patients to all mental institutions. They had to be filled out for every single patient. They were then sent back to the organization, which passed them on to fifty psychiatrists, among them ten university professors (de Crinis, Heyde, Mauz, Nitsche, Panse, Pohlisch, Reisch, C. Schneider, Villinger, and Zucker). These psychiatrists then checked the questionnaires for a fee of a few *Pfennig* per patient. A cross meant death. The public soon coined the word *Kreuzelschreiber* ('cross-writers') for these, and for all psychiatrists. Babies and children who were supposedly incurably ill from psychiatric disease were dealt with by a special commission of two professors and one doctor, who decided whether they should live.

What started in high secrecy soon became general knowledge. The patients whose fate had been decided were transferred to another asylum, and from there to one of the five regional extermination centres (Brandenburg, Bernburg, Hartheim, Sonnenstein, Hadamar), some of them inside, others outside psychiatric institutions. There patients waited naked to be killed in a room camouflaged as a wash-room. It was the duty of a psychiatrist to open the valve of the cylinder containing carbon monoxide. Everybody knew. Relatives, Protestant and Catholic priests, and bishops protested openly. However, almost all psychiatrists remained silent. Only one professor (Ewald) protested. Nothing happened to him. Nothing happened to the very few psychiatrists who refused to participate in the killing. There were too many applicants for the job.

The absence of a law legitimizing the killing worried some psychiatrists. At least five university professors of psychiatry (de Crinis, Mauz, Kihn, Pohlisch, and C. Schneider), together with *the* leading German (eu)geneticist (Lenz) tried to draft a law. 'The life of a patient, who otherwise would need lifelong care, may be ended by medical measures of which he remains unaware' was the suggestion of Lenz.[2] It was all in vain. The law was never passed.

## The fate of the remaining patients[2,5]

German opinion was against the uncontrolled killing of German psychiatric patients. The war against the Soviet Union demanded a truly united effort; so the killing by gas was stopped in August 1941—the killers were needed to kill Jews in Poland and the Soviet Union. But quiet death—'discreet euthanasia'—continued in the institutions. The food rations of the patients were shortened to the uttermost, and the hospitals remained unheated during winter. In some institutions psychiatrists and nurses helped to speed up the death of their patients by giving them low doses of barbiturates over prolonged periods. The pneumonia which invariably followed was usually terminal, and looked innocent. In other places less discrete killings went on with the injection of various drugs. The exact number of surviving patients is not known. The number of 40 000 survivors has been cited.[16] At the beginning of the war about 280 000 beds had been available in public and private institutions. In Poland and the occupied parts of the USSR almost all psychiatric patients were murdered: by hunger in the institutions, by gas after transportation to Auschwitz, or by shooting on the spot.[17] In Vichy France 40 000 psychiatric patients died from hunger, almost unnoticed by the profession: the death from hunger of a psychiatric patient seemed apparently normal when the official food rations for patients and other civilians were the same.[18] The fact that the other civilians had various means to improve their rations was simply overlooked.

## Patients as a resource for brain research[2,5]

If patients had to die anyhow following the expert opinion of one's colleagues, why not make use of them—alive and dead—for research? Two large research projects about various forms of feeble-mindedness and epilepsy were begun by C. Schneider (Professor at Heidelberg University) and Professor Heinze (director of the Mental Asylum of Goerden/ Brandenburg). The idea was to test the patients exhaustively, psychologically and physiologically, possibly over years, then to have them killed discreetly at one of the killing-centres, and finally to crown the research by studying their brain anatomy. The work did not get far, since, after the Soviet victory at Stalingrad, most of the doctors involved in the project were called into military service. From the correspondence of C. Schneider it becomes quite clear that he was most eager to receive specific permission for the killing of his patients from the experts who had previously evaluated the questionnaires.[2] After getting it, the patients were transferred to a killing-centre and killed. It is less clear how far the work in Goerden/ Brandenburg progressed. In the third case, Professor Hallervorden, subdirector (*Abteilungsleiter*) of the *Kaiser-Wilhelm Institut für Hirnforschung* ('Institute for Brain Research') in Berlin–Buch went in person to one of the killing-centres (the one in the Brandenburg gaol close to the Goerden hospital) to take out the brains of those just killed. The diagnoses of patients were available to him before they were killed. So he was actually sure that they were of relevance to his research. He invited the psychiatrist in charge of the killing-centre to work for a while in his Berlin institute to learn techniques, and he transferred one of his technicians to the killing-centre to speed up the work. After the war C. Schneider committed suicide, Heinze became director of a psychiatric institution for children in West Germany, and Hallervorden remained the honoured sub-director of his institute.

## Expansion of the killing of psychiatric patients to the murder of the Jews[6,19]

The killing by gas of German psychiatric patients was stopped in August 1941. At that time the *Einsatztruppen* of the SS had already begun to murder the Jews of the USSR. It may be added here as a symbolic fact that about half the leaders of these murder squads had doctoral degrees, mostly in law. It was soon realized that individual killing was inefficient, and, at least for some of the killers, a great strain. So the experienced killers of the 'euthanasia programme' were asked to set up the first killing-centre, where the Jews would be killed with the same technology (carbon monoxide) which was found to be so effective in the killing of the psychiatric patients. Thus the staff of Belzec, Sobibor, and Treblinka consisted of the old experienced killers; the first commander of Treblinka was indeed a psychiatrist. The white coats, signifying the presence of medical doctors, played a significant part in deceiving the arriving Jews. A place where one is received by medical doctors cannot be all bad. But obviously no further psychiatric knowledge was required to murder the Jews *en masse*. In fact the psychiatrist who headed Treblinka (Eberl) was replaced when it became clear that he was unable to organize the effective disposal of the corpses of those murdered. In Auschwitz, which far surpassed all the other killing-facilities, again only medical doctors (but not just psychiatrists) had the right to select and to supervise killing with gas. Again, no particular medical knowledge was needed to single out children and the aged: anyone else could have replaced them. It was a symbolic fact that medical doctors had obtained this right.

## 'Normal' psychiatry[2,20,21]

It would be erroneous to see the above-mentioned psychiatrists, for example Heinze or C. Schneider, just as killers pure and simple, or as persons who simply consented to the deaths of all their patients. Many of those doctors active in the killing programme strongly advocated the best possible care for new patients after all the chronic patients had disappeared. In 1941 or 1942 C. Schneider presumably wrote the bulk of a memorandum,[2] co-authored by de Crinis, Heinze, Nitsche, and Rüdin, which today reads as most progressive, with just one tiny exception: a little sentence mentioning 'discreet euthanasia' in hopeless chronic cases. In fact, German psychiatrists were seriously worried that they would lose the respect of the public and medical students altogether because of the ongoing killings. Thus the proposals for intensive individual care for every new patient, including work and shock-therapy, sound perfect. Yet serious doubts remain in the mind of the non-psychiatric[2,5] and psychiatric[20] observer. It seems to me that the two compartments of 'psychiatric science' and 'crime' cannot coexist in one person without a slow merger. The easy coexistence of both in one person, moreover, signals that something was deeply wrong in the former.

I can summarize my doubts by observing that psychiatrists then, as often today, viewed the 'delusions' of their patients in a context-free manner. Let me begin with the most extreme case: it is reported that quite a number of the *Einsatztruppen* murderers had severe mental breakdowns, which required psychiatric and/or psychotherapeutic help. And true enough such help was given. The anxieties of the mass murderers were dealt with in a context-free way. Apparently, therapy worked sufficiently well in many cases to send them back with fresh energy and spirit to their murderous business.[8]

A case in which therapy failed is described in detail in a dissertation of a student of Professor de Crinis from Berlin University on the typical 'end-of-the-world syndrome' (*Weltuntergangssyndrome*) of acute schizophrenia.[22]

An acute attack of schizophrenia supposedly leads patients to believe that they experience the falling apart and end of the world. In the thesis three such patients are described. The first, a young SS-soldier, had a nervous breakdown in Poland. We do not hear about the crucial event. He is quoted as saying to the psychiatrist 'The war is wrong ... it will be a war where everybody shoots everybody. Nobody will survive it.' Shock-therapy does not seem to have helped him. When the SS took him out of the hospital (presumably to shoot him) he was regarded as uncured.

The two other cases described in the dissertation are interesting too. One is a young Catholic girl. 'She believed [in 1941: BMH] that the end of the Jews was coming ... In the night she saw the letter J [the sign all Jews had to wear: BMH] glowing on the wall. She felt physically and spiritually dead. She had always wanted to help the people, and she suddenly realized that she was bad like the others.' We do not know what happened to this sensitive girl. The other patient was a young half-Jew, a decorated army officer, who had to quit the army after the Jewishness of his father was discovered. On 2 January 1942 he tells his non-Jewish mother 'Gangs of murderers are around to kill all peaceful people, the streets swim in blood. It is my duty to fight the murderers, who may come at any moment.' Shock-therapy calmed both down. We do not learn whether the young man was eventually deported to Theresienstadt or Auschwitz. All three cases show people revolted and distressed by the persecution of the Jews. Psychiatrists tried to cure them of their 'schizophrenic', humanitarian delusion. There is no hint in the literature after 1945 that psychiatrists undertook treatment in order to save these and similar patients from political persecution. They saw them as truly medical cases.

The psychiatrists who served in the army had a similar general problem. What was to be done with soldiers who had breakdowns? In the First World War many psychiatrists readily attested to soldiers' nervous breakdowns at the front. Thus soldiers who deserted could get away with it. The German army hospitals were full of such deserters, who spread anti-war propaganda. This resulted finally in 1918 in a general uprising, and the breakdown of the front. As a consequence the Kaiser had to flee, and democracy was installed. This time—1942—the German army psychiatrists decided collectively not to accord any more such diagnoses. Whoever suffered a nervous breakdown would in fact be treated as a coward. At best he would be treated with electricity, in the manner made popular by the Nobel prize-winner, Wagner-Jauregg.[23] Few soldiers resisted this torture, and this time no mutinies were recorded in the German army until the end of the war.

This attitude of looking at psychiatric phenotypes without reference to their context did not change with the end of the Second World War. Professor Bürger-Prinz, for example, describes the rare and curious case of a high Nazi government official who experienced extreme guilt feelings after the war. Electroshock eventually delivered the man from his 'pathological conscience'.[24] In general, psychiatrists very rarely honoured the legal complaints of former patients who were sterilized or who had suffered in other ways.[25] Sterilization after all had been legal, and every decision had been covered by the law. At Cologne University the medical faculty voted in 1946 that the law allowing sterilization should be upheld without any changes. Most of those psychiatrists involved in the murder of patients got off free, and continued practising. Most of them could produce patients they had saved, and even those who had killed all their patients were believed when they said that they actually thought it to be a good therapeutic act to free those poor creatures from their suffering.[21] When expert reports had to be written about patients who claimed to have reacted with depression or schizophrenia to the treatment they had received in the concentration camps the general German expert opinion was, for a long time, that such claims were phoney.[25] According to this view, mental disease develops via genetics, irrespective of particular circumstances. The psychiatrists were safe. Until recently all diagnosis could be withheld from the psychiatric patient. I may mention in this context a dissertation on electroshock from the respected institute of Kurt Schneider, which lists the disastrously high incidence of broken bones during the treatment. It summarizes for the psychiatrist: 'Never tell a depressed patient that he suffered such a complication, it might keep him in the depressed mood.'[26]

One aspect which may have been particularly Germanic has only been touched on briefly: language. The German psychiatrists were adept in coining and accepting degrading terms for their patients. For example, it was common to call schizophrenic patients 'inferior' (*minderwertig*). The German word is much stronger than its English counterpart. The imagination of German psychiatrists was extremely productive in creating other demeaning words, for example *Ballastexistenzen* ('human ballast'), *leere Menschenhülsen* ('empty human shells'), and *lebensunwertes Leben* ('lives not worth living), which were immediately understood; these terms almost demanded of society that it had to get rid of people who had been labelled in such a way.

## What can be learned from the events of this period in German psychiatry

This sudden descent from the former high level of psychiatry to the lowest possible depths presents us with the question of what went wrong and what can be learned. I will try to summarize my conclusions here, while conceding that other observers may arrive at different ones:

1. The abandonment of the individual patient in favour of the group (community, nation) should always be resisted.

2. The wishes of the patient should always be respected.

3. The (poetic, metaphorical) description of reality which the patient gives should be understood and accepted.

4. If a patient claims that the psychiatric treatment offered him is inadequate or undesirable this view should be honoured, and new alternative options should be explored.

5. Psychiatrists should question their terminology: it creates reality.

6. Psychiatrists should question themselves as to why they did not want to face the truth about the crimes of their colleagues in Germany during the following half-century. A profession which obliterates its past is not to be trusted.

## Worries of a geneticist

The Nazis were successful because they could rely on the widespread feeling that differences in the genes (the blood, they said metaphorically) were unchangeable. Now we all know how shaky the evidence was for these supposedly genetic differences. It relied on poor phenotypical analysis and poor statistics for small pedigrees. The term pseudoscience may apply to these types of analysis. The notion of DNA as the basis of heredity, and the advent of techniques like hybridization, DNA sequencing, and PCR-reaction have changed human genetics radically. Sooner or later this change will hit psychiatry.

At the moment the claims for DNA-linkage of affective disorders[27] and schizophrenia[28] are uncertain. In fact the evidence for linkage in manic depression mysteriously disappeared when this article went into press.[29] But I am confident that this will change in the first half of the next century. I predict that frequent dominant alleles will be found which make their carriers unable to bear the hardships of modern industrialized life. Some of the carriers of these alleles will show a phenotype resembling schizophrenia and other psychiatric conditions.

This raises serious questions. On the one hand psychiatrists (and employers and insurance companies) will be happy that predictive diagnosis will then be much safer, when DNA evidence is being used. On the other hand the patient will see the diagnosis as a condemnation. He will feel that his essence, his genotype, is robbed and exploited. I have discussed this problem with several people involved in the Human Genome Project, and am astonished at their *laissez faire* attitude. They seriously believe that it is not their business to declare that the patient and nobody but the patient should have the right to know his phenotype, and that before he agrees not even his psychiatrist should be allowed to determine his relevant genotype; and that no employer or insurance company has *even the right to ask him* about his relevant genotype. The disasters of the future may differ sufficiently from those of the past to escape attention now while they can still be averted. It would be very bad indeed if scientists eventually lost the trust of the public simply by being unaware of the human and civil rights of their patients.

# References

1 Musto, D.: A historical perspective, in *Psychiatric ethics*, ed. S. Bloch and P. Chodoff. Oxford, Oxford University Press, 1981, pp. 13–30.

2 Müller-Hill, B.: *Murderous science. Elimination by scientific selection of Jews, Gypsies, and others in Germany 1933–1945.* Oxford, Oxford University Press, 1988.

3 Proctor, R. N.: *Racial hygiene medicine under the Nazis.* Cambridge Mass., Harvard University Press, 1988.

4 Kenrik, D. and Puxon, G.: *The destiny of Europe's Gypsies.* Heinemann, London, 1972.

5 Klee, E.: *'Euthanasie' im NS-Staat. Die 'Vernichtung lebensunwerten Lebens'.* Hamburg, S. Fischer, 1983.

6 Friedländer, H.: Jüdische Anstaltspatienten im NS-Deutschland, in *Aktion T4 1939–1945. Die 'Euthanasie-' Zentrale in der Tiergartenstrasse 4*, ed. G. Aly. Berlin, Edition Hentrich, 1988.

7 Lapon, L.: *Mass murderers in white coats. Psychiatric genocide in Nazi Germany and the United States.* PO Box 80071, Springfield, Il, Psychiatric Genocide Research Institute, 1986.

8 Lifton, R. J.: *The Nazi doctors. Medical killing and the psychology of genocide.* New York, Basic Books, 1986.

9 Breggin, P. R.: How and why psychiatry became a death machine. Unpublished manuscript, presented at the Cologne Autumn Meeting, 1988, on 'Medical science without compassion: past and present'.

10 Vogel, F. and Motulsky, A. G.: *Human genetics. Problems and approaches.* Berlin, Springer-Verlag, 1986.

11 Anonymous: It's over, Debbie. *Journal of the American Medical Association* **259**:272, 1988.

12 Kevles, D. L.: *In the name of eugenics. Genetics and the uses of human heredity.* New York, Knopf, 1985.

13 Gütt, A., Rüdin, E., and Ruttke, F.: *Gesetz zur Verhütung erbkranken Nachwuchses vom 14. Juli 1933 mit Auszug aus dem Gesetz gegen gefährliche Gewohnheitsverbrecher und über Massregeln der Sicherung und Besserung vom 24. Nov. 1933.* Munich, Lehmanns Verlag, 1934.

14 Hitler, A.: *Mein Kampf.* Munich, Franz Eher, 1930, p. 448.

15 Binding, K. and Hoche, A.: *Die Freigabe lebensunwerten Lebens, ihr Mass und ihre Form.* F. Meiner, Leipzig, 1920.

16 Wertham, F.: *A sign for Cain.* Macmillan, New York, 1969, p. 155.

17 Szarejko, P., Wasilewski, B., and Glinski, J.: Die Vernichtung der psychiatrischen Kranken in Polen während der deutschen Okkupation. Die Methoden der Durchführung der Vernichtung und die Versuche ihrer Geheimhaltung. Unpublished manuscript for the international symposium 'Das Schicksal der Medizin unter dem deutschen Faschismus', Erfurt/Weimar,, 1988.

18 Lafont, M.: *L'extermination douce. La mort de 40 000 malades mentaux dans les hôpitaux psychiatriques en France sous le régime de Vichy.* Ligne, France, editions de l'AREFPPI, 1987.
19 Hilberg, R.: *The destruction of the European Jews.* Chicago, Quadrangle, 1967.
20 Dörner, K.: *Tödliches Mitleid. Zur Frage der Unerträglichkeit des Lebens oder: die Soziale Frage: Entstehung, Medizinierung, NS-Endlösung heute, morgen.* Gütersloh, Verlag Jakob van Hoddis, 1988.
21 Klee, E.: *Was sie taten—was sie wurden. Ärzte, Juristen und andere Beteiligte am Kranken-oder Judenmord.* Frankfurt, Fischer, 1986.
22 Metzig, E.: *Das Weltuntergangserlebnis als Initialsymptom der Schizophrenie.* Medical Dissertation, Berlin, 1944.
23 Eissler, K. R.: *Freud und Wagner-Jauregg vor der Kommission zur Erhebung militärischer Pflichtverletzungen.* Vienna, Löcker, 1979.
24 Büger-Prinz, H.: *Ein Psychiater berichtet.* Hamburg, Hoffmann u. Campe, 1971.
25 Pross, C.: *Wiedergutmachung: Oder der Kleinkrieg gegen die Opfer.* Frankfurt-on-Main, Athenäum Verlag, 1988.
26 Gerhart, A.: *Über die Häufigkeit chirurgischer Komplikationen beim Elektro-Krampf-Verfahren.* Medical Dissertation, Heidelberg, 1946.
27 Egeland, J. A., Gerhards, D. G., Pauls, D. L., *et al.*: Bipolar affective disorders linked to DNA markers on chromosome 11. *Nature* 325:783–7, 1987.
28 Sherrington, R., Brynjolfsson, I., Petursson, H., *et al.*: Localization of a susceptibility locus for schizophrenia on chromosome 5. *Nature* 336:164–7, 1988.
29 Kelsoe, J. R., Ginns, E. I., Egeland, J. A., *et al.*: Re-evaluation of the linkage relationship between chromosome 11p loci and the gene for bipolar affective disorder in the Old Order Amish. *Nature* 342:238–43, 1989.

# 23

# Ethical issues in the delivery of mental health services: abuses in Japan

*Timothy Harding*

The examination of ethical issues in psychiatry must start with an analysis of the relationship between the psychiatrist and the individual patient. However, ethical issues arising in the macro-environment of mental health service-delivery cannot be regarded simply as a multiplication of individual ethical issues. Large institutions, resource-allocation, government policy, legislation, professional associations, training, and human resources are crucial elements encountered in the psychiatric macro-environment. The purpose of this chapter is to show that in interacting with these elements the mental health professional faces ethical choices, just as in relating with individual patients. Failure to analyse these ethical issues or to respect basic ethical principles in the macro-environment can lead to abuses and suffering on a large scale.

An underlying theme in this chapter is the relationship which exists between the State and the psychiatrist. This is part of a larger question of the individual's ethical duties in relation to the State. What should a psychiatrist do when confronted with bad laws and inadequate services which cause suffering to his patients? This dilemma was addressed, but not resolved, in the *Nuremberg Declaration*.[1] There is, indeed, an inherent conflict between the interests of the State and the interests of an individual patient in any real world. This is not only the opposition between group and individual interests, but a conflict of values between that espoused by psychiatrists in their work—health—and the diverse values which underlie the actions of the State: justice, security, economic growth, etc., and the role of the law.[2] Psychiatrists should beware of utopian models of the role of the State or of definitions of health, which tend to obscure the inherent conflict of interests and values. Failure to recognize and react to such conflicts was a crucial element in the genesis of abuses in mental health service-delivery in Japan.

The doctor–patient relationship is traditionally highly privileged, protected and hermetic; the State intervening in a rather distant and limited manner to regulate certain interventions, such as the prescription of narcotic drugs or interruption of pregnancy, and to require a limited amount of essential information relating to births, deaths, and infectious diseases.

Once the doctor–patient relationship loses its consensual nature, the ethical basis of the relationship changes dramatically, and the relationship can no longer be secluded and exempt from outside regard. Thus, while a hermetic doctor–patient relationship is an essential element in ethical medical practice, hermetic institutions are extremely dangerous. A different set of ethical principles must be applied to the institutional setting, although the doctor–patient relationship should be preserved within the institution. While ethics and law should be clearly distinguished, mental health personnel have a duty to be concerned about the legal rights and protection of their patients, especially in the setting of involuntary hospitalization and treatment. This point is particularly important in the macro-environment of mental health service-delivery.

The system of mental health care in Japan is described, to illustrate how large-scale abuses can arise, how the causes can be analysed, and what remedial action can be undertaken.

## Historical development of mental health care in Japan

The ways of caring for and healing the mentally sick in Japan have diverse historical origins. Traditional Japanese medicine, influenced by Chinese medicine, used herbal remedies, diet, acupuncture, and moxibustion (the localized application of heat) to achieve a balance between the *yin* and *yang* among the body's elements and to relieve fluid congestion. Buddhist temples were often places of healing and asylum for the mentally ill, and the Daiun-ji Temple in Iwakura, Kyoto served a role similar to the village of Gheel in Belgium, with hostels in the local community. The system persisted for eight hundred years before being incorporated into a mental hospital. Some traditional elements still exist in care for the mentally ill: Morita therapy is a refinement of Buddhist meditation techniques, and non-Western approaches are sometimes tried in the early stages of illness.

Following the Meiji restoration in 1868 Western ideas became accepted and respected, and modern Japanese psychiatry was born, strongly influenced by German psychiatry and oriented towards neuropathology. Treatment was largely biologically oriented, and psychiatric teaching and research were concerned mainly with genetics, neuropathology, and physical treatments.

Although psychiatry was established as a medical discipline at the beginning of the twentieth century, there were relatively few psychiatric hospital beds before the end of the Second World War. Most mental patients were kept in seclusion by their own families, without being seen by psychiatric specialists. Physical restraints were often used and accepted by society, and police supervision was sometimes required for such domiciliary forms of confinement.

Following the Second World War, the predominant external influence was from the United States of America. Psychiatric teaching was influenced by many of the currents in US psychiatry, but most academic chairs were still held by conservative, biologically oriented psychiatrists. The ideological tensions between younger and older psychiatrists grew steadily in the post-war years, to culminate in open conflict at the annual meeting of the Japanese Society of Psychiatry and Neurology in 1969. The younger psychiatrists pressed for an eclectic approach to psychiatric treatments, and for more academic freedom within University departments. For many years, these conflicts caused turmoil in University Departments of Psychiatry, and paralysed both teaching and services. As a result, Japanese academic psychiatry had no significant influence on service development, and the general level of postgraduate training is still mediocre. There is no official certification or registration of psychiatrists.

The economic and social changes in post-war Japan meant that home care of the mentally ill became more difficult. Family units were smaller and more mobile, and a greater proportion of women worked. Housing shortages were severe in all urban areas. The development of institutional care became an increasingly felt need. Successive Liberal party governments were opposed to developing public medicine, and therefore the main growth was in the private sector. Service-delivery thus developed in an environment in which economic factors predominated, neither government health authorities nor academic psychiatry having much influence.

Central government has played a very limited role in the mental health field. Some government activity is devolved to the next governmental tier: the prefectures. Most prefectures have established a public mental hospital, and prefectural authorities are meant to supervise staffing levels and conditions in both public and private hospitals. In most prefectures, the supervision has been perfunctory, and widespread non-observance of required staffing ratios has been reported.

This was the background to the period of growth of the private mental hospitals which was to lead to large-scale abuses: a lack of professional leadership and standard-setting; a liberal, *laissez faire* government policy; and a strong degree of stigmatization and rejection of the mentally ill. This last factor was to be reinforced in 1964, when a psychiatric patient attempted to assassinate the US ambassador in Japan, provoking a feeling of national shame and increasing negative attitudes to the mentally ill.

## The growth of private mental hospitals

Two laws laid the foundation for the rapid growth of the private sector.

The *Medical Service Law* of 1948[3] allowed any registered medical practitioner to establish a private clinic. A public finance corporation provided subsidies and low-interest loans to encourage private investment. The governmental support was based on the number of beds established, with little or no control of the quality of care, virtually no incentives for the creation of community and out-patient services, and no encouragement for the integration of psychiatric care into general hospitals or community public health services. The result of this policy was to provoke sustained growth of the private sector. The number of patients in psychiatric hospitals rose from 3/10 000 population in 1953 to 28/10 000 in 1983.[4] In nearly every other industrialized country there was a steady decrease over the same period. The proportion of psychiatric beds in private hospitals rose over the same period: in fact 96 per cent of the increase in beds over the period 1970 to 1986 was accounted for by growth in the private sector. The geographical distribution of beds in different prefectures is very uneven, and over 80 per cent of private mental hospitals are located in rural areas. Economic factors are responsible, since land prices are much lower in these rural areas. As a result many patients are hospitalized at great distances from their homes. Visits are infrequent, and contacts with families difficult to sustain.

The *Mental Health Act* of 1950[5] provided for three forms of admission, none of which was voluntary. The most widely used form, which in 1985 accounted for over 80 per cent of hospitalizations, is misleadingly known as 'consent' admission (article 33). It is in fact closely modelled on the *placement volontaire* of the 1838 French *Mental Health Law*, by which a family member requests admission, which is accepted by the hospital director.[6] There was no outside control of the admission criteria, and no possibility of appeal by the patient. The defenders of this system described it as a benevolent form of paternalism, respecting the needs, wishes, and autonomy of the family, and preventing unnecessary outside interference. Otherwise, about 15 per cent of patients were admitted by order of the prefectural governor (article 29), and a small number under provisional compulsory admission (article 34), which allowed for temporary hospitalization for observation.

A revision of the *Mental Health Act* in 1965 was meant to encourage community care. Mental Health Centres were established in each prefecture, and more financial incentives were given to out-patient care. The result was a steep rise in out-patient attendances (an 86 per cent increase between 1972 and 1982). However, over the same period the number of in-patients rose by 23 per cent. It seems clear that the policy created a new class of patients consulting for less serious disorders, while those with chronic psychotic disorders remained in hospital.

The *Mental Health Act* prior to 1988 offered no effective protection to individual patients and minimal inspection to ensure standards of care. The *Medical Service Law* of 1948 provided for a minimum level of one physician (not necessarily a psychiatrist) per 48 beds, and one nurse for 6 beds, in psychiatric hospitals. These ratios of staff to patients are three times lower than for non-psychiatric hospitals. There are no legal norms for the numbers of occupational therapists and social workers, and they are extremely few in numbers (0.1 and 0.3 per 100 beds respectively). Overall a comparison between staff for all kinds of mental health facilities in Japan and Scotland has shown that, whereas there were about one and a half times the number of physicians in Scotland, there were three times as many nurses, four times as many social workers, and nearly fifty times as many occupational therapists.[7]

The lack of legal protections, the understaffing, and the insufficient rehabilitation services encouraged custodial care and lengthy admissions. According to figures provided by the Association of Psychiatric Hospitals, based on a survey covering 80 per cent of all private hospitals, most patients (64 per cent) are kept in wards locked 24 hours a day, and only 25 per cent were nursed on wards which were not locked more than 5 hours a day (so-called 'open wards'). In fact one-fifth of private mental hospitals had *no* open wards. Data on the length of stay of all discharged patients and the duration of stay of all hospitalized patients indicate clearly that patients remain for unusually long periods in Japanese hospitals, and that there is no trend to shorter admissions, as in other countries. In 1983 over half the in-patients had been hospitalized for more than five years. The turnover of patients is low, since such a high proportion of beds is occupied by long-stay patients.[4] Thus in Japan there are approximately 0.7 admissions per annum for every psychiatric bed, whereas in European countries the figure is in general three or four times higher (2.9 for England and Wales; 2.5 for the Federal Republic of Germany; 2.0 for Ireland; 5.5 for Sweden).[8] Short-term admissions of up to one month, accompanied by mobilization of community resources and followed by day care or intensive out-patient care, are rarely used in Japan, whereas in European countries they are regarded as an important part of mental health care.

These data are presented to demonstrate that custodial mental health care, unintegrated with general health services, and lacking in community-based care, became the norm in Japan, and was widely accepted until 1984. The Japanese Association of Psychiatric Hospitals defends the interests of 90 per cent of private-hospital managers. The Association lobbies for maintaining government subsidies, and warns against changing the system by referring to the homelessness among the mentally ill in the United States following deinstitutionalization. In fact, in the mental health sector only 12 per cent of the budget is devoted to out-patient care, whereas almost 50 per cent of the total health budget is spent on out-patient care.

It was this sytem of financing and service-development which created conditions conducive to inappropriate forms of care and serious human-rights violations. Neither the health authorities nor the courts intervened to any significant degree. The former have adopted an essentially passive role in developing mental health services. Decisions are taken by individuals and corporations which own hospitals, and there is no centrally organized system of standard-setting, quality-control, or inspection. The courts had virtually no basis for action under the *Mental Health Law* before 1988, and the potential application of the Japanese *Habeas Corpus Act* was severely limited in regard to hospitalized psychiatric patients by a Supreme Court decision in 1971. In a 12-year period only five appeals were brought to court. Article 9, paragraph 4 of the United Nations Covenant on Civil and Political Rights, of which Japan is a State party, guarantees the right of persons deprived of liberty to take proceedings without delay before a court to decide on the lawfulness of their detention. Clearly, this provision was completely denied to hundreds of thousands of Japanese psychiatric patients until 1988.

## Bringing abuses to light

### Early reactions

The structural weaknesses of Japan's mental health services were outlined as early as 1953 by Blain and Lemkau, two public-health-oriented psychiatrists, who carried out a consultancy at the request of the health authorities.

In 1968 the Ministry of Health requested the assistance of the World Health Organization in reviewing mental health services. Dr D. H. Clark undertook the consultancy, and made a thorough and detailed evaluation through visits to hospitals, discussions with interested parties, and analysis of statistical information. In what has come to be known as the *Clark Report*[9] he showed the trend towards increasing use of hospitalization and custodial care. He expressed 'alarm' about the situation, and called for legal reforms, the development of community services, and improved training for psychiatrists, nurses, and other mental health personnel. Since 1968 the *Clark Report* has been cited as the basis for government policy on service-development. A systematic check of government action against Dr Clark's recommendations shows that no significant implementation has taken place. The report is however of great importance for two reasons: firstly, the most pessimistic projections in Dr Clark's analysis of trends have been fully confirmed; and secondly, the existence of the report means that the health authorities and the psychiatric profession were fully aware of the risks being taken in pursuing the policy of private hospital development with insufficient mental health personnel and inadequate community services. A number of Japanese authorities also drew attention to these structural weaknesses in subsequent years.[10–12]

## The Utsunomiya scandal

Professional and public opinion was, however, not widely alerted to the existence of abuses until 1984, when two patients in the Hotukai Hospital, Utsunomiya City, died of maltreatment. Investigations revealed horrendous conditions in the hospital, and a large number of suspect deaths over the previous three years. Financial irregularities were also uncovered, in particular reimbursement of nursing fees from the prefectural government based on false information about the number of nurses employed. Dr Ishikawa, the medical director of the hospital, was tried on a number of charges, and sentenced to a year's imprisonment and a 300 000 yen fine. In his judgement, the judge of the Tokyo district court stated 'Ishikawa has considered profits first and foremost in the management of the hospital and ignored the fundamental human rights of patients.' The prefectural health authorities carried out psychiatric examinations of the patients hospitalized at the Utsonomiya hospital under article 33 ('consent' admission), which revealed that two-fifths of the patients did not require treatment in hospital.

Public opinion was aroused. Questions were asked in the Diet. International concern was expressed through a letter from the International Commission of Jurists to the Japanese Prime Minister in May 1984, and through criticism at the 1984 session of the UN Sub-Commission on the Prevention of Discrimination and Protection of Minorities. The representative of the Japanese government replied that 'although a few cases of ill-treatment in mental hospitals have been reported in Japan, these cases are extremely exceptional . . .'.

However, it soon became apparent that the Utsonomiya scandal was symptomatic of widespread *malaise* in mental hospitals. A medical journal listed seven other hospitals as having unacceptable standards, and the press reported incidents of abuse at further hospitals.

Etsuro Totsuka, a lawyer known for his commitment to human-rights causes, had already in 1983 drawn attention to the high proportion of involuntary patients in Japanese psychiatric hospitals.[13] He and Dr I. Hirota, a psychiatrist working at the Tokyo University Department of Psychiatry, started a campaign to investigate the extent of abuses. With a group of activist lawyers and psychiatrists, they founded the Japanese Fund for Mental Health and Human Rights.

## The investigation by the International Commission of Jurists

The active involvement of an international non-governmental organization, the International Commission of Jurists (ICJ), was a striking feature of the reaction to the revelations concerning abuses. The ICJ had been contacted by human-rights activists in Japan. Its first strategy was to suggest to the Japanese government the appointment of an independent committee of enquiry to investigate allegations of abuses and to make appropriate recommendations. When no response was forthcoming the ICJ's Secretary-General decided to take the initiative and to mandate a small group of experts.[14] This was certainly a risky enterprise, since the expert mission could easily be seen as outside interference. Indeed, in the early stage of the mission's first visit, the collaboration of the Ministries of Health and Justice was far from enthusiastic. The strongest official support came from the Ministry of Foreign Affairs, no doubt because of its awareness of Japan's obligations under international human-rights law and its sensitivity to Japan's image in relation to human-rights abuses. The mission was able to meet officials of the three ministries, representatives of Japanese medical, nursing, and psychiatric associations (including the influential Association of Psychiatric Hospitals), patients' groups, and the association of patients' families. The mission also visited a number of psychiatric hospitals. As the work of the mission progressed, it was apparent that many officials and organizations came to see this 'outside interference' as a valuable lever to bring about changes.

The conclusions of this investigative mission[15] were in agreement with the views which were being reached by many Japanese parliamentarians, journalists, and progressive psychiatrists. Abuses in mental hospitals were indeed widespread. Staff, patients' families, and even patients themselves had become anaesthetized to the abuses, and accepted them passively. With a few notable exceptions, conditions in hospitals reflected the custodial and static nature of the care provided. Patients spent most of their time in overcrowded wards with few activities. They often had no personal possessions. Writing materials and stamps were not available. Few patients had access to telephones. Many had no visits, and never received letters. The main component of therapy was medication, principally with neuroleptic drugs.

Behind these conditions were consistent cost-cutting and financial irregularities, stimulated by the need to make profits. Many hospitals did not have the minimum number of staff required. Patients' labour was sometimes exploited.

When the findings of the ICJ mission were submitted confidentially to the government, the existence of widespread abuses was no longer contested, and the intention to introduce a major reform of the Japanese *Mental Health Law* was announced by the Minister of Health. The ICJ mission had in fact recommended the creation of an independent tribunal system at prefectural level, regular review of all cases of involuntary hospitalization, freedom of communication for patients by letter and telephone, and the possibility of legal assistance. The mission also recommended a reform of the system of reimbursement of health costs to encourage the development of community care and rehabilitation services.

The recommendations, however, went much further than suggesting legal and administrative reforms. While the law could provide both concrete and symbolic support to service-development, no significant change could take place without a shift in both professional and public attitudes. It was pointed out that mental health professionals should provide leadership in breaking down the stigma attached to mental illness. The system of 'consent admission' had the opposite effect, since it sanctioned and legitimized families' sense of shame and the need to hide mental illness. The psychiatric establishment collaborated, thereby reinforcing prejudices. Arguments based on cultural relativism are dangerous for the protection of human rights and the promotion of ethical standards. Thus, the 'cultural specificity' of negative attitudes towards the mentally ill and of family responsibilities was often advanced by those defending the Japanese system of hospital care and 'consent admission'. Criticisms were considered as an 'imposition of alien ideas'. Such reactions place a foreign observer in a delicate position. It requires courage and persistence to affirm that certain values and human rights transcend cultural barriers.

## The case of Dr Matsuda

An illustrative individual example is provided by Dr Michiko Matsuda, a young psychiatrist, who realized during the course of her work at a private hospital in Gunma province that she was participating in systematic abuses. For many months she kept detailed notes on conditions prevailing in the hospital. The bed-occupancy rate was maintained at over 100 per cent. The medical director discouraged contacts between patients and their families, and preparing discharges was extremely difficult. Psychopharmacological treatments were extensively used, many patients being treated with more than six different psychotropic drugs at high doses. Entries in the patients' files, however, were strikingly sparse—in a sample of 76 case records in a ward taken over by Dr Matsuda, she found that there was an average of 2.2 notes recorded annually in the patients' records. The patients were housed in unhygienic, overcrowded surroundings, with no organized activities. Seclusion rooms were used for disturbed patients, who could remain in isolation for periods of many months. Unqualified staff were employed as nurses, and there was often no doctor on call at night. Dr Matsuda describes the patients as apathetic and lethargic, and in a poor state of health, many being underweight.

In 1985 Dr Matsuda confronted the medical director, who was also the owner, and put forward a plan for improving care. She also tried to organize the hospital staff in a trade union. She was dismissed within a few weeks. She found it extremely difficult to find new employment as a psychiatrist in any other hospital. Finally, she brought a civil action for wrongful dismissal, and after a long legal battle was awarded substantial damages.

Dr Matsuda realized that her dismissal was inevitable, since her actions had provoked criticisms of the hospital in newspapers and an inspection by the prefectural health authorities, which had ordered a reduction in the number of patients by 20 per cent. She reflects bitterly on the lack of solidarity shown by psychiatric colleagues, and on the distorting effect of economic pressures on a medical director who is also the owner of the hospital. She believes that many psychiatrists find themselves in comparable positions and are afraid to speak out. She expresses the need for a greater degree of sensitivity to ethical issues, and for a forum where young psychiatrists can express their concerns: 'If psychiatry is run as a business, profits come before patients. It took me many years to realize what was wrong.'

## The Osaka case-study

Dr Matsuda provided detailed information from inside one hospital. Her experience shows how individual doctors face painful ethical dilemmas alone and without support. Another insight into the nature of abuses in Japanese hospitals was provided by a small group of psychiatrists working in both the public sector and private hospitals in Osaka prefecture in association with the Osaka Human Rights Centre. They decided to prepare a descriptive account of mental health services in the prefecture in order to understand the structural weaknesses which were responsible for the development of abuses. They submitted this report anonymously to the members of the ICJ mission, who were able to verify much of the data.

Osaka prefecture typifies modern Japanese development. Its 31 cities, with a population of nearly 9 million, have coalesced to form a gigantic metropolitan area of industrial and commercial development. The centre and most densely populated area, with a population of 2.7 million, has no psychiatric hospital and only 390 psychiatric beds attached to general hospitals (1.4 beds/10000 population). Almost all patients dwelling in this area are sent to distant hospitals. In the more outlying areas (Toyono, Mishima, Kita-Kawachi, Naka-Kawachi, and Minami-Kawachi) there are 27 mental hospitals, and the bed/population ratio varies between 19.5 and 28.0 beds/10000 population. There is only one public mental hospital in the prefecture.[16]

A survey of hospitalized patients showed that 82.8 per cent were long-stay patients of over one year; 24.5 per cent were admitted by governor's order (article 29 of the Mental Health Law); and 65.6 per cent by 'consent admission'.

Mental health consultants (mainly psychiatric social workers) have been attached to Public Health Centres. They organize support systems for the mentally disabled in the community. However, this system is under-financed because of lack of funds for public health. At present there is no concrete programme to stem the rise in hospitalization of the mentally ill (the number of beds in the prefecture rose from 4000 in 1953 to 20 000 in 1985).

A series of apparently isolated incidents reported over the years can now be seen as symptomatic of abuses:

- *1968:* The medical director and several nurses at Kurioka hospital committed acts of violence on several patients attempting to abscond. A patient was killed. News of the incident only became known publicly two years later when a patient threw a letter out of a hospital window.
- *1969 and 1979:* Two serious episodes of violence occurred at Yasuda hospital. In 1969 three male nurses killed a patient with baseball bats. A second patient was killed by nurses in 1979.
- *1971:* Patients rioted in Izumigaoko Hospital.
- *1984:* Misappropriation of patients' money and dismissal of a doctor advocating open wards and active rehabilitation at Hichiyama hospital.
- *1985:* A further incident at Izumigaoko Hospital, in which a patient presenting psychomotor excitement was forcibly restrained and gagged; he choked to death.
- *1986:* A case of corruption by the director of Kijama hospital, who bribed welfare staff to send patients to his hospital.

The group of psychiatrists working with the Osaka Human Rights Centre believes that these scandals represent the tip of the iceberg. They point to two factors to support this contention: the low staffing ratio of psychiatric hospitals and the closedness and secrecy which characterizes hospitals. The Ministry of Health operates a ranking system of mental hospitals according to the staff–patient ratios. For first-rank hospitals there are 2.5 patients per nurse; for fifth-rank hospitals there are 6 patients per nurse. In Osaka prefecture 37 per cent of hospitals fall below the minimum level of the fifth rank. It is consistently in these hospitals that scandals occur.

The Osaka Human Rights Centre, with which the group of psychiatrists who made this study are associated, requested that data on the number of beds, the number of open wards, the development of rehabilitation services, and staffing ratios should be made public. The authorities refused this request, assimilating such information to the commercial secrets of private companies.

The members of the ICJ mission were able to visit a limited number of hospitals in the Osaka area. Access was refused to two hospitals. They were able to confirm that serious overcrowding, prolonged use of seclusion rooms, and lack of activities prevailed in certain hospitals, and that lack of staff was a major factor in bad hospital conditions.

*The study of seclusion*

Both Dr Matsuda's observations and the Osaka study concluded that prolonged and abusive use of seclusion is one of the major forms of abuse in Japanese psychiatric hospitals. This impression was confirmed by members of the ICJ mission, who found that isolation in punitive settings was widely regarded as a legitimate and necessary element in psychiatric hospital care. In a number of hospitals, separate blocks of isolation rooms are set aside; the size of the rooms, their amenities, and the system of care used fall far below the UN *Minimum rules for prisoners*. In other hospitals, seclusion rooms are linked to most wards, and some have sophisticated forms of electronic surveillance.

Dr K. Nakayama, former Director of the Japanese Society for Psychiatry and Neurology, and a keen advocate of reform, has recently reported a survey on the management of 'refractory patients' in Japanese hospitals.[17] The sample consists partly of offender patients and partly of civilly committed patients with disturbed behaviour. For both groups the lack of trained nursing staff, extreme overcrowding, and the lack of therapeutic activities enhance disruptive behaviour. Seclusion accompanied by heavy and repeated doses of neuroleptic drugs is seen as the only effective response. Nakayama obtained information on 950 patients whose management caused 'considerable difficulties' to the hospital. Two hundred and fifty of these patients (27 per cent) were kept continuously in seclusion rooms, and 587 continuously in closed wards. Information on the duration of seclusion was available for 207 patients: 133 (64 per cent) had been in solitary confinement for more than a year, and 52 had spent more than six years in more or less continuous seclusion. When these results were presented to the authorities, the Public Hygiene Council immediately established a committee on refractory patients and the use of seclusion in psychiatric hospitals.

## Reform of the Mental Health Law

By 1986 the political will to bring about mental health reform was established. The pressure came from criticism voiced in a sub-commission of the UN Commission on Human Rights, the ICJ report, commentaries in international medical journals, and newspapers within Japan. What was remarkable was the rapidity and efficiency of the consultation process and the parliamentary procedure. An advisory committee was set up by the Public Hygiene Council, which included Professor Ryniche Hirano, a distinguished academic jurist. This committee was extremely energetic in provoking debate, and was able to draw up detailed recommendations to the Ministry of Health for reform early in 1987. It is apparent that the advisory committee was quickly aware of the gravity of problems and abuses, and determined to adopt a pragmatic approach designed to bring about a real change in patients' conditions and prospects. The committee drew heavily on experience in other countries, and on the case-law of the European Court of Human Rights in defining legal protections for patients and promotion of service-development in a realistic manner.

By 1986 senior officials in the Ministry of Health had also become convinced of the need for change, and they actively supported the legislative process. With the committed support of Diet members from both the government and opposition parties, certain objections from the Association of Psychiatric Hospitals were resisted, and the amendment law was accepted by the Diet on 26 September 1987. The new provisions came into force on 1 July 1988.[18]

Under the general provisions of the law, rehabilitation is introduced as a duty for national and local government authorities. There is also an interesting innovation under the heading 'the duties of the people', embracing the idea of tolerance and social acceptance of the mentally ill. These general principles are given a concrete form in the chapter on institutions, where prefectures and local authorities are given the power to establish rehabilitation programmes. These measures should help to shift the emphasis of services from custodial, long-term care towards a mobilization and resocialization of chronic patients. It should be noted, however, that the provisions are enabling rather than mandatory, only the establishment of prefectural mental hospitals being the latter.

Perhaps the single most important change is the introduction of voluntary hospitalization. The text makes it clear that this is the preferred form of entry: the medical superintendent 'shall endeavour to hospitalize [the patient] voluntarily'. There are, as in most jurisdictions, provisions for detaining the voluntary patient who requests discharge. However, such a measure is implicitly regarded as exceptional, since the law states clearly that a voluntary patient who requests his discharge 'shall be discharged'. The exception requires the intervention of an independent psychiatrist ('the designated physician') who has undergone a prescribed course of training. The criterion is the fact of being in need of care and protection rather than dangerousness. This criterion is also used for admissions, at the request of a family member without the informed consent of the patient (formerly known as 'consent admission'). This latter form of admission, now explicitly defined as a form of involuntary admission, will presumably be used less frequently than previously.

The establishment of Psychiatric Review Boards is a key provision in terms of the International Covenant on Civil and Political Rights. The boards have been set up in each prefecture, and will include psychiatrists, jurists, and 'other learned and experienced persons'. The boards have two main functions:

1. To carry out *periodic reviews* of all hospitalized patients on the basis of reports provided by the medical superintendent of every hospital. This review procedure is independent of the patient's or family's initiative. The frequency of review is not defined, but will presumably be laid down in a ministerial regulation. In order to carry out the review the board may interview the medical administrator, the patient, or the family. On the basis of the review the board can recommend discharge of the patient.

2. To consider *requests for discharge or for better treatment* made by the patient or the person liable for his protection (normally a close family member). In this case the board must decide not only whether continued hospitalization is necessary, but also whether current treatment is adequate. The latter implies a form of quality control of hospital therapeutic programmes which could have a stimulating effect on the development of services. Thus, in certain circumstances, the board may consider that a patient is not ready for discharge, but that his condition justifies an intensive rehabilitation programme in order to prepare for a discharge. The board may require access to such a programme in its decision following a patient's request for discharge. This is an imaginative provision, which seems highly relevant in the Japanese context.

In international law, the psychiatric review set up by the new legal provisions would appear to possess the characteristics of a court, for the purpose of article 9, paragraph 4, of the International Covenant of Civil and Political Rights.[19]

Those psychiatrists who reject legalistic approaches to defending patients' interests should reflect on the relevance and importance of these provisions. In practical terms, the boards, of which a majority of the members will be psychiatrists, should be autonomous of local government authorities, and should hear the patient personally. These would appear to be eminently desirable conditions, which can only facilitate high ethical standards in the work of boards.

Japanese psychiatrists are aware of the problems in the care of the chronic mentally ill in other industrialized countries, and have warned against dismantling the present system of institutionalized psychiatric care. The new law appears to strike a balance between those who wish to move rapidly to prevent the abuses associated with custodial care and those who fear a problem of the stigmatization, rejection, and homelessness of the de-institutionalized mentally ill. The Japanese Diet has opted clearly for changes in the mental health care system, with an emphasis on rehabilitation services. Adequate resources will be needed to bring about such change progressively while ensuring effective patient care. The speed and direction of the change will depend to a large extent on the cumulative effect of the multiple decisions to be taken by the Psychiatric Review Boards.

A follow up mission of the ICJ[20] expressed guarded optimism in April 1988, and referred to the improved legal protection of patients as well as to 'increased awareness of the scope and seriousness of the problems on the part of officials, mental health professionals, and parliamentarians and a remarkable mobilization by patients' family groups, lawyers, psychiatrists, and patients themselves'. The mission's report stressed the need for improved training of mental health professionals and for special programmes to mobilize the chronic mental-patient population.[21]

A further legal handicap affecting the mentally ill is the existence of over 400 national, prefectural, and local laws and regulations discriminating against the mentally ill. By 1987, in the climate created by the debate over the proposed amendment of the *Mental Health Law*, it became possible to repeal the law excluding psychiatric patients from public baths. In view of the popularity of such baths in Japan, this was a symbolically significant step. However, psychiatric patients (that is, all people who have been psychiatrically hospitalized in the past) are still restricted in their access to many public places, such as libraries and sporting facilities. They are also prohibited from taking up certain employment. Psychiatric patients also do not benefit from the social welfare provision available to physically handicapped persons. These issues call for sustained public education and advocacy of patients' rights, both of which should be regarded as ethical duties for the psychiatrist confronted with the unjustified discrimination described.

The ICJ mission reports have both stressed the need for increased awareness of ethical principles among Japanese psychiatrists. Indeed, the priority given to training in medical ethics in Japanese medical schools is generally low.

### Analysis of the legal and ethical issues

The case of Japan as described in this chapter is a striking example of large-scale abuses involving hospitalized psychiatric patients over a long period. The origins of the abuse were: (i) inadequate legal protection of patients; (ii) low professional standards, reflecting lack of leadership from professional associations and academic departments; (iii) stigmatization of the mentally ill, reinforced by custodial forms of care; and (iv) economic factors, with profitability of private hospital care directly related to the number of patients entering the system and the length of stay, and inversely related to the cost of the care provided. This form of abuse can be termed 'psychiatric abuse for economic motives'.

This is by no means a unique example of abuses arising in a mental health delivery system. Well-documented examples of individual abuses are to be found in judgments of the European Commission and Court of Human Rights.[22] On the basis of cases heard before the European Commission and Court of Human Rights, the following risk-factors for abuse in psychiatric hospitals have been identified: large hospitals (over 500 patients); a high proportion of patients detained following criminal proceedings;

most frequent duration of hospitalization over three years; infrequent visits by relatives; lack of individual treatment programmes; and insufficient numbers of and inadequately trained staff.

Systematic abuses have also been documented previously. The English mental hospital scandal provoked by the publication of Dr Montagu Lomax's book *The experiences of an asylum doctor*[23] is one historical example. Like Dr Matsuda forty-five years later, Dr Lomax was shocked by his participation in an evil system, and felt impelled to write an exposure. He was personally condemned by the psychiatric establishment. The health authorities chose to deny his allegations, although senior civil servants realized that Lomax's charges were fully justified.[24] Vested interests led to the persistence of an iniquitous system for several further years before a Royal Commission prepared the way for major legal reforms in the English and Welsh *Mental Treatment Act* of 1930. Many of the reforms had been advocated by Lomax ten years previously. The role of 'whistle-blowers', individuals who feel impelled to speak out when they find themselves involved in systematic abuses in which their colleagues acquiesce, deserves more attention. Support for whistle-blowers at both a national and an international level should be regarded as an ethical duty of professional organizations.

Abuses undoubtedly occurred in many US State hospitals in the 1950s and 1960s. The US system was characterized by striking inequalities of care according to social class.[25] The judgements in a series of decisions in the case of *Wyatt*, a patient in the Alabama State Hospital, revealed overcrowding, dehumanized relationships, humiliation, and lack of basic hygiene which manifestly exceeded any reasonable definition of inhuman or degrading treatment.[26]

Jurists would see these abuses as being due to inadequate legal protection. Indeed, this account of the Japanese abuses has stressed the legal context created by the 1950 *Mental Health Act*, the failure to comply with international legal instruments, and the major legal reform enacted in response to revelation of the abuses. Whereas in the Soviet Union abuses occurred because of a fusion of psychiatry with the State, and the willingness of certain psychiatrists to participate actively in the suppression of dissent, the Japanese abuses came about in a very different legal context. The psychiatrist was given unimpeded power. The State failed in its duty to protect the individual. A legal vacuum was created in which abuses developed insidiously in the absence of professional standards and under the pressure of economic motives. This situation can be termed: State abdication in the field of mental health care.

Although the abuses in Japan arose from economic motives, it would obviously be a mistake to imply that private care-provision necessarily leads to abuses. The other examples of abuses in mental health service delivery quoted above all occurred in public systems. Decent care, respectful of individual rights, can be provided in private hospitals; indeed, several such hospitals exist in Japan.

Legal remedies can best be described as necessary but insufficient. Stone[27] describes how the US courts reacted to 'shockingly low standards of care' in hospitals by making it harder for patients to get into hospital. Stromberg and Stone[28] argue that removing psychiatrists' discretionary authority, restricting involuntary commitment to demonstrably dangerous persons, and applying due-process safeguards from the criminal-justice system ('the criminalization of civil commitment') led to a social disaster. Stone[27] further emphasizes the dangers of responding to abuse solely by legal reforms. He maintains that de-institutionalization brought about by legal criteria, and in particular the almost universal application of the dangerousness criterion to civil commitment, is counter-productive and against patients' interests. There is however equally a danger in rejecting legal processes as a way of stimulating social change. Such processes may be particularly significant in Japan, where Upham[29] suggests that '. . . the tripartite élite coalition identifies litigation as a threat to the political and social status quo . . . self-interest has led the Japanese élite to take deliberate steps to discourage litigation'. In the campaign to secure rights for the *barakumin* (former outcast communities in Japanese society, who are still subject to widespread stigmatization and discrimination) the fact that the *burakumin* leaders resort to 'denunciation' (*kyudan*: active campaigning and agitation outside the normal political arena), rather than demanding legal reforms, has allowed the government to keep control of the pace of reform. Legal protection corresponding to international standards are necessary in defining the relationship and the distance between the State, the psychiatrist, and the patient. It is only when this framework is established that ethical issues can be defined and resolved. The recent legal reforms in Japan have followed European models more closely than US legislation, with limited use of normal court systems through the establishment of special review boards. Stone's warnings may therefore be less relevant.

What then are the *ethical* issues to be considered? Cannot these problems be resolved simply by improving standards and providing adequate legal safeguards? The cases of Dr Ishikawa, Dr Matsuda, and many others show that there is indeed a major ethical dilemma for psychiatrists caught up in a system of bad care and institutional abuses.

Ethical issues are particularly acute in the practice of psychiatry, as compared to medicine as a whole, because of the acceptance of involuntary forms of treatment as necessary and legitimate. This creates a potential for abuse which, in turn, calls for a high degree of vigilance and sensitivity to ethical and human-rights issues among psychiatric personnel.

In Japan, as elsewhere, individual psychiatrists are concerned with a limited number of patients. They could remain unaware of ethical issues because their patients are not treated worse than tens of thousands of other patients. Furthermore, the failure of the law to provide any meaningful safeguards for patients reinforced psychiatrists' beliefs that the system was implicitly accepted by society and sanctioned by the State.

Psychiatrists, psychiatric nurses, and other mental health professionals have an ethical duty to reveal all instances of abuses in service-provision which come to their notice. They should be supported by their colleagues; professional leaders and associations have a special responsibility in this respect. Psychiatrists have also an ethical duty to ensure that patients have adequate legal safeguards. This is not in conflict with an attitude of benevolent paternalism. Psychiatrists can believe that involuntary treatment is justified by the imperative need for care; but this in no way precludes the need for outside control. Every psychiatrist knows that abuses can occur in mental health service-delivery systems. The Japanese case shows how this has happened over a long period and on a large scale in a modern industrialized society. Other examples certainly exist. Mental health professionals have an ethical duty to prevent and, if necessary, expose such abuses in the psychiatric macro-environment, and not to limit their concern to their own individual practices.

## References

1 Luban, D.: The legacies of Nuremberg. *Social Research* **54**:779–829, 1987.
2 Gray, J. C.: *Nature and sources of law.* New York, Columbia University Press, 1909.
3 Japan: Law no. 205 of 30 July 1948 (with amendments 1949–62).
4 National data on psychiatric patients hospitalized in Japan are available from surveys conducted on an annual census day and from occasional surveys published by the Ministry of Health; see, for example: Koseisho Tokei Joho Kyoku (1960–1986): *Kanja Chosa (Patient Survey)* (in Japanese) Ministry of Health, Tokyo; and Koseisho (1983): *Seishin Esei Jittai Chosa hokoku no Gaiyo* (in Japanese), Ministry of Health, Tokyo.
5 For an English version of the 1950s law, see *International Digest of Health Legislation*, **3**:340, 1951–2.
6 For an account of the 1838 French law, see *International Digest of Health Legislation*, **39**(2):513–28, 1988.
7 This comparison is based on data gathered by Dr I. Hirota in an unpublished study (1985) and on McCreadine, R. G., Affleck, J. W., and Robinson, A. D.: The Scottish survey of psychiatric rehabilitation and support services. *British Journal of Psychiatry*, **147**:289–94, 1985.
8 Freeman, H. L, Fryers, T., and Henderson, J. H.: *Mental health services in Europe: 10 years on.* Public health in Europe, no. 25. Copenhagen, WHO Regional Office for Europe, 1985.

9 Clark, D. H.: *Assignment report, November 1967–February 1968*. Manila, World Health Organization, Regional Office for the Western Pacific, 1968.

10 Toida, S.: Forced hospitalisation and psychiatrists. *Psychiatria et neurologica Japonica* **76**:816–18, 1974.

11 Nakayama, K.: Psychiatric care delivery patterns and economic policy after World War II in Japan. Paper delivered at the World Psychiatric Regional Symposium, Kyoto, Japan, 1982.

12 Aoyama, H.: Public health, medical treatment and administrative psychiatry. *Seishin-iryo* **11**:4–14, 1983.

13 Totsuka, E., Mitsuishi, T., and Kitamura, Y.: Mental health and human rights: illegal detention in Japan, in *Psychiatry, law and ethics*, ed. A. Carmi, S. Schneider, and A. Hefez. Berlin, Springer-Verlag, 1986.

14 The first of the two missions was co-sponsored by the International Commission of Health Professionals, whose Executive Secretary, Dr C. L. Graves, acted as secretary to the mission.

15 Harding, T. W., Schneider, J., and Visotsky, H. M.: *Human rights and mental patients in Japan*. Geneva, International Commission of Jurists, 1986.

16 Asao, H.: Current situation of mental health services in Osaka prefecture. Paper prepared for the Osaka Human Rights Centre, 1986.

17 Nakayama, K.: *Refractory patients in mental hospitals in Japan* (unpublished text, 1989). Preliminary report of a research group established by the Mental Health Division of the Ministry of Health and led by Dr C. Mitishita.

18 Amendment by law no. 98 of 26 September 1987—summarized in *International Digest of Health Legislation*, **40**:214–17, 1989.

19 United Nations: Human rights: a compilation of international instruments. New York, UNO, 1983.

20 The second ICJ mission visited Japan in April 1988, and was accompanied by Mr Niall MacDermot, Secretary-General of the ICJ.

21 International Commission of Jurists' Mission to Japan, April 1988: *Preliminary report and recommendations*. Geneva, ICJ, 1988.

22 Harding, T. W.: The application of the European Convention of Human Rights in the field of psychiatry. *International Journal of Law and Psychiatry* **12**:245–62, 1989.

23 Lomax, M.: *The experiences of an asylum doctor*. London, Allen and Unwin, 1921.

24 Harding, T. W.: 'Not worth powder and shot': a re-appraisal of Montagu Lomax's contribution to mental health reform. *British Journal of Psychiatry* **156**:180–7, 1990.

25 Hollingshead, A. B. and Redlich, F. C.: *Social class and mental illness*. New York, Wiley, 1958.

26 See for example *Wyatt* v. *Stickney*, **344** F. Supp. 373 (MD Ala 1972).

27 Stone, A.: The social and medical consequences of recent legal reforms of mental health law in the U.S.A.: the criminalization of mental disorder, in M. Roth and R. Bluglass (ed.): *Psychiatry, human rights and the law*. Cambridge, Cambridge University Press, 1985.

28 Stromberg, C. D. and Stone, A.: A model state law on commitment of the mentally ill. *Harvard Journal on Legislation* **20**:275–396, 1983.

29 Upham, F. K.: *Law and social change in postwar Japan*. Cambridge, Mass., Harvard University Press, 1988.

# 24

# The political misuse of psychiatry in the Soviet Union

*Sidney Bloch*

That psychiatry is bedevilled by complex ethical problems is abundantly clear from the mushrooming literature on the subject in recent years, and from the other contributions to this book. The vast majority of psychiatrists strive to practise their profession as ethically as they can, guided chiefly by the principle that they do all in their power to serve the interests and needs of the patient. Unfortunately, these interests and needs are sometimes neglected, or even intentionally ignored. Here, we need to distinguish between poor practice—the inept or inconsiderate actions and attitudes of psychiatrists who, because of inadequate training or poor working conditions or disturbed personal functioning, cause patients to suffer rather than to benefit—and misuse of psychiatric theory and treatment for purposes other than medical.

In this chapter I am concerned with psychiatry's improper use, and then with a quite specific form of misuse: the suppression of political and other forms of dissent through their designation as mental illness. Although there is evidence that such abuse has occurred in a number of countries,[1] the most notable example of it is in the Soviet Union. The Soviet case can also serve to illustrate most pertinently the ethical complexity of the psychiatrist's position wherever he works. I hope this chapter will therefore enable the reader to reflect on how the many thorny issues raised by other contributors to this book are involved in the political abuse of psychiatry as it currently occurs in the Soviet Union.

The features of the abuse, having been described in detail by several observers, are well known (see for example refs. 2–11), and it would serve little purpose to recount them here. My concern rather is with the *underlying causes of the abuse—how is it possible that Soviet psychiatry came to be exploited as a punitive weapon of the state?* To answer this question we need to consider (1) the role of the professional generally, and the psychiatrist specifically, in a totalitarian state; (2) the features of the Soviet system in which, on the one hand, deviance has until the advent of *perestroika* and *glasnost*, been abhorred and suspected, and on the other, conformism has been valued; and (3) the effects of these attitudes on the definition and treatment of psychiatric illness.

Before embarking on a consideration of the underlying causes of Soviet psychiatric abuse, it would be well to sketch out the facts. The abuse can be summarized thus: since the late 1950s a small, but nevertheless significant proportion of dissenters in the Soviet Union were* diagnosed, although mentally well, as suffering from such serious psychiatric conditions as schizophrenia and paranoid personality disorder. As a result of their 'illness', they were detained involuntarily in ordinary or prison psychiatric hospitals for periods ranging from weeks to many years. While in hospital some were given tranquillizing and other drugs for which they had no need; the purpose rather was to use medication as a form of social control. All experienced the trauma of being placed alongside genuinely ill patients, and the fear of not knowing when, and indeed whether, they would ever be released; and some the indignity of being pressed to recant their dissenting views, often held with considerable conviction and over many years, in order to signify their 'recovery' and expedite their release.

Those detained in this way were loosely termed dissenters or dissidents; they shared the characteristic that they had deviated in some way from social norms and conventions laid down, and regarded as obligatory, by the Soviet state. The dissenters fell into five main groups:

1. *Advocates of human rights and democratization*. Through various peaceful and legal means they called on the regime to respect citizens' rights as accorded in the Soviet Constitution and to permit democratic processes to operate.

2. *Nationalists*. Those dissenters who protested about the lack of rights of ethnic groups—for example, the Crimean Tartars, the Ukrainians, the Estonians, the Lithuanians—and appealed for the granting of political and economic autonomy to each of the Soviet Union's 15 national republics, again in accordance with the Constitution.

3. *Would-be emigrants*. Those who applied, or tried physically, to leave the Soviet Union.

4. *Religious believers*. People belonging to a variety of religious groups, who were detained solely because of their religious convictions; they wished to practise their religion freely and to see an end to the state's domination and restriction of the church.

---

* It is problematic at the time of writing determining what tense should be used. Although the abuse is being brought to an end, there is evidence that some 50 cases of psychiatric oppression exist. In March 1989 an authoritative delegation of American psychiatrists to the USSR found firm evidence of abuse in 17 of the 27 cases they examined. Since I will discuss the practice as it occurred from the 1950s to the 1980s, it is more convenient for me to use the past tense (I also do so in the hope that, by the time of publication, the abuse will indeed have terminated).

5. *Citizens inconvenient to the State.* A more amorphous group, comprising those who were inconvenient to Party or State officials because of their obdurate complaints about bureaucratic excesses and abuses.

The repression of representatives of these dissenter groups by 'political psychiatry' was only one of several State strategies—the mental hospital joined the labour camp, the prison, and exile as means of social control and punishment. Why did the authorities resort to psychiatry when the alternatives available were well established and more than adequate? The psychiatric gambit had certain attractive features.

With the dawn of *détente*, during the Krushchev era, the Government sought to portray the Soviet Union as a state which respected the rule of law and where the arbitrariness and excesses of the Stalin period no longer applied. Political trials in which the defendant could proclaim his innocence and highlight the abuses of the legal system had to be avoided. Psychiatry was a convenient ally: by declaring the defendant ill, and therefore not responsible, the trial became a mere formality, with no opportunity for the dissenter—who was deemed too disturbed to attend the proceedings—to defend himself. Once he had been declared not responsible and placed in a mental hospital, the dissenter's release could result—in many cases—only from his recantation, that is, from an admission that his 'dissenting behaviour' was a product of a diseased mind, with his promise not to 'relapse' into such behaviour after his discharge. Along with the indignity and distress of recantation came other unpleasant experiences mentioned earlier: in some respects these were even more tormenting than those suffered in prison or labour camp. One other key advantage of the psychiatric option was the opportunity it provided to the regime to discredit ideas which it regarded as heterodox and dangerous; such 'crazy' ideas were therefore, not worth consideration. The human-rights campaign of figures like a Red Army Major-General (Pyotr Grigorenko)[12] or a Marxist academic (Leonid Plyushch)[13] were especially threatening in so far as they suggested serious 'internal' flaws in the system. Such criticism could not be brooked and had to be quashed as the rantings of the insane. Potential critics could be deterred from expressing their views publicly.

Hitherto I have referred to a system of psychiatric misuse which was inspired and manipulated by the State. In the Soviet context this meant the Communist Party-State. I have not commented on how the psychiatrist fitted into the picture. Clearly the State authorities could not have executed 'political psychiatry' without the collaboration and connivance of the practising psychiatrist. We can now turn to the question posed at the outset: *how was Soviet psychiatry deflected from its customary professional pursuits?* Although the explanation is neither straightforward nor clear-cut,

I would like to offer an analysis based on evidence from several different sources, including the testimony of dissenters who were dealt with psychiatrically; the reports of Soviet psychiatrists who have spoken out against the abuse; the attitudes expressed by the Soviet psychiatric establishment in its defence of the profession against allegations of its unethical character;[14] the voluminous documentation that has reached the West over the past two decades; the observations by social scientists of the dominant role of the State and Party in the supposedly autonomous profession of psychiatry throughout most of the post-Revolutionary period, and the reports of Western psychiatrists who have had the opportunity to inspect Soviet psychiatric institutions (especially important here is the official visit by a United States delegation in February–March 1989).[15]

## The psychiatrist in the Soviet system

The most appropriate first step in our analysis is a consideration of the relationship between the psychiatrist and the Soviet state. In a totalitarian system of government such as that of the Soviet Union, the interlocked State and Party are supreme: every aspect of life is subordinate to them, and no one and nothing escapes their control.* And so it is with a profession like psychiatry. Whether the individual psychiatrist wishes it or not, he is faced with the reality that he is not a member of an independent profession and that his actions are guided by political overlords. This position is to be contrasted with the psychiatric profession in Western states. There, governments, through legislation, also exert some control of psychiatrists' activities. For example, in England the 1983 Mental Health Act governs the way in which psychiatrists can and cannot deprive a person of his liberty, while a statutory body, the General Medical Council, has the power to strip a psychiatrist of his right to practise if he is found to have acted unethically. Similarly, in the United States the professional activities of the psychiatrist must be carried out within a framework of limiting laws. But in both countries these forms of control do not prevent the psychiatrist from practising his profession according to his own clinical and ethical judgements. True, there are other subtle social and political pressures that face the psychiatrist, and against which he needs to be vigilant. However, he is in a much stronger position than his Soviet colleague to fend off the pressures (see Chapter 4).

This is because the Soviet situation has differed in several crucial respects. Probably the most significant has been the *omnipresence of*

---

* Under the leadership of Mikhail Gorbachev since April 1985, and in the context of *perestroika* and *glasnost*, this socio-political pattern is being subjected to radical change. We will address this later in the chapter. For the moment, the analysis that follows remains relevant to contemporary psychiatry in the USSR and its position through the Soviet period.

*political ideology*. This begins in the psychiatrist's professional life whilst he is still a medical student. Political studies—Marxism-Leninism, political economy, dialectical materialism, historical materialism, history of the Communist Party, and scientific atheism are the subjects involved—are an obligatory part of the curriculum.[16] Later, he will be reminded of their relevance by comments like the following, which appeared in *Medical Worker*, the organ of the Ministry of Health: 'In order to be a working representative of the physician's noble profession, it is necessary not only to have an excellent professional education, but also to be well acquainted with the principles of Marxism-Leninism' [p. 33].[17] The medical student, therefore, graduates with two interwoven qualifications—medical and political. The oath he then takes strengthens this medico-political link, since, in addition to the customary patient-directed ethical promises, he also declares, 'That I will in all my actions be *guided by the principles of communist morality*, ever to bear in mind the high calling of the Soviet physician and of *my responsibility to the people and the Soviet State*.'[18] The 'principles of communist morality' are not elaborated upon; but the mere inclusion of such a phrase in the oath, coupled with the statement about the doctor's responsibility to the people and State, introduces a political tone into what should, ideally, be a document exclusively concerned with the care and welfare of patients.

That political studies are included in the medical course and that the physician's oath contains political elements are not surprising in the light of the dominance of ideology in Soviet Union, a dominance which had its roots in Stalin's view of the place of professions in Soviet society. This view is clearly seen in Stalin's attitudes to professional qualifications:

There is one branch of science which Bolsheviks in all branches of science are in duty bound to know, that is the Marxist-Leninist science of society ... a Leninist cannot just be a specialist in his favourite science; he must also be a political and social worker, keenly interested in the destinies of his country, acquainted with the laws of social development, capable of applying these laws, and striving to be an actual participant in the political guidance of the country [p. 74].[16]

Stalin's emphasis on political qualifications has always been associated in the first place with Party membership, with its attendant loyalties, acceptance of Party policy and a preparedness to obey directives. Generally, professionals who have occupied positions of power, such as heads of institutions or senior officials in government bodies, have been Party members. This pattern has held for the medical profession too, and doctors who have been members of the Party have tended to occupy posts of influence and authority in medical institutions and in the Ministry of Health [p. 126].[16] We can assume that in this regard the specialty of psychiatry has been no different from the rest of medicine.

There has been good reason for the concentration of Party members in the top echelons, since their presence there has enabled the regime to monitor the working of the system and to manipulate it. The implementation of Party policy through its 'loyal' membership has been guaranteed; not to comply with directives has been hazardous and has promptly resulted in demotion or worse. It can be readily seen that the psychiatrist in a senior position has been obliged to function as 'double agent': on the one hand he has been duty-bound to the Party, and on the other his allegiance has been supposedly to his patients and psychiatric colleagues (see Chapter 4). Lest the impression be gained that senior psychiatrists have glided into their positions, there is reason to believe that many of them join the Party in the first place for careerist reasons, in order to fulfil personal ambitions. And, even for those whose professional integrity might have been intact at the outset, the need, for career purposes, to subordinate themselves to the political and ideological demands of the regime has led inexorably to its erosion.

This decline in integrity has been well described by Dr Yury Novikov, a young Moscow psychiatrist, who defected to the West in 1977.[19] In a series of illuminating articles, he used his own case to illustrate his 'slide' into potentially unprofessional conduct. He concluded that defection was his only option to avoid becoming corrupt. As a promising forensic psychiatrist on the staff of The Serbsky Institute for Forensic Psychiatry, he became the protégé of its Director, Professor G. Morozov (a central figure in political psychiatry). Novikov was clearly being groomed to become a senior psychiatrist at the Serbsky. This process entailed a role for Novikov in the manipulation of visiting Western psychiatrists in order to convince them that hospitalized dissenters were mentally ill. He also turned a blind eye to the diagnosis of political dissenters as disturbed (which he knew to be occurring, although he was hardly involved himself), so as not to disturb his privileged status.

The structure of the Soviet health service has certainly also contributed to the erosion of a physician's integrity. The Ministry of Health is the sole employer of psychiatrists (apart from the military, and prison psychiatrists, who are under the Ministry of the Interior) and for professional advancement and promotion they are limited to the institutions controlled by the Ministry. Following the 1917 Revolution, the model of local government, the zemstvo—which had existed for fifty years and which had exercised some control over medical services—was entirely revamped and replaced by a tightly directed, pyramidal, central-government model. The newly formed Federal Ministry of Health assumed, and has maintained since, a dominant role in the setting and implementation of all aspects of health policy. Although each of the Soviet Republics has its own Health Ministry, all major decisions emanate from Moscow. The Federal Minister of

Health, therefore, has wielded enormous power. This includes the determination of psychiatric policy, for which the responsible subordinate is the
Chief Psychiatrist.* The latter is an influential figure, since all decisions
regarding the practice of psychiatry have required his approval. Both
officials, in turn, have been advised by the Institute of Psychiatry, a branch
of the prestigious Academy of Medical Sciences. (In 1987 the Institute
became part of the All-Union Research Centre on Mental Health.) The
Director of the Institute has had considerable power, and played a key role
in shaping virtually every facet of psychiatry, including clinical practice,
training, and research (it is noteworthy that the former Director, Andrei
Snezhnevsky; his successor, Marat Vartanyan; and an ex-Chief Psychiatrist, Zoya Serebryakova have all been involved in one way or another in
the psychiatric repression of dissent.)

Concentration of power and influence in the hands of a small group and
the rigid hierarchical system have gone hand-in-glove with the disproportionate number of Communist Party members who have occupied top
positions. By these means control has been efficiently exercised, and any
unorthodoxy among rank-and-file psychiatrists checked. Rank-and-file
psychiatrists as a result have had to submit to official policies, and have had
little freedom to initiate or experiment. No wonder that clinical innovation
in Soviet psychiatry has been slow.

The best illustration of this system of tight control has been the
domination of diagnostic theory by Professor Snezhnevsky and his colleagues. To appreciate his monopoly we need to return to 1950. In that
year a battle was waged at a special joint session of the Academy of
Medical Sciences and the Academy of Sciences between the advocates and
opponents of the thesis that Pavlovian theory was central to psychiatric
practice. Snezhnevsky, at that time a senior academic and Chief of the
Serbsky Institute, successfully led the pro-Pavlov forces. His achievement
was another step in a rapidly developing career which included his
appointment at the relatively young age of twenty-eight as head of a
psychiatric hospital. Ten years later, in 1938, he had become a Deputy
Director of the prestigious Gannushkin Institute. Snezhnevsky, it
appeared, was an ambitious man, talented as a psychiatrist and astute as a
politician. Thus, in the intense ideological turmoil that characterized the
1950 conference, having confirmed his readiness to serve the political
machine, he was the obvious person to promote the 'Party' line. The
conference took place in the context of an extensive purge in science, the
rise of dogma, strong anti-Semitism, and the repudiation of opponents to

---

* It comes as no surprise that Dr Alexander Karpov, the Acting Chief Psychiatrist, took a
prominent part in defending Soviet psychiatry at the World Congress of the World Psychiatric
Association in Athens in October 1989, when the thorny issue of the readmission of the Soviet
Psychiatric Society was under consideration.[20]

Pavlov. Pavlovian ideas were approved as the only right approach, and the entire psychiatric profession was remoulded to fit the new dogma. Anti-Pavlovian psychiatrists were removed from any important jobs they held, and forced into retirement or transferred to lesser assignments.

Snezhnevsky's triumph led to his progressive elevation to supreme power; he was soon appointed to the chair of psychiatry at the Central Post-Graduate Medical Institute in Moscow, and in 1962 reached the acme of his career when he was admitted to full membership of the esteemed Academy of Medical Sciences, a rare honour for a psychiatrist. He also took over the directorship of the Institute of Psychiatry.

In the course of Snezhnevsky's rise to power he fought a second battle, this time over the concept of schizophrenia. This campaign, and Snezhnevsky's ultimate victory, illustrate further the immense power of the Soviet psychiatric establishment and its capacity to curb critics and independently-minded psychiatrists. Soon after the adoption of the Pavlovian doctrine, Snezhnevsky began to promote his theories on schizophrenia. We shall turn to these later. For the moment suffice it to say that his views amounted to a broadening of the concept of schizophrenia sufficient to encompass even relatively minor behavioural change as evidence of the condition. His theories were vehemently rejected by other schools of psychiatry, particularly those based in Leningrad and Kiev. Opposition, however, gradually declined—some critical psychiatrists died, others were demoted—and Snezhnevsky, with official support, and in command of the Institute of Psychiatry and also of the country's only psychiatric journal, gained almost complete control. This control, apart from the odd abortive revolt, remained intact for virtually the next three decades.

It is perhaps facile to suggest that Snezhnevsky was, in effect, a Party *apparatchik*. But the centralization of professional power, the dominance of the Party, and the pervasiveness of ideology all point to the politicization of psychiatry and to Snezhnevsky's career as an example. It would appear that a requisite for advancement is 'political-mindedness', a quality obviously demonstrated by Professor Snezhnevsky.

One might reasonably ponder over the value of waging these battles for professional power. What propelled Snezhnevsky (and his colleagues) to battle over several years for complete power? His motives, undoubtedly complex and manifold, were probably a blend of the following. First, an ideological motive, its strength difficult to assess, may apply: namely, a conviction that the Party is supreme and its interests paramount; the psychiatrist, like any other loyal citizen, recognizes that the Party knows best and that it must be respected. Secondly, careerist ambition—the knowledge early on in a person like Snezhnevsky that, like all other professions in the Soviet Union, psychiatry was hierarchical in nature, with much power wielded from the top, made clear to him the means whereby personal ambition could be satisfied. Thirdly, the rewards that result from loyalty to the Party and adherence to its directives have been substantial and varied. For example, only a minuscule group of Soviet psychiatrists have received permission to attend foreign conferences. Inevitably the same psychiatrists have arrived no matter whether the subject of the meeting has been schizophrenia or psychosomatic disorders or genetics or social psychiatry. One might infer that all expertise in Soviet psychiatry has been limited to a handful of psychiatrists; but it soon becomes obvious that repeated opportunities for international travel have been granted only to the small coteries of 'trusted' psychiatrists who have occupied top administrative or hospital positions, and rarely to anyone else.

The rewards have also been ample at a material level, and have included salaries about three times those of ordinary psychiatrists, access to special stores selling luxury goods at moderate prices, the possibility of owning a country cottage, and the opportunity to holiday at special sanatoria or abroad. The reward system has remained intact so long as the recipient has satisfied the donor by acting with loyalty to the Party and obeying its directives. It is obvious that a psychiatrist who has wished to receive these rewards has been vulnerable to manipulation by his political masters, and that the way has been greased for his entry into the role of double agent: the Party-State on the one hand and the patient on the other.

The problem of multiple allegiance, as discussed by David Mechanic in Chapter 4 on the social context of psychiatric practice affects any psychiatrist. As he puts it: 'When psychiatrists work for organizations other than the patient, their loyalties are split.' And he cites as the most dramatic example of this the psychiatrist who serves as State bureaucrat in a totalitarian society. This as we have seen earlier in this chapter, is precisely the situation that has obtained in the Soviet Union, and that has enabled psychiatry to perform the function of social control at the State's bidding.

How does this pattern link up with the political misuse of psychiatry? Peter Reddaway and I[5] have suggested elsewhere that Soviet psychiatrists can be categorized into three groups *vis-à-vis* their involvement in, and attitudes to, the misuse. The *core* group of psychiatrists has probably been no more than several dozen in number. They have occupied senior hospital or administrative positions, and have participated in the assessment of moderately known or well-known dissenters, or at least consulted in some way about them.

The second group has consisted of *average* psychiatrists—the vast majority of the profession who, after they became aware of the abuse (it only began to become common knowledge in the 1970s) tried to steer clear of any dealings with 'the complicated cases' of political patients. Motivated by fear and a strong need to conform they went along with the system, probably using denial and rationalization to avoid their entrapment in ethical dilemmas. Conformism is a most crucial aspect, as suggested earlier in the chapter. Semyon Gluzman has captured the essence of the average psychiatrist's position well in pointing out that:

Psychiatrists are ordinary people, products of their time and the State in which they live. As a group, they share the 'standard' attitude of their time and place. Soviet psychiatry is the offspring of a totalitarian system. Its representatives are standard citizens who happened to choose medicine as their profession . . . . Living and working within the confines of thought and behaviour allowed by the totalitarian State, psychiatrists, like their fellow citizens, are 'cogs' in the totalitarian machine, which inexorably and harshly punishes unsanctioned deviations from 'standard' behaviour.[21]

The third group has comprised a very small number of *dissenting psychiatrists*, who openly criticized some of their colleagues for perpetrating the non-medical use of psychiatry. Some of them, like Semyon Gluzman and Anatoly Koryagin, were punished severely for their criticism; others—Yury Novikov, Marina Voikhanskaya, Boris Zoubok, Avtandil Papiashvili, Alexander Voloshanovich among them—emigrated to the West and there expressed their condemnation of the Soviet practices. Voloshanovich and Koryagin are particularly interesting members of the dissenting group in that they served, as psychiatric consultants to the Moscow-based Working Commission, a small body, composed of human-rights activists seeking to publicize political psychiatry and bring it to an end. In this consultant capacity, they undertook a remarkable task: to assess and prepare reports on dissenters who had been previously hospitalized and on others who had reason to fear that they might become the victims of psychiatric abuse. Their motive for submitting to psychiatric examination was simple—they hoped that a clean bill of mental health, publicized widely both in the Soviet Union and abroad, might deter the authorities from applying the psychiatric gambit to them (and perhaps to others) in future.

Another form of dissent has appeared among Soviet psychiatrists—the challenge to the Snezhnevsky school, to both its theoretical tenets and its practical implications. An example of this development is the paper by Etely Kazanetz, published in a western psychiatric journal in 1979.[22] Dr Kazanetz, then a psychiatrist at the Serbsky Institute, took issue with Snezhnevsky's diagnostic schema, and argued that it led to an excessive use of schizophrenia as a diagnosis, and consequently to undesirable labelling effects on the patient from the diagnosis itself. It is significant that Kazanetz openly criticized Snezhnevsky's hegemony. But he paid for this by being dismissed from his post.

The era of *perestroika* has witnessed the formation of new associations of psychiatrists, which explicitly or implicitly reject Snezhnevskyism. The most notable group is the Independent Psychiatric Association, founded in March 1989, in Moscow. Its introductory charter refers to the need to develop and improve the science and practice of psychiatry, to defend doctors against social and political pressure, and to protect people from 'extreme socio-political and psychiatric arbitrariness'. The Association has since developed into an alternative professional organization, and gained membership of the World Psychiatric Association.[23]

The attitudes of psychiatrists have probably been more complex than the above classification suggests. With the school of Snezhnevsky so entrenched over the last three decades, it is likely that a younger generation of psychiatrists, who have known no other diagnostic system, have been influenced by his position. Thus, they could have been sincere in viewing dissent in a serious light, and the boundaries of mental illness as more widely extended than do their Western counterparts. They could well have been influenced by senior colleagues such as Professor N. Timofeyev, who maintained that: 'dissent is a different way of thinking . . . a way of thinking which is in disagreement with that of other people. It can be of various origins . . . it may also be determined by a disease of the brain in which the morbid process develops very slowly (sluggish form of schizophrenia) so that its other manifestations remain imperceptible . . . diagnostic difficulties increase if the subject relates in a formally correct way to the environment.'[24]

This does not rule out that these psychiatrists' intrinsic conformity and their reluctance to 'rock the boat' lest they jeopardized their careers have also affected their professional attitudes to dissenters. It would appear that average Soviet psychiatrists have not been encouraged to think about ethical issues for themselves, and, even with personal or second-hand knowledge of improper conduct among their colleagues, have been likely to avoid the issue of their profession's accountability to the public.

We now turn to a more detailed consideration of Snezhnevsky's theories to note their place in the overall picture of psychiatric abuse.

## The Soviet attitude to mental illness.

The labelling of political and other modes of dissent in the Soviet Union as severe mental illness is a recent phenomenon, linked with the theories promoted by the Snezhnevsky school. But intolerance of dissent has always been a hallmark of Soviet society, and indeed of the Tsarist era too. The authoritarian nature of both Soviet and Tsarist rule has embodied a concern that dissent always spelled danger and threat.

A society's concern about unorthodox ideas and behaviour amid its members appears to be universal, although varying widely in degree. The essence of this anxiety is summarized by the British sociologist, Kathleen Jones, when she comments:

without the stigmatization of some acts and some people as 'abnormal' or 'antisocial', there would be no idea of the normal, no rules to govern social behaviour . . . it follows that people whose behaviour is labelled as schizophrenic, criminal, inadequate or otherwise anti-social provide the yardstick by which acceptable conduct is measured. Society is making use of them for its own ends, the orthodox depend on the unorthodox to define their own orthodoxy; but the labels tend to be attached to people haphazardly. Behaviour which is seen as psychiatric disturbance in one society may be regarded as criminal in another, and simply tolerated in a third.[25]

Since the 1917 Revolution unorthodoxy has been labelled both as a criminal offence and a psychiatric illness, undoubtedly with the main purpose of defusing its potential to shake the fragile equilibrium of Soviet society. The threshold for deviance from conventionally accepted norms has been low, the level of conformity high. Conformity became deeply entrenched in Soviet citizens for good reason: during the Stalin's Great Terror it was a means to survival. Any demonstration of independent thinking could bring Stalin's repressive machine into action, with death or long-term imprisonment the result. A wide range of behaviour—social practices like homosexuality, certain attitudes to religion, particular styles in personal appearance, a love of certain music, art, or literature, and the like—was readily viewed as deviant, and the person who exhibited it labelled as 'different' and therefore suspect. Moreover, in a society where the collective has been paramount, and the group has taken priority, the individual could not afford to act unconventionally. Rather, he has had to adhere to the collective and its norms.

Thus deviance, troubling and unwelcome to the average, strongly conformist, Soviet citizen (and this has included most psychiatrists) could be explained away as stemming from a disturbed mind. Bukovsky and Gluzman have portrayed this attitude vividly in their *Manual on psychiatry for dissenters*,[26] when they advise the dissenter liable to a psychiatric interview to reply thus:

Unless your studies or your profession require it, you show no interest (and never have) in philosophical problems (for there is a term 'metaphysical intoxication') in psychiatry, parapsychology, or mathematics ... do not display any interest in modern art and especially any understanding of it [p. 109].

In sum, act the complete conformist!

The tendency to label deviant behaviour as illness escalated considerably with the advent of Snezhnevsky's diagnostic scheme. Earlier we noted his triumph in the medico-ideological upheaval of 1950. In the subsequent two decades he achieved another victory in the successful dissemination of his theories on schizophrenia. As chief psychiatric adviser to the Minister of Health, Director of the Institute of Psychiatry, and therefore the architect of training and research throughout the profession, and editor of the only psychiatric journal in the Soviet Union, he was powerfully placed to emasculate all opposition to his theories. The ascendancy of his school probably constitutes the most significant milestone in Soviet psychiatry since the Second World War, in terms of reshaping the diagnostic practice of an entire profession, and of facilitating the exploitation of psychiatry for political purposes.

Let us turn briefly to Snezhnevsky's diagnostic approach, which has had such profound effects on Soviet psychiatry. Walter Reich, in Chapter 7 on 'Psychiatric diagnosis as an ethical problem', provides additional details on the Snezhnevsky schema. He also shows convincingly in his discussion of the 'power of diagnostic theory to shape psychiatric vision' that diagnosis is a social act, affected by what the psychiatrist views as the society's norms; and how easily—particularly in the absence of competing theories of diagnosis—illness categories can become reified. His observations are most cogent in our consideration of the Snezhnevsky school of psychiatry and its approach to dissent. The most radical element is the prominence given to schizophrenia. This condition is considered to be basically genetic in origin, and to lead ineluctably to personality deterioration. Thus the diagnosis has very serious import. Once a patient is diagnosed as schizophrenic he is regarded as a lifelong victim of the illness, and this is true even if he does not show features of it. The Snezhnevsky school postulates the existence of three forms of schizophrenia: continuous, shift-like, and periodic, with subtypes in each form. In the continuous form the patient's course is progressively downhill, and no remission occurs, this differentiating it from the periodic form, where attacks of the illness are followed by remission, and the shift-like form, which is a cross between the continuous and the periodic. Subtypes of the continuous form—rapid or malignant, moderate, and sluggish or mild—are distinguishable by the rate of progression of the illness. In all subtypes the onset may be so gradual that the disease is not at all obvious—so-called 'seeming normality', of which more later. The early behavioural changes are often subtle, for example, the patient tends to withdraw, lose interest, and become apathetic. Thereafter follow the 'positive' and obviously psychotic features, such as delusions and hallucinations.

The mild, sluggish variety is all-important to our purposes in so far as it reflects a broadening of the schizophrenic concept so extensive as to allow even the mildest and subtlest behavioural change to be readily labelled as one of the most severe psychiatric conditions. And it is also the diagnosis of sluggish schizophrenia that has been commonly applied to dissenters who have been the victims of political psychiatry. Typical of this form of schizophrenia is its slow, insidious development and a picture of 'pseudoneurotic' symptoms, which may be obsessional, hysterical, or hypochondriacal. Other clinical manifestations include psychopathic or paranoid symptoms. Although the patient often retains insight into his illness, he overvalues his own importance, and may develop unrealistic plans for reforming society or for inventions of extraordinary significance.

## The Snezhnevsky school and dissent

'Delusional reformism', 'overestimation of the personality', and 'poor adaptation to society' have been some of the criteria encountered in the diagnostic reports of dissenters. Two alternative possibilities exist: (1) these 'patients' genuinely exhibit reformist ideas which are unrealistic, irrational, grandiose, and extraordinary; and (2) Snezhnevsky and his colleagues—following 'official albeit implicit pressure'—intentionally widened the schizophrenic net so as to entrap political and other dissenters. The extension of the criteria for schizophrenia is indisputable (it was shown clearly in the 1972 International Study on Schizophrenia[27] conducted by the World Health Organization); but Snezhnevsky could have averred that, based on his extensive clinical research (the study of thousands of cases at the Institute of Psychiatry), milder forms of the psychosis occur. That other Soviet schools of psychiatry and most western psychiatrists fail to subscribe to his views is neither here nor there. The concept of schizophrenia has, since its creation by Kraepelin, attracted much controversy over the extent of its boundaries, the primary criteria required for the use of the label, its cause and its treatment—indeed, every facet of this illness remains cluttered with uncertainties. With no objective yardstick to confirm the presence or absence of schizophrenia in a patient, the Snezhnevsky view of how the concept should be applied is arguably as valid as any other. In any event, most psychiatrists would subscribe to the notion that the belief tenaciously held by a person that he, and only he, has exceptional plans to reshape society or the world, may point to a psychotic disorder. The patient claiming to be Jesus Christ, a prophet, or some other exalted personage is familiar to most clinicians. But, the question remains, have Soviet dissenters belonged in this group? The voluminous evidence indicates that they have not. While not an easy matter for research, sufficient examples exist of prominent Soviet dissenters once labelled as schizophrenic who have enjoyed mental health since their emigration to the West. The Soviet psychiatric establishment's retort that such 'patients' were actively treated while in the Soviet Union and are now experiencing a remission lacks credibility. Is it mere concidence that Zhores Medvedev, Pyotr Grigorenko,[28] Vladimir Bukovsky, Leonid Plyushch, Natalya Gorbanevskaya, Ilya Rips, Alexander Volpin, Viktor Davydov, and Algirdas Statkevicius among others have remained 'free of relapse' for periods of up to two decades or longer?*

* I have had occasion to meet with all these dissenters, and have been struck by their integrity, both psychological and moral. Dr Statkevicius is a noteworthy example of the group. Himself a psychiatrist, he spent seven years in a prison psychiatric hospital until his release and emigration to the West in 1987. His insightfulness, sense of humour, and generosity of spirit were impressively obvious during the several days I associated with him at the World Psychiatric Association's World Congress in Athens in 1989.

One approach to the issue is to examine closely the criteria used by Soviet diagnosticians. Peter Reddaway and I have done this in detail in *Russia's political hospitals*, and the reader is referred to the accounts in Chapters 5 and 6. Our study led us to the following conclusion: that even within the context of Snezhnevsky's model of schizophrenia 'the application of a diagnosis to dissenters is unwarranted, at least as regards those whose detailed case histories were sent to the west by Bukovsky' [p. 251]. Let us consider some of the key criteria used to make the diagnosis in these dissenters. Commonly used phrases are 'paranoid delusion of reforming society or of reorganizing the state or of revising Marxism-Leninism'. In fact, dissenters acted in ways which in a Western democratic society would be regarded as completely reasonable, that is, they protested about the State's neglect of basic rights as set out in the Constitution; they called for a separation of Church and State so as to permit a person to practise his religion freely according to his own conviction; they criticized legitimately the severe restrictions imposed by the regime on scientists; they appealed for the abolition of cults of personality amongst the Soviet leadership; and so on.

Such views were usually expressed through letters and telegrams and peaceful demonstrations. Furthermore, dissenters fought for the promotion of human rights within an international framework. This is reflected in the support that was given to the most prominent member of the Soviet movement, the late Dr Andrei Sakharov (who was not dealt with by political psychiatry, but was always a potential target and the object of repeated official rumours that he was mentally ill) by distinguished figures in the West who recognized the justice and validity of various forms of Soviet dissent. If the Russian diagnostic system is valid, many of them would presumably find themselves tagged with a label of sluggish schizophrenia! The supreme irony is that President Gorbachev himself would be suspect. He has been the foremost architect of political and social reform, and in his advocacy of the policy of *perestroika* has proposed many of the very changes in Soviet society which dissenters sought during the era of Brezhnev and his predecessors.

Another criterion used in the psychiatric case-reports of dissenters was 'over-estimation of the personality'—usually a companion criterion to 'paranoid delusions of reformism'. Grandiosity certainly suggests a serious psychiatric condition; but the concept, it would seem, was distorted and perverted in the case of dissenters, who were aware of the task they undertook. They did not believe that their actions would automatically bear fruit or that the regime would necessarily heed their protests, and none were messianic in their messages. They recognized the frustrating, and, above all, hazardous nature of their struggle. The passage into dissident territory was fraught with danger—demotion or loss of job, expulsion from the Party, mental hospitalization, internment in a prison or labour camp, exile—the penalties were obvious and well known. Yet dissenters considered the risk worth taking because of the importance of their objectives. They were not out to prove their courage, but rather were convinced, justifiably, that they had the right, granted by the country's Constitution, to express views about the State's lack of respect for that very right and for many other rights.

'Poor social adjustment' was another presumptive symptom of schizophrenia in dissenters' diagnostic reports. Social adjustment is regarded, reasonably, as one indicator, among others, of mental health. Inadequate adjustment may well suggest the presence of a psychiatric condition. Ironically, Soviet citizens who assumed a dissenting role were, in a way, maladjusted to their social environment. They deviated from the social conventions so characteristic of a totalitarian society—complete conformity stemming from a fear of the State's retaliation against unorthodoxy, and lifelong social conditioning. Dissenters, unlike the 'loyal' citizen, proclaimed their independence and autonomy, since their actions steered them away from the compliant collective. They did not, however, withdraw from society. On the contrary, they were much concerned with its welfare and ultimate fate. Moreover, dissent was not an exclusive preoccupation: they might work as a mathematician, artist, labourer, engineer, physicist, or doctor; and they might have achieved much success in their careers; for example, Grigorenko as a Red Army Major-General, Medvedev as a biologist, Plyushch as a mathematician, Rafalsky as a headmaster, Ponamaryov as a research engineer (it should be noted that many dissenters were dismissed from their positions as part of the State's policy of harrassment, and were prevented from continuing to work in their professions).

We can now return to the questions posed earlier. First, have the reformist ideas of dissenter 'patients' been delusional, and have they been accompanied by other features of illness? The evidence from case-reports smuggled out of the Soviet Union and from clinical assessments of dissenters made by Western psychiatrists is persuasive. It would appear that the behaviour of dissenters has been distorted in such a way as to fulfil the criteria for schizophrenia set down by the Snezhnevsky school. While these criteria are in and of themselves not unreasonable, when cut to fit the dissenter the fit simply did not match. As for the second question, evidence that the Snezhnevsky school's extension of the schizophrenic concept resulted from 'official pressure' or was originally engineered to provide a psychiatric weapon against the growing tide of dissent in the 1960s remains equivocal. In any event, the extremely broad boundary of the diagnosis paved the way for a subtle collusion between a political authority, determined to stamp out dissent by any available means, and a compliant and intimidated psychiatric establishment, willing to apply the newly established diagnosis of schizophrenia to dissenters. The most likely pattern therefore probably amounted to mostly implicit pressure by the State on psychiatrists to use their theories to place deviance within the orbit of mental illness. Snezhnevsky and his colleagues managed to satisfy the political authorities by applying their comprehensively developed diagnostic package.

Interestingly, in the wake of international publicity about Soviet political psychiatry and protest against it from both professional and lay sources—in the Soviet Union and in the West—this diagnostic scheme came to contain other ingredients. The most striking addition to the Soviet psychiatric lexicon was 'seeming normality', a concept promulgated by leading Soviet physicians in a letter defending their country's psychiatric profession.[29] The signatories adamantly rebutted allegations that Soviet psychiatry was unethical, and argued that:

> There is a small number of mental cases whose disease, as a result of a mental derangement, paranoia, and other psycho-pathological symptoms, can lead them to anti-social actions which fall in the category of those that are prohibited by law, such as disturbance of public order, dissemination of slander, manifestation of aggressive intentions, etc. It is noteworthy that they can do this after preliminary preparations, with 'a cunningly calculated plan of action' . . . To the people around them such mental cases do not create the impression of being obviously 'insane'. Most often, these are people suffering from schizophrenia or a paranoid pathological development of the personality. Such cases are known well both by Soviet and foreign psychiatrists. The seeming normality of such sick persons when they commit socially dangerous actions is used by anti-Soviet propaganda for slanderous contentions that these persons are not suffering from a mental disorder.

The trial of Natalya Gorbanevskaya illustrates the use to which this concept has been put. The expert psychiatric witness, in defence of his diagnosis of sluggish schizophrenia, argued that well-defined clinical features of psychosis, such as delusions and hallucinations, did not have to be characteristically present for the diagnosis. Moreover, this form of schizophrenia did not require clear symptoms, but was present 'from the theoretical point of view' [p. 140].[5] Professor Lunts seemed to be saying that a condition like schizophrenia could exist theoretically but not clinically in a patient—a diagnosis of mental illness in the absence of any features of mental illness! Or, as Dr Martynenko put it in the case of the dissenter Olga Iofe: 'The presence of this form of schizophrenia does not presuppose changes in the personality noticeable to others' [p. 250].[5] Via 'seeming normality', schizophrenia has become an Orwellian and forbidding creature—a giant amoeba which has swallowed up anything that lies across its path.

The Russian writer Chekhov, in his story *Ward number six*, portrays a chilling situation in which the boundaries of psychiatric illness become so utterly diffuse and blurred that the distinction between normality and abnormality evaporates. The Snezhnevsky doctrine has brought us uncomfortably close to fiction.

## Soviet psychiatry in the era of *perestroika* and *glasnost*

Revealing certain key developments in Soviet psychiatry since the advent of *perestroika* and *glasnost* in the mid-1980s provides new insights into the nature of the abuse of psychiatry.

The practice continued more or less unabated until 1983. When, in that year, the World Psychiatric Association was due to debate several resolutions from member societies calling for the suspension or expulsion of the Soviet Psychiatric Society at its World Congress in Vienna, the Russians preempted the decision by submitting its resignation.[6] They did so adamantly maintaining that the Western accusations were nothing but anti-Soviet slander. Similar references to slanderous attacks had been made during the previous decade by the Soviet psychiatric establishment; and indeed, throughout this period, there was no hint of an acknowledgement that something was amiss.

The ascendancy of Gorbachev in April 1985 did not herald any shift in the customary Soviet retorts. Clearly, Soviet society had other weighty issues to deal with. But then, rather dramatically, in July 1987 the Soviet press as part of the process of *glasnost* or openness permitted the first publication of a critique of the misapplication of psychiatry. In an article published in *Izvestia*,[30] a journalist and lawyer described two clinical cases in order to assert that psychiatry was being deployed to suppress dissent. Moreover, they attacked the previously invincible Snezhnevsky school of psychiatry with a reference to its improper application of the diagnosis of schizophrenia. They also highlighted the limitations of mental health law, which had failed to provide a detained patient with the right of appeal.

Other critical articles soon followed. For instance, it was argued in November 1987[31] that the dominance of the Snezhnevsky school had facilitated the diagnosis as schizophrenia of people generally considered sane, by the construing as signs of mental illness of such qualities as a strong sense of justice and consistency. In the same month[32] even a senior figure like Dr Anatoly Potapov, the Minister for Health of the Russian Republic, conceded that involuntary psychiatric hospitalization occurred too frequently, and that the diagnosis of schizophrenia was applied too arbitrarily.

A series of critiques of a similar kind have been published at regular intervals since 1987, a pattern evidently reflecting the intention of the reformists in government to utilize the media as a means of discarding former unjust policies and practices.[33] This strategy became even more pronounced in 1989, when criticism was levelled at named psychiatrists, with the implication that they should be removed from office. A particularly incisive attack appeared in the prestigious journal *Literaturnaya Gazeta*.[34] Dr Alexander Churkin, then Chief Psychiatrist in the Federal Ministry of Health; Professor Marat Vartanyan, Director of the All-Union Centre for Mental Health Research; and Professor Georgy Morozov, Director of the Serbsky Institute for Forensic Psychiatry (we have previously encountered the latter pair in this chapter) were all accused of conniving with an abusive system.

Dr Churkin was subsequently removed from his post, in October 1989 (personal communication: Dr Alexander Karpov, Athens, October 1989). This may have resulted, in part, from his clumsy effort to defend Soviet psychiatry a year earlier. Then, he had added a new term to the Soviet psychiatric lexicon, namely that of *hyperdiagnosis*. In referring to the 300 clinical case histories of dissenters that he had analysed, he denied that any intentional political misuse of psychiatry had occurred, but conceded that he had '... sometimes stumbled on cases of so-called hyperdiagnosis, where the symptoms and severity of the mental disturbance were less pronounced than those diagnosed by the psychiatrist.'[35]

This form of defence against criticism of abuse remained the standard tactic of the psychiatric establishment until the momentous events that unfolded at the World Congress of the World Psychiatric Association in Athens in October 1989.[20] The Russians were resolved to regain membership, and thus, symbolically, to be deemed acceptable by world psychiatry. During the days leading up to the meeting of the governing body which would vote on the issue of readmission, the Soviet delegation repeatedly prevaricated when challenged by Western psychiatrists who were insisting upon an unambiguous acknowledgement that political misuse of psychiatry had taken place.

Indeed, it was only with this relentless pressure that, at the eleventh hour, the Soviet representatives admitted: '... that previous political conditions created an environment in which psychiatric abuse occurred for non-medical, including political, reasons'. Moreover, 'victims of abuse [would] have their cases reviewed within the USSR and, also in co-operation with the World Psychiatric Association ...' Thus, after eighteen years of repeated denial and constant evasiveness (allegations of abuse were initially made at the World Congress in 1971) came the first official admission. This development and the form it assumed provide clear evidence of the political nature of Soviet psychiatry and its facilitation of abuse. As we have commented earlier, the psychiatric leadership had colluded with the political authorities over many years, and were deeply immersed in improper practices. To expect an expression of *mea culpa* with all the attendant risks, such as professional demotion or worse, would have been far too sanguine. It was only with State pressure of a new kind, as part of *perestroika*, that the psychiatric delegation grudgingly gave way.

The pressure, in Athens, came in the form of Yuri Reschetov, a lawyer and director of the Department of Humanitarian Problems and Human Rights of the USSR's Ministry of Foreign Affairs. He himself had obviously been assigned by high political authority, chiefly from within his own ministry, to negotiate Soviet readmission. Given the resistance of establishment psychiatry (in association with senior figures in the federal Ministry of Health, and especially the Minister, Dr E. Chazov) to acknowledging the issue of abuse, and the Foreign Affairs Ministry's own pressing need to eliminate this 'black spot' from the country's previously tarnished human-rights record, Reschetov's central role in Athens was designed to accomplish readmission at virtually any cost, including the possible loss of high-ranking jobs for those psychiatrists in the official delegation itself.

The chief 'diplomatic' strategy came in the form of a memorandum (this was undated but signed by Professor G. Lukacher, the scientific Secretary-General of the Soviet Psychiatry Society). The memorandum, like Reschetov's crucial role in the proceedings in Athens, provides further insights into aspects of Soviet psychiatry which facilitated its abuse. The material covered recently introduced reforms in Soviet psychiatry, including new mental health legislation, the transfer of the special (prison) psychiatric hospitals from the Ministry of the Interior (also concerned with the police, the security police, and security in general) to the Ministry of Health; and the plan to establish an independent commission consisting of psychiatrists, lawyers, and social workers which would monitor cases of psychiatric abuse.

The reform of mental health legislation is especially noteworthy, in that several articles deal specifically with the prevention of the improper deployment of psychiatry. (The legislation was published as a decree of the Presidium of the USSR Supreme Soviet on 5 January 1988.) Thus the detention in a psychiatric hospital of a person known to be mentally healthy, is a 'criminal offence punishable in accordance with the law of the Union Republics'. A person detained in a psychiatric hospital is entitled 'to appeal to the chief psychiatrist of the health authority ... where the diagnosis was carried out'. The chief psychiatrist is then obliged to seek a second opinion from an entirely new psychiatric commission. The rules governing the diagnostic process and treatment must be 'available for inspection' [by patients and their relatives, one assumes]. Finally, the chief psychiatrist is legally accountable, and appeals against his actions may be made to a court, while the federal Procurator-General (prosecutor) and his subordinates are obliged to check that psychiatrists are observing the law.

It had long been argued by leading Soviet psychiatrists that laws of this type, including the right of appeal, were unnecessary in the USSR, since psychiatrists acted objectively, and from an independent base. (It is indeed the case that the adversarial system has not been a feature of Soviet forensic psychiatry.) While this held in theory, the absence of legal safeguards for patients made them vulnerable to psychiatrists, who were in turn subject to external influences contrary to the patient's interests. Some contemporary commentators, particularly Alexander Podrabinek, who has been a long-standing proponent of ethical psychiatry in the Soviet Union, are dubious that the new law will prevent abuse, on the premise that there have been articles in the previous criminal code which could have been used to deter psychiatrists from acting improperly.[36] Podrabinek contends that in a totalitarian system the law cannot serve to guarantee the protection of society from repressive psychiatry. Several additional changes are required, such as a means of enforcing the accountability of State officials, the presence of lay people on monitoring bodies, and an independent press.

Thus, while progress in mental health law-reform is to be applauded, other fundamental changes in Soviet society will be required before the spectre of Soviet abuse can be laid to rest.

## Conclusion

The political misuse of psychiatry in the Soviet Union is a flagrant example of unethical practice, but obviously it is not the only example. The euthanasia programme of Nazi psychiatrists, for example—responsible for the death of thousands of mentally disabled and handicapped patients—constitutes one of the most unsavoury chapters in twentieth-century psychiatry (see Chapter 22). It could be argued that the inequitable distribution of mental health care to poor members of some Western societies, especially the United States (see Chapter 21) is another case of grossly unethical conduct.

The Soviet case, however, is of extraordinary significance for psychiatrists because it demonstrates, in bold relief, the vulnerabilities to which their profession is subject, and how complex are the ethical dilemmas which face them in practice. Many of these vulnerabilities and dilemmas have been dealt with in earlier chapters, where more often than not questions have been posed, rather than solutions offered. This, it seems to me, is how it should be. The Soviet abuse has preoccupied the profession in the 1970s and 1980s; tomorrow other ethical problems will no doubt present themselves. Remedies for these future problems will prove as elusive and demanding as for those we grapple with now. What we as a profession can, and should, strive for are two interrelated goals: to commit ourselves to the task of facing the ethical dimensions of our work, and to try to clarify as clearly as possible the nature of these ethical dimensions.

Should we succeed in reaching these two goals, the chance of an unethical system of practice like the Soviet one may decline; happily, even vanish.

## References and Notes

1 Human rights organizations such as Amnesty International and the International Association on the Political Use of Psychiatry have documented cases, albeit sporadic, in several countries, for instance Romania, Czechoslovakia, Yugoslavia, Bulgaria, Hungary, Turkey, and Cuba.
2 Fireside, H.: *Soviet psychoprisons*. New York, Norton, 1979.
3 Nekipelov, V.: *Institute of fools: notes from the Serbsky*. London, Gollancz, 1980.
4 Lader, M.: *Psychiatry on trial*. Harmondsworth, Penguin, 1977.
5 Bloch, S. and Reddaway, P.: *Russia's political hospitals: the abuse of psychiatry in the Soviet Union*. London, Gollancz, 1977. (In US: *Psychiatric terror: how Soviet psychiatry is used to suppress dissent*. New York, Basic Books, 1977.)
6 Bloch, S. and Reddaway, P.: *Soviet psychiatric abuse. The shadow over world psychiatry*. London, Gollancz, 1984.
7 Medvedev, Z. and Medvedev, R.: *A question of madness*. London, Macmillan, 1971.
8 Podrabinek, A.: *Punitive medicine*. Ann Arbor, Karoma, 1980.
9 Gorbanevskaya, N.: *Red Square at noon*. London, Deutsch, 1972.
10 Bukovsky, V.: *To build a castle: my life as a dissenter*. London, Deutsch, 1978.
11 Plyushch, L.: *History's carnival*. London, Collins and Harvill Press, 1979.
12 Grigorenko, P.: *The Grigorenko papers*. London, Hurst, 1976.
13 Khodorovich, T. (ed.): *The case of Leonid Plyushch*. London, Hurst, 1976.
14 See for example *The Guardian*, 29 September 1973; *British Medical Journal*, 10 August 1974.
15 *Report of the US delegation to assess recent changes in Soviet psychiatry*. Washington DC, 12 July 1989.
16 Quoted in Field, M. G.: *Doctor and patient in Soviet Russia*. Cambridge, Mass., Harvard University Press, 1957.
17 Quoted in Field, M. G.: *Soviet socialized medicine; an introduction*. New York, Free Press, 1967.
18 Survey, No. 81, p. 114, 1971. Translation of Soviet Physician's Oath originally published in *Meditsinskaya Gazeta*, 20 April, 1971. (See Appendix for complete text.)
19 Novikov, J.: Kronzeuge Gegen den KGB. *Der Stern*, 22 March–26 April 1978.
20 Bloch, S.: Athens and beyond: Soviet psychiatric abuse and the World Psychiatric Association. *Psychiatric Bulletin* 14:129–133, 1990.
21 Gluzman, S.: *On Soviet totalitarian psychiatry*. Amsterdam, International Association on the Political Use of Psychiatry, 1989.
22 Kazanetz, E.: Differentiating exogenous psychiatric illness from schizophrenia. *Archives of General Psychiatry* 36:740–5, 1979. See also Kazanetz, E.: The delineation of schizophrenia from other psychiatric illnesses. *British Journal of Psychiatry* 155:160–5, 1989.
23 *Information Bulletin* No. 21 pp. 9–10. Amsterdam, International Association on the Political Use of Psychiatry, 1989.

24 Timofeyev, I. N.: Deontological aspects of diagnosing schizophrenia. *Zhurnal Nevropat. i. Psikhiatrii* **74**:1065–9, 1974.
25 Jones, K.: Society looks at the psychiatrist. *British Journal of Psychiatry* **132**:321–32, 1978.
26 Bukovsky, V. and Gluzman, S.: A manual on psychiatry for dissidents. Appendix 1 in Fireside, H.: *Soviet psychoprisons*. New York, Norton, 1979.
27 *The international pilot study of schizophrenia*, Vol. 1. Geneva, World Health Organization, 1972.
28 Reich, W.: Grigorenko gets a second opinion. *New York Times Magazine* 13 May 1979. Dr Reich summarizes the results of a comprehensive psychiatric examination carried out by Drs A. Stone, L. C. Kolb, and himself, as well as the results of psychological and neurological testing. See also *Moscow News*, 10 December 1989.
29 *The Guardian*, 29 September, 1973.
30 *Izvestia*, 11 July 1987.
31 *Komsomolskaya Pravda*, 11 November 1987.
32 *Sovietskaya Rossiya*, 20 November 1987.
33 Van Voren, R.: Soviet psychiatry criticized in the Soviet press, in *Soviet psychiatric abuse in the Gorbachev era*, ed. R. Van Voren. Amsterdam, International Association on the Political Use of Psychiatry, 1989.
34 *Literaturnaya Gazeta*, 28 June 1989.
35 *Novoye Vrema*, **No. 43**, 1988.
36 Podrabinek, A.: Punitive psychiatry during the period of perestroika, in *Soviet psychiatric abuse in the Gorbachev era*, ed. R. Van Voren. Amsterdam, International Association on the Political Use of Psychiatry, 1989.

# Appendix

## Codes of ethics

Codes for the ethical guidance of physicians have been promulgated over many centuries and in many different countries. In this appendix we offer a selection which we believe are relevant to the psychiatrist. Included are the hallowed Hippocratic Oath and the revised *Principles of medical ethics* of the American Medical Association. Also included is the well-known *Declaration of Geneva* of the World Medical Association and, because of its relevance to the chapter on the political misuse of psychiatry in the Soviet Union, the *Oath of Soviet physicians*.

Two codes for the ethical conduct of biomedical research in general are provided—the World Medical Association's *Declaration of Helsinki* and the *Principles of experimental research on human beings* of the British Medical Association.

It is of interest that there are few specific codes of ethics for psychiatrists. We are aware of only two of them—*The Principles of medical ethics with annotations especially applicable to psychiatry* of the American Psychiatric Association and the World Psychiatric Association's *Declaration of Hawaii*.

## The Hippocratic Oath

I swear by Apollo Physician and Asclepius and Hygieia and Panaceia and all the gods and goddesses, making them my witnesses, that I will fulfil according to my ability and judgment this oath and this covenant:

To hold him who has taught me this art as equal to my parents and to live my life in partnership with him, and if he is in need of money to give him a share of mine, and to regard his offspring as equal to my brothers in male lineage and to teach them this art—if they desire to learn it—without fee and covenant; to give a share of precepts and oral instruction and all the other learning to my sons and to the sons of him who has instructed me and to pupils who have signed the covenant and have taken an oath according to the medical law, but to no one else.

I will apply dietetic measures for the benefit of the sick according to my ability and judgment; I will keep them from harm and injustice.

I will neither give a deadly drug to anybody if asked for it, nor will I make a suggestion to this effect. Similarly I will not give to a woman an abortive remedy. In purity and holiness I will guard my life and my art.

I will not use the knife, not even on sufferers from stone, but will withdraw in favor of such men as are engaged in this work.

Whatever houses I may visit, I will come for the benefit of the sick, remaining free of all intentional injustice, of all mischief and in particular of sexual relations with both female and male persons, be they free or slaves.

What I may see or hear in the course of the treatment or even outside of the treatment in regard to the life of men, which on no account one must spread abroad, I will keep to myself holding such things shameful to be spoken about.

If I fulfil this oath and do not violate it, may it be granted to me to enjoy life and art, being honored with fame among all men for all time to come; if I transgress it and swear falsely, may the opposite of all this be my lot.

[Reprinted by permission from *Ancient Medicine*: Selected Papers of Ludwig Edelstein edited by Oswei Temkin and C. Temkin, Baltimore: Johns Hopkins University Press, 1967.]

## The Declaration of Geneva

*Physician's Oath*

At the time of being admitted as a member of the medical profession:

I solemnly pledge myself to consecrate my life to the service of humanity;

I will give to my teachers the respect and gratitude which is their due;

I will practise my profession with conscience and dignity; the health of my patient will be my first consideration;

I will maintain by all the means in my power, the honor and the noble traditions of the medical profession; my colleagues will be my brothers;

I will not permit considerations of religion, nationality, race, party politics or social standing to intervene between my duty and my patient;

I will maintain the utmost respect for human life from the time of conception, even under threat, I will not use my medical knowledge contrary to the laws of humanity;

I make these promises solemnly, freely and upon my honor.

[Adopted by the General Assembly of the World Medical Association, Geneva, 1948, amended 1968. Reprinted by permission.]

## The Physician's Oath of the Soviet Union

Having attained the high calling of physician and entering medical practice I solemnly swear:

to devote all my knowledge and strength to the preservation and improvement of the health of man, to the curing and prevention of diseases, to work conscientiously wherever the interests of society demand;

to be ever ready to render medical aid, to be attentive and thoughtful of the patient, to maintain medical confidence;

constantly to perfect my medical knowledge and physician's skills, to further by my work the development of medical science and practice;

to turn, if the patient's interests demand it, for advice to my professional colleagues and that I myself will never refuse advice and help to them;

to preserve and further the noble traditions of our native medicine, that I will in all my actions be guided by the principles of communist morality, ever to bear in mind the high calling of the Soviet physician, and of my responsibility to the people and the Soviet State.

I swear that I will be faithful to this oath throughout the rest of my life. [Originally published in *Meditsinskaya Gazeta*, 20 April 1971. English translation in *Survey* No. 4 (81) Autumn 1971, p. 114. Reprinted by permission.]

## Principles of Medical Ethics of the American Medical Association

Preamble: the medical profession has long subscribed to a body of ethical statements developed primarily for the benefit of the patient. As a member of this profession, a physician must recognize responsibility not only to patients, but also to society, to other health professionals, and to self. The following Principles adopted by the American Medical Association are not laws, but standards of conduct which define the essentials of honorable behaviour for the physician.

I. A physician shall be dedicated to providing competent medical service with compassion and respect for human dignity.

II. A physician shall deal honestly with patients and colleagues, and strive to expose those physicians deficient in character or competence, or who engage in fraud or deception.

III. A physician shall respect the law and also recognize a responsibility to seek changes in those requirements which are contrary to the best interests of the patient.

IV. A physician shall respect the rights of patients, of colleagues, and of other health professionals, and shall safeguard patient confidences within the constraints of the law.

V. A physician shall continue to study, apply and advance scientific knowledge, make relevant information available to patients, colleagues, and the public, obtain consultation, and use the talents of other health professionals when indicated.

VI. A physician shall, in the provision of appropriate patient care, except in emergencies, be free to choose whom to serve, with whom to associate, and the environment in which to provide medical services.

VII. A physician shall recognize a responsibility to participate in activities contributing to an improved community.

[Adopted by the American Medical Association, Chicago, 1980. Reprinted by permission.]

## The Declaration of Helsinki

*Introduction*

It is the mission of the medical doctor to safeguard the health of the people. His or her knowledge and conscience are dedicated to the fulfilment of this mission.

The Declaration of Geneva of the World Medical Association binds the doctor with the words, 'The health of my patient will be my first consideration,' and the International Code of Medical Ethics declares that, 'Any act or advice which could weaken physical or mental resistance of a human being may be used only in his interest.'

The purpose of biomedical research involving human subjects must to be improve diagnostic, therapeutic and prophylactic procedures and the understanding of the aetiology and pathogenesis of disease.

In current medical practice most diagnostic, therapeutic or prophylactic procedures involve hazards. This applies *a fortiori* to biomedical research.

Medical progress is based on research which ultimately must rest in part on experimentation involving human subjects.

In the field of biomedical research a fundamental distinction must be recognized between medical research in which the aim is essentially diagnostic or therapeutic for a patient, and medical research, the essential object of which is purely scientific and without direct diagnostic or therapeutic value to the person subjected to the research.

Special caution must be exercised in the conduct of research which may affect the environment, and the welfare of animals used for research must be respected.

Because it is essential that the results of laboratory experiments be applied to human beings to further scientific knowledge and to help suffering humanity, the World Medical Association has prepared the following recommendations as a guide to every doctor in biomedical research involving human subjects. They should be kept under review in the future. It must be stressed that the standards as drafted are only a guide to physicians all over the world. Doctors are not relieved from criminal, civil and ethical responsibilities under the laws of their own countries.

## I. Basic principles

1. Biomedical research involving human subjects must conform to generally accepted scientific principles and should be based on adequately performed laboratory and animal experimentation and on a thorough knowledge of the scientific literature.

2. The design and performance of each experimental procedure involving human subjects should be clearly formulated in an experimental protocol which should be transmitted to a specially appointed independent committee for consideration, comment and guidance.

3. Biomedical research involving human subjects should be conducted only by scientifically qualified persons and under the supervision of a clinically competent medical person. The responsibility for the human subject must always rest with a medically qualified person and never rest on the subject of the research, even though the subject has given his or her consent.

4. Biomedical research involving human subjects cannot legitimately be carried out unless the importance of the objective is in proportion to the inherent risk to the subject.

5. Every biomedical research project involving human subjects should be preceded by careful assessment of predictable risks in comparison with foreseeable benefits to the subject or to others. Concern for the interests of the subject must always prevail over the interests of science and society.

6. The right of the research subject to safeguard his or her integrity must always be respected. Every precaution should be taken to respect the privacy of the subject and to minimize the impact of the study on the subject's physical and mental integrity and on the personality of the subject.

7. Doctors should abstain from engaging in research projects involving human subjects unless they are satisfied that the hazards involved are believed to be predictable. Doctors should cease any investigation if the hazards are found to outweigh the potential benefits.

8. In publication of the results of his or her research, the doctor is obliged to preserve the accuracy of the results. Reports of experimentation not in accordance with the principles laid down in this Declaration should not be accepted for publication.

9. In any research on human beings, each potential subject must be

adequately informed of the aims, methods, anticipated benefits and potential hazards of the study and the discomfort it may entail. He or she should be informed that he or she is at liberty to abstain from participation in the study and that he or she is free to withdraw his or her consent to participation at any time. The doctors should then obtain the subject's freely-given informed consent, preferably in writing.

10. When obtaining informed consent for the research project the doctor should be particularly cautious if the subject is in a dependent relationship to him or her or may consent under duress. In that case the informed consent should be obtained by a doctor who is not engaged in the investigation and who is completely independent of this official relationship.

11. In case of legal incompetence, informed consent should be obtained from the legal guardian in accordance with national legislation. Where physical or mental incapacity makes it impossible to obtain informed consent, or when the subject is a minor, permission from the responsible relative replaces that of the subject in accordance with national legislation.

12. The research protocol should always contain a statement of the ethical considerations involved and should indicate that the principles enunciated in the present Declaration are complied with.

## II. Medical research combined with professional care (clinical research)

1. In the treatment of the sick person, the doctor must be free to use a new diagnostic and therapeutic measure, if in his or her judgement it offers hope of saving life, reestablishing health or alleviating suffering.

2. The potential benefits, hazards and discomfort of a new method should be weighed against the advantages of the best current diagnostic and therapeutic methods.

3. In any medical study, every patient—including those of a control group, if any—should be assured of the best proven diagnostic and therapeutic method.

4. The refusal of the patient to participate in a study must never interfere with the doctor–patient relationship.

5. If the doctor considers it essential not to obtain informed consent, the specific reasons for this proposal should be stated in the experimental protocol for transmission to the independent committee.

6. The doctor can combine medical research with professional care, the objective being the acquisition of new medical knowledge, only to the extent that medical research is justified by its potential diagnostic or therapeutic value for the patient.

## III. Non-therapeutic biomedical research involving human subjects (non-clinical biomedical research)

1. In the purely scientific application of medical research carried out on

a human being, it is the duty of the doctor to remain the protector of the life and health of that person on whom biomedical research is being carried out.

2. The subjects should be volunteers—either healthy persons or patients for whom the experimental design is not related to the patient's illness.

3. The investigator or the investigating team should discontinue the research if in his/her or their judgement it may, if continued, be harmful to the individual.

4. In research on man, the interest of science and society should never take precedence over considerations related to the well-being of the subject.

[Adopted by the General Assembly of the World Medical Association, Helsinki 1964; revised Tokyo 1975. Reprinted by permission.]

## Principles of Experimental Research on Human Beings

1. New drugs or other therapy should not be prescribed unless prior investigation as to the possible effects upon the human body has been fully adequate.

2. Before a new drug is used in treatment, the clinician should ensure that the distributors of the drug are reputable and the claims made for the products include reference to independent evidence of its effects.

3. No new technique or investigation shall be undertaken on a patient unless it is strictly necessary for the treatment of the patient, or, alternatively, that following a full explanation the doctor has obtained the patient's free and valid consent to his actions, preferably in writing.

4. A doctor wholly engaged in clinical research must be at special pains to remember the responsibility to the individual patient when his experimental work is conducted through the medium of a consultant who has clinical responsibility for the patient.

5. The patient must never take second place to a research project nor should he be given any such impression. Before embarking upon any research the doctor should ask himself these questions:

   (a) Does the patient know what it is I propose to do?
   (b) Have I explained fully and honestly to him the risks I am asking him to run?
   (c) Am I satisfied that his consent has been freely given and is legally valid?
   (d) Is this procedure one which I would not hesitate to advise, or in which I would readily acquiesce, if it were to be undertaken upon my own wife or children?

[Adopted by the British Medical Association, 1963. Reprinted by permission.]

## The Declaration of Hawaii

Ever since the dawn of culture, ethics has been an essential part of the healing art. It is the view of the World Psychiatric Association that due to conflicting loyalties and expectations of both physicians and patients in contemporary society and the delicate nature of the therapist–patient relationship, high ethical standards are especially important for those involved in the science and practice of psychiatry as a medical specialty. These guidelines have been delineated in order to promote close adherence to those standards and to prevent misuse of psychiatric concepts, knowledge and technology.

Since the psychiatrist is a member of society as well as a practitioner of medicine, he or she must consider the ethical implications specific to psychiatry as well as the ethical demands on all physicians and the societal responsibility of every man and woman.

Even though ethical behaviour is based on the individual psychiatrist's conscience and personal judgement, written guidelines are needed to clarify the profession's ethical implications.

Therefore, the General Assembly of the World Psychiatric Association has approved these ethical guidelines for psychiatrists, having in mind the great differences in cultural backgrounds, and in legal, social and economic conditions which exist in the various countries of the world. It should be understood that the World Psychiatric Association views these guidelines to be minimal requirements for ethical standards of the psychiatric profession.

1. The aim of psychiatry is to treat mental illness and to promote mental health. To the best of his or her ability, consistent with accepted scientific knowledge and ethical principles, the psychiatrist shall serve the best interests of the patient and be also concerned for the common good and a just allocation of health resources. To fulfil these aims requires continuous research and continual education of health care personnel, patients and the public.

2. Every psychiatrist should offer to the patient the best available therapy to his knowledge and if accepted must treat him or her with the solicitude and respect due to the dignity of all human beings. When the psychiatrist is responsible for treatment given by others he owes them competent supervision and education. Whenever there is a need, or whenever a reasonable request is forthcoming from the patient, the psychiatrist should seek the help of another colleague.

3. The psychiatrist aspires for a therapeutic relationship that is founded on mutual agreement. At its optimum it requires trust, confidentiality, cooperation and mutual responsibility. Such a relationship may not be possible to establish with some patients. In that case, contact should be

established with a relative or other person close to the patient. If and when a relationship is established for purposes other than therapeutic, such as in forensic psychiatry, its nature must be thoroughly explained to the person concerned.

4. The psychiatrist should inform the patient of the nature of the condition, therapeutic procedures, including possible alternatives, and of the possible outcome. This information must be offered in a considerate way and the patient must be given the opportunity to choose between appropriate and available methods.

5. No procedure shall be performed nor treatment given against or independent of a patient's own will, unless because of mental illness, the patient cannot form a judgement as to what is in his or her own best interest and without which treatment serious impairment is likely to occur to the patient or others.

6. As soon as the conditions for compulsory treatment no longer apply, the psychiatrist should release the patient from the compulsory nature of the treatment and if further therapy is necessary should obtain voluntary consent. The psychiatrist should inform the patient and/or relatives or meaningful others, of the existence of mechanisms of appeal for the detention and for any other complaints related to his or her well being.

7. The psychiatrist must never use his professional possibilities to violate the dignity or human rights of any individual or group and should never let inappropriate personal desires, feelings, prejudices or beliefs interfere with the treatment. The psychiatrist must on no account utilize the tools of his profession, once the absence of psychiatric illness has been established. If a patient or some third party demands actions contrary to scientific knowledge or ethical principles the psychiatrist must refuse to cooperate.

8. Whatever the psychiatrist has been told by the patient, or has noted during examination or treatment, must be kept confidential unless the patient relieves the psychiatrist from this obligation, or to prevent serious harm to self or others makes disclosure necessary. In these cases however, the patient should be informed of the breach of confidentiality.

9. To increase and propagate psychiatric knowledge and skill requires participation of the patients. Informed consent must, however, be obtained before presenting a patient to a class and, if possible, also when a case-history is released for scientific publication, whereby all reasonable measures must be taken to preserve the dignity and anonymity of the patient and to safeguard the personal reputation of the subject. The patient's participation must be voluntary, after full information has been given of the aim, procedures, risks and inconveniences of a research project and there must always be a reasonable relationship between calculated risks or inconveniences and the benefit of the study. In clinical research every subject must retain and exert all his rights as a patient. For children and

other patients who cannot themselves give informed consent, this should be obtained from the legal next-of-kin. Every patient or research subject is free to withdraw for any reason at any time from any voluntary treatment and from any teaching or research programme in which he or she participates. This withdrawal, as well as any refusal to enter a programme, must never influence the psychiatrist's efforts to help the patient or subject.

10. The psychiatrist should stop all therapeutic, teaching or research programmes that may evolve contrary to the principles of this Declaration. [Adopted by the General Assembly of the World Psychiatric Association, 1977, revised, 1983. Reprinted by permission.]

## Principles of Medical Ethics with Annotations Especially Applicable to Psychiatry of the American Psychiatric Association

### Preamble

*The medical profession has long subscribed to a body of ethical statements developed primarily for the benefit of the patient. As a member of this profession, a physician must recognize responsibility not only to patients, but also to society, to other health professionals, and to self. The following Principles, adopted by the American Medical Association, are not laws, but standards of conduct which define the essentials of honourable behaviour for the physician.*

### Section 1

*A physician shall be dedicated to providing competent medical service with compassion and respect for human dignity.*

1. The patient may place his/her trust in his/her psychiatrist knowing that the psychiatrist's ethics and professional responsibilities preclude him/her gratifying his/her own needs by exploiting the patient. This becomes particularly important because of the essentially private, highly personal, and sometimes intensely emotional nature of the relationship established with the psychiatrist.

2. A psychiatrist should not be a party to any type of policy that excludes, segregates, or demeans the dignity of any patient because of ethnic origin, race, sex, creed, age, socioeconomic status, or sexual orientation.

3. In accord with the requirement of law and accepted medical practice, it is ethical for a physician to submit his/her work to peer review and to the ultimate authority of the medical staff executive body and the hospital administration and its governing body. In case of dispute, the ethical psychiatrist has the following steps available:

(a) Seek appeal from the medical staff decision to a joint conference committee, including members of the medical staff executive committee, and the executive committee of the governing board. At this appeal, the ethical psychiatrist could request that outside opinions be considered.
(b) Appeal to the governing body itself.
(c) Appeal to state agencies regulating licensure of hospitals if, in the particular state, they concern themselves with matters of professional competency and quality of care.
(d) Attempt to educate colleagues through development of research projects and data and presentations at professionals meetings and in professional journals.
(e) Seek redress in local courts, perhaps through an enjoining injunction against the governing body.
(f) Public education as carried out by an ethical psychiatrist would not utilize appeals based solely upon emotion, but would be presented in a professional way and without any potential exploitation of patients through testimonials.

4. A psychiatrist should not be a participant in a legally authorized execution.

## Section 2

*A physician shall deal honestly with patients and colleagues, and strive to expose those physicians deficient in character or competence, or who engage in fraud or deception.*

1. The requirement that the physician conduct himself with propriety in his/her profession and in all the actions of his/her life is especially important in the case of the psychiatrist because the patient tends to model his/her behaviour after that of his/her therapist by identification. Further, the necessary intensity of the therapeutic relationship may tend to activate sexual and other needs and fantasies on the part of both patient and therapist, while weakening the objectivity necessary for control. Sexual activity with a patient is unethical. Sexual involvement with one's former patients generally exploits emotions deriving from treatment and therefore almost always is unethical.

2. The psychiatrist should diligently guard against exploiting information furnished by the patient and should not use the unique position of power afforded him/her by the psychotherapeutic situation to influence the patient in any way not directly relevant to the treatment goals.

3. A psychiatrist who regularly practices outside his/her area of professional competence should be considered unethical. Determination of professional competence should be made by peer review boards or other appropriate bodies.

4. Special consideration should be given to those psychiatrists who, because of mental illness, jeopardize the welfare of their patients and their own reputations and practices. It is ethical, even encouraged, for another psychiatrist to intercede in such situations.

5. Psychiatric services, like all medical services, are dispensed in the context of a contractual arrangement between the patient and the treating physician. The provisions of the contractual arrangement, which are binding on the physician as well as on the patient, should be explicitly established.

6. It is ethical for the psychiatrist to make a charge for a missed appointment when this falls within the terms of the specific contractual agreement with the patient. Charging for a missed appointment or for one not cancelled 24 hours in advance need not, in itself, be considered unethical if a patient is fully advised that the physician will make such a charge. The practice, however, should be resorted to infrequently and always with the utmost consideration for the patient and his/her circumstances.

7. An arrangement in which a psychiatrist provides supervision or administration to other physicians or nonmedical persons for a percentage of their fees or gross income is not acceptable; this would constitute fee-splitting. In a team of practitioners, or a multidisciplinary team, it is ethical for the psychiatrist to receive income for administration, research, education, or consultation. This should be based upon a mutually agreed upon and set fee or salary, open to renegotiation when a change in the time demand occurs. (See also Section 5, Annotations 2, 3, and 4.)

8. When a member has been found to have behaved unethically by the American Psychiatric Association or one of its constituent district branches, there should not be automatic reporting to the local authorities responsible for medical licensure, but the decision to report should be decided upon the merits of the case.

## Section 3

*A physician shall respect the law and also recognize a responsibility to seek changes in those requirements which are contrary to the best interests of the patient.*

1. It would seem self-evident that a psychiatrist who is a law-breaker might be ethically unsuited to practice his/her profession. When such illegal activities bear directly upon his/her practice, this would obviously be the case. However, in other instances, illegal activities such as those concerning the right to protest social injustices might not bear on either the image of the psychiatrist or the ability of the specific psychiatrist to treat his/her patient ethically and well. While no committee or board could offer prior assurance that any illegal activity would not be considered unethical,

it is conceivable that an individual could violate a law without being guilty of professionally unethical behaviour. Physicians lose no right of citizenship on entry into the profession of medicine.

2. Where not specifically prohibited by local laws governing medical practice, the practice of acupuncture by a psychiatrist is not unethical per se. The psychiatrist should have professional competence in the use of acupuncture. Or, if he/she is supervising the use of acupuncture by non-medical individuals, he/she should provide proper medical supervision. (See also Section 5, Annotations 3 and 4.)

## Section 4

*A physician shall respect the rights of patients, of colleagues, and of other health professionals, and shall safeguard patient confidences within the constraints of the law.*

1. Psychiatric records, including even the identification of a person as a patient, must be protected with extreme care. Confidentiality is essential to psychiatric treatment. This is based in part on the special nature of psychiatric therapy as well as on the traditional ethical relationship between physician and patient. Growing concern regarding the civil rights of patients and the possible adverse effects of computerization, duplication equipment, and data banks makes the dissemination of confidential information an increasing hazard. Because of the sensitive and private nature of the information with which the psychiatrist deals, he/she must be circumspect in the information that he/she chooses to disclose to others about a patient. The welfare of the patient must be a continuing consideration.

2. A psychiatrist may release confidential information only with the authorization of the patient or under proper legal compulsion. The continuing duty of the psychiatrist to protect the patient includes fully apprising him/her of the connotations of waiving the privilege of privacy. This may become an issue when the patient is being investigated by a government agency, is applying for a position, or is involved in legal action. The same principles apply to the release of information concerning treatment to medical departments of government agencies, business organizations, labour unions, and insurance companies. Information gained in confidence about patients seen in student health services should not be released without the student's explicit permission.

3. Clinical and other materials used in teaching and writing must be adequately disguised in order to preserve the anonymity of the individuals involved.

4. The ethical responsibility of maintaining confidentiality holds equally for the consultations in which the patient may not have been present and in

which the consultee was not a physician. In such instances, the physician consultant should alert the consultee to his/her duty of confidentiality.

5. Ethically the psychiatrist may disclose only that information which is relevant to a given situation. He/she should avoid offering speculation as fact. Sensitive information such as an individual's sexual orientation or fantasy material is usually unnecessary.

6. Psychiatrists are often asked to examine individuals for security purposes, to determine suitability for various jobs, and to determine legal competence. The psychiatrist must fully describe the nature and purpose and lack of confidentiality of the examination to the examinee at the beginning of the examination.

7. Careful judgment must be exercised by the psychiatrist in order to include, when appropriate, the parents or guardian in the treatment of a minor. At the same time the psychiatrist must assure the minor proper confidentiality.

8. Psychiatrists at times may find it necessary, in order to protect the patient or the community from imminent danger, to reveal confidential information disclosed by the patient.

9 .When the psychiatrist is ordered by the court to reveal the confidences entrusted to him/her by patients he/she may comply or he/she may ethically hold the right to dissent within the framework of the law. When the psychiatrist is in doubt, the right of the patient to confidentiality and, by extension, to unimpaired treatment, should be given priority. The psychiatrist should reserve the right to raise the question of adequate need for disclosure. In the event that the necessity for legal disclosure is demonstrated by the court, the psychiatrist may request the right to disclosure of only that information which is relevant to the legal question at hand.

10. With regard for the person's dignity and privacy and with truly informed consent, it is ethical to present a patient to a scientific gathering, if the confidentiality of the presentation is understood and accepted by the audience.

11. It is ethical to present a patient or former patient to a public gathering or to the news media only if the patient is fully informed of enduring loss of confidentiality, is competent, and consents in writing without coercion.

12. When involved in funded research, the ethical psychiatrist will advise human subjects of the funding source, retain his/her freedom to reveal data and results, and follow all appropriate and current guidelines relative to human subject protection.

13. Ethical considerations in medical practice preclude the psychiatric evaluation of any adult charged with criminal acts prior to access to, or availability of, legal counsel. The only exception is the rendering of care to the person for the sole purpose of medical treatment.

## Section 5

*A physician shall continue to study, apply, and advance scientific knowledge, make relevant information available to patients, colleagues, and the public, obtain consultation, and use the talents of other health professionals when indicated.*

1. Psychiatrists are responsible for their own continuing education and should be mindful of the fact that theirs must be a lifetime of learning.

2. In the practice of his/her specialty, the psychiatrist consults, associates, collaborates, or integrates his/her work with that of many professionals, including psychologists, psychometricians, social workers, alcoholism counselors, marriage counselors, public health nurses, etc. Furthermore, the nature of modern psychiatric practice extends his/her contacts to such people as teachers, juvenile and adult probation officers, attorneys, welfare workers, agency volunteers, and neighbourhood aides. In referring patients for treatment, counselling, or rehabilitation to any of these practitioners, the psychiatrist should ensure that the allied professional or paraprofessional with whom he/she is dealing is a recognized member of his/her own discipline and is competent to carry out the therapeutic task required. The psychiatrist should have the same attitude toward members of the medical profession to whom he/she refers patients. Whenever he/she has reason to doubt the training, skill, or ethical qualifications of the allied professional, the psychiatrist should not refer cases to him/her.

3. When the psychiatrist assumes a collaborative or supervisory role with another mental health worker, he/she must expend sufficient time to assure that proper care is given. It is contrary to the interests of the patient and to patient care if he/she allows himself/herself to be used as a figurehead.

4. In relationships between psychiatrists and practicing licensed psychologists, the physician should not delegate to the psychologist or, in fact, to any nonmedical person any matter requiring the exercise of professional medical judgment.

5. The psychiatrist should agree to the request of a patient for consultation or to such a request from the family of an incompetent or minor patient. The psychiatrist may suggest possible consultants, but the patient or family should be given free choice of the consultant. If the psychiatrist disapproves of the professional qualifications of the consultant or if there is a difference of opinion that the primary therapist cannot resolve, he/she may, after suitable notice, withdraw from the case. If this disagreement occurs within an institution or agency framework, the differences should be resolved by the mediation or arbitration of higher professional authority within the institution or agency.

## Section 6

*A physician shall, in the provision of appropriate patient care, except in emergencies, be free to choose whom to serve, with whom to associate, and the environment in which to provide medical services.*

1. Physicians generally agree that the doctor–patient relationship is such a vital factor in effective treatment of the patient that preservation of optimal conditions for development of a sound working relationship between a doctor and his/her patient should take precedence over all other considerations. Professional courtesy may lead to poor psychiatric care for physicians and their families because of embarrassment over the lack of a complete give-and-take contract.

2. An ethical psychiatrist may refuse to provide psychiatric treatment to a person who, in the psychiatrist's opinion, cannot be diagnosed as having a mental illness amenable to psychiatric treatment.

## Section 7

*A physician shall recognize a responsibility to participate in activities contributing to an improved community.*

1. Psychiatrists should foster the cooperation of those legitimately concerned with the medical, psychological, social and legal aspects of mental health and illness. Psychiatrists are encouraged to serve society by advising and consulting with the executive, legislative, and judiciary branches of the government. A psychiatrist should clarify whether he/she speaks as an individual or as a representative of an organization. Furthermore, psychiatrists should avoid cloaking their public statements with the authority of the profession (e.g., 'Psychiatrists know that . . .').

2. Psychiatrists may interpret and share with the public their expertise in the various psychosocial issues that may affect mental health and illness. Psychiatrists should always be mindful of their separate roles as dedicated citizens and as experts in psychological medicine.

3. On occasion psychiatrists are asked for an opinion about an individual who is in the light of public attention, or who has disclosed information about himself/herself through public media. It is unethical for a psychiatrist to offer a professional opinion unless he/she has conducted an examination and has been granted proper authorization for such a statement.

4. The psychiatrist may permit his/her certification to be used for the involuntary treatment of any person only following his/her personal examination of that person. To do so, he/she must find that the person, because of mental illness, cannot form a judgement as to what is in his/her own best

interests and that, without such treatment, substantial impairment is likely to occur to the person or others.

[Adopted by the American Psychiatric Association, 1973, revised 1988. Reprinted by permission.]

# Name Index

*Page numbers followed by 'n' refer to footnotes or endnotes to chapters.*

# Subject Index

*Page numbers followed by 'n' refer to footnotes or endnotes to chapters.*